9-12-03

Atlas of Nuclear Cardiology

Atlas of Nuclear Cardiology

Volume Editors

VASKEN DILSIZIAN, MD
*Professor of Medicine and Radiology
University of Maryland School of Medicine
Director of Cardiovascular Nuclear Medicine and
 Cardiac Positron Emission Tomography
University of Maryland Medical Center
Baltimore, Maryland*

JAGAT NARULA, MD, DM, PHD
*Thomas J. Vischer Professor of Medicine
Drexel University College of Medicine
Chief, Division of Cardiology
Director, Heart Failure and Transplant Center
Director, Center for Molecular Cardiology
Hahnemann University Hospital
Philadelphia, Pennsylvania*

Series Editor

EUGENE BRAUNWALD, MD, MD (HON), ScD (HON)
*Distinguished Hersey Professor of Medicine
Harvard Medical School
Faculty Dean for Academic Programs at Brigham and Women's
 Hospital and Massachusetts General Hospital
Harvard Medical School
Chief Academic Officer
Partners HealthCare System
Boston, Massachusetts*

WITH 17 CONTRIBUTORS

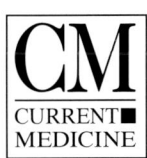

Developed by Current Medicine, Inc.
Philadelphia

CURRENT MEDICINE, INC.

400 Market Street, Suite 700 • Philadelphia, PA 19106

Developmental Editor	Teresa M. Giuliana and Elise M. Paxson
Commissioning Supervisor	Annmarie D'Ortona
Cover Design	William C. Whitman, Jr.
Cover Illustration	Wieslawa Langenfeld
Design and Layout	William C. Whitman, Jr.
Illustrators	Wieslawa Langenfeld and Maureen Looney
Assistant Production Manager	Margaret La Mare
Index	Dorothy Hoffman

Library of Congress Cataloging-in-Publication Data

Atlas of nuclear cardiology / edited by Vasken Dilsizian, Jagat Narula ;
with 17 contributors.
    p. ; cm.
Includes bibliographical references and index.
  ISBN 1-57340-185-4 (alk. paper)
  1. Cardiovascular system—Radionuclide imaging—Atlases.
  [DNLM: 1. Cardiovascular Diseases—radionuclide imaging—Atlases. 2.
Heart—radionuclide imaging—Atlases. WG 17 A884394 2003] I. Title:
Nuclear cardiology. II. Dilsizian, Vasken. III. Narula, Jagat.
  RC670.5.R32A86 2003
  616.1'07575—dc21

                     2002034791

ISBN 1-57340-185-4

Although every effort has been made to ensure that drug doses and other information are presented accurately in this publication, the ultimate responsibility rests with the prescribing physician. Neither the publishers nor the authors can be held responsible for errors or for any consequences arising from the use of information contained herein. Products mentioned in this publication should be used in accordance with the prescribing information prepared by the manufacturers. No claims or endorsements are made for any drug or compound at present under clinical investigation.

© Copyright 2003 by Current Medicine, Inc. All rights reserved. No part of this publication may be reproduced, stored in a retrieval system, or transmitted in any form by any means electronic, mechanical, photocopying, recording, or otherwise, without prior written consent of the publisher.

Printed in Singapore by Imago

10 9 8 7 6 5 4 3 2 1

PREFACE

Nuclear cardiology is one of the fastest growing subspecialties in the field of cardiovascular diseases. During the past three decades, the field has evolved from a research tool to a well-established clinical discipline. Approximately 5 million nuclear cardiology procedures are performed annually, representing nearly one third of all nuclear medicine studies performed in the United States. The field has excelled in the noninvasive evaluation and quantification of myocardial perfusion, function, and metabolism. Unlike anatomically oriented approaches to medicine, the strengths of nuclear techniques are based on physiologic, biochemical, and molecular properties. The ability to define myocardial perfusion, viability, and ventricular function from a single study has become a powerful diagnostic and prognostic tool. Because of its important contribution to the management and care of cardiac patients, nuclear cardiology is now recognized as a distinct clinical entity.

Nuclear cardiology first became a discipline in the early 1970s. A major breakthrough in the field came with the development of myocardial perfusion radiotracers, such as ^{201}Tl, which permitted noninvasive detection and physiologic characterization of anatomic coronary artery lesions. The development of first-pass and equilibrium radionuclide angiography allowed for the noninvasive assessment of regional and global left ventricular function. The field blossomed further as concepts of exercise physiology, demand-supply mismatch, coronary vasodilator reserve, and systolic and diastolic left ventricular dysfunction became a clinical reality. Pharmacologic vasodilators, such as dipyridamole and adenosine, widened the application of myocardial perfusion studies to patients who were unable to exercise, had uncomplicated acute coronary syndromes, or were undergoing intermediate to high-risk noncardiac surgical procedures. Subsequently, the field advanced from detection of coronary artery disease to risk stratification and prognosis. Now that great reliance has been placed on the clinical cardiologist to appropriately select patients for medical or interventional therapy, as well as monitoring the effectiveness of that therapy, nuclear cardiology procedures have become the cornerstone of the decision-making process. Parallel advances in both radiopharmaceuticals and instrumentation have fostered further the growth of nuclear cardiology. The introduction of ^{99m}Tc-labeled perfusion tracers in the 1990s improved the count rate and image quality of myocardial perfusion studies, which allowed for ECG-gated acquisition and simultaneous assessment of regional myocardial perfusion and function with a single radiotracer. Because some ^{99m}Tc-labeled perfusion tracers demonstrate minimal redistribution over time after injection, they have been used in the emergency room and in the early hours of an infarct to estimate the extent of myocardium in jeopardy. A follow-up study, performed several days later, provides information on final infarct size and myocardial salvage. The introduction of PET has widened the scope of the cardiac examination from perfusion and function alone to assessment of metabolic substrate utilization, cardiac receptor occupancy, and adrenergic neuronal function. The ability to image the shift in the primary source of myocardial energy production from fatty acids toward glucose utilization in the setting of reduced blood flow has helped explain the pathophysiology of hibernation. The therapeutic impact of PET has broadened the utility of nuclear cardiology procedures to include patients with chronic ischemic left ventricular dysfunction and heart failure for the assessment of myocardial viability.

The aim of the *Atlas of Nuclear Cardiology* is to elucidate the role of cardiovascular nuclear procedures in the clinical practice of cardiology. Diagnostic algorithms and schematic diagrams integrated with nuclear cardiology procedures are generously interspersed with color illustrations to emphasize key concepts in cardiovascular physiology and metabolism. In the first chapter, a brief historical perspective of the development of the field along with an introduction to the principles of radiotracers, instrumentation, and image acquisition are reviewed. The next five chapters detail SPECT and PET techniques for the detection of coronary artery disease, assessment of myocardial viability, risk stratification, and prognosis. Chapters 7 and 8 address the role of radionuclide imaging in the diagnosis and risk stratification of patients suffering from acute and chronic ischemic coronary syndromes. Chapters 9 and 10 review the techniques of first-pass and equilibrium radionuclide angiography and gated myocardial perfusion SPECT. The last three chapters examine the latest approaches of radionuclide techniques for advancement of cardiovascular research: myocardial innervation, imaging myocardial necrosis and apoptosis, and imaging atherosclerotic lesions.

In the next century, innovative imaging strategies in nuclear cardiology will propel the field into molecular imaging while it continues to build on its already well-defined strengths of myocardial perfusion, function, and metabolism. Realization of these ideas and progress in the diagnosis, treatment, and prevention of cardiovascular disease will depend not only on new discoveries but also on meaningful interactions between clinicians and investigators. It is our hope that the *Atlas of Nuclear Cardiology* will serve as a foundation for clinicians and a reference guide for scientists within the field.

VASKEN DILSIZIAN, MD
JAGAT NARULA, MD, DM, PHD

CONTRIBUTORS

DANIEL S. BERMAN, MD
Professor
Department of Medicine
University of California, Los Angeles
Director, Nuclear Cardiology
Cedars-Sinai Medical Center
Los Angeles, California

JEFFREY S. BORER, MD
Gladys and Roland Harriman Professor of Cardiovascular Medicine
Division of Cardiovascular Pathophysiology
Weill Medical College of Cornell University
Chief, Division of Cardiovascular Pathophysiology
Director, The Howard Gilman Institute for Valvular Heart Diseases
The New York-Presbyterian Hospital/Weill Cornell Medical Center
New York, New York

VASKEN DILSIZIAN, MD
Professor of Medicine and Radiology
University of Maryland School of Medicine
Director of Cardiovascular Nuclear Medicine and Cardiac Positron Emission Tomography
University of Maryland Medical Center
Baltimore, Maryland

GUIDO GERMANO, PhD
Professor
Departments of Medicine and Radiological Sciences
University of California Los Angeles School of Medicine
Director, Artificial Intelligence and Nuclear Medicine Physics
Cedars-Sinai Medical Center
Los Angeles, California

RORY HACHAMOVITCH, MD, MSc
Division of Nuclear Cardiology
University of Southern California Keck School of Medicine
Los Angeles, California

LEO HOFSTRA, MD, PhD
Staff Cardiologist
University Hospital
Maastricht, The Netherlands

DIWAKAR JAIN, MD
Professor of Medicine
Director of Nuclear Cardiology
Drexel University College of Medicine
Philadelphia, Pennsylvania

D. DOUGLAS MILLER, MD, CM, MBA
Professor and Chairman
Department of Internal Medicine
Saint Louis University Hospital
St. Louis, Missouri

JAGAT NARULA, MD, DM, PhD
Thomas J. Vischer Professor of Medicine
Drexel University College of Medicine
Chief, Division of Cardiology
Director, Heart Failure and Transplant Center
Director, Center for Molecular Cardiology
Hahnemann University Hospital
Philadelphia, Pennsylvania

MARIA ANGELA OXILIA-ESTIGARRIBIA, MD
Post Graduate Researcher
Department of Molecular and Medical Pharmacology
Geffen School of Medicine at University of California, Los Angeles
Los Angeles, California

HEINRICH R. SCHELBERT, MD, PhD
The George V. Taplin Professor
Department of Molecular and Medical Pharmacology
Geffen School of Medicine at University of California, Los Angeles
Los Angeles, California

MARKUS SCHWAIGER, MD
Professor
Department of Nuclear Medicine
Technische Universitaet
Munich, Germany

H. WILLIAM STRAUSS, MD
Professor
Department of Radiology
Weill Medical College of Cornell University
Chief, Clinical Service
Nuclear Medicine
Memorial-Sloan Kettering Hospital
New York, New York

JAMES E. UDELSON, MD
Associate Professor
Department of Medicine
Tufts University School of Medicine
Associate Chief
Division of Cardiology
Tufts-New England Medical Center
Boston, Massachusetts

RENU VIRMANI, MD
Chair, Department of Cardiovascular Pathology
Armed Forces Institute of Pathology
Clinical Professor
Department of Pathology
Georgetown University
Washington, DC

FRANS J. TH. WACKERS, MD, PHD
Professor
Departments of Medicine/Diagnostic Radiology
Yale University School of Medicine
Attending Physician
Yale-New Haven Hospital
New Haven, Connecticut

BARRY L. ZARET, MD
Robert W. Berliner Professor of Medicine
Chief, Section of Cardiovascular Medicine
Vice Chairman, Department of Internal Medicine
Yale University School of Medicine
New Haven, Connecticut

Contents

CHAPTER 1
PRINCIPLES OF CARDIOVASCULAR NUCLEAR IMAGING 1
Diwakar Jain and H. William Strauss
Basic Physics and Chemistry 2
Historical Perspective 5
Instrumentation 9
Image Acquisition and Processing 12
Novel Applications of Radionuclide Techniques for Advancement of Cardiovascular Research 15

CHAPTER 2
SPECT AND PET TECHNIQUES 19
Vasken Dilsizian
SPECT Techniques: Thallium-201 21
SPECT Techniques: ^{99m}Tc-labeled Perfusion Tracers 28
PET Techniques: Flow, Metabolism, and Prognosis 34

CHAPTER 3
PHARMACOLOGIC STRESSORS IN CORONARY ARTERY DISEASE 47
D. Douglas Miller

CHAPTER 4
SPECT DETECTION OF CORONARY ARTERY DISEASE 63
Frans J. Th. Wackers
Clinical Imaging 65
Image Interpretation and Quantification 69
Cardiomyopathy 74
Clinical Indications for SPECT Imaging and Diagnostic Yield 76

CHAPTER 5
PET QUANTITATION OF MYOCARDIAL BLOOD FLOW 79
Heinrich R. Schelbert and Maria Angela Oxilia-Estigarribia
Methodology 80
Findings in the Normal Heart 84
Myocardial Blood Flow in Cardiovascular Disease 87

CHAPTER 6
RISK STRATIFICATION AND PATIENT MANAGEMENT 97
Daniel S. Berman, Rory Hachamovitch, and Guido Germano

CHAPTER 7
DIAGNOSIS AND RISK STRATIFICATION IN ACUTE CORONARY SYNDROMES 115
James E. Udelson
Assessment of Patients with Suspected Acute Coronary Syndrome 117
Assessment of Patients with ST Segment Elevation Myocardial Infarction 121
Assessment of Patients with Non–ST Segment Elevation Myocardial Infarction/Unstable Angina 127

CHAPTER 8

MYOCARDIAL VIABILITY: REVERSIBLE LEFT VENTRICULAR DYSFUNCTION 131
Vasken Dilsizian
Myocardial Ischemia and Viability 132
Left Ventricular Dysfunction and Heart Failure 133
Contraction–Perfusion Mismatch and Match: Stunning and Hibernation 135
Histomorphologic and Structural Changes Underlying Left Ventricular Dysfunction 139
Left Ventricular Remodeling 140

CHAPTER 9

FIRST-PASS AND EQUILIBRIUM RADIONUCLIDE ANGIOGRAPHY 147
Jeffrey S. Borer
First-pass Radionuclide Angiography 151
Equilibrium Radionuclide Angiography 152
Valvular Heart Disease 158
Cardiomyopathic Disorders 162

CHAPTER 10

GATED MYOCARDIAL PERFUSION SPECT 167
Guido Germano and Daniel S. Berman

CHAPTER 11

MYOCARDIAL INNERVATION 183
Markus Schwaiger
Autonomic Nervous System 185
Adrenergic Nerve Terminals 187
Radiopharmaceuticals 188
Myocardial Infarction 191
Cardiomyopathy and Arrhythmias 193

CHAPTER 12

IMAGING MYOCARDIAL NECROSIS AND APOPTOSIS 197
Jagat Narula and Leo Hofstra
Imaging Necrotic Cell Death 198
Apoptotic Cell Death 208

CHAPTER 13

RADIONUCLIDE IMAGING OF ATHEROSCLEROTIC LESIONS 217
Jagat Narula, Renu Virmani, and Barry L. Zaret
Evolution of Atherosclerotic Lesions 218
Targeting Macrophage Infiltration in Atherosclerotic Lesions 219
Targeting Large Lipid Cores in Atherosclerotic Lesions 225
Targeting Proliferating Smooth Muscle Cells 227
Future Directions 233

INDEX 237

CHAPTER 1

PRINCIPLES OF CARDIOVASCULAR NUCLEAR IMAGING

Diwakar Jain and H. William Strauss

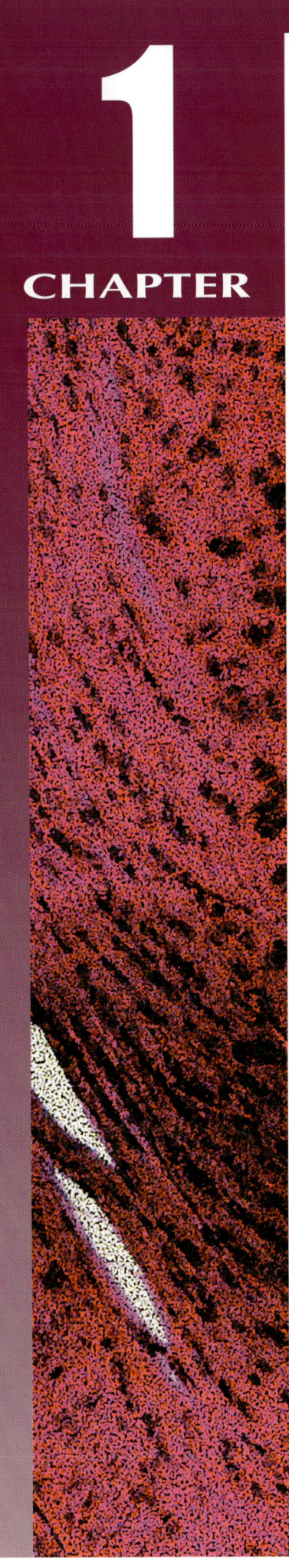

The field of nuclear medicine is built on its ability to harness the unique properties of radiopharmaceuticals in elucidating the pathophysiology of heart diseases. These radiopharmaceuticals can localize in specific receptors, serve as substrates for pumps or metabolic reactions, or equilibrate in a specific compartment, pool, or space. Advances in instrumentation permit imaging or graphic representation of these processes.

Cardiovascular nuclear imaging employs radioisotopes and pharmaceutical agents labeled with radioisotopes for the imaging of the cardiovascular system. The role of nuclear medicine in cardiology is primarily in the area of diagnostic imaging. Recently, therapeutic radiation has been used successfully for the prevention of coronary artery restenosis following percutaneous interventions. This chapter presents a brief historical perspective of the development of this field, the principles of radioactivity, radioisotopes, radiopharmaceuticals, instrumentation for imaging the cardiovascular system, the process of imaging, and image processing, reconstruction, and interpretation.

In 1927, Blumgart *et al.* were the first to use radionuclides in vivo to study the circulation [1]. They used radium C (^{214}Bi) to study pulmonary vascular volume and transit time. This was followed by several landmark discoveries in all aspects of cardiovascular nuclear imaging. Blumgart's technique was followed, in 1948, by Prinzmetal's work on the radiocardiogram, a tracing of the passage of a radioactive substance through the heart, using a simple radiation detector after intravenous injection of radiolabeled albumin. The study of myocardial perfusion gained interest in 1964. Inert gases dissolved in saline were injected directly into the coronary arteries. Washout curves of these agents from the myocardium provided an index of myocardial blood flow. The innovative use of sodium iodide crystal as a scintillation detector was a major turning point in the development of scintillation imaging devices. Up to that point, nuclear studies were composed only of curves for radioactive clearance and washout from various organs or tissues. The initial imaging device consisted of a small sodium iodide crystal with a single photomultiplier tube mounted on a device that would move across, or scan, the organ to be imaged. This prototype imaging device was soon replaced with a gamma camera, which increased in sophistication and complexity.

A major breakthrough in cardiovascular nuclear imaging came with the development of myocardial perfusion imaging using radiopharmaceuticals. This was the first noninvasive imaging technique for the detection of coronary artery disease. Despite the development of a number of other competing modalities, myocardial perfusion imaging using radiopharmaceuticals continues to be the most widely used noninvasive test for the detection of coronary artery disease and remains the gold standard for comparison with emerging new imaging modalities. Development of equilibrium radionuclide angiocardiography, or gated blood pool imaging, in the 1970s was another landmark development in cardiology. This was the first noninvasive modality for the assessment of left ventricular wall motion and ejection fraction. This technique has, to a large extent, been replaced by other imaging modalities. However, gated blood pool imaging continues to be the most reliable, reproducible, and objective technique for the assessment of left ventricular wall motion and ejection fraction. Currently, cardiovascular nuclear imaging is an integral part of the evaluation of patients with suspected or known coronary artery disease. Nuclear imaging techniques allow precise and reproducible quantitative assessment of myocardial perfusion, metabolism, and necrosis and regional and global left ventricular wall motion and ejection fraction. Nuclear imaging techniques have also played a critical role in improving our understanding of important phenomena in the fields of cardiovascular physiology, cell biology, and pathology.

BASIC PHYSICS AND CHEMISTRY

RADIOACTIVITY

Radioactivity: Spontaneous transformation (decay or disintegration) of unstable atoms that results in the emission of radiation

Radiation: Energy in transit in the form of high-speed particles and electromagnetic waves

Ionizing radiation: Radiation with enough energy to knock tightly bound electrons from their orbits around the nucleus, causing the atoms to become charged or ionized, *eg*, gamma rays and neutrons

Nonionizing radiation: Radiation without enough energy to knock tightly bound electrons from their orbits around the nucleus, *eg*, microwaves and visible light

FIGURE 1-1. Radioactivity. *Radioactivity* is the process of spontaneous transformation of an unstable element into a more stable form that results in the emission of energy in the form of radiation. During this process, the mass of the parent element decreases with the release of energy. The time it takes to reduce a radionuclide to half of its mass is termed *half-life*. Elements that are unstable and decay spontaneously are called *radionuclides*. Whereas elements are characterized by their atomic number (Z) alone (the number of protons in the nucleus), radionuclides are characterized by their mass number (A) and atomic number (Z). The mass number (A) is the sum of the number of protons (Z) and neutrons (N). Radionuclides having the same number of protons (Z) are termed *isotopes*. Radionuclides attempt to stabilize over time by emitting charged particles, or electromagnetic radiation. Transmutation describes a process by which the nucleus of a radioactive atom undergoes decay into an atom with a different number of protons, until such time as a stable nucleus is produced. Nearly 60 naturally occurring radioisotopes are found in the crust of the earth. These radioisotopes have been present in the earth since its formation or are the products of decay of the original radioisotopes, which have since decayed. These radioisotopes have a very long half-life—millions of years. A few examples of these are ^{226}Ra (half-life 1.6×10^3 years; found in limestone and igneous rocks), ^{238}U (half-life 4.5×10^9 years; found in rocks), ^{232}Th (half-life 1.4×10^{10} years; found in rocks), ^{222}Rn (half-life 3.8 days; found in air), and ^{40}K (half-life 1.3×10^9 years; found in soil). The agents with long half-lives are not suitable for use in diagnostic imaging. Some of these agents have industrial uses, such as in power plants or in atomic weapons.

Radiation is energy in the process of transfer or transit in the form of charged particles and electromagnetic waves. Based on their interaction with matter, radiation can be grouped as ionizing or nonionizing. Radiation energy that is high enough to knock tightly bound electrons from their orbits around the nucleus and cause the atoms to become charged or ionized (*eg*, x-rays, gamma rays, and neutrons) is known as *ionizing radiation*. Radiation energy that is low and unable to knock tightly bound electrons from their orbits (*eg*, microwaves and visible light) is termed *nonionizing radiation*. Interaction of x-rays or gamma rays with matter results in the production of negatively charged electrons and positively charged ions. Electrons travel some distance and produce further ionization. Absorption of radiation by water molecules results in the ejection of electrons and dissociation of water molecules into hydrogen ions and hydroxyl ions (free radicals).

RADIOACTIVE DECAY

Alpha decay
$$^{238}_{92}U \rightarrow {}^{234}_{90}Th + {}^{4}_{2}He$$
Beta decay
$$^{234}_{90}Th \rightarrow {}^{234}_{91}Pa + {}^{0}_{-1}e$$
Gamma decay
$$^{99m}_{43}Tc \rightarrow {}^{99}_{43}Tc + {}^{0}_{0}\gamma$$

FIGURE 1-2. Radioactive decay. There are three processes by which radionuclides attempt to stabilize over time while conforming to the conservation laws of energy, mass number, and electric charge. These processes are alpha, beta, and gamma decay. In *alpha decay*, the nuclide emits an alpha particle, which is a stable nuclide with an atomic mass number (A) of 4 and atomic number (Z) of 2 (the same as the nucleus of a helium atom). *Beta decay* occurs through 1) β⁻, or electron emission (the conversion of a neutron into a proton inside the nucleus of a radionuclide), 2) β⁺, or positron emission (the conversion of a proton into a neutron), or 3) electron capture (the conversion of a proton into a neutron by capturing an electron from one of the atomic shells). In all three processes, the mass number (A) remains unchanged (also called *isobaric transition*). In *gamma decay*, the excited radionuclide (isomer) decays to a lower-energy ground state (isomeric transition). This process is accomplished through either emission of high-energy photons known as gamma rays or internal conversion (transfer of the released energy directly to an orbital electron). A gamma ray cannot be distinguished from an x-ray of the same energy (> 100 KeV) because both interact with matter in exactly the same way. They differ with regard to the origin of the emitted energy. Gamma rays are emitted from the nucleus, and x-rays are emitted from the atom. In clinical practice, gamma ray–emitting radioisotopes are used for diagnostic imaging, whereas alpha wave– and beta wave–emitting radioisotopes are used for local therapy, *eg*, brachytherapy and obliteration of tumor cells. (The superscript on the left is the atomic mass, and the subscript on the right reflects the atomic number of the element.)

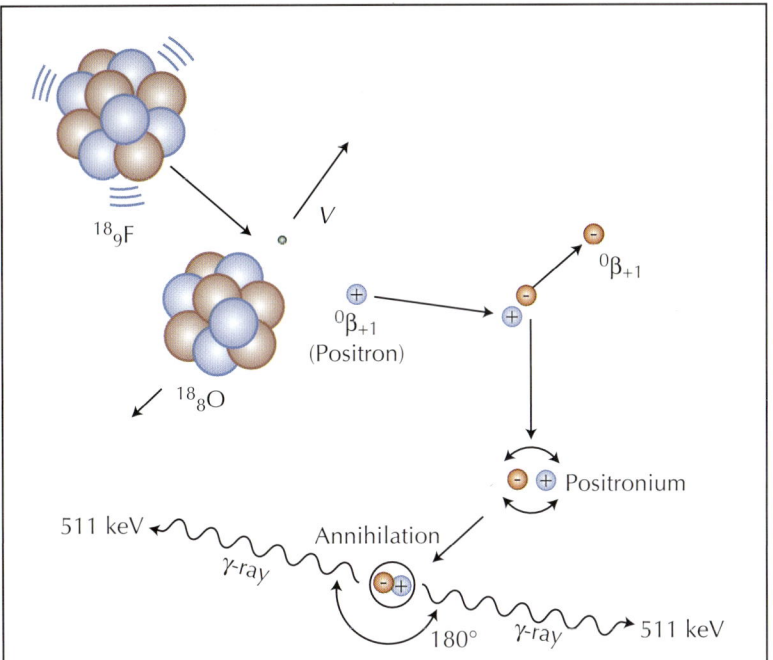

FIGURE 1-3. Positron decay. An example of isobaric transition (beta decay) of ^{18}F to ^{18}O, in which a proton inside the nucleus is converted into a neutron, and the excess energy is released as a positron (β^+) and a neutrino (V). A neutrino is a particle with no electric charge or mass. After being ejected from the nucleus, a high-energy positron travels a short distance and, once it has lost almost all of its energy, collides with an electron and is quickly annihilated. The combined mass energy of the positron and electron is converted into electromagnetic radiation (2 gamma rays; 511 keV of energy each). The gamma rays travel in opposite directions, discharged at an angle of 180 degrees to each other.

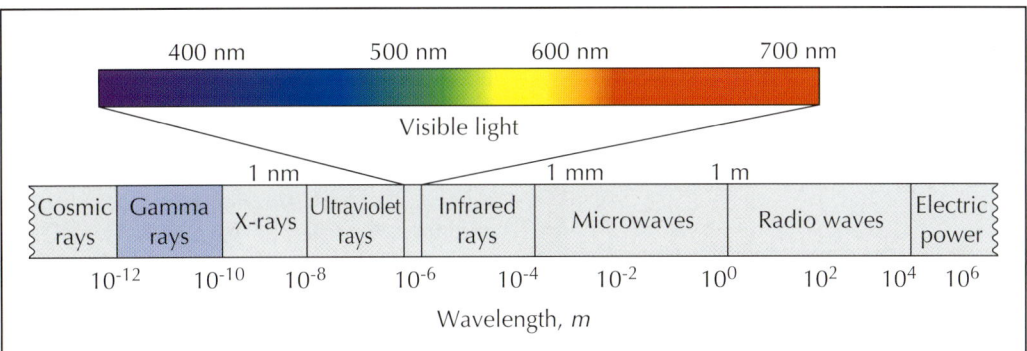

FIGURE 1-4. The spectrum of electromagnetic waves. Gamma rays are part of the spectrum of the electromagnetic waves. The range of electromagnetic waves is wide. All of these waves travel at the speed of light (3×10^{10} cm/s, or 186,000 mile/s in a vacuum). At one end of the spectrum are the waves with extremely long wavelengths, measured in meters, such as radio and television waves. At the other end are the cosmic rays, with extremely short wavelengths—smaller than the size of the nucleus of an atom. These waves also have energy, which is measured in electron volts (eV). Electromagnetic waves with long wavelengths have very low energy (on the order of 10^{-8} to 10^{-10} eV), whereas electromagnetic waves with short wavelengths have very high energy (10^3 to 10^5 eV for gamma rays and 10^8 eV for cosmic rays). The electromagnetic waves are also classified as ionizing and nonionizing radiation, depending on their interaction with matter. (*Courtesy of Thinkquest, http://library.thinkquest.org*).

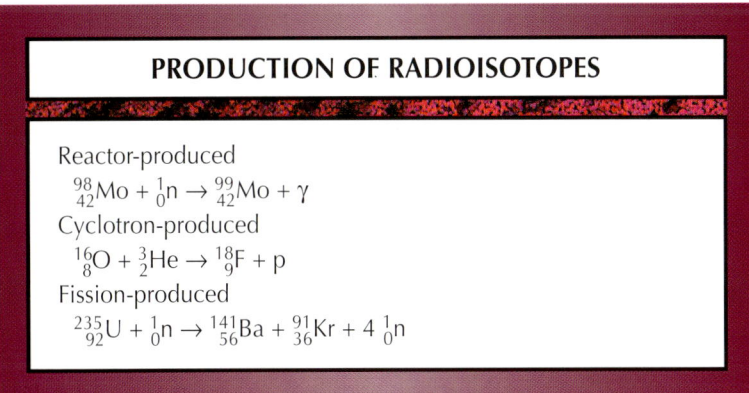

FIGURE 1-5. Production of radioisotopes. Most of the naturally occurring radionuclides (^{40}K, ^{14}C, and elements with higher atomic numbers and larger nuclei) have long half-lives and are not used in medicine. The radionuclides commonly used in medicine are manmade and are produced by a nuclear reactor or cyclotron (accelerator), or by fission. Alteration of the nuclear configuration results in an unstable nucleus, which tends to regain stability by the emission of radioactivity. Some radioisotopes used in medicine are the daughter products of other radioisotopes, which have been produced in a nuclear reactor or a cyclotron. For example, ^{99m}Tc, which accounts for nearly 80% of the radiotracers used in nuclear imaging, is the decay product of ^{99}Mo, which is produced in a nuclear reactor by capture reaction of neutrons (n). ^{99m}Tc is produced by the elution of a generator containing ^{99}Mo. ^{99m}Tc exists as a polyvalent ion, which can be incorporated into a large number of organic and inorganic molecules. In cyclotron-produced radionuclides, high-energy charged particles, such as proton (p) and helium (He) particles, are captured by stable nuclides. For example, ^{18}F, which is used for labeling deoxyglucose in the study of myocardial viability and tumor imaging, is produced by nuclear reaction between ^{3}He and ^{16}O. In fission, a heavier nucleus is split into two smaller nuclei, with the production of a large number of neutrons. For example, when ^{235}U captures a neutron, it results in the production of ^{141}Ba and ^{91}Kr, along with four neutrons. In fission, a captured neutron initiates the process, with the production of more than one neutron. The additional neutrons that are produced incite further fission. The mechanism of the atomic bomb is the process of uncontrolled chain reaction until the supply of fissionable material is exhausted.

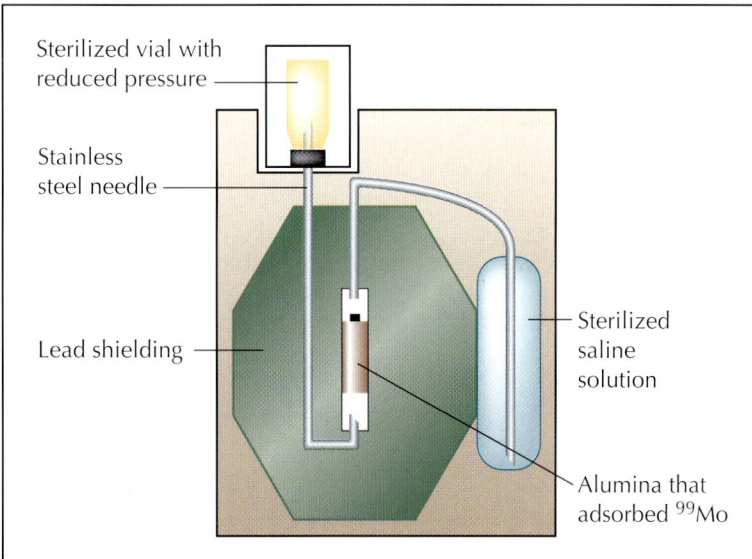

FIGURE 1-6. Cross-sectional view of a ^{99}Mo-^{99m}Tc generator. ^{99m}Tc, a short-lived radionuclide (6-hour half-life), is produced from the elution of a generator that contains ^{99}Mo, a long-lived reactor-produced radionuclide (67-hour half-life). The generator is used in routine clinical practice to obtain a continuous supply of the radiotracer. ^{99}Mo is adsorbed on a column filled with alumina as sodium molybdate. ^{99m}Tc is eluted by oxidant-free physiologic saline in the form of sodium pertechnetate. The generator has a usable life of 1 week, after which the ^{99}Mo source needs to be replenished.

A. UNITS OF RADIOACTIVITY

Curie (Ci)	$= 37 \times 10^9$ dps
Millicurie (mCi)	$= 37 \times 10^6$ dps
Becquerel (Bq)	$= 1$ dps
Megabecquerel (MBq)	$= 10^6$ dps
1 mCi	$= 37$ MBq

B. UNITS OF RADIOACTIVITY EXPOSURE

Roentgen (R): A measure of the ionization of molecules caused by x-rays or gamma rays
Rad (radiation absorbed dose): Measure of absorbed dose of any type of radiation
  Gray (Gy): SI unit of absorbed dose
    1 Gy = 100 rads
Rem (roentgen equivalent man): Unit of absorbed dose in human tissue equivalent to its biologic damage
  Sievert (Sv): SI unit of equivalent dose
    1 Sv = 100 rem

FIGURE 1-7. Units of radioactivity. **A,** The activity of radionuclides is measured in terms of the rate at which the radioactive atoms within the nuclei disintegrate. The two commonly applied units of radioactivity that describe disintegrations per second (dps) are the Curie (Ci), which is the most commonly used unit in the United States, and the becquerel (Bq), which has been adopted as the standard international (Systeme Internationale, SI) unit. One Ci represents 3.7×10^9 dps, while 1 Bq represents 1 dps. The radionuclides commonly used in clinical practice are measured in millicurie (mCi) or megabecquerel (MBq) units. A quantity of 1 MBq represents 10^6 dps, and therefore 1 mCi equals 37 MBq. *Specific activity* provides a relationship between mass and radioactivity. This is expressed as mCi/g or Bq/L. Highly purified forms of short-lived radiotracer have very high specific activity. Lower specific activity of these radiotracers indicates the presence of impurities. **B,** The basic unit of radioactivity exposure is the roentgen (R), which is a measure of the ionization of molecules caused by x-rays or gamma rays in dry air. Roentgen is used to describe radiation levels in the environment, which are measured by radiation detectors, such as Geiger counters. The amount of radiation absorbed by irradiated material is termed *radiation dose* and is expressed either in rads (radiation absorbed dose) or grays (Gy). One rad is defined as the absorption of 100 ergs of energy per gram of material; 1 gray is defined as 1 joule of energy deposited in 1 kilogram of material and is equivalent to 100 rads. Beyond the rad, the biologic effect of radiation also depends on the density of ionizations produced by the radiation, known as *linear energy transfer*. For example, for a similar path length, alpha particles and neutrons produce 10- to 20-fold more ionizations than gamma rays, x-rays, or beta particles. In order to account for the variable biologic effects of different types of radiation, the radiation dose in rads or grays is multiplied by a quality factor that is unique to the incidental radiation. The result is a new measurement termed *rem* (roentgen-equivalent-man), which relates the radiation dose in rads or grays to the biologic damage produced by the radiation in human tissue. For gamma rays, x-rays, and beta particles, the quality factor is 1; as a result, rads and rems turn out to be numerically equivalent. Similarly, grays and sieverts (Sv) are numerically equivalent. Sievert is the Systeme Internationale (SI) unit of equivalent dose, and 1 Sv is equal to 100 rems.

POPULATION RADIATION EXPOSURE		
	AVERAGE ANNUAL EFFECTIVE DOSE EQUIVALENT	
SOURCE	µSV	MREM
Inhaled (radon and decay products)	2000	200
Other internally deposited radionuclides	390	39
Terrestrial radiation	280	28
Cosmic radiation	280	28
Total from natural sources	3000	300
Total from artificial sources*	600	60
Total	3600	360

*Mostly from diagnostic sources such as x-rays, nuclear scans; < 1% comes from power plants.

FIGURE 1-8. Natural radiation exposure. The human species is exposed constantly to naturally occurring radiation from the earth as well as from extraterrestrial sources. The soil and rocks contain small quantities of natural radioactivity. Radon gas is released during radioactive decay of uranium in rocks and seeps into water and our living environment. This is the single most important source of natural radiation. Small quantities of radioactive potassium (^{40}K) and carbon (^{14}C) also occur in the environment and are ingested with food and incorporated into the body. Certain areas have higher naturally occurring radioactivity. At higher altitudes and during air travel, there is greater exposure to cosmic radiation. Manmade sources such as diagnostic procedures (x-rays and radioisotope scans) constitute only a very small source of radiation exposure. (*Adapted from* National Council on Radiation Protection and Measurements Reports.)

HISTORICAL PERSPECTIVE

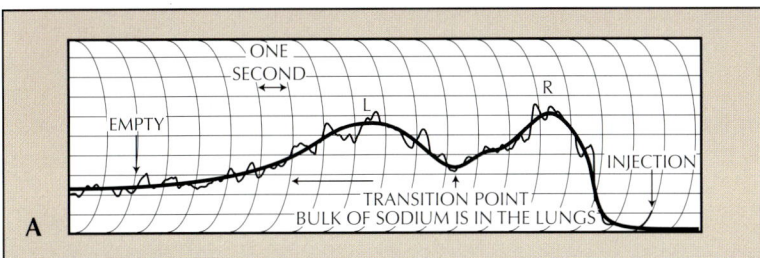

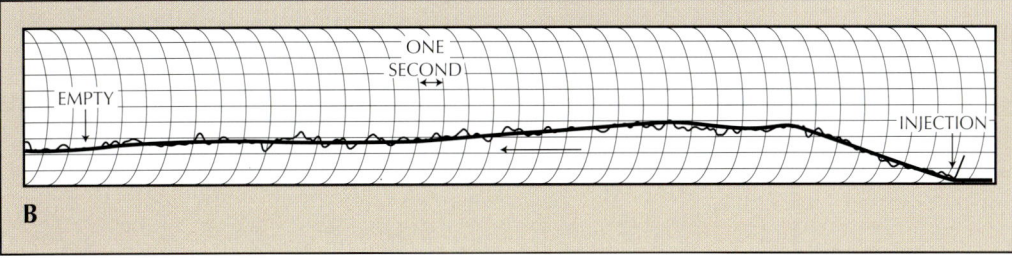

FIGURE 1-9. First use of radionuclides in humans. **A**, Radiocardiogram of a healthy patient. **B**, Radiocardiogram of a patient with rheumatic heart disease. In 1948, Prinzmetal *et al.* described the radiocardiogram, a tracing recorded by a Geiger detector placed over the heart to record the time-activity curve following intravenous administration of radiolabeled albumin. The tracing could be analyzed for transit times, identification of shunts, determination of cardiac output, and calculation of pulmonary and ventricular blood volumes. The clinical applications of this technique are summarized in the work of several investigators, including that of the famous Italian cardiovascular physiologist Luigi Donato [2]. The initial studies of Prinzmetal utilized a shielded Geiger-Mueller detector and an analog ratemeter to record passage of the bolus through the heart and lungs. In 1952, investigators applying this technique had replaced the Geiger-Mueller detector with a sodium iodide scintillation detector. This change resulted in higher fidelity of the data recording because of the higher count rate capacity of the detector. (*Adapted from* Prinzmetal *et al.* [3].)

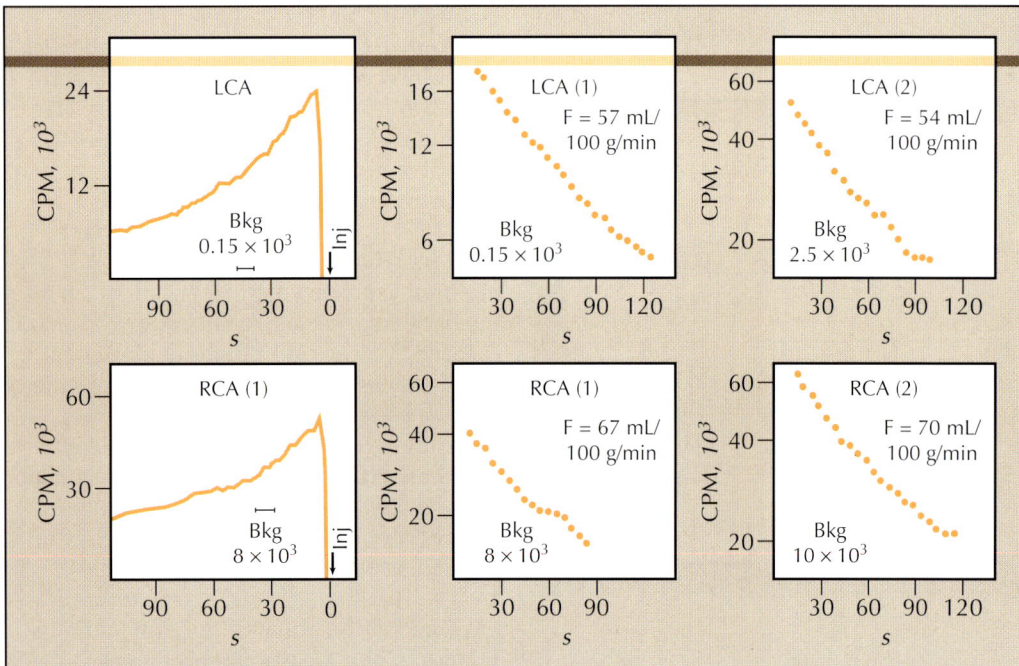

FIGURE 1-10. Direct measurement of myocardial perfusion. The direct measurement of myocardial perfusion began in 1964, with the intracoronary studies of Ross. Ross applied principles of the inert gas clearance technique, as originally described by Kety [4], to the study of the cerebral circulation. During coronary catheterization, ^{133}Xe or ^{85}Kr dissolved in saline was injected directly into each coronary artery. Coronary blood flow in the territory perfused by each artery was calculated from the rate of clearance of the tracer. This technique occasionally produced puzzling results—in some patients with infarction tracer clearance was normal. This occurred because the infarct territory had little mass and very low flow—the clearance was dominated by the normal tissue. When validation studies were performed in animals, this limitation became a driving force for the development of multi-detector counting and imaging systems. In the panels at *left*, kymographs, time is an x axis and moves from right to left, with 0 as the injection (Inj) time and 30, 60, and 90 seconds to the left of the injection arrow. BKG—background; CPM—counts per minute; F—flow; LCA—left coronary artery; RCA—right coronary artery. (*Adapted from* Ross *et al.* [5].)

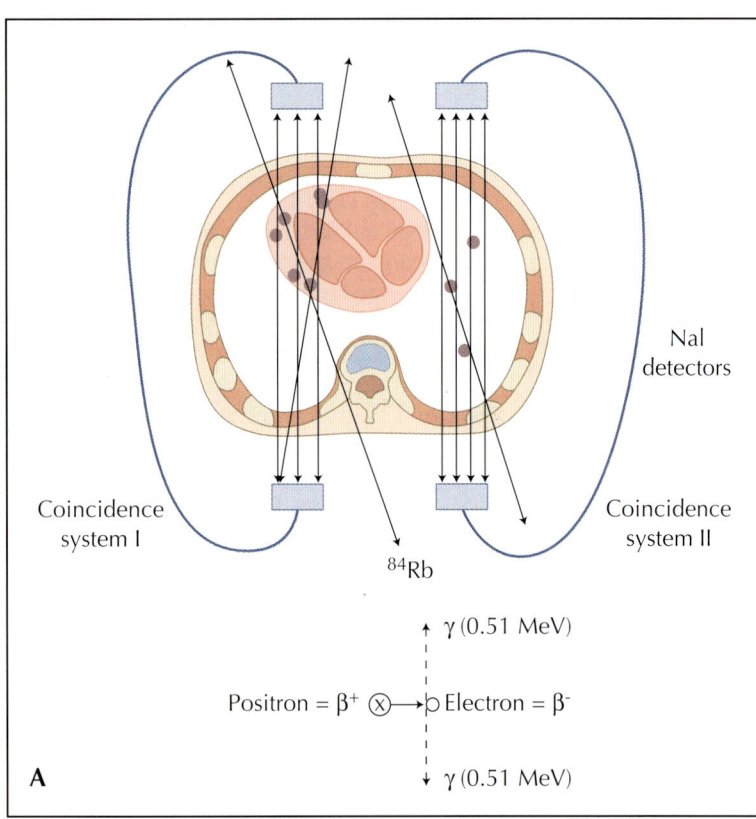

FIGURE 1-11. Early scintigraphic detection of myocardial perfusion. **A,** In 1964, Bing *et al.* [6] described the use of the positron-emitting radionuclide ^{84}Rb and multidetector coincidence counting for the determination of total myocardial perfusion in humans. Myocardial washout of ^{84}Rb was determined by two pairs of sodium iodide (NaI) detectors functioning in coincidence mode, after the injection of radiotracer at rest and after nitroglycerin (NTG) administration.

Continued on next page

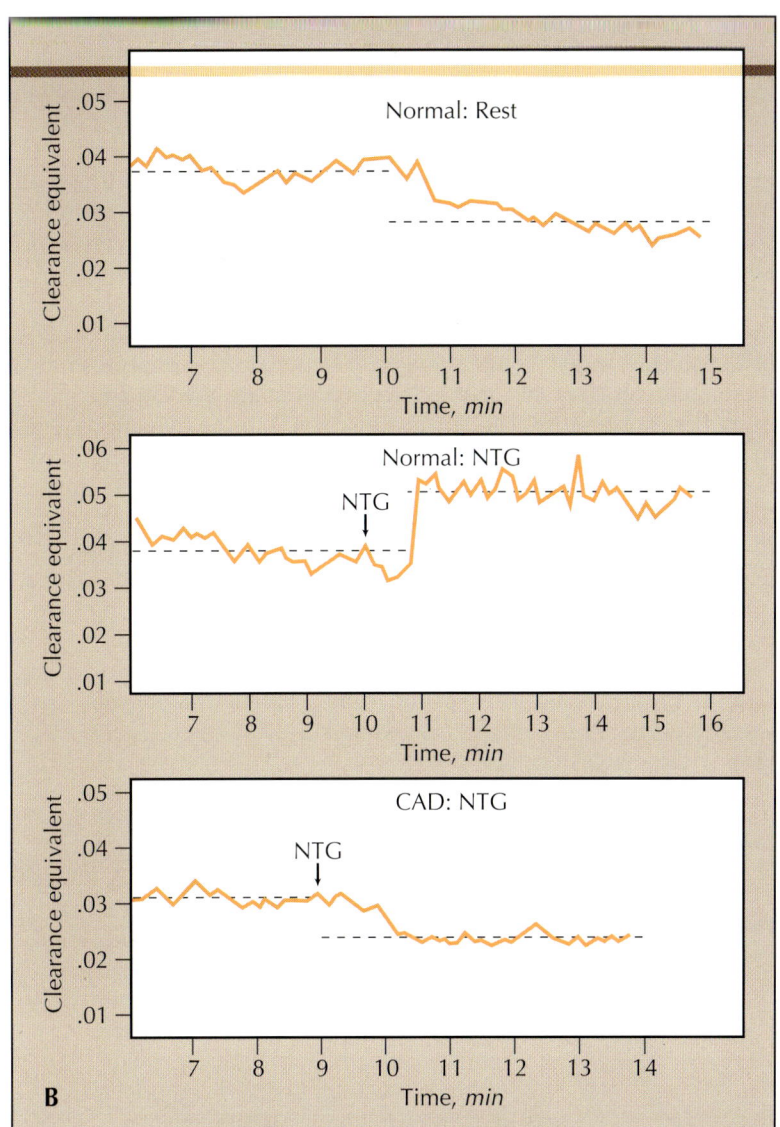

Figure 1-11. *(Continued) B*, These studies were followed by the work of Knoebel describing the findings in patients with coronary artery disease (CAD). These examinations were limited by the variability of probe placement, and the global values that were observed, rather than the regional determinations that were desired. (*Adapted from* Bing *et al.* [6].)

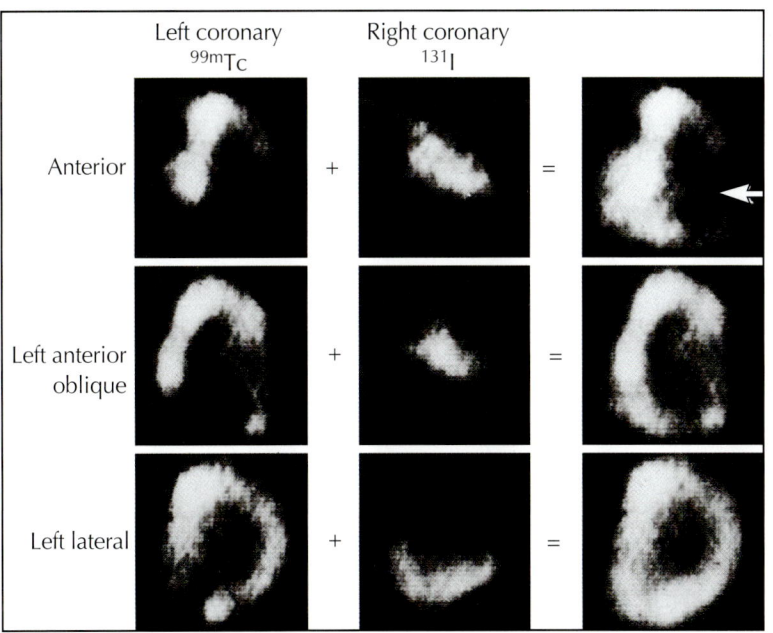

Figure 1-12. Direct assessment of myocardial perfusion. Rudolph and Heymann [10], in their classic studies of the fetal circulation, developed the radiolabeled microsphere technique to determine regional perfusion in tissues. Prior to their work, investigators had injected glass beads to evaluate the arterial circulation. The animals were killed and the beads counted to determine regional flow. Labeling the particles (carbonized microspheres) with multiple radiotracers allowed repeated determinations of myocardial perfusion in animals. This work was extended to humans when Jansen and Judkins [8,9] injected degradable particles (albumin aggregates) into the right and left coronary arteries. Studies with these agents provided insights into control of myocardial perfusion, distribution of cardiac output, and the role of collateral circulation. Microspheres of human albumin labeled with ^{99m}Tc or ^{131}I were injected directly into the left and right coronary arteries to define myocardial perfusion in the vascular territories of each vessel. Shown in this figure are images from a patient in Ashburn's original study. Of remarkable high quality, these images show a perfusion abnormality in the lateral wall. Radiolabeled microspheres are still commonly used for studying myocardial perfusion in experimental animal studies [7–10]. (*From* Ashburn *et al.* [7]; with permission.)

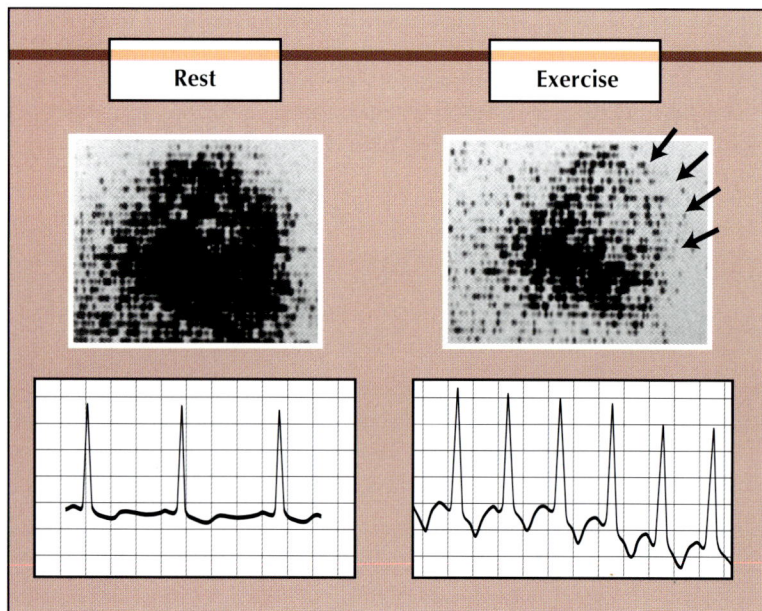

FIGURE 1-13. Evolution of present-day myocardial perfusion imaging. Four major radionuclide imaging devices, the rectilinear scanner, the single photon multicrystal gamma camera of Bender and Blau, and the single-crystal gamma camera of Anger as well as the initial planar positron camera designed by Brownell, allowed the evolution of probe-based determinations to imaging techniques, which extended the information available from global determinations to small regions of the heart. This technological advance was rapidly applied to determinations of global and regional cardiac function, myocardial perfusion, and identification of acute necrosis. In 1963, initial studies by Carr *et al.* [11] using ^{131}Cs demonstrated myocardial infarction as an area of decreased perfusion when the tracer was injected at rest. ^{131}Cs had slow clearance from the blood pool and was not an ideal agent for myocardial perfusion imaging. In 1969, Hurley *et al.* [12] described initial studies with ^{43}K, an agent with better photon energies for the rectilinear scanner, for the detection of acute myocardial infarction in humans. The application of ^{43}K to the detection of myocardial ischemia in the clinical setting was described by Zaret *et al.* [13–15]. ^{43}K was administered on two occasions, once at rest (*left*) and once during stress (*right*), with rectilinear scanner imaging after each injection. A reduction in myocardial tracer uptake during stress, which improved at rest, represented an area of ischemia (*arrows*). This technique was used for detection of patients with false-positive findings on exercise electrocardiography. Despite a relatively coarse image quality, these studies laid the foundation of present-day scintigraphic imaging of exercise-induced myocardial ischemia [13–15]. (*From* Zaret *et al.* [13]; with permission.)

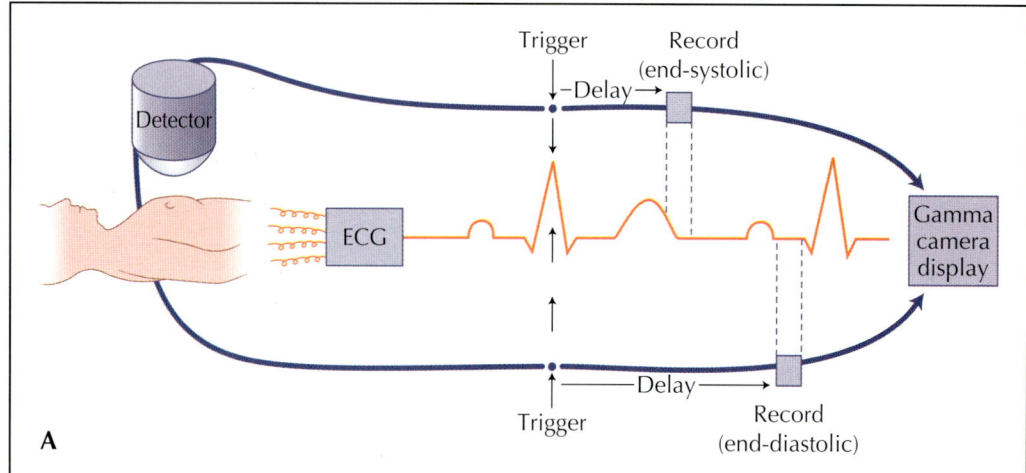

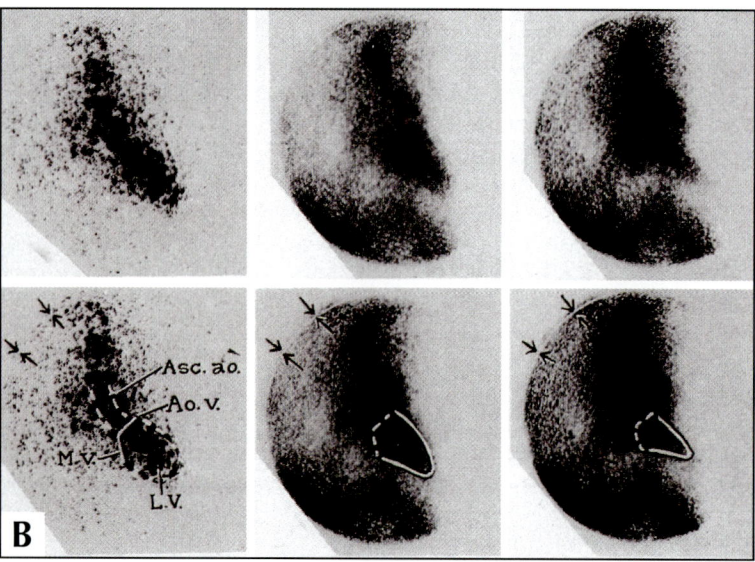

FIGURE 1-14. Assessment of myocardial function. First-pass studies of the heart were performed with the Anger camera. **A**, Images at the end of systole and the end of diastole during the first pass of tracer were recorded by Ashburn *et al.* [7] in 1968. These images were very count limited, making determination of regional wall motion abnormalities difficult. **B**, In 1969, the gating technique was applied to blood pool tracers that had equilibrated in the circulation, which permitted high-quality images of the cardiac blood pool to be recorded at end-diastole and end-systole. This technique was applied to the calculation of left ventricular ejection fraction and to the identification of regional wall motion abnormalities [16]. (*Panel B from* Strauss *et al.* [17]; with permission.)

Instrumentation

FIGURE 1-15. Radiation detectors. The detectors currently used for cardiac radionuclide studies have evolved from the following:

The cloud chamber detector used by Blumgart. The cloud chamber was designed by Charles Wilson and produced in 1927. Wilson was awarded the Nobel Prize for his discovery.

The Geiger-Mueller counter employed by Prinzmetal. The Geiger counter had a limited count rate capability and had limited sensitivity—because the detector is filled with gas, a low Z material that allowed the majority of gamma photons to pass through without an interaction.

Sodium iodide scintillation crystal used by rectilinear scanners and by single-photon gamma cameras. This was developed independently by Kallman in Germany and by Hofstadter in the United States.

Gas-filled detectors. These operate on the principle that when voltage is applied across two electrodes in a gas-filled space, an ionization event results in flow of current across the electrodes. Gas-filled detectors include ionization chambers, proportional counters, and Geiger-Mueller counters. These detectors differ primarily in the voltage applied between the electrodes. Gas-filled counters have low efficiency for gamma rays.

Scintillation detectors. These detectors operate on the principle that because denser media (both liquids and solids) have greater stopping power than gas-filled models, the energy released by the absorption of ionizing radiation by inorganic crystals such as sodium iodide is converted into visible light or ultraviolet rays, which can be converted into electrical signals. Sodium iodide crystal is used extensively as a scintillation detector. The presence of slight impurities greatly increases the light output by sodium iodide crystal. Therefore, sodium iodide crystal in gamma cameras is impregnated with thallium. Sodium iodide crystals are universally used in conventional gamma cameras. Conventional gamma cameras traditionally use sodium iodide crystals one-quarter inch to three-eighths inch thick. However, they have less stopping power for high-energy photons, such as those produced by PET tracers. Bismuth germanate (BGO) is most commonly used in PET cameras because it is denser than sodium iodide. Lutetium orthosilicate (LSO) is also dense and has higher sensitivity than BGO for the detection of high-energy photons; therefore, it is a promising new scintillator for use in PET cameras. Recently, thicker sodium iodide crystals (three quarters of an inch to 1-inch thick) have also been used for imaging high-energy positron tracers with SPECT. Several organic crystals and liquids, primarily hydrocarbons such as naphthalene and ordinary plastics and polystyrenes, emit fluorescence in response to ionizing radiation. Organic detectors are faster than inorganic crystals but are less efficient. They are used in well counters and in counting chambers.

Semiconductor detectors. These are used in solid-state detectors in which ionizing radiation is directly converted into an electric current. Several tetravalent elements such as silicone and germanium, when mixed with another element, generate weak electric current during exposure to ionizing radiation. Therefore, these detectors can be used for imaging ionizing radiation.

RADIATION DETECTORS

Gas-filled detectors
  Ionization chamber
  Proportional counter
  Geiger-Mueller counter
Scintillation detectors
  Inorganic crystals
    Sodium iodide
    Bismuth germanate (BGO)
    Gadolinium orthosilicate (GSO)
    Lutetium orthosilicate (LSO)
    Barium fluoride, cesium iodide
  Organic scintillators
    PPO (diphenyloxazole)
    BBOT (butyl-benzoxazolyl-thiophene)
Semiconductor detectors
  Silicon-lithium
  Germanium-lithium
  Cadmium-telluride

IMAGING DEVICES

Rectilinear scanner
Multicrystal camera
Anger camera
   Rotating Anger camera—SPECT
Coincidence detection—PET scanners
Nonimaging detectors
Small animal imaging cameras
Intravascular detectors

FIGURE 1-16. Radionuclide imaging devices. *Rectilinear scanners* were the first imaging devices for obtaining images with the use of radioisotopes. This scanner contained a small sodium iodide crystal with a single photomultiplier tube. Images were obtained by scanning the area of interest with these scanners. These were soon replaced with larger gamma cameras.

The *multicrystal camera* contains several sodium iodide crystals, each with a separate photomultiplier tube. These cameras have limited spatial resolution but very high count sensitivity. Currently, they are used only for dynamic first-pass imaging study.

The *Anger camera* is the most commonly used gamma camera in clinical practice. This contains a single large sodium iodide crystal with a large number of photomultiplier tubes for high spatial resolution. These detectors can be stationary or mounted on a gantry for obtaining tomographic images. The present generation of gamma cameras have multiple detectors that simultaneously acquire images at various projections of the heart—simultaneously, thereby decreasing the imaging time.

Coincidence detection is the principle on which PET cameras were developed. Each positron decays into two gamma rays that are released at 180 degrees to each other; thus, a positron decay event can be detected and localized in space when two opposing detectors capture photons simultaneously. Recently, conventional SPECT cameras have also been used in coincidence mode for imaging positron-emitting tracers after making several modifications.

Small animal imaging cameras. Both PET and SPECT cameras have been produced in highly miniaturized form for imaging small animals, such as rats and mice, for experimental animal studies. These devices have excellent spatial resolution. The SPECT equipment has two sodium iodide detectors with pinhole collimators. The animal to be imaged is placed in a plastic or glass tube and is rotated in front of the detectors to obtain very high resolution (on the order of 1 mm) SPECT images. Both PET and SPECT systems have been used successfully for mapping gene expression in various organ systems and for studying various biologic processes in small animals.

Nonimaging detectors. The field of nuclear cardiology started with nonimaging probes. A sophisticated, upgraded version of these probes continues to play an important role in cardiology for studying left ventricular function.

Intravascular detectors. Highly miniaturized catheter-mounted detectors are used in experimental studies for intravascular imaging.

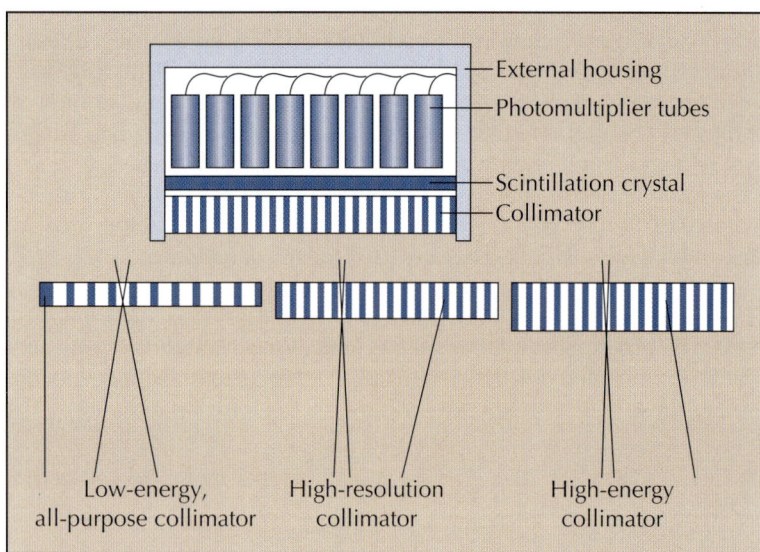

FIGURE 1-17. Structure of a gamma camera. The components of a gamma camera include the 1) scintillation detector, 2) photomultiplier tubes, 3) collimator, and 4) computer and electronics.

Scintillation detector. The scintillation detector, made up of sodium iodide or bismuth germanate (BGO), absorbs gamma rays and converts them into visible light. A gamma ray travels through the collimator and strikes the crystal, causing a scintillation, and this light is converted into an electrical signal. The intensity of the signal depends on the energy of the gamma ray. A pulse-height analyzer determines the energy of the incident gamma ray from the intensity of the light produced by its interaction with the crystal.

Photomultiplier tubes. The photomultiplier tubes amplify the light signal and convert it into an electrical signal for further processing. Photomultiplier tubes receive light signal from the crystal. They augment the signals of light and locate them spatially along the x and y axis. The modern scintillation camera has grown from seven phototubes to 91 phototubes viewing crystals that are now as large as 40×60 cm. The increasing number of phototubes translates into greater accuracy in locating the exact point on the crystal at which the gamma ray impinges. This constitutes the intrinsic resolution of the scintillation camera and is defined by the full width at half-maximum (FWHM). The intrinsic resolution has improved from its original 4 to 16 mm to the current 3 to 4 mm.

Collimator. The collimator is a sheet of lead, tungsten, or other heavy metal. It is interposed between the patient and the scintillation detector and allows only parallel gamma rays to reach the scintillation detector through holes in the sheet. Thicker sheets of metal are required for the use of tracers with high-energy gamma rays.

Computer and electronics. A computer and electronics process the electrical signals to reconstruct a spatial image of the organ of interest, such as the heart.

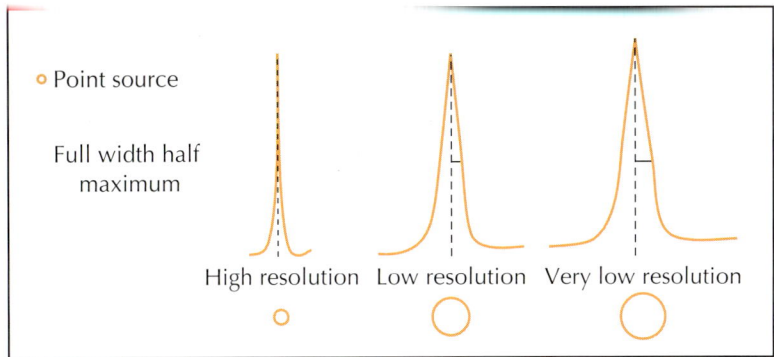

FIGURE 1-18. Spatial resolution and point spread function. Three parameters contribute to the technical adequacy of the radionuclide images: 1) spatial resolution, 2) noise, and 3) contrast.

Spatial resolution is instrument or hardware-dependent. The limitations of spatial resolution make a point source appear as a dot, rather than a point, during imaging with a gamma camera. The intrinsic resolution of an imaging system is described by point spread function or by obtaining the full width at half-maximum. With improvements in detector and collimator design and electronics, the intrinsic resolution of the gamma cameras has improved significantly over the last decade. Currently, this resolution is on the order of 3 to 4 mm.

Noise is irrelevant information or a disturbance of the useful data in the image. Noise can be filtered out by applying appropriate filters.

Contrast is a measure of the intensity or counts in a target organ compared with the intensity in the background region, and is often measured as a difference in the counts between the target organ and the background divided by the background counts. The higher the contrast, the more visible the organ of interest.

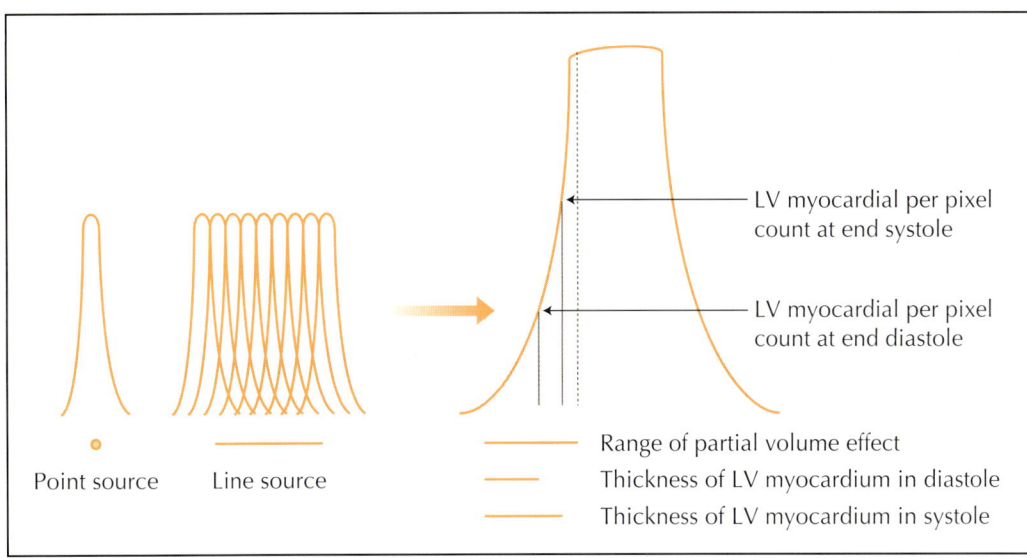

FIGURE 1-19. Partial volume effect. The inherent limitation of the resolution of the nuclear imaging systems makes the image of a point source appears as a dot of variable size, depending on the resolution of the system. Each point appears as a gaussian curve. An object being imaged (which can be considered to be made up of multiple, successive points) appears as overlapping dots. As a result of this overlap, the object appears brighter at the center than at the periphery, even when the imaged object has uniform distribution of the radiotracer. An important resultant of this phenomenon occurs during gated SPECT imaging. The left ventricular (LV) myocardial thickness varies during the cardiac cycle. The myocardium is thicker during systole than during diastole. Consequently, the myocardium appears brighter during systole than during diastole. The increase in myocardial brightness during systole compared with the myocardial brightness in diastole is an artifact of partial volume effect. However, this technique is used quite successfully in nuclear imaging to assess regional myocardial thickening during the cardiac cycle.

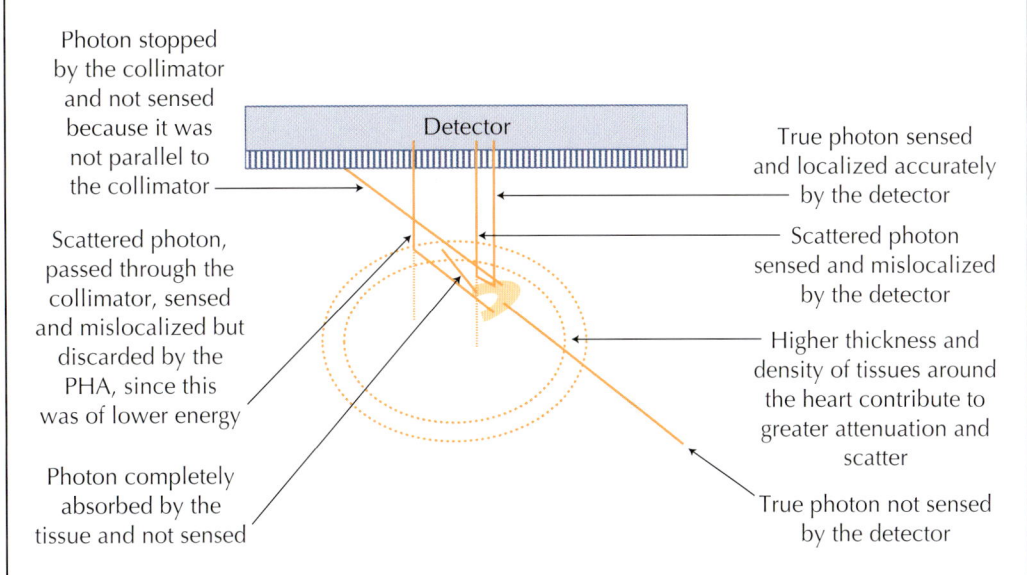

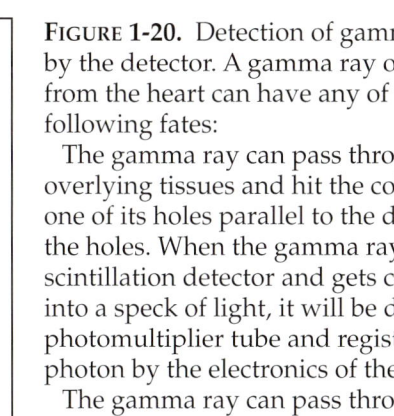

FIGURE 1-20. Detection of gamma rays by the detector. A gamma ray originating from the heart can have any of the following fates:

The gamma ray can pass through the overlying tissues and hit the collimator on one of its holes parallel to the direction of the holes. When the gamma ray falls on the scintillation detector and gets converted into a speck of light, it will be detected by a photomultiplier tube and registered as a photon by the electronics of the system.

The gamma ray can pass through the body and exit in a space that is not facing the gamma camera. This is a wasted photon. Use of multiple detectors maximizes photon detection.

Continued on next page

FIGURE 1-20. *(Continued)* The gamma ray can pass through the body and hit the collimator at an angle to the direction of the holes. Such photons are absorbed by the collimator. Depending on the width of the collimator holes and thickness of the lead sheet, only 0.5% to 2.0% of the photons reaching the collimator surface are able to pass through the collimator to the scintillation crystal.

The gamma ray can get absorbed while passing through the body tissues. This results in attenuation artifact. The thicker and denser the overlying tissue, the higher the chances of attenuation. Attenuation correction programs rely on deriving a three-dimensional pixel-by-pixel map of attenuation coefficient of the body using an external source of gamma radiation or x-rays.

The gamma ray may hit another atom in the body while passing through the tissues, bounce off this atom, and change its course, but eventually it will make its way to the collimator surface and to the scintillation detector. In this process, the photon loses a part of its energy. The gamma ray will be registered by the electronics, but if there was a significant loss of energy to a level below the chosen energy window (typically 20%), the pulse-height analyzer (PHA) will discard the photon as below the range of acceptance. If the energy loss was minimal and the photon still had energy in the accepted energy window, it will be accepted. However, the photon will be spatially mislocalized. These scattered and mislocalized photons degrade the quality of the image. Such photons can be avoided by decreasing the acceptance energy window of the photons.

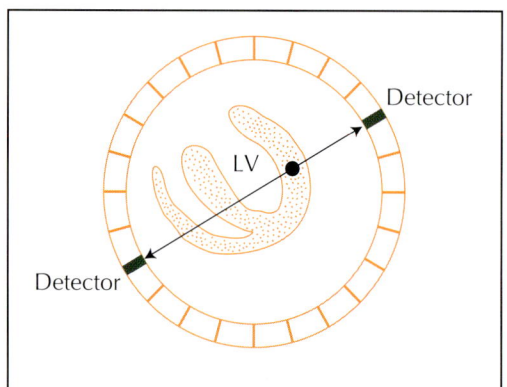

FIGURE 1-21. Coincidence detection. PET cameras use a principle for photon detection different from that used by the conventional gamma cameras. Two gamma rays (511 keV of energy each) are produced by the annihilation of positrons, which travel in opposite directions discharged at a 180-degree angle to each other; thus, positron decay can be localized by the electronics with the use of the principles of coincidence detection. These imaging systems do not require collimators and consequently have a very high count rate compared with standard SPECT equipment. The count rates with PET cameras are at least tenfold higher with SPECT cameras. LV—left ventricle.

IMAGE ACQUISITION AND PROCESSING

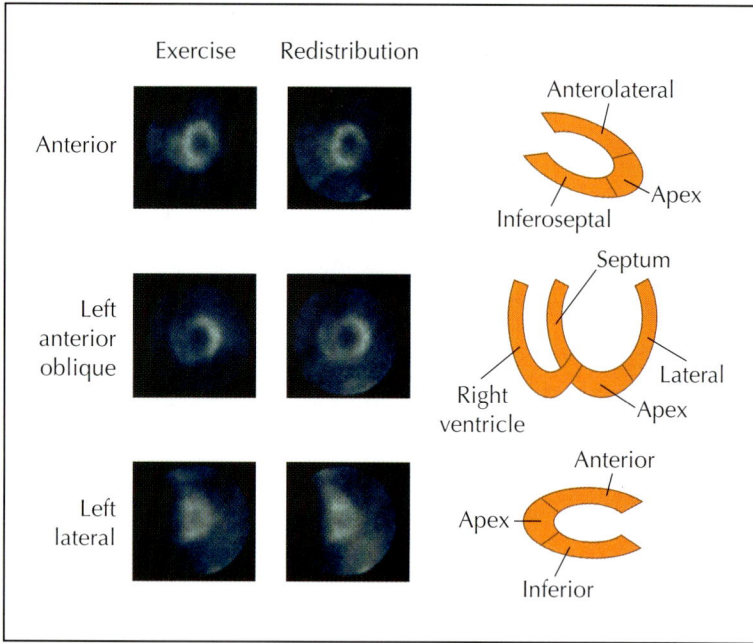

FIGURE 1-22. Planar imaging technique. Planar images of the heart are obtained in three standard views: anterior, left anterior oblique, and left lateral. For studying myocardial perfusion, these images are acquired for myocardial perfusion following exercise or pharmacologic stress and, again, following thallium redistribution or at rest. Areas of ischemia appear as reversible perfusion abnormality, whereas areas of scar appear as fixed perfusion abnormality, as shown in this example. Apart from visual examination, these images can also be analyzed with the use of a quantitative circumferential analysis program, in which the counts in each sector of the left ventricular myocardium are compared using the stress and rest images and with a normal database. Planar imaging is simple; however, it has the drawback of overlapping of structures.

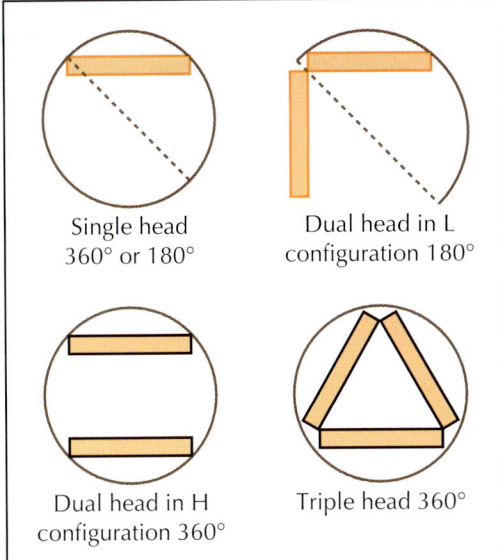

FIGURE 1-23. SPECT imaging camera head configuration. With SPECT, a series of planar images are obtained in an orbit around the patient. The images can be obtained over a full orbit of 360 degrees or over half of that (180 degrees). The asymmetric position of the heart in the thorax means that a 180-degree orbit can suffice in most clinical instances. However, a 180-degree orbit may sometimes result in artifacts. With the use of multihead detectors, data are acquired at various projections of the heart simultaneously, thereby shortening the time of image acquisition or improving image count density. Imaging with dual- and triple-head detectors can be completed in half or one third of the time taken by a single-head detector. With dual-head cameras, the detectors can be arranged parallel to each other or at right angles to each other. The latter configuration is preferable if simultaneous attenuation correction is applied.

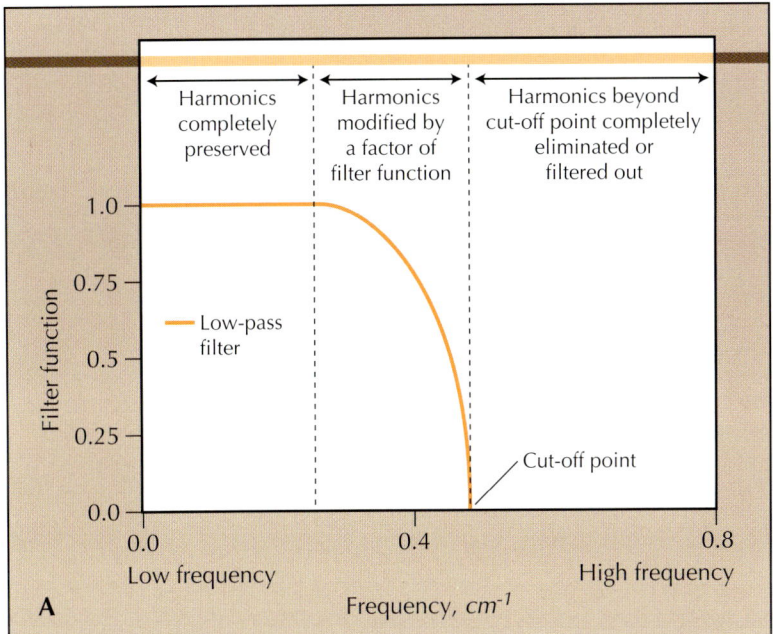
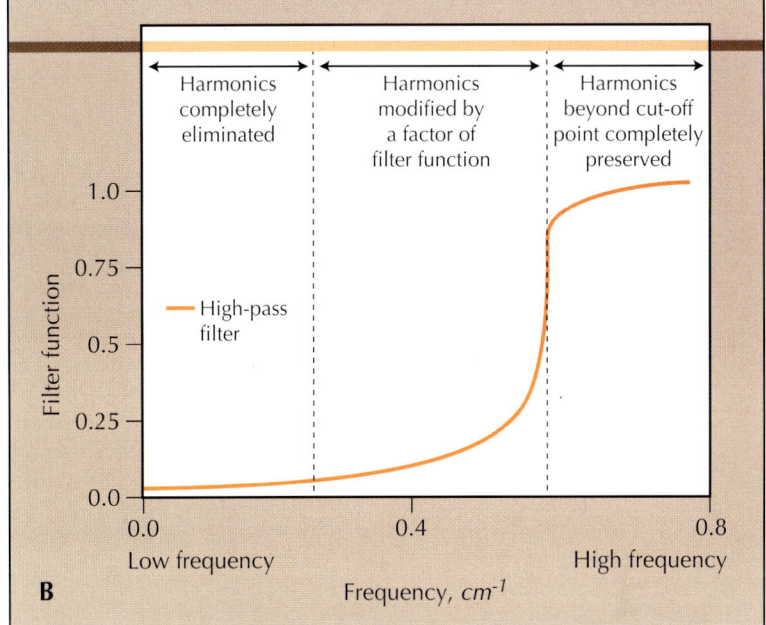

FIGURE 1-24. Filtering of SPECT images. The acquired raw images are somewhat noisy, and so filtering is required to eliminate or reduce the noise. There are several ways of filtering out the noise. The most common way is by Fourier transformation of the raw images, in which the image data are transformed into a series of frequencies. The relevant data are present in the low-frequency range, whereas noise is present in the high-frequency range. **A**, Low-pass filter allows the low frequencies to be retained unaltered and eliminates completely the high frequencies above the cut-off range. The frequencies in the intermediate range are altered by a function depicted by the slope of the cut-off curve. If too much filtering is used, even the useful data may be lost. **B**, The high-pass filter retains the high frequencies and eliminates the low frequencies. This filter is used primarily for edge enhancement.

Continued on next page

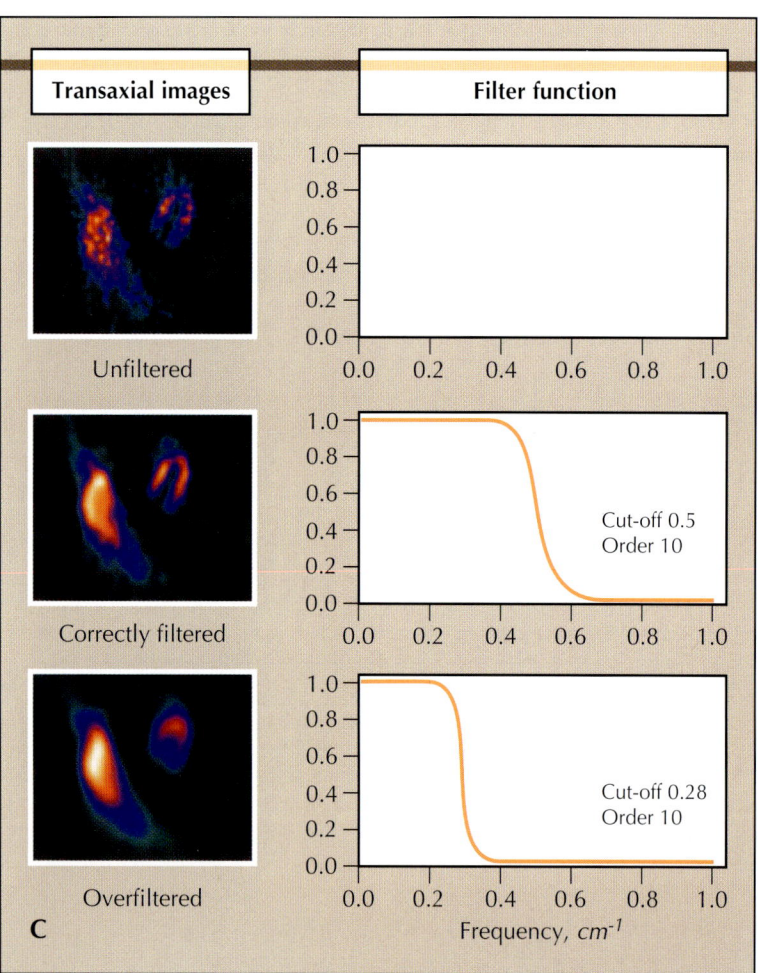

FIGURE 1-24. *(Continued)* **C,** A patient example in which low-pass filter (Butterworth filter) is applied to transaxial images of the heart is shown. The unfiltered images *(top)* are of poor quality and very noisy. The background noise is eliminated in the properly filtered images *(center)*. However, overfiltering results in distortion of the myocardial contour *(bottom)*.

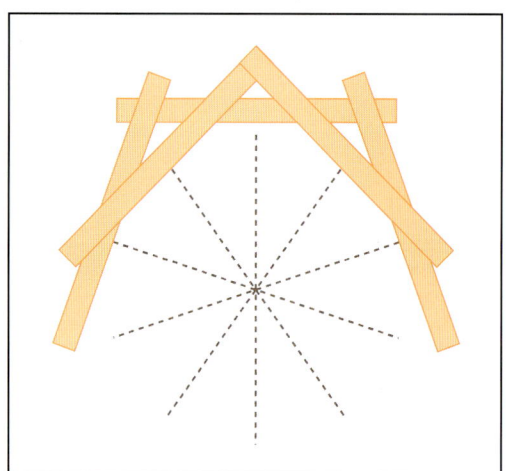

FIGURE 1-25. Backprojection of filtered data. The data from the raw SPECT images are localized in three-dimensional space by backprojection of the filtered data. Each photon is localized along a line on the z axis from a single planar image. The point where the z axes from the different planar images transect determines the location of the photon along the z axis.

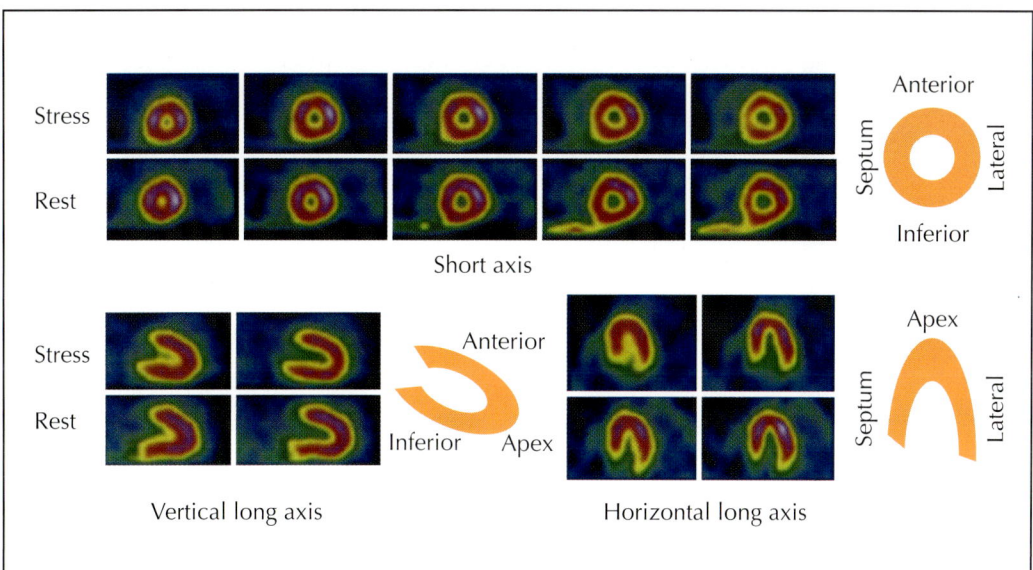

FIGURE 1-26. Display of SPECT slices. The SPECT perfusion images of the heart are displayed as a series of slices (usually 1 pixel thick) in short-axis, vertical long-axis, and horizontal long-axis views. The short-axis slices *(top row)* are displayed starting from the apex *(left)* and proceeding toward the base *(right)* of the heart. The corresponding stress and rest perfusion slices are displayed in a paired manner. Similarly paired vertical long-axis slices *(bottom row, left)* are displayed from the anterior *(left)* to the posterior *(right)* aspect of the heart, and paired horizontal long-axis slices *(bottom row, right)* are displayed from the inferior *(left)* to the superior *(right)* aspect of the heart. The left ventricular myocardium is divided into anterior, septal, inferior, and lateral walls and apex (shown in the schematic representation of the heart). In normal hearts, the radiotracer distribution should appear uniform in the left ventricular myocardium. However, normally, the most proximal part of the septum is membranous and appears thin compared with the rest of the septum. The inferior wall also has fewer counts compared with the lateral wall and anterior wall because of attenuation from the diaphragm. The example shown here is a normal study.

Novel Applications of Radionuclide Techniques for Advancement of Cardiovascular Research

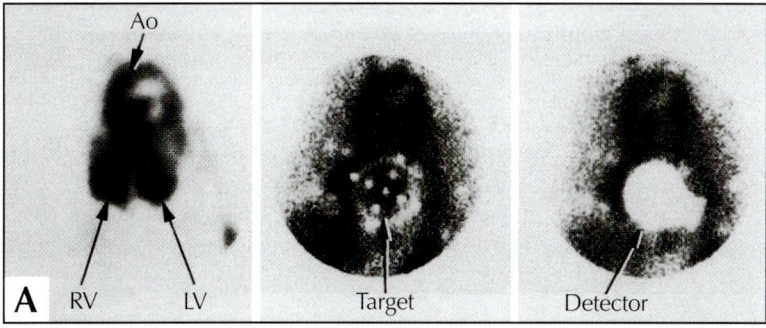

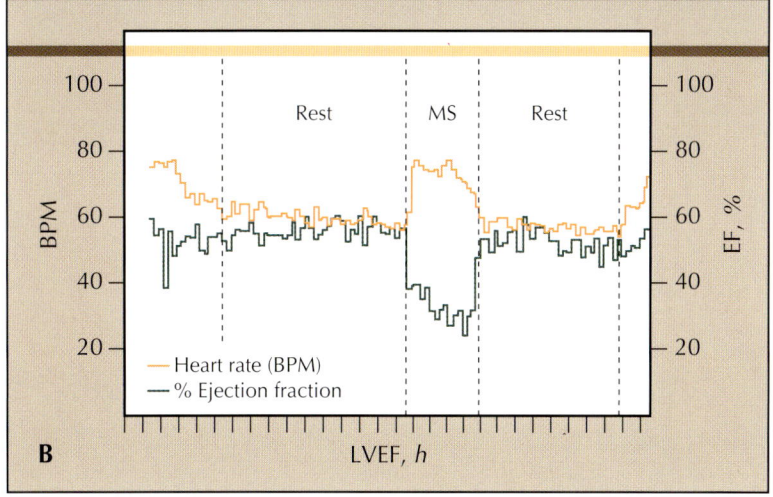

FIGURE 1-27. Ambulatory left ventricular function monitoring. A highly miniaturized nonimaging detector with high count sensitivity and high temporal resolution (C-Vest [Capintec, Inc., Ramsey, NJ]) has been developed for continuous ambulatory left ventricular (LV) function monitoring. After blood pool labeling with ^{99m}Tc, similar to that in radionuclide angiocardiography, the miniature detector is positioned on the chest over the left ventricular blood pool under gamma camera control. The detector obtains counts from the left ventricular blood pool at a rate of 32/s and records them digitally on a solid-state modified Holter monitor. An ECG is also recorded simultaneously. A continuous trend of heart rate, relative end-diastolic and end-systolic volumes, left ventricular ejection fraction (LVEF), and relative cardiac output is obtained. **A,** A picture of the cardiac blood pool obtained in the left anterior oblique view after blood pool labeling with ^{99m}Tc is shown. In this view, the left and right ventricular (RV) blood pools are well separated. A positioning target device with lead markers and ring is used to determine the optimal position for the detector. Once an optimal position is obtained, the positioning target is removed from the ring and is replaced with the detector, which is held in place with the help of a semirigid plastic vest-like garment [18–21]. **B,** Changes in left ventricular function in response to a mental stress (MS) task (mental arithmetic) in a patient with coronary artery disease are shown. There is more than a 20% point drop in LVEF in response to mental arithmetic, which recovers promptly on cessation of the task. Coronary artery disease patients with mental stress–induced left ventricular dysfunction have a threefold higher incidence of adverse cardiac events on follow-up compared with coronary artery disease patients with no decrease in LVEF with mental stress [22–24]. BPM—beats per minute.

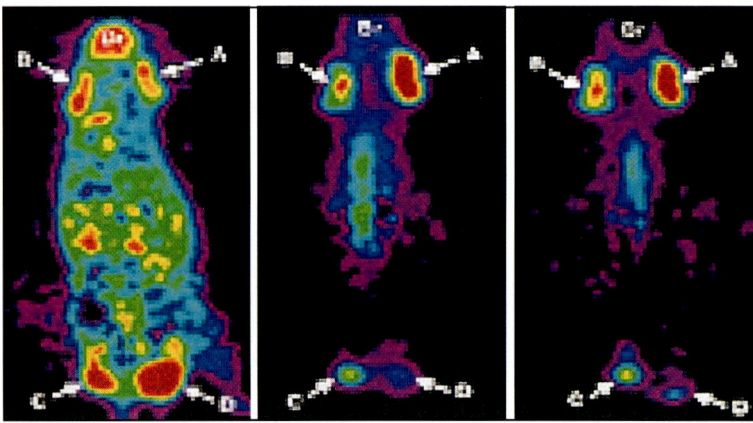

FIGURE 1-28. Small animal imaging systems. Highly miniaturized PET and SPECT cameras for imaging small animals have been developed [25–29]. The miniaturized PET system has a ring of lutetium oxyorthosilicate detectors with a spatial resolution of less than 2 mm. This system has been used for imaging gene expression and assessment of the metabolic activity of the heart in rats and mice. The miniaturized SPECT camera has two sodium iodide detectors with pinhole collimators. The animal to be imaged is placed in a plastic or glass tube and is rotated in front of the detectors to obtain very high-resolution SPECT images. This system has a resolution of 1 mm. The development of transgenic animals has revolutionized biomedical research. Small imaging systems provide the capacity to image various molecular subcellular processes as well as gene expression in small animals. These images show miniaturized PET images of bi-cistronic reporter gene expression in nude mice implanted with tumor cell lines (C6) infected with reporter genes (HSV1-sr39tk and rl). This is referred to as pCMV-D2R-IRES-sr39tk C6 tumor cell line. The cell lines were injected in four different positions: infected cell lines in positions A, B, and C, and the parent cell line in position D. When each tumor had grown to approximately 6 mm, whole-body images were obtained with FDG ([^{18}F]–fluorodeoxyglucose) (*left*), FESP (^{18}F–labeled ethylspiperone) (*center*), and FPCV (^{18}F–labeled penciclovir) (*right*) on separate occasions. FDG accumulated in all four tumor sites, but FESV and FPCV accumulated in sites A, B, and C, which had genes for the substrates for these ligands. Moreover, the intensity of FESV and FPCV uptake in sites A, B, and C correlated with the concentration of corresponding mRNA in each tumor site [25–29]. (*Courtesy of* S.S. Gambhir; *from* Yu *et al.* [30]; with permission.)

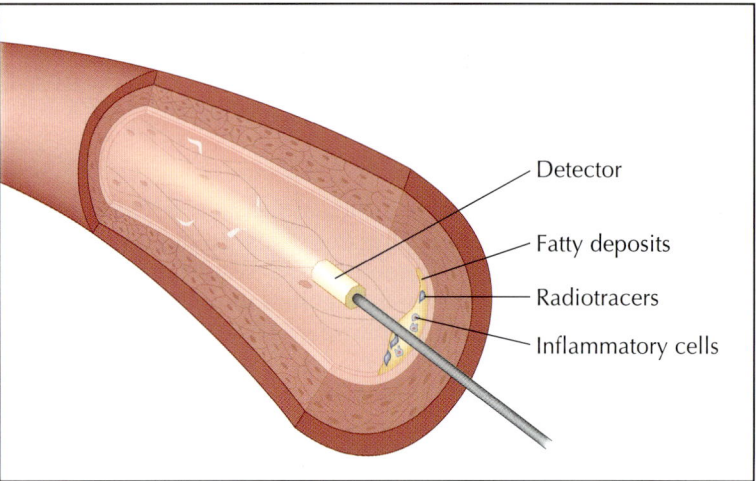

FIGURE 1-29. Intravascular radiation probe. The intravascular radiation detector probe currently under development is a highly miniaturized, catheter tip–mounted nuclear probe system. The probe has a plastic scintillation detector at its tip for the detection of beta rays. The light produced by the scintillation detector is transmitted via optical fibers to a point where it is converted into electrical signals for further processing. A catheter tip–mounted solid-state detector, which directly converts beta rays into electrical signals, is also under development. These detectors are used in experimental animal studies of the biology of atheromatous plaques after the injection of radiopharmaceuticals with affinity for various components of the plaque. In a recent study, Tawakol *et al.* [31] successfully used intravascular radiation probes to map aortic [^{18}F]-fluorodeoxyglucose uptake in rabbits with experimental atherosclerosis [31].

References

1. Blumgart H: *The Velocity of Blood Flow in Health and Disease*. Baltimore: Williams & Wilkins; 1931.

2. Donato L: Basic concepts of radiocardiography. *Semin Nucl Med* 1973, 3:111–130.

3. Prinzmetal M, Corday E, Bergman HC, *et al.*: Radiocardiography: a new method for studying the blood flow through the chambers of the heart in human beings. *Science* 1948, 108:143.

4. Kety SS, Schmidt CF: The determination of cerebral blood flow in man by the use of nitrous oxide in low concentration. *Am J Physiol* 1945, 143:53.

5. Ross RS, Ueda K, Lichtlen PR, Rees JR: Measurement of myocardial blood flow in animals and man by selective injection of radioactive inert gas into the coronary arteries. *Circ Res* 1964, 15:28.

6. Bing RJ, Bennish A, Bluemchen G, *et al.*: The determination of coronary flow equivalent with coincidence counting technic. *Circulation* 1964, 39:833.

7. Ashburn WL, Braunwald E, Simon AL, *et al.*: Myocardial perfusion imaging with radioactive-labeled particles injected directly into the coronary circulation of patients with coronary artery disease. *Circulation* 1971, 44:851–865.

8. Grames GM, Jansen C, Gander M, *et al.*: Safety of the direct coronary injection of radiolabeled particles. *J Nucl Med* 1974, 15:2–6.

9. Kirk GA, Adams R, Jansen C, Judkins MP: Particulate myocardial perfusion scintigraphy: Its clinical usefulness in evaluation of coronary artery disease. *Semin Nucl Med* 1977, 7:67–84.

10. Heymann MA, Payne BD, Hoffman JI, Rudolph AM: Blood flow measurements with radionuclide-labeled particles. *Prog Cardiovasc Dis* 1977, 20:55–79.

11. Carr EA, Gleason G, Shaw J, *et al.*: Direct imaging of myocardial infarction by photoscanning after administration of cesium-131. *Am Heart J* 1964, 68:627–630.

12. Hurley PJ, Cooper M, Reba RC, *et al.*: ^{43}KCl: a new radiopharmaceutical for imaging the heart. *J Nucl Med* 1971, 12:516–519.

13. Zaret BL, Strauss BL, Martin ND, *et al.*: Noninvasive evaluation of regional myocardial perfusion with radioactive potassium: study of patients at rest, exercise and during angina pectoris. *N Engl J Med* 1973, 288:809–812.

14. Zaret BL, Stenson RE, Martin NE, *et al.*: Potassium-43 myocardial perfusion scanning for the noninvasive evaluation of patients with false-positive exercise tests. *Circulation* 1973, 48:1234–1240.

15. Strauss HW, Zaret BL, Martin ND, *et al.*: Non-invasive evaluation of regional myocardial perfusion with potassium-43. *Radiology* 1973, 108:85–90.

16. Zaret BL, Strauss HW, Hurley PJ, *et al.*: A noninvasive scintigraphic method for detecting regional ventricular dysfunction in man. *N Engl J Med* 1971, 284:1165–1170.

17. Strauss HW, Zaret BL, Hurley PJ, *et al.*: A scintiphotographic method for measuring left ventricular ejection fraction in man without cardiac catheterization. *Am J Cardiol* 1971, 28:575–580.

18. Zaret BL, Jain D: Monitoring of left ventricular function with miniaturized non-imaging detectors. In *Nuclear Cardiology: State of the Art and Future Directions*, edn 2. Edited by Zaret BL, Beller GA. St. Louis: Mosby–Year Book; 1999:191–200.

19. Jain D, Zaret BL: Ambulatory monitoring of left ventricular function. In *Cardiac Nuclear Medicine*, edn 3. Edited by Gerson MC. New York: McGraw-Hill; 1996:415–426.

20. Jain D, Wagner HN Jr, Zaret BL: Miniature probes for continuous monitoring of left ventricular function. In *Principles of Nuclear Medicine*, edn 2. Edited by Wagner HN Jr, Szabo Z, Buchanan JW. Philadelphia: WB Saunders; 1995:286–291.

21. Kayden DS, Wackers FJ, Zaret BL: Silent left ventricular dysfunction during routine activity after thrombolytic therapy for acute myocardial infarction. *J Am Coll Cardiol* 1990, 15:1500–1507.

22. Burg MM, Jain D, Soufer R, *et al.*: Role of behavioral and psychological factors in mental stress–induced silent left ventricular dysfunction in coronary artery disease. *J Am Coll Cardiol* 1993, 22:440–448.

23. Jain D, Burg MM, Soufer RS, Zaret BL: Prognostic significance of mental stress–induced left ventricular dysfunction in patients with coronary artery disease. *Am J Cardiol* 1995, 76:31–35.

24. Jain D, Shaker SM, Burg M, *et al.*: Effects of mental stress on left ventricular and peripheral vascular performance in patients with coronary artery disease. *J Am Coll Cardiol* 1998, 31:1314–1322.

25. Cherry SR, Shao Y, Silverman RW, *et al.*: Micro PET: a high-resolution PET scanner for imaging small animals. *IEEE Trans Nucl Sci* 1997, 44:1161–1166.

26. Chatziioannou AF, Cherry SR, Shao Y, *et al.*: Performance evaluation of micro PET: a high-resolution lutetium-oxyorthosilicate PET scanner for animal imaging. *J Nucl Med* 1999, 40:1164–1175.

27. Weber DA, Ivanovic M, Franceschi D, *et al.*: Pinhole SPECT: an approach to in vivo high resolution SPECT imaging in small laboratory animals. *J Nucl Med* 1994, 35:342–348.

28. Strand SE, Ivanovic M, Erlandsson K, *et al.*: Small animal imaging with pinhole single-photon emission computed tomography. *Cancer* 1994, 73:981–984.

29. Ishizu K, Mukai T, Yonekura Y, *et al.*: Ultra-high resolution SPECT system using four pinhole collimators for small animal studies. *J Nucl Med* 1995, 36:2282–2287.

30. Yu Y, Annala AJ, Barrio J, *et al.*: Quantification of target gene expression by imaging reporter gene expression in living animals. *Nat Med* 2000, 6:933–937.

31. Tawakol A, Elmaleh D, Gewirtz H, *et al.*: Detection of macrophage-rich atherosclerotic lesions with ^{18}FDG and a novel catheter-mounted beta probe. *Circulation* 2002, 106(suppl II):II-331.

CHAPTER 2

SPECT AND PET TECHNIQUES

Vasken Dilsizian

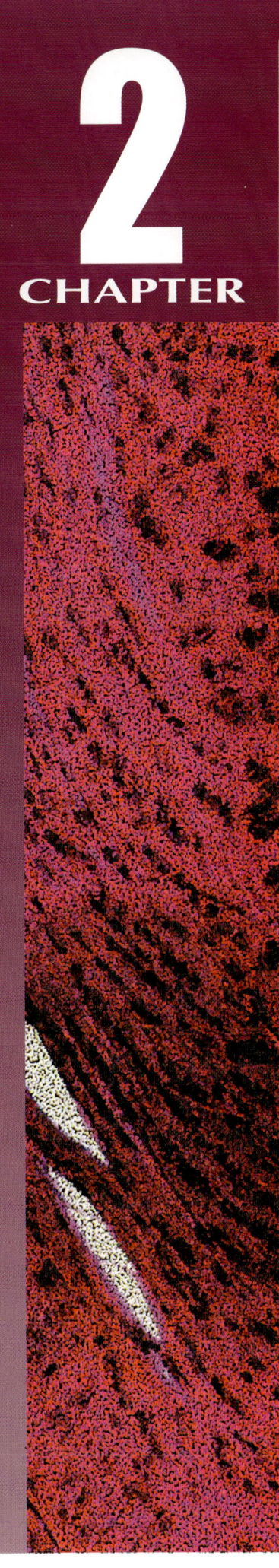

The advent of SPECT in the late 1970s and PET in the 1980s changed dramatically the clinical utility of radiotracer technique for the assessment of myocardial perfusion and viability. Both SPECT and PET technologies use a similar reconstruction process to obtain tomographic images of the heart. However, they differ in the type of radiopharmaceuticals and the kind of instrumentation used to acquire cardiac images. SPECT allows noninvasive evaluation of myocardial blood flow by extractable tracers such as ^{201}Tl and ^{99m}Tc-labeled perfusion tracers. PET, on the other hand, allows noninvasive assessment of regional blood flow, function, and metabolism using physiologic substrates prepared with positron-emitting isotopes, *eg*, carbon, oxygen, nitrogen, and fluorine. After acute myocardial injury and coronary reperfusion, SPECT and PET techniques allow the noninvasive determination of the extent of myocardial salvage by distinguishing stunned from necrotic myocardium. Similarly, in patients with chronic coronary artery disease and left ventricular dysfunction, these techniques allow the noninvasive differentiation between hypoperfused but viable myocardium (hibernation) and hypoperfused and scarred myocardium in dysfunctional regions. Such differentiation of viable (reversible) from nonviable (irreversibly injured) myocardium with SPECT and PET techniques has been used to guide therapeutic decisions for revascularization.

Radioisotopes commonly used with SPECT emit gamma rays of varying energies and have relatively long physical half-lives. Localization of gamma rays emitted by single photon-emitting radiotracers in the heart is accomplished by an Anger scintillation camera (gamma camera) which converts the gamma rays to light photons via sodium iodide scintillation detectors. The gamma camera limits the direction of photons entering the detector by a collimator and then positions each event electronically. Thus, the radioisotopes used for optimal scintigraphic registration with SPECT are limited to those that emit gamma rays with an energy range suitable for the gamma camera and related single photon devices, *eg*, ^{201}Tl, ^{99m}Tc, and ^{123}I. The spatial resolution of the SPECT system is between 12 and 15 mm. Although clinically useful, estimates of relative myocardial blood flow by SPECT are significantly affected by attenuation artifacts.

Positron-emitting radioisotopes commonly used with PET emit two gamma rays, 511 keV each, and have relatively short physical half-lives. When the high-energy positron is emitted from a nucleus, it travels a short distance and collides with an electron. The result is complete annihilation of both the positron and the electron, and conversion of the combined mass to energy in the form of electromagnetic radiation (two gamma rays, 511 keV each). Because the gamma rays are perfectly collinear (discharged at 180° to each other) and travel in opposite directions, the PET detectors can be programmed to register only events with temporal coincidence of photons that strike directly at opposing detectors. This results in improved spatial (4 to 6 mm) and temporal resolution. Moreover, the PET system is more sensitive than the SPECT system (higher count rate) and affords the possibility of attenuation correction. The consequence of these advantages with PET is the possibility for quantitation of tracer concentration in absolute units.

The radioisotopes commonly used with SPECT are not naturally occurring elements used for physiologic building blocks. Although ^{99m}Tc is the best-suited radioisotope for scintigraphic work with the gamma camera, it does not covalently bind to oxygen, carbon, and nitrogen in organic molecules and usually demands more complicated linkage systems to tag it onto organic substrates in chelated form. In contrast, isotopes of naturally occurring elements, *eg*, ^{11}C, ^{15}O, and ^{13}N, are all positron emitters, and therefore tagging molecular substrates with such elements can be accomplished without significant alteration of substrate specificity. The positron emitter ^{18}F can displace molecular hydrogen without altering substrate specificity for an enzyme-catalyzed reaction. Thus, a serious distinction between PET and SPECT is in the development of radioligands in the future that label primary substrates for energy metabolism and membrane receptor subtypes in the heart without significantly altering substrate specificity.

SPECT AND PET TECHNIQUES

SEVERITY OF REDUCTION IN MYOCARDIAL PERFUSION
SPECT tracers
 ^{201}Tl, ^{99m}Tc-labeled tracers (with and without nitrates)
PET tracers
 ^{82}Rubidium, ^{13}N-ammonia, ^{15}O-water

SARCOLEMAL CELL MEMBRANE INTEGRITY
SPECT techniques
 ^{201}Tl redistribution
PET techniques
 ^{82}Rubidium washout

CONTRACTILE RESERVE
Dobutamine echocardiography
Dobutamine MRI
Exercise or dobutamine radionuclide angiography
Gated SPECT with dobutamine
Gated PET with dobutamine

METABOLISM
SPECT techniques
 ^{123}I-labeled fatty acids
PET techniques
 [^{18}F]-fluorodeoxyglucose
 ^{11}C-acetate
 ^{11}C-palmitate
 Metabolic trapping of ^{13}N-ammonia

FIGURE 2-1. SPECT and PET techniques. The use of radiotracers that interrogate severity of reduction in myocardial blood flow, cell membrane integrity, contractile reserve, or cellular metabolism could enable the differentiation between viable and scarred myocardium among patients with chronic ischemic left ventricular dysfunction. Therapeutic interventions that improve dysfunctional but viable myocardial regions may significantly increase left ventricular ejection fraction and impact left ventricular remodeling and patient outcome.

SPECT TECHNIQUES: THALLIUM-201

SPECT TECHNIQUES: ^{201}Tl

- Monovalent cation with biologic properties similar to potassium
- 80 keV mercury x-ray emission, 74-h physical half-life
- High first-pass extraction fraction ($\approx 85\%$)
- Transported across myocyte sarcolemmal membrane via the Na-K ATPase transport system and by facilitative diffusion
- Peak myocardial concentration within 5 min of intravenous injection
- Rapid clearance from the intravascular compartment
- Redistribution begins 10 to 15 min after injection

FIGURE 2-2. SPECT techniques: ^{201}Tl. Myocardial extraction of ^{201}Tl is dependent on energy utilization, membrane adenosine triphosphate (ATPase), and active transport. ^{201}Tl does not actively concentrate in regions of infarcted or scarred myocardium. Thus, decreased myocardial ^{201}Tl uptake early after injection could be caused either by reduced regional blood flow or by infarction. Experimental studies with ^{201}Tl have shown that the cellular extraction of ^{201}Tl across the cell membrane is unaffected by hypoxia unless irreversible injury is present. Similarly, pathophysiologic conditions of chronic hypoperfusion (hibernation) and postischemic dysfunction (stunning), in which regional contractile function is impaired in the presence of myocardial viability, do not adversely alter extraction of ^{201}Tl.

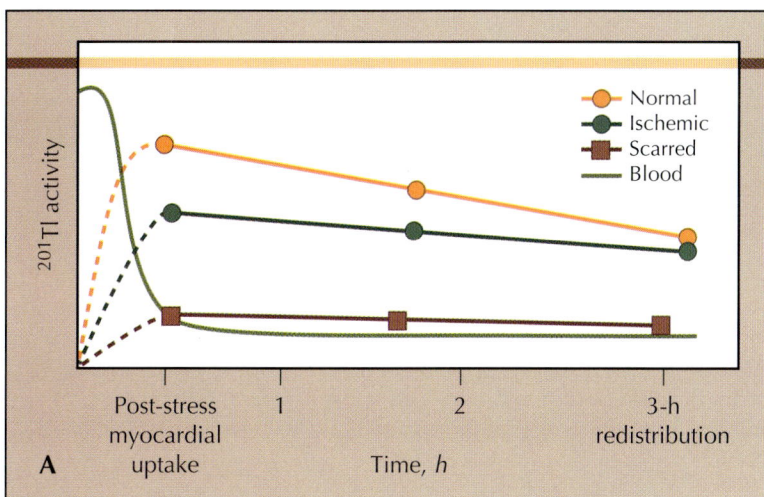 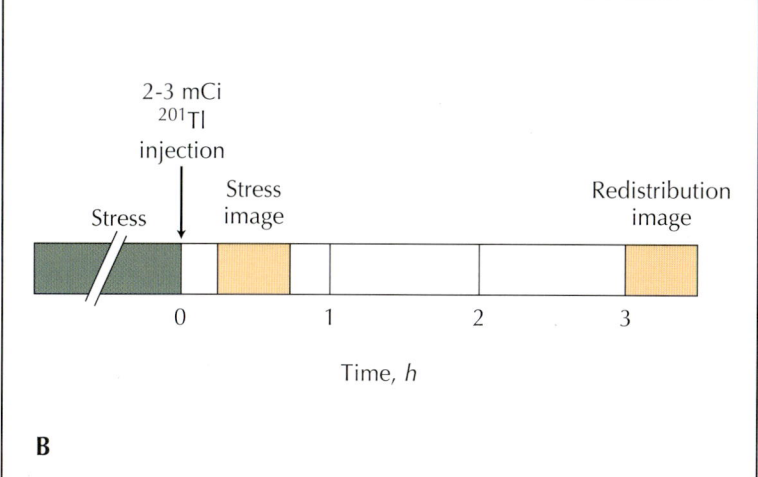

FIGURE 2-3. Stress-redistribution ^{201}Tl protocol. Schematic diagrams of ^{201}Tl uptake and redistribution in normal and ischemic myocardium, **A**, and a stress-redistribution protocol, **B**, are shown. While the initial distribution of ^{201}Tl (early after intravenous injection) is proportional to regional blood flow, the later distribution of ^{201}Tl over a 3- to 4-hour period, the redistribution phase, is a function of regional blood volume and is unrelated to flow. During the redistribution phase, there is a continuous exchange of ^{201}Tl between the myocardium and the extracardiac compartments, driven by the concentration gradient of tracer and myocyte viability. Thus, the extent to defect resolution, from the initial to delayed redistribution images over time (a reversible defect), reflects one index of myocardial viability. When only nonviable, scarred myocardium is present, the initial ^{201}Tl defect (an irreversible defect) persists over time without redistribution. When both viable and scarred myocardium are present, ^{201}Tl redistribution is incomplete, giving the appearance of partial reversibility. Thus, the initial phase of ^{201}Tl studies reflect reductions in flow caused by coronary artery narrowing, while the delayed, redistribution phase of ^{201}Tl studies reflect myocardial potassium space, differentiating viable from scarred myocardium.

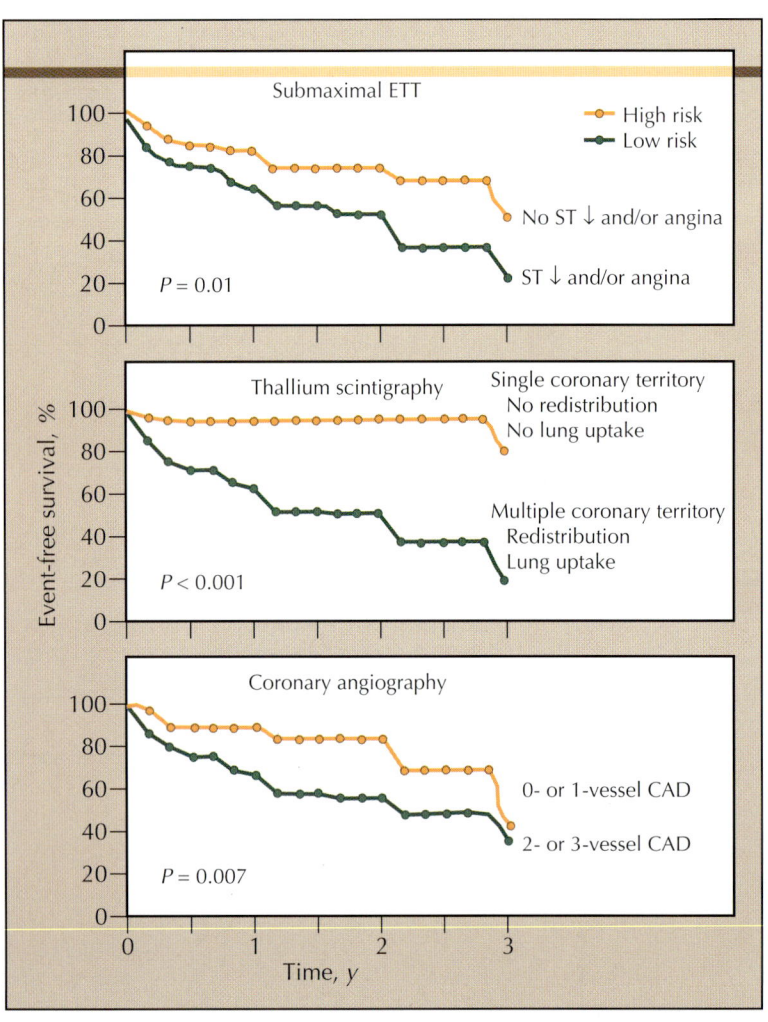

FIGURE 2-4. Prognostic value of thallium scintigraphy. Beyond its value as a perfusion and viability tracer, the stress-redistribution ^{201}Tl studies provide useful information regarding patient outcome and prognosis. In patients with chronic ischemic heart disease, increased lung-to-heart ratio after stress, transient left ventricular cavity dilatation, and extensive reversible and irreversible ^{201}Tl defects have been shown to be important predictors of adverse outcome. Similarly, the combination of reversible ^{201}Tl defects and increased lung-to-heart ratio has been shown to differentiate between low-risk and high-risk patients after an acute myocardial infarction. Among patients with acute myocardial infarction who underwent a predischarge submaximal exercise treadmill test (ETT), ^{201}Tl scintigraphy, and coronary angiography, ^{201}Tl identified the low-risk subgroup much better than submaximal exercise treadmill testing or coronary angiography. (*Adapted from* Gibson *et al*. [1].)

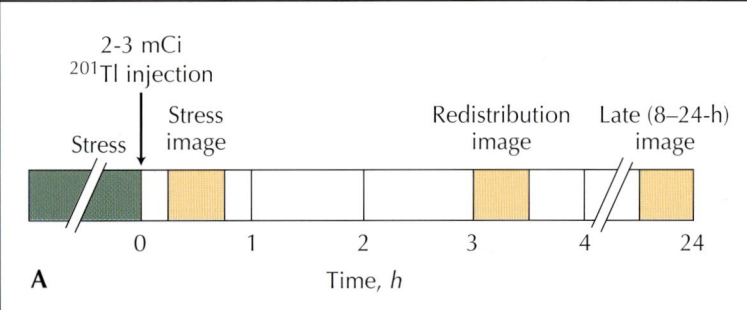

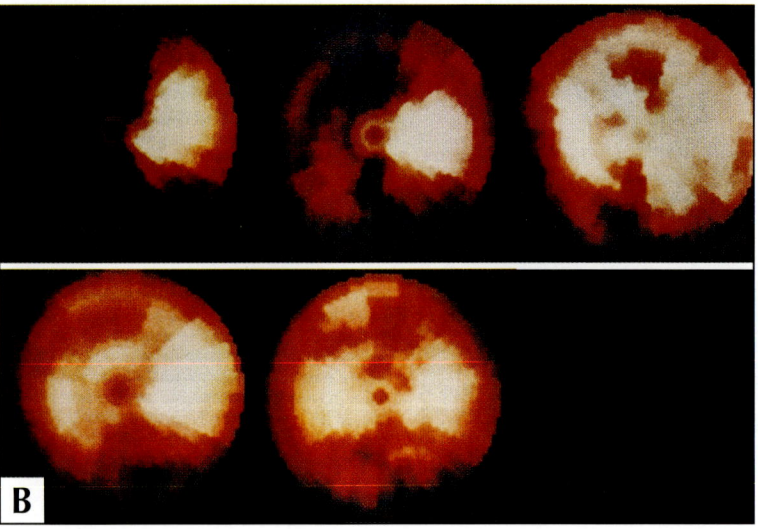

FIGURE 2-5. Late (24-hour) ^{201}Tl redistribution. **A,** Late redistribution protocol after stress-redistribution ^{201}Tl imaging. In some patients with critically stenosed coronary arteries, the initial uptake of ^{201}Tl in the ischemic region is low and the accumulation of the tracer from the recirculating ^{201}Tl in the blood is slow. Consequently, ischemic but viable myocardium may appear irreversible over the 3- to 4-hour redistribution period and may mimic the appearance of scarred myocardium. However, if more time is allowed for redistribution, a greater number of viable myocardial regions may be differentiated from scarred myocardium.

B, Polar maps demonstrating the effect of late ^{201}Tl redistribution. Bull's-eye image of ^{201}Tl immediately after exercise (*top panel, left*) shows marked decrease in tracer uptake throughout the anterior, septal, apical, and inferoapical regions, with partial redistribution on the 4-hour delayed image (*center*). However, on the late (17-hour) redistribution image (*right*), there is complete reversibility in all myocardial regions, suggestive of extensive myocardial ischemia rather than scar. After successful percutaneous transluminal coronary angioplasty (PTCA), bull's-eye image of ^{201}Tl immediately after exercise (*bottom panel, left*) shows normal distribution of the tracer throughout all myocardial regions, documenting the accuracy of late redistribution ^{201}Tl and the absence of myocardial scarring. In patients undergoing revascularization, 95% of segments that demonstrated late redistribution showed improved ^{201}Tl uptake after revascularization. However, as with early (3–4 hour) redistribution, the absence of late redistribution underestimates the presence of viable myocardium (*right*). Up to 37% of segments that remained irreversible on both early and late redistribution studies showed improvement in function after revascularization [2]. Moreover, despite implementing longer imaging time, a number of late redistribution studies had suboptimal counts statistics at 24 hours. The data suggest that although late ^{201}Tl imaging improves the identification of viable myocardium when compared with early redistribution imaging, it continues to underestimate segmental improvement after revascularization. (*Panel B from* Cloninger *et al*. [3]; with permission.)

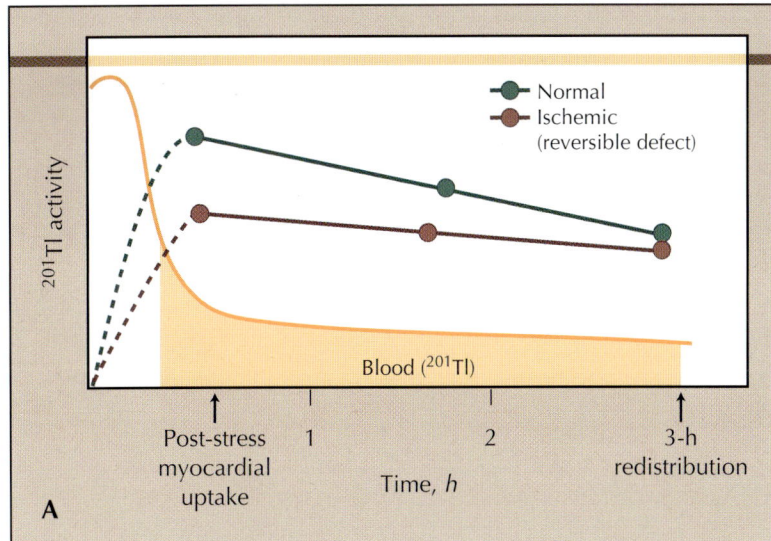
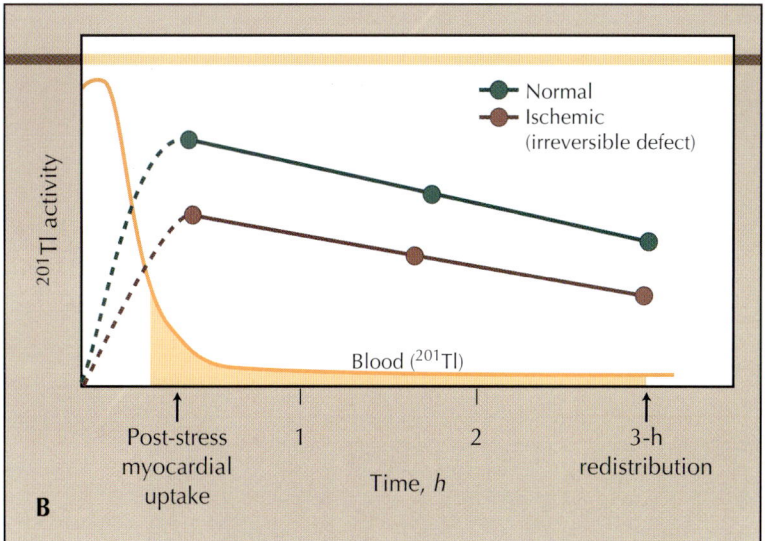

FIGURE 2-6. Myocardial thallium uptake and clearance in relation to blood activity of thallium. Redistribution of ^{201}Tl is dependent, in part, on blood levels of ^{201}Tl. Redistribution of ^{201}Tl in a given myocardial region depends not only on the severity of the initial defect post-stress, but also on the presence of viable myocytes, the concentration of the tracer in the blood, and the rate of decline of ^{201}Tl levels in the blood. During the redistribution phase, there is continuous exchange of ^{201}Tl between the myocardium and the extracardiac compartments, driven by the concentration gradient of the radiotracer across the myocytes and blood and myocyte viability. **A,** If the blood level of ^{201}Tl remains the same (or increases) during the period between stress and redistribution imaging, then a stress-induced defect in a region with viable myocytes that can accumulate ^{201}Tl on the redistribution phase will appear reversible. **B,** If the blood level of ^{201}Tl is low (or decreases) during the imaging interval, the delivery of ^{201}Tl may be insufficient and the stress-induced ^{201}Tl defect may remain irreversible even though the underlying myocardium is viable. Thus, some ischemic but viable regions may show no redistribution on either early (3- to 4-hour) or late (24-hour) imaging, unless blood levels of ^{201}Tl are increased. (*Adapted from* Dilsizian [4].)

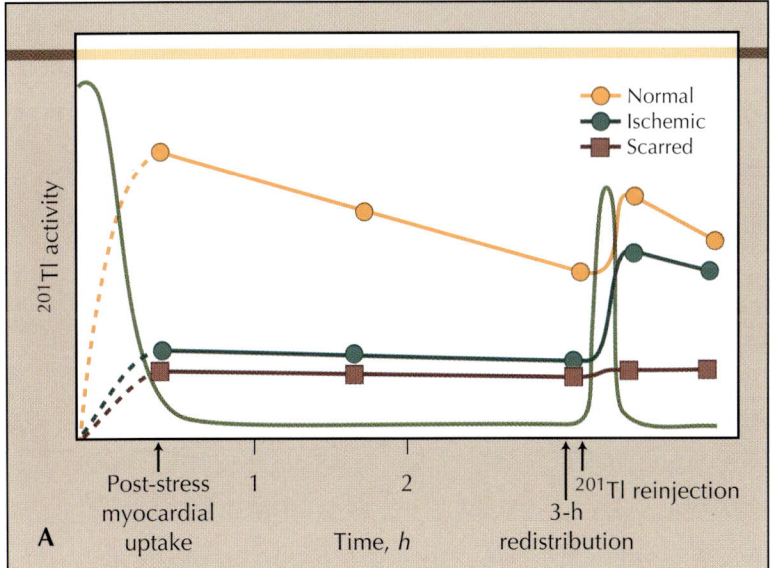

FIGURE 2-7. Thallium reinjection. **A,** ^{201}Tl reinjection differentiates ischemic but viable myocardium from scarred myocardium by augmenting the blood levels of ^{201}Tl at rest. A viable segment may be asynergic on the basis of repetitive stunning and hibernation. Thus, an asynergic but viable region may have reduced (but not absent) blood flow at rest (hibernation) or transient reduction in blood flow after a period of ischemia (stunning). Although standard stress–3- to 4-hour redistribution ^{201}Tl scintigraphy may underestimate the presence of ischemic but viable myocardium in many patients with coronary artery disease, reinjection of ^{201}Tl at rest after stress–3- to 4-hour redistribution imaging substantially improves the assessment of myocardial ischemia and viability in up to 49% of patients with apparently irreversible defects [5]. The theory that myocardial regions identified by ^{201}Tl uptake following ^{201}Tl reinjection represent viable myocardium is supported by improved regional function after revascularization and preserved metabolic activity by [^{18}F]-fluorodeoxyglucose PET. In addition, a significant inverse correlation between the magnitude of ^{201}Tl activity after reinjection and regional volume fraction of interstitial fibrosis has been demonstrated in comparative clinicopathologic studies [6]. It is possible that the initial myocardial uptake of ^{201}Tl (postinjection) reflects regional blood flow while redistribution of ^{201}Tl in a given defect depends not only on the severity of the initial defect but also on the presence of viable myocytes, the concentration of the tracer in the blood, and the rate of decline of ^{201}Tl levels in the blood. Thus, the heterogeneity of regional blood flow observed on the initial stress-induced ^{201}Tl defects may be independent of the subsequent extent of ^{201}Tl redistribution. If the blood level of ^{201}Tl remains the same (or increases) during the period between stress and 3- to 4-hour redistribution imaging, then an apparent defect in a region with viable myocytes that can retain ^{201}Tl should improve. On the other hand, if the serum ^{201}Tl concentration decreases during the imaging interval, the delivery of ^{201}Tl may be insufficient, and the ^{201}Tl defect may remain irreversible although the underlying myocardium is viable. This suggests that some ischemic but viable regions may never redistribute, even with late (24-hour) imaging, unless serum levels of ^{201}Tl are increased.

(Continued on next page)

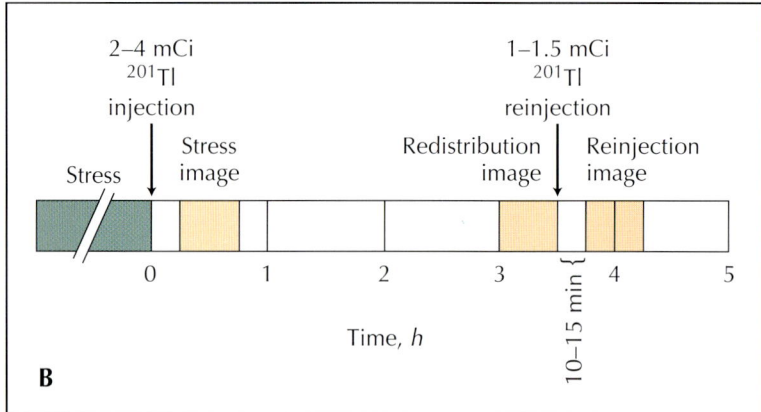

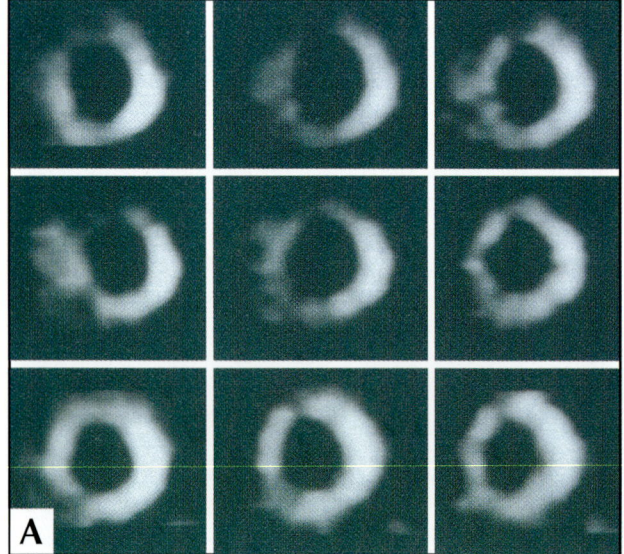

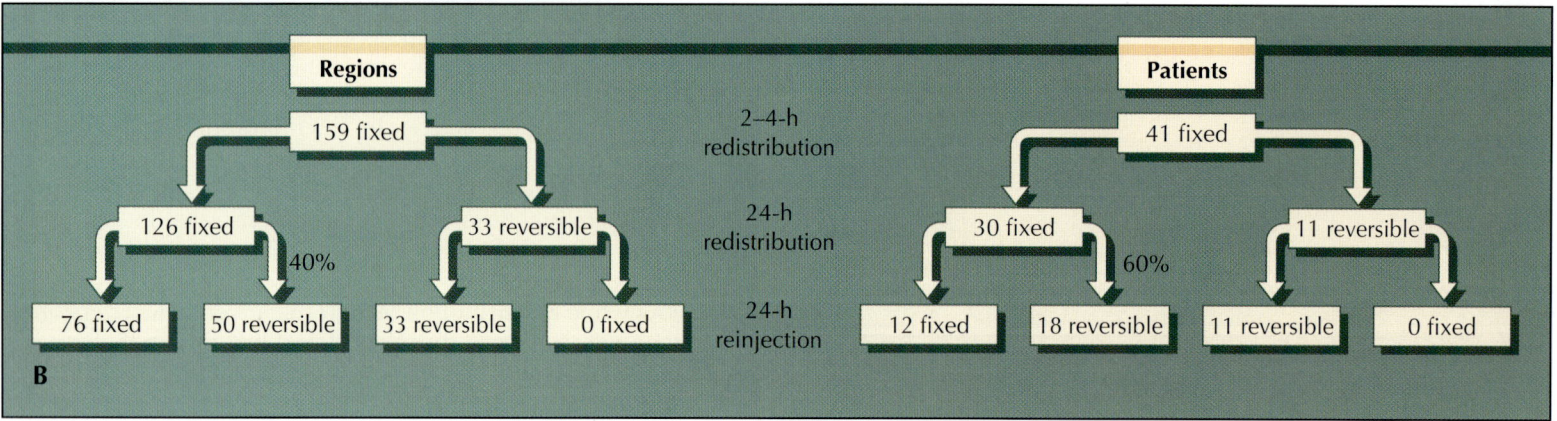

FIGURE 2-7. *(Continued)* **B**, This hypothesis is supported by a study where ^{201}Tl reinjection was performed immediately after 24-hour redistribution images were obtained [7]. Improved ^{201}Tl uptake after reinjection occurred in 40% of defects that appeared irreversible on late (24-hour) redistribution images. Thus, reinjection of 1 mCi of ^{201}Tl at rest immediately after either stress–3- to 4-hour redistribution or stress–24-hour redistribution studies, followed by image acquisition 10 to 15 minutes later, improves significantly the assessment of myocardial ischemia and viability. (*Adapted from* Dilsizian [4].)

FIGURE 2-8. The beneficial effect of ^{201}Tl reinjection in the clinical setting. **A**, Short-axis tomograms demonstrate extensive ^{201}Tl defects in the anterior and septal regions on stress images (*top row*) that persist on redistribution images (*center row*) but improve markedly on reinjection images (*bottom row*). Among patients who underwent coronary artery revascularization, 87% of myocardial regions identified as viable by reinjection studies had normal ^{201}Tl uptake and improved regional wall motion after revascularization. In contrast, all regions with irreversible defects on reinjection imaging before revascularization had persistent wall motion abnormality after revascularization [5].

B, Similar results were obtained when ^{201}Tl reinjection was performed immediately after late (24-hour) redistribution imaging. Improved ^{201}Tl uptake after reinjection occurred in 40% of regions (involving 60% of patients) that appeared fixed on late redistribution imaging. (Panel A *courtesy of* Vasken Dilsizian, National Institutes of Health, Bethesda, MD; *panel B adapted from* Kayden *et al.* [7].)

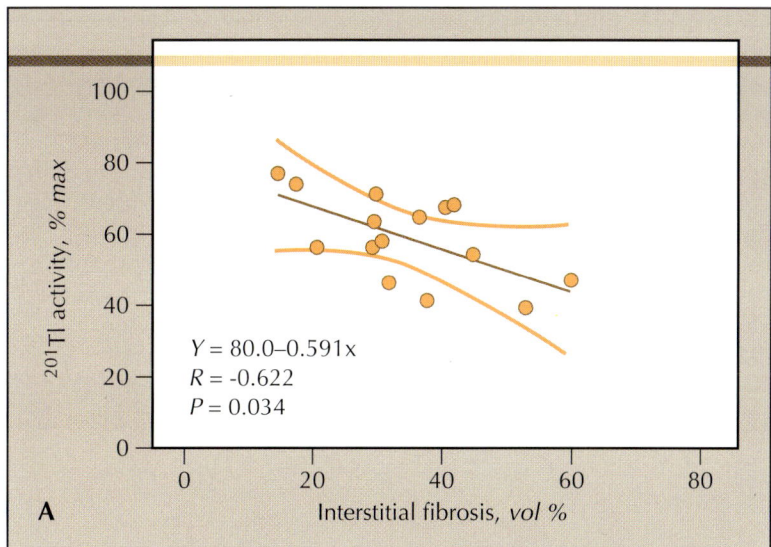
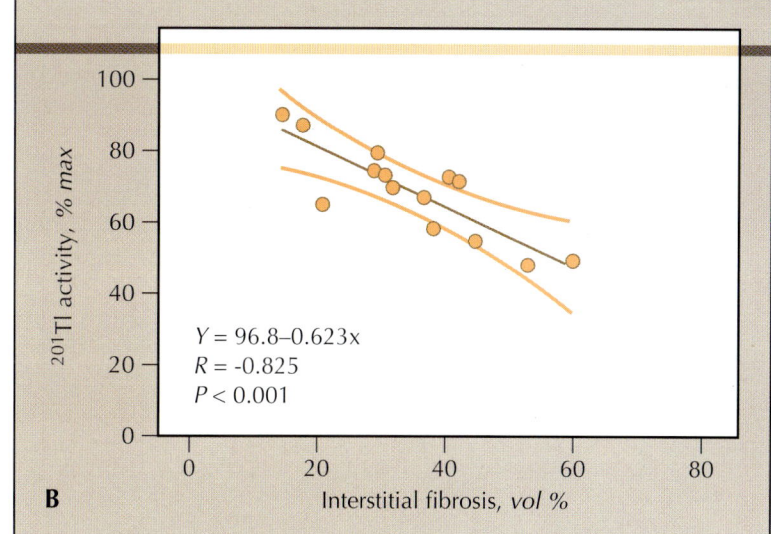

FIGURE 2-9. Relation between regional ^{201}Tl activity and regional volume fraction of interstitial fibrosis. In comparative clinicopathologic studies, a significant inverse correlation is shown between the magnitude of ^{201}Tl uptake after reinjection and regional volume fraction of collagen. Two transmural biopsies were taken from patients undergoing coronary artery bypass surgery, and volume fraction of interstitial fibrosis was assessed by use of light microscopic morphometry. **A,** When compared to redistribution images, regression analysis shows a significantly improved correlation ($P < 0.01$) between ^{201}Tl reinjection and regional volume fraction of interstitial fibrosis, **B**. *Orange lines indicate 95% confidence limits for the regression line. (Adapted from* Zimmermann *et al.* [6].)

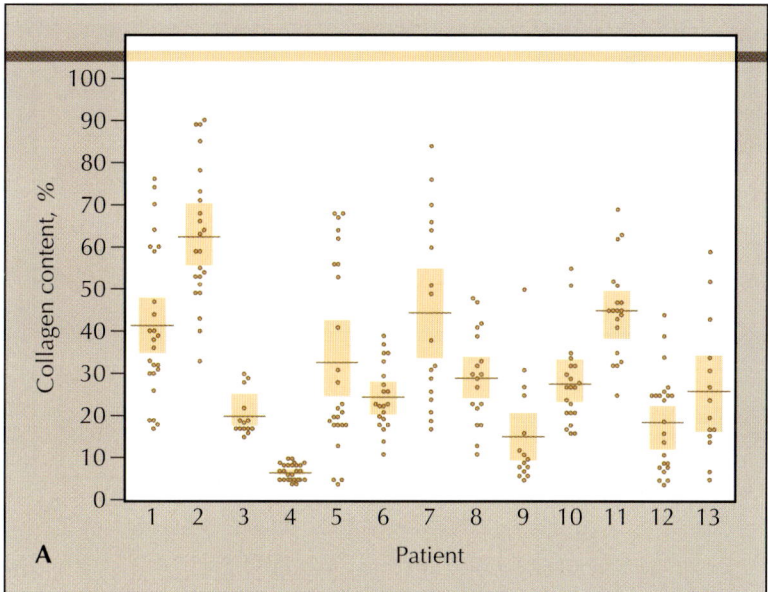
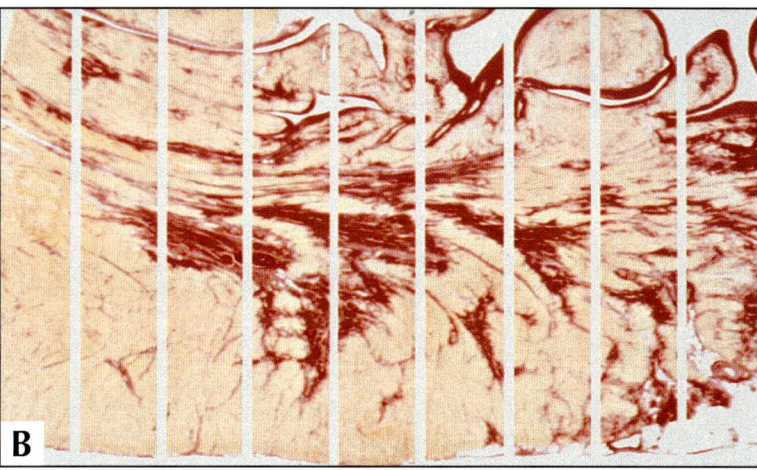

FIGURE 2-10. Heterogeneous nature of structural damage in chronic ischemic heart disease. **A,** Variations in collagen content of small, 2-mm–wide (biopsy equivalent) transmural sections from the mid left ventricular anterior wall are shown in 13 explanted hearts of patients with chronic ischemic heart disease. The degree of myocardial fibrosis from such small biopsy samples obtained at the time of coronary artery bypass surgery have been used to correlate with the results of various noninvasive tests for assessment of preoperative regional myocardial viability. However, when compared with large anterior myocardial segments of explanted hearts, differences in collagen content of the 2-mm–wide biopsy-equivalent sections ranged from 2% to 65% (mean, 28% ± 17%). Hence, classification of asynergic regions as viable or nonviable based on small left ventricular biopsy samples may be an oversimplification of the rather heterogeneous nature of structural damage in chronic ischemic heart disease [8].

B, A representative mid left ventricular transverse anterior region of an explanted heart demonstrates wide variations in collagen content of consecutive 2-mm–wide sections. Volume fraction of the red-staining collagen in these sections ranged from 5.4% to 69.7% (picrosirius red stain, × 4)[8]. (*Panel B courtesy of* Jamshid Shirani, Albert Einstein College of Medicine, Bronx, NY.)

SPECT AND PET TECHNIQUES 25

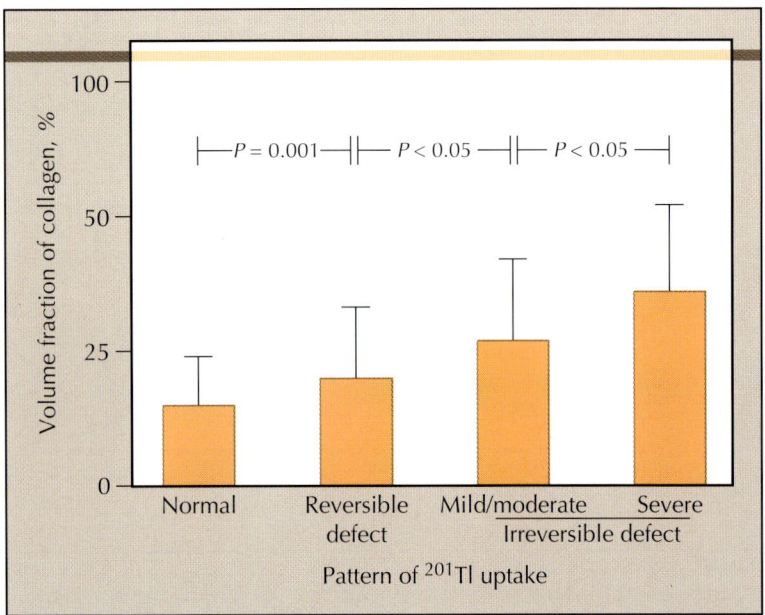

FIGURE 2-11. Histomorphologic confirmation of clinical observations with ^{201}Tl. In patients with chronic ischemic cardiomyopathy undergoing pretransplantation stress-redistribution-reinjection ^{201}Tl imaging, patterns of normal, reversible, mild to moderate irreversible, and severe irreversible defects correlate with the post-transplantation extent and distribution of collagen replacement. Percent collagen replacement is significantly higher in regions with irreversible defects compared with reversible or normal ^{201}Tl regions. The higher collagen content in irreversible ^{201}Tl regions is associated with lower wall thickness and more severe cross-sectional coronary artery narrowing (9.7 ± 2.8 mm and 95 ± 8%) when compared with reversible (11.7 ± 2.7 mm and 87 ± 13%) and normal (12.8 ± 2.6 mm and 80 ± 14%) ^{201}Tl regions. (*Adapted from* Shirani *et al.* [9].)

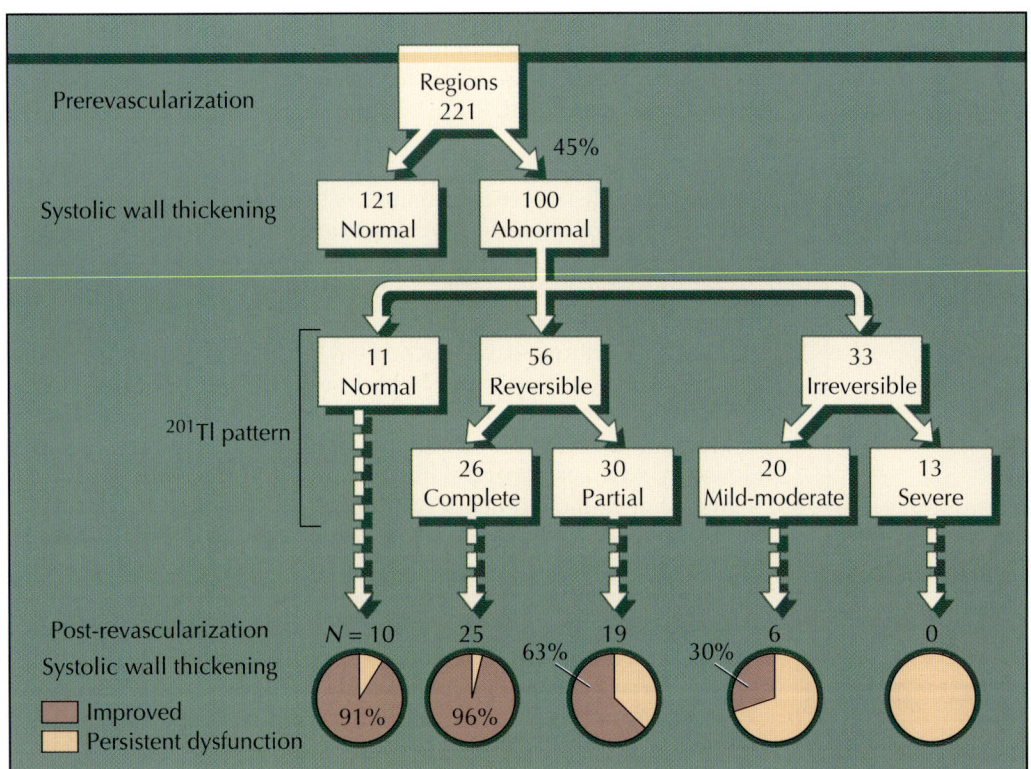

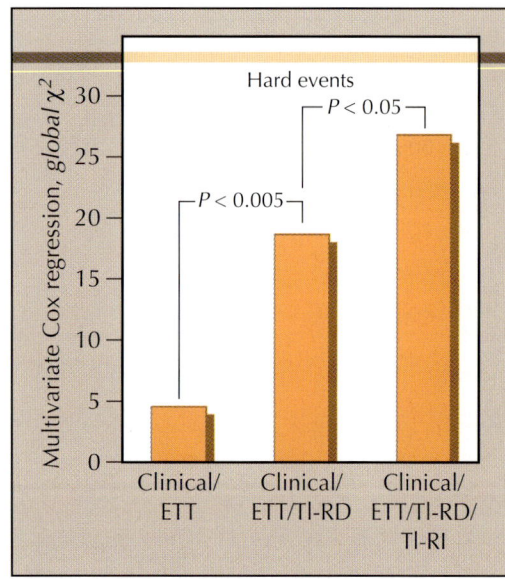

FIGURE 2-12. Post-revascularization functional outcome of asynergic regions in relation to prerevascularization ^{201}Tl patterns of normal, reversible, partially reversible, mild to moderate irreversible, and severe irreversible defects using stress-redistribution-reinjection ^{201}Tl protocol. The probabilities of functional recovery after revascularization were over 90% in normal or completely reversible defects, 63% in partially reversible defects, 30% in mild to moderate irreversible defects, and 0% in severe irreversible defects. Asynergic regions with reversible defects (complete or partial) on the prerevascularization ^{201}Tl study were shown more likely to improve function after revascularization when compared with asynergic regions with mild-to-moderate irreversible defects (79% vs 30%, respectively; $P < 0.001$). Even at a similar mass of viable myocardial tissue (as reflected by the final ^{201}Tl content), the presence of inducible ischemia (reversible defect) was associated with an increased likelihood of functional recovery. (*Adapted from* Kitsiou *et al.* [10].)

FIGURE 2-13. Incremental prognostic value of ^{201}Tl reinjection. In patients with prior myocardial infarction and left ventricular dysfunction in whom the assessment of myocardial viability is of clinical relevance, ^{201}Tl reinjection (Tl-RI) imaging provides incremental prognostic information to clinical, ECG stress testing (ETT), and ^{201}Tl stress-redistribution (Tl-RD) imaging. Similarly, in patients with chronic coronary artery disease and prior myocardial infarction, the scintigraphic variable that was the strongest predictor of hard events (cardiac death or myocardial infarction) was the presence of more than three irreversible defects that remained irreversible after ^{201}Tl reinjection. (*Adapted from* Petretta *et al.* [11].)

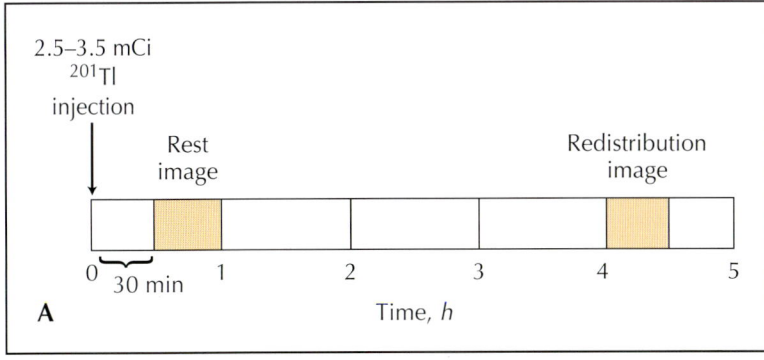

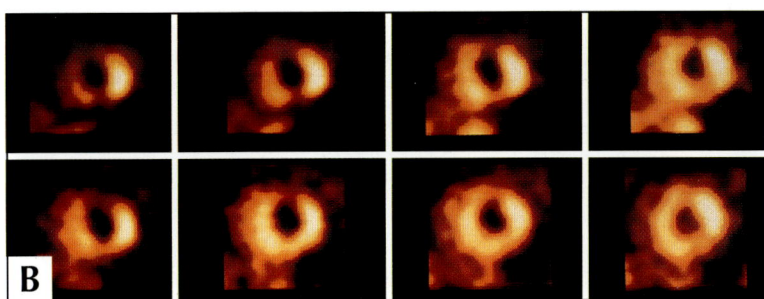

FIGURE 2-14. Rest-redistribution ^{201}Tl protocol. **A,** The stress-redistribution-reinjection ^{201}Tl protocol provides important diagnostic information regarding both inducible ischemia and myocardial viability. In most cases, the identification of myocardial ischemia is much more important clinically in terms of patient management and risk stratification than knowledge of myocardial viability. However, if the clinical question is one of the presence and extent of viable myocardium within a dysfunctional region and not inducible ischemia, then it is reasonable to perform rest-redistribution ^{201}Tl imaging only.

B, Rest-redistribution short-axis ^{201}Tl tomograms are shown from a patient with chronic coronary artery disease. There are extensive ^{201}Tl perfusion defects in the anteroapical, anteroseptal, and inferior regions on the initial rest images (*top row*). On the delayed (3- to 4-hour) redistribution images (*bottom row*), the inferior region remains fixed (scarred myocardium), while the anteroapical and anteroseptal regions show significant reversibility, suggestive of viable myocardium [12]. (*Panel B courtesy of Vasken Dilsizian, National Institutes of Health, Bethesda, MD.*)

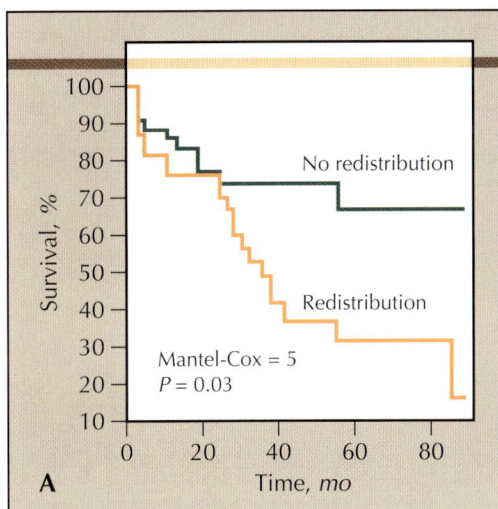

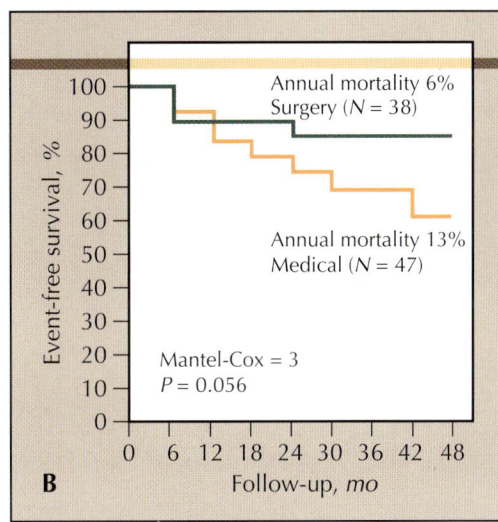

FIGURE 2-15. Prognostic value of rest-redistribution ^{201}Tl SPECT. In patients with chronic ischemic left ventricular dysfunction, the demonstration of redistribution on rest ^{201}Tl imaging protocols portend a higher mortality rate with medical therapy than do patients with a comparable degree of left ventricular dysfunction without evidence of redistribution. **A,** Actuarial survival curve in 81 medically treated patients is shown; 38 patients (mean left ventricular ejection fraction [LVEF] = 26% ± 7%) showed redistribution on rest ^{201}Tl images and 43 patients (mean LVEF = 27% ± 8%) showed no redistribution. Moreover, in a nonrandomized, retrospective study with rest-redistribution ^{201}Tl, survival and survival without myocardial infarction tended to be significantly higher in patients with chronic ischemic left ventricular dysfunction treated with coronary artery revascularization compared with those treated with medical therapy alone. **B,** Actuarial survival curve in 85 patients with evidence of myocardial viability by rest-redistribution ^{201}Tl is shown; 38 patients underwent coronary artery revascularization and 47 patients were treated medically. (*Adapted from* Gioia *et al.* [13,14].)

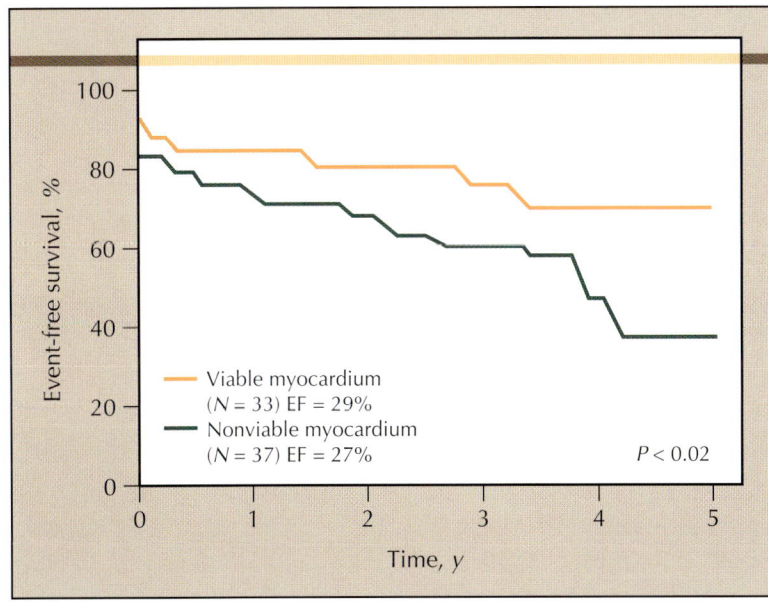

FIGURE 2-16. Extent of myocardial viability assessed by rest-redistribution ^{201}Tl and patient outcome. Considering the survival advantage of coronary artery revascularization when compared with medical therapy in patients with chronic ischemic left ventricular dysfunction, one might question whether preoperative assessment of myocardial viability is necessary in making revascularization decisions. Should coronary artery revascularization be considered in all patients with chronic ischemic left ventricular dysfunction with or without evidence of myocardial viability? Event-free survival in a retrospective study in patients with preoperative rest-redistribution ^{201}Tl testing undergoing coronary artery bypass surgery is shown. Perioperative and long-term postoperative survival is significantly better in patients with evidence of significant myocardial viability on rest-redistribution ^{201}Tl compared with those patients with less evidence of myocardial viability. The prognostic significance of rest-redistribution ^{201}Tl in large-scale, randomized, prospective studies is the subject of ongoing investigation. EF—ejection fraction. (*Adapted from* Pagley *et al.* [15].)

SPECT Techniques: ^{99m}Tc-Labeled Perfusion Tracers

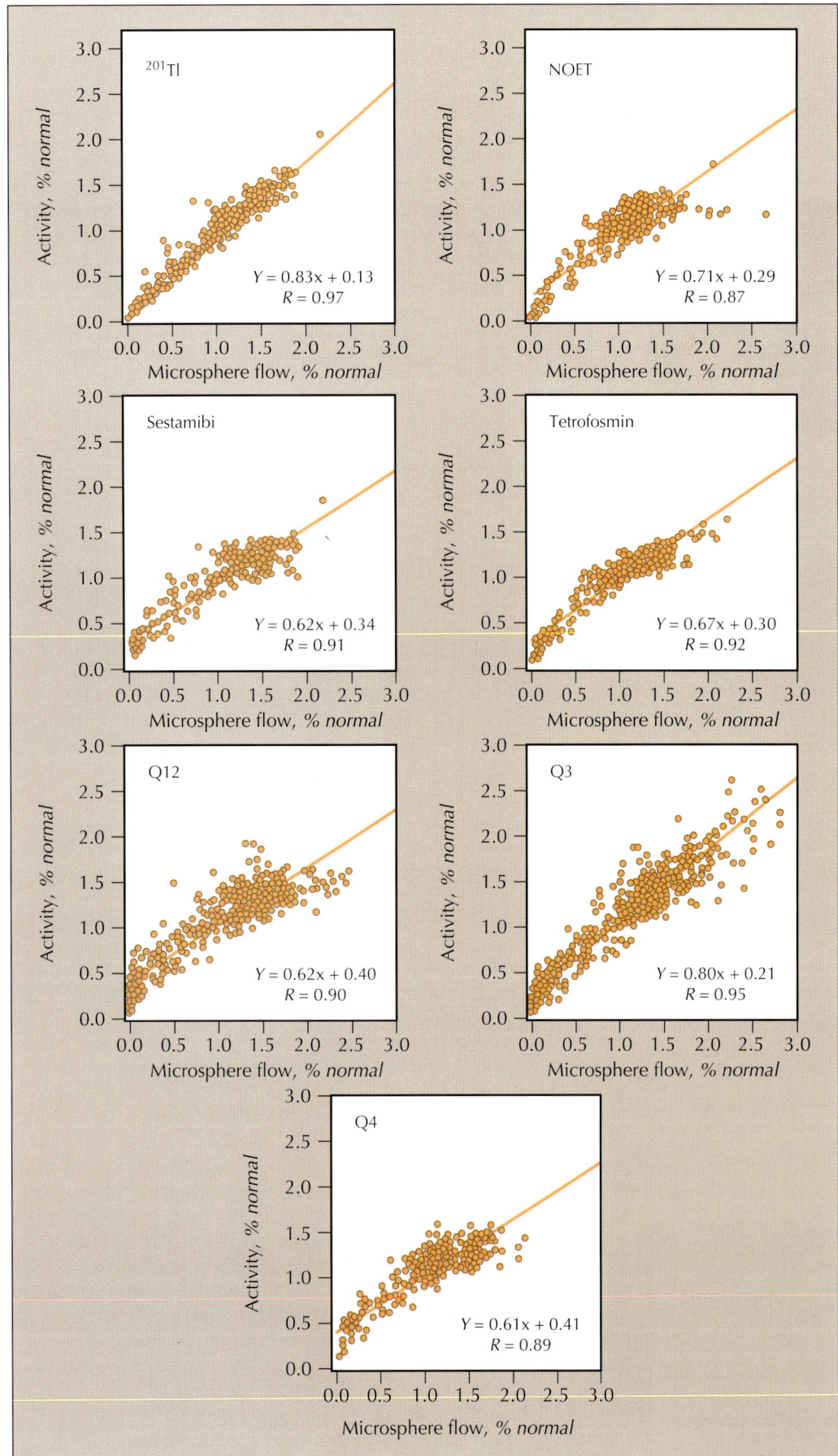

FIGURE 2-17. Myocardial perfusion tracers. Several new classes of ^{99m}Tc-labeled complexes have been developed since 1981 for myocardial perfusion imaging. These tracers are taken up by the myocardium in proportion to regional blood flow, as shown in the plots of myocardial tracer activity versus myocardial blood flow assessed by radioactive microspheres. Multicenter clinical trials have indicated that the accuracy of ^{99m}Tc-sestamibi, teboroxime, and tetrofosmin for detection of coronary artery disease is similar to that of ^{201}Tl. Whether these ^{99m}Tc-labeled perfusion tracers also provide similar information to ^{201}Tl with regard to myocardial viability is controversial. Clinical experience with teboroxime, tetrofosmin, and NOET [bis(N-etoxy, N-ethyl dithiocarbamato) nitrido technetium (V)] for the assessment of myocardial viability is limited. (*Adapted from* Meleca *et al.* [16].)

A. SPECT TECHNIQUES: ^{99m}Tc-LABELED SESTAMIBI AND TETROFOSMIN

- Lipid-soluble cationic compounds
- 140 keV photopeak energy, 6-h physical half-life
- First-pass extraction fraction ≈ 60%
- Uptake is passive across mitochondrial membranes
- At equilibrium, they are retained within the mitochondria because of a large negative transmembrane potential
- Clearance from the intravascular compartment via hepatobiliary excretion
- Minimal redistribution when compared with ^{201}Tl

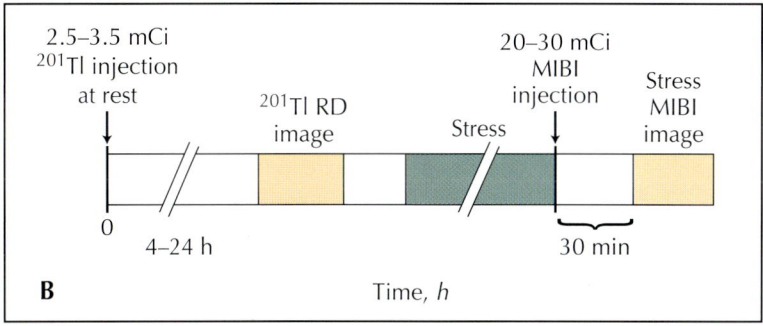

FIGURE 2-18. SPECT techniques: ^{99m}Tc-labeled sestamibi and tetrofosmin. **A,** ^{99m}Tc-sestamibi (isonitrile) (MIBI) and ^{99m}Tc-tetrofosmin (diphosphine) are both lipophilic cationic complexes with similar myocardial uptake and blood clearance kinetics. However, the clearance of tetrofosmin from the lungs and the liver is faster than ^{99m}Tc-sestamibi, which may improve the resolution of cardiac images and reduce the overall radiation burden. Both ^{99m}Tc-sestamibi and tetrofosmin are taken up across sarcolemmal and mitochondrial membranes of myocytes by passive distribution, and retained within the mitochondria at equilibrium because of a large negative transmembrane potential. Experimental studies with ^{99m}Tc-sestamibi have shown that myocardial uptake and clearance of ^{99m}Tc-sestamibi are related to the mitochondrial transmembrane potential and do not differ from ischemic to nonischemic regions. In addition, experimental studies of myocardial infarction, with and without reperfusion, have fueled optimism in the use of ^{99m}Tc-sestamibi clinically for myocardial viability assessment. In the clinical setting, however, with the exception of a few studies, both ^{99m}Tc-sestamibi and tetrofosmin appear to underestimate myocardial viability. Compared with ^{201}Tl and PET tracers, factors that may contribute to the impaired ^{99m}Tc-sestamibi or tetrofosmin accumulation in viable regions at rest include differences in 1) extraction fraction, 2) blood clearance, 3) redistribution (RD), and 4) response to altered metabolic states. Perhaps a likely improvement in viability assessment with ^{99m}Tc-sestamibi and tetrofosmin could be achieved through nitrate administration before rest ^{99m}Tc-sestamibi injection and quantitation of regional radiotracer uptake. **B,** Alternatively, dual-isotope gated SPECT imaging could be performed, which combines rest-redistribution ^{201}Tl (for viability) with stress ^{99m}Tc-sestamibi or tetrofosmin (for perfusion), thereby taking advantage of the favorable properties of each of the two tracers.

SPECT TECHNIQUES: ^{99m}Tc-TEBOROXIME

- Neutral, lipophilic compound
- 140 keV photopeak energy, 6-h physical half-life
- High first-pass extraction fraction under hyperemic conditions (≈ 91%)
- Extraction by the myocardium remains linear even at high-flow conditions
- Rapid clearance from the myocardium at a rate proportional to regional blood flow
- Uptake and washout are independent of the metabolic status of the myocardial cells

FIGURE 2-19. SPECT techniques: ^{99m}Tc-teboroxime. ^{99m}Tc-teboroxime is a neutral, lipophilic BATO (boronic acid adducts of technetium dioxime) compound with a reported first-pass extraction of 88% at rest and 91% under hyperemic conditions. Unlike ^{99m}Tc-sestamibi and tetrofosmin, clearance of teboroxime from the myocardium is rapid and the washout rate is proportional to blood flow. In experimental studies, approximately two thirds of the teboroxime activity has been shown to clear from the heart, with a half-life of 3.6 minutes. Thus, both uptake and clearance of teboroxime from the myocardium are proportional to regional blood flow and are not confounded by tissue metabolism or other binding characteristics within the myocardium. Therefore, teboroxime is particularly more suitable as a blood flow tracer rather than as a viability tracer.

SPECT TECHNIQUES: ^{99m}Tc-N-NOET

Neutral, lipophilic compound
High first-pass extraction under hyperemic conditions (≈ 85%)
After passive diffusion, it links to proteins bound in the lipid membrane of myocytes
Binding is associated with L-type calcium channels and is independent of ATP content
Does not accumulate in the cytosolic or mitochondrial fractions
Slow myocardial clearance and long retention in normal myocardium
Clearance from the intravascular compartment via urinary and fecal excretion
Redistribution over time predominantly by differential washout

FIGURE 2-20. SPECT techniques: ^{99m}Tc-N-NOET. ^{99m}Tc-N-NOET (bis[N-etoxy, N-ethyl dithiocarbamato] nitrido technetium [V]) is a neutral, lipophilic compound characterized by the presence of a Tc-N triple bond group. The first-pass extraction fraction of NOET is 75% at rest and 85% under hyperemic conditions. After passive diffusion, the mechanism of NOET uptake is thought to be through linkage to proteins bound in the lipid membrane of isolated myocytes. Similar to ^{99m}Tc-sestamibi and tetrofosmin, clearance of NOET from the myocardium is slow, with longer retention in normal myocardium. However, unlike ^{99m}Tc-sestamibi and tetrofosmin, NOET demonstrates significant redistribution over time predominantly by differential washout. Because uptake and retention of NOET is dependent on the structural integrity of cell membrane, NOET may be a potentially useful tracer to assess both regional blood flow (early images) and myocardial viability (redistribution images).

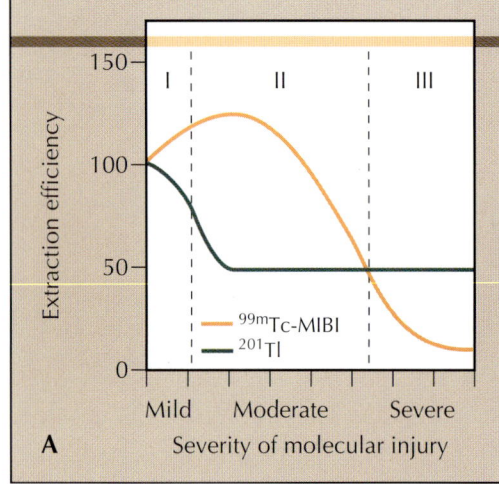
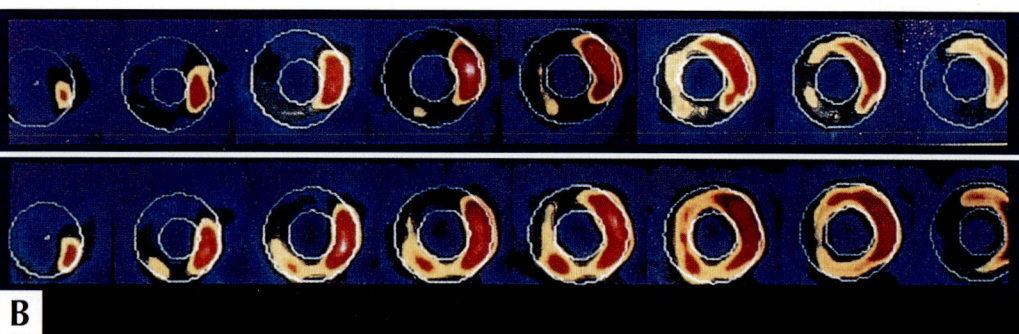

FIGURE 2-21. Cellular kinetics of ^{201}Tl and ^{99m}Tc-sestamibi (^{99m}Tc-MIBI) during metabolic inhibition in cultured chick embryo cardiac myocytes, independent of perfusion. **A**, Oxidative phosphorylation and glycolysis were inhibited simultaneously by rotenone (10 μm) and iodoacetate (1 mmol/L), respectively, producing a decline in myocellular ATP content. Under these conditions, initial extraction efficiency of ^{201}Tl and ^{99m}Tc-sestamibi responded in divergent ways to ATP depletion. Extraction efficiency of ^{201}Tl declined within 20 minutes of metabolic inhibition by 50% to 70%, while extraction efficiency of ^{99m}Tc-sestamibi increased significantly by 10 to 20 minutes and remained elevated for the first 40 to 60 minutes of metabolic inhibition. The observed disparity in initial uptake rates between ^{201}Tl and ^{99m}Tc-sestamibi during mild-to-moderate metabolic injury may explain on metabolic basis alone the clinical observation that ^{99m}Tc-sestamibi defects are smaller than those assessed by ^{201}Tl. **B**, Images taken with ^{201}Tl 5 to 10 minutes after stress (*top row*) and with ^{99m}Tc-sestamibi 2 hours after stress (*bottom row*) are shown from a patient who performed the same level of exercise with both tracers. Quantitative left ventricular mass algorithm provided similar measures of total mass for ^{201}Tl (197 g) and for ^{99m}Tc-sestamibi (189 g). However, the stress-induced defect mass derived from ^{201}Tl imaging (41 g) is significantly larger than that detected by ^{99m}Tc-sestamibi (3 g). No transmural defects are present on the ^{99m}Tc-sestamibi images. (*Panel A adapted from* Piwnica-Worms *et al.* [17]; *panel B from* Narahara *et al.* [18]; with permission.)

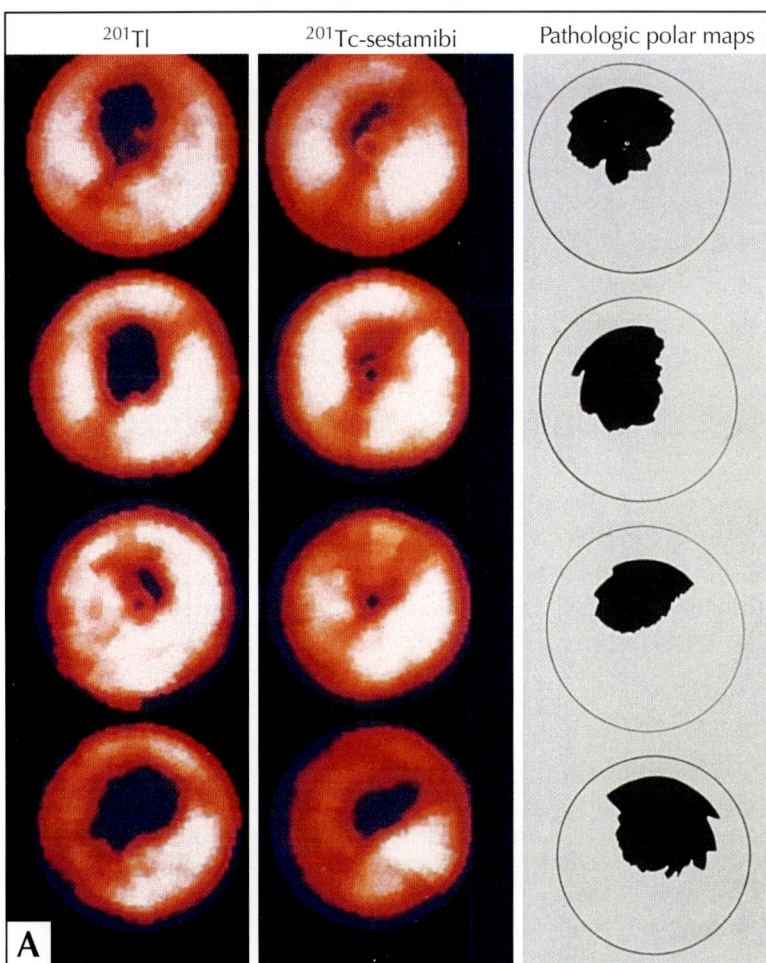
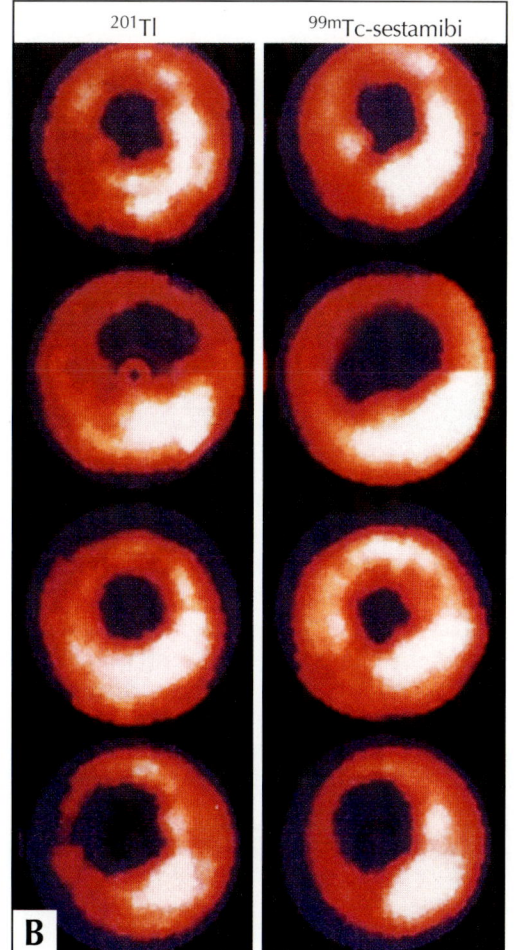

FIGURE 2-22. Pharmacologic stress. In canine models of **A**, moderate and **B**, severe coronary artery occlusion, ^{201}Tl and ^{99m}Tc-sestamibi myocardial perfusion defect size are compared during pharmacologic stimulation and with postmortem staining to define the extent of the hypoperfused region. Bull's-eye displays from four representative experiments of moderate coronary artery stenosis during pharmacologic stimulation for ^{201}Tl and ^{99m}Tc-sestamibi and corresponding pathologic polar displays from the same four experiments are shown. The extent of ^{201}Tl myocardial perfusion defect size (but not ^{99m}Tc-sestamibi) approaches the hypoperfused area on the corresponding pathologic display. The ^{99m}Tc-sestamibi defect size occupies only 37% of the area of the defect on the ^{201}Tl images of the same dog, and the counts within the defects are 39% higher for ^{99m}Tc-sestamibi compared to ^{201}Tl (*panel A*). On the other hand, when coronary artery occlusion is near total (severe), ^{201}Tl and ^{99m}Tc-sestamibi show similar defect contrast and areas (*panel B*). These observations in canines are similar to the experimental observations made in cultured myocytes. (*From* Leon *et al.* [19]; with permission).

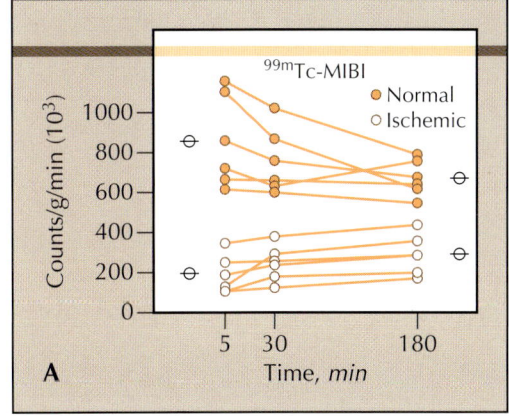
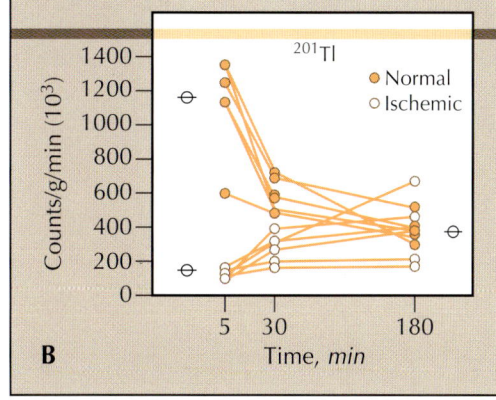

FIGURE 2-23. ^{99m}Tc-sestamibi and ^{201}Tl activities in myocardial biopsies. Change in defect size of ^{99m}Tc-sestamibi (MIBI) with time (redistribution) has been shown both in animal models and in patients with chronic coronary artery disease [20,21]. Depending on the level of blood activity of ^{99m}Tc-sestamibi after stress, continued uptake by the myocardium after the first pass may reduce the defect severity and area in the hypoperfused region. In the early comparative studies of ^{201}Tl and ^{99m}Tc-sestamibi, ^{201}Tl images were acquired 5 to 10 minutes after injection, while ^{99m}Tc-sestamibi images were acquired 1 to 2 hours after injection. The 1- to 2-hour delay between ^{99m}Tc-sestamibi injection and imaging was based on the best compromise between a high myocardial count rate and low background activity and on the assumption that ^{99m}Tc-sestamibi does not "redistribute" over time.

A, Following transient ischemia and reperfusion after 5 minutes in a canine model, there was evidence for change in defect size of ^{99m}Tc-sestamibi with time, albeit more slowly and less completely when compared to ^{201}Tl redistribution (**B**). For both ^{99m}Tc-sestamibi and ^{201}Tl, the consistent fall in normal zone activity and rise in ischemic zone activity over the 3-hour time interval, consistent with redistribution, is noted. It is important to point out, however, that there is no change in ^{99m}Tc-sestamibi defect size between the 5-minute and 30-minute time intervals. In view of these and other similar reports, it is now recommended that ^{99m}Tc-sestamibi images be acquired earlier, approximately 30 minutes after injection of the tracer. (*Adapted from* Li *et al.* [20].)

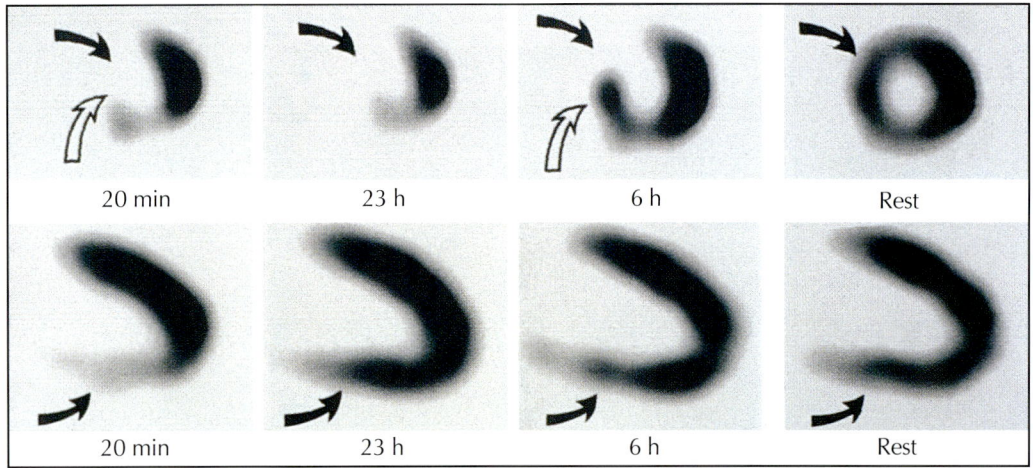

FIGURE 2-24. Clinically relevant change in defect size of ^{99m}Tc-sestamibi with time (redistribution) in two patients undergoing exercise ^{99m}Tc-sestamibi studies. Myocardial SPECT images obtained from two different patients are presented in the short-axis plane (*top row*) and in the vertical long-axis plane (*bottom row*) after exercise and at rest. In the short-axis plane, there is no change in ^{99m}Tc-sestamibi defect size from 20 minutes to 2 hours after exercise. However, by 6 hours there is significant change in defect size in the inferoseptal region (*open arrow*) but not in the anteroseptal region (*closed arrow*). On the injected image taken at rest, complete normalization of all perfusion defects is seen, which suggests that delayed ^{99m}Tc-sestamibi images alone do not provide accurate information regarding defect reversibility. In the vertical long-axis plane, there is significant change in ^{99m}Tc-sestamibi defect in the inferior region (*closed arrow*) from 20 minutes to 2 hours after exercise (redistribution), without further fill-in at 6 hours or on rest-injected ^{99m}Tc-sestamibi images. Although interpretation of ^{99m}Tc-sestamibi data should be viewed cautiously when imaging is delayed by 2 hours or more after stress (underestimation of defect size and extent of myocardial ischemia), the same concept does not apply for rest-injected ^{99m}Tc-sestamibi studies. On the contrary, delaying ^{99m}Tc-sestamibi images by 2 hours or more after rest injection may improve myocardial viability assessment. (*From Franceschi et al.* [22]; *with permission.*)

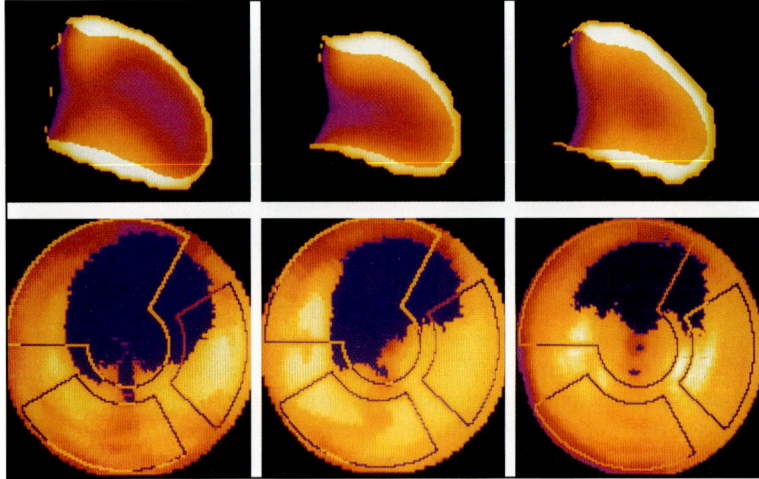

FIGURE 2-25. Nitrate administration before rest ^{99m}Tc-sestamibi or ^{99m}Tc-tetrofosmin injection. Considering the kinetics of ^{99m}Tc-sestamibi and ^{99m}Tc-tetrofosmin, uptake of these radiotracers in myocardial regions with reduced perfusion and partially impaired viability appear to be influenced by regional perfusion rather than myocyte viability. In view of the limitations in the clinical setting of rest-injected ^{99m}Tc-sestamibi and ^{99m}Tc-tetrofosmin for assessing myocardial viability, some investigators have proposed injection of the radiotracers during nitrate infusion. In addition to lowering preload and afterload, nitrates may cause vasodilatation of the flow, limiting epicardial coronary arteries as well as collateral vessels. The injection of ^{99m}Tc-sestamibi during nitrate infusion (10 mg of isosorbide dinitrate in 100 mL solution of isotonic saline solution infused over 20 minutes) is shown to improve the accuracy of ^{99m}Tc-sestamibi for predicting recovery of regional and global left ventricular function after revascularization. In this patient example with anterior myocardial infarction and single vessel left anterior descending (LAD) coronary artery disease, prerevascularization baseline images (*left*) show anteroapical akinesis and global left ventricular ejection fraction (LVEF) of 38% on first-pass radionuclide angiography associated with a large anterior and apical ^{99m}Tc-sestamibi perfusion defect (63% of the LAD vascular territory in the bull's-eye image at rest). ^{99m}Tc-sestamibi images acquired after nitrate infusion (*center*) show improvement in the anteroapical wall motion associated with an increase in global LVEF to 42% and a decrease in the extent of ^{99m}Tc-sestamibi perfusion defect size to 42% of the LAD vascular territory. After revascularization of the LAD (*right*), there is improvement in the anteroapical wall motion at rest, increase in global LVEF to 45%, and decrease in the extent of ^{99m}Tc-sestamibi perfusion defect to 38% of the LAD vascular territory [23]. (*Courtesy of Roberto Sciagra.*)

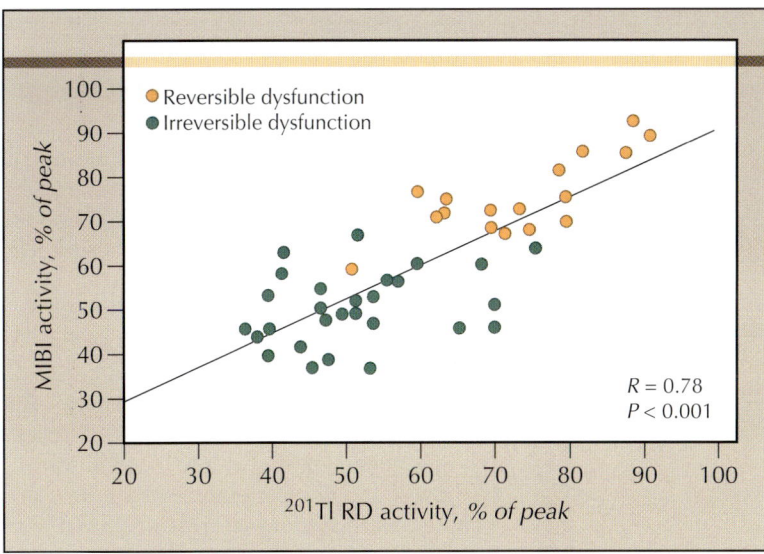

FIGURE 2-26. Quantitation of severity of reduction in myocardial perfusion at rest. Unlike ^{201}Tl studies, there are a growing number of studies in the literature to suggest that ^{99m}Tc-sestamibi and tetrofosmin studies underestimate defect reversibility and myocardial viability in patients with chronic coronary artery disease. One approach that may overcome, in part, the limitations of ^{99m}Tc-sestamibi and tetrofosmin in assessing myocardial viability is to quantify the severity of regional tracer activity, *ie*, severity of myocardial perfusion at rest. Among 18 patients with coronary artery disease undergoing revascularization, good correlation between quantitative regional activities of ^{201}Tl (on redistribution imaging after rest injection) and ^{99m}Tc-sestamibi (at rest) is shown. Moreover, the scatterplot shows that at 60% threshold level for both radiotracers, dysfunctional myocardial regions that improve function after revascularization (*green circles*) can be differentiated from dysfunctional myocardial regions that do not improve function after revascularization (*orange circles*). The positive and negative predictive accuracies attained when the severity of radiotracer defects were quantitated are 80% and 96%, respectively. Considering the kinetics of ^{99m}Tc-sestamibi, in myocardial regions with decreased blood flow and partially impaired viability, uptake of ^{99m}Tc-sestamibi appears to be influenced by regional perfusion rather than myocyte viability [24]. (*Adapted from* Udelson et al. [25].)

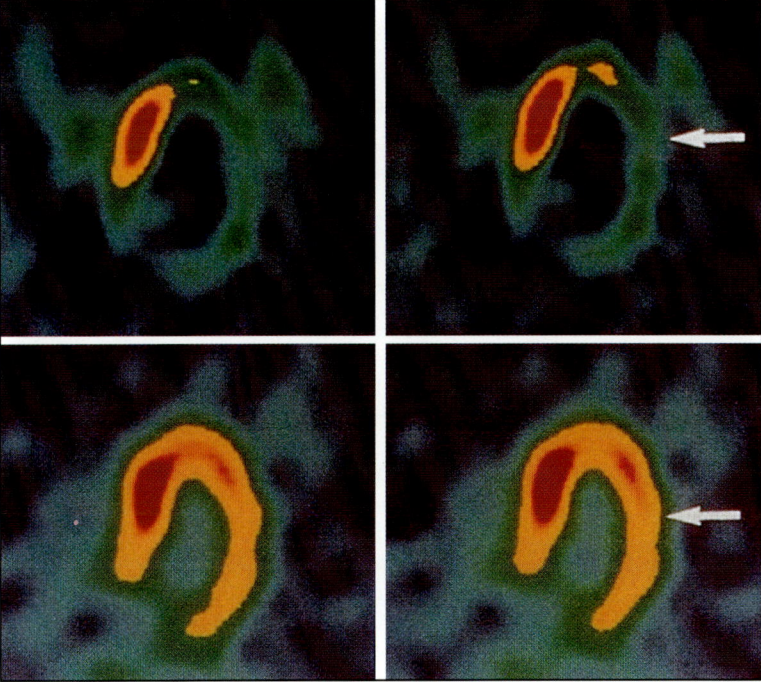

FIGURE 2-27. Underestimation of myocardial viability by rest ^{99m}Tc-sestamibi SPECT. Using dual-isotope injection at rest (same physiologic state) and simultaneous acquisition using SPECT (accurate anatomical alignment), these images show mismatch between rest cardiac perfusion assessed by ^{99m}Tc-sestamibi and metabolism assessed by [^{18}F]-fluorodeoxyglucose (FDG). After oral glucose loading, the patient was injected with 10 mCi of FDG and 25 mCi of ^{99m}Tc-sestamibi at rest. Dual-isotope single acquisition SPECT was performed approximately 60 minutes later by positioning two 20% pulse-height analyzer windows symmetrically around the 140 keV photopeak of ^{99m}Tc and the 511 keV photopeak of FDG. The digital electronics of the camera permitted frame-by-frame decay correction for short-lived FDG. Thus, two separate sets of slices mapping the ^{99m}Tc-sestamibi and FDG distribution were simultaneously obtained, resulting in one-to-one correspondence in spatial registration. Rest ^{99m}Tc-sestamibi images in the horizontal long-axis plane (*top row*) show reduced perfusion in the apical and lateral regions (*arrow*). Corresponding FDG images (*bottom row*) show preserved metabolism in the apical and lateral regions suggestive of viable myocardium (*arrow*). (*From* Delbeke et al. [26]; with permission.)

PET Techniques: Flow, Metabolism, and Prognosis

CARDIAC PET APPLICATIONS AND POSITRON-EMITTING RADIOTRACERS

MYOCARDIAL BLOOD FLOW

Rubidium-82	75 s half-life; produced from strontium-82 generator
^{15}O-water	2 min half-life; cyclotron-produced
^{13}N-ammonia	10 min half-life; cyclotron-produced

MYOCARDIAL METABOLISM

^{11}C-palmitate	20 min half-life; cyclotron-produced
^{11}C-acetate	20 min half-life; cyclotron-produced
[^{18}F]-fluorodeoxyglucose	110 min half-life; cyclotron-produced

FIGURE 2-28. Cardiac PET applications and positron-emitting radiotracers. Advantages of PET over SPECT include accepted method for attenuation correction, high spatial resolution, and increased count density images. Clinically available cardiac PET radiotracers fall within two broad categories: those that evaluate myocardial blood flow and those that evaluate specific metabolic pathways. By labeling various compounds of physiologic interest, valuable insights into biochemical pathways and tissue metabolism can be obtained in functional and dysfunctional myocardium. Because estimates of both myocardial blood flow and metabolism can be obtained in absolute terms, beyond the diagnosis of ischemic left ventricular dysfunction, PET may allow monitoring of both the progression of disease and the effect of various treatments in such patients.

MYOCARDIAL BLOOD FLOW AND VIABILITY

A. PET TECHNIQUES: RUBIDIUM-82

Positron-emitting cation with biologic properties similar to potassium
Emits two gamma rays, 511 keV each, with a short physical half-life of 75 s
Transported across the sarcolemmal membrane via the Na-K ATPase system
Initial uptake reflects myocardial blood flow
Kinetics of washout phase may be used as an index of viability

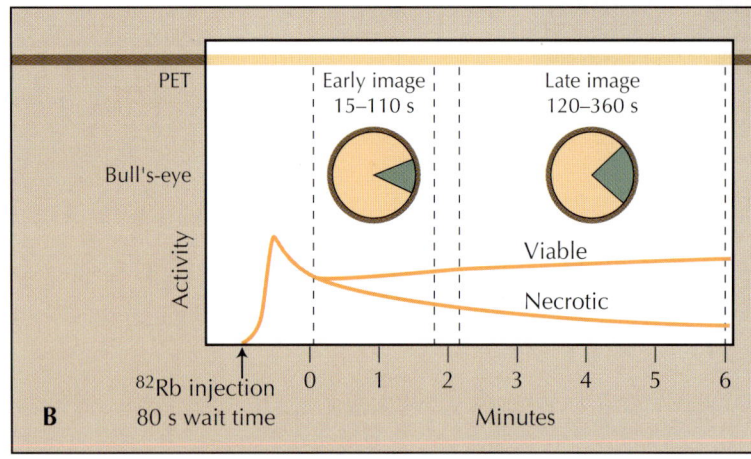

FIGURE 2-29. PET techniques: rubidium-82. **A**, ^{82}Rb is a generator-produced, short-lived, positron-emitting cation with biologic properties that are similar to potassium and ^{201}Tl. As with potassium and ^{201}Tl, intracellular uptake of ^{82}Rb across the sarcolemmal membrane reflects active cation transport via the Na-K ATPase transport system. In patients with chronic coronary artery disease, myocardial uptake of ^{82}Rb is preserved in viable regions and severely reduced in scarred regions. In the setting of acute myocardial injury and reperfusion, initial uptake of ^{82}Rb reflects blood flow. **B**, Because necrotic myocardium cannot retain ^{82}Rb, the kinetics of ^{82}Rb washout may be used as an index of myocardial viability. This is demonstrated in the schematic bull's-eye diagram of ^{82}Rb on early and late image. Such application of ^{82}Rb washout kinetics provides myocardial viability information comparable to metabolic imaging with PET. In the clinical setting, 40 to 60 mCi of ^{82}Rb is administered intravenously. (*Panel B adapted from Gould et al.* [27].)

34 ATLAS OF NUCLEAR CARDIOLOGY

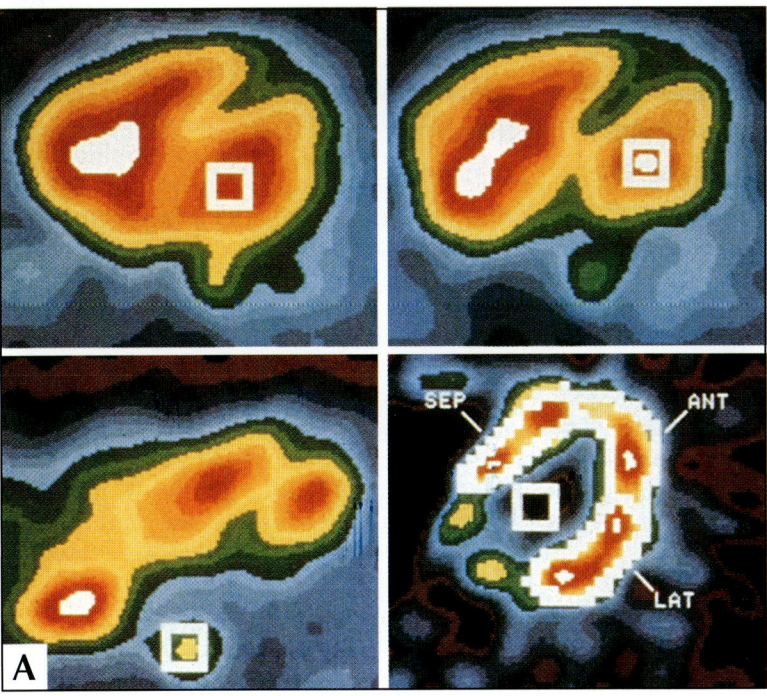

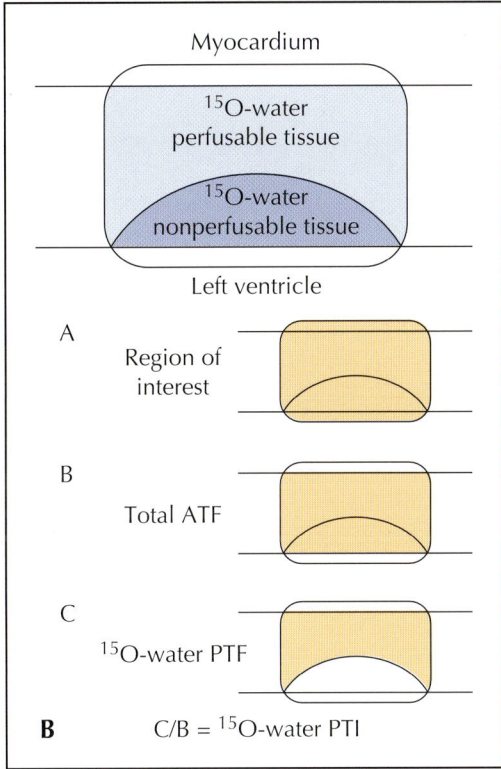

FIGURE 2-30. PET techniques: ^{15}O-water. ^{15}O-water is a freely diffusable tracer that correlates closely with perfusion as assessed by microspheres with a first-pass extraction fraction approaching unity. Because ^{15}O-water is both in the vascular space and myocardium, visualization of myocardial activity requires correction for activity in the vascular compartment. **A**, Correction for activity in the left atrium (*top left*), left ventricle (*top right*), and thoracic aorta (*bottom left*) is shown in a healthy patient after inhalation of 30 to 40 mCi of ^{15}O-carbon monoxide, which labels erythrocytes in vivo. *Bottom right*, the distribution of ^{15}O-water is shown in the left ventricular myocardium after correction for vascular space.

B, The ability of ^{15}O-water to assess myocardial viability through modification of the blood flow information is shown. This method, termed *water perfusable tissue index* (PTI), is based on measurement of perfusable tissue fraction (PTF) as a method to correct for the partial volume effects in ^{15}O-water studies [28]. PTF is defined as the fractional volume of a given region of interest occupied by myocardium that is capable of exchanging water rapidly. Using transmission and ^{15}O-blood pool images, the anatomical tissue fraction (ATF), a quantitative estimate of extravascular tissue density, is derived. The ratio of PTF to ATF thus represents the proportion of the extravascular tissue that is perfusable by ^{15}O-water. Because water can freely exchange across all normal tissue cells, the PTF should approach unity in normal myocardium and be reduced in scarred myocardium.

A myocardial region of interest containing a mixture of ^{15}O-water perfusable and nonperfusable tissue is diagrammed. *A*, Volume of the region of interest. *B*, ATF for the region of interest produced by subtraction of the blood pool (^{15}O-carbon monoxide) from the transmission images after normalization of the latter to tissue density (1.04 g/mL). Total ATF represents the total extravascular tissue and contains both perfusable and nonperfusable tissue components. *C*, ^{15}O-water PTF for the region of interest calculated from the ^{15}O-water data set identifies the mass of tissue within the region of interest that is capable of rapid trans-sarcolemmal exchange of water. Note that the nonperfusable or necrotic region is excluded from this parameter. The ^{15}O-water PTI is calculated by dividing ^{15}O-water PTF (*C*) by the total anatomic tissue fraction (*B*), and represents the fraction of the total anatomic tissue that is perfusable by water. ANT—anterior; LAT—lateral; SEP—septal. (*Panel A from* Bergmann *et al.*; with permission [29]; *panel B adapted from* Yamamoto *et al.* [30].)

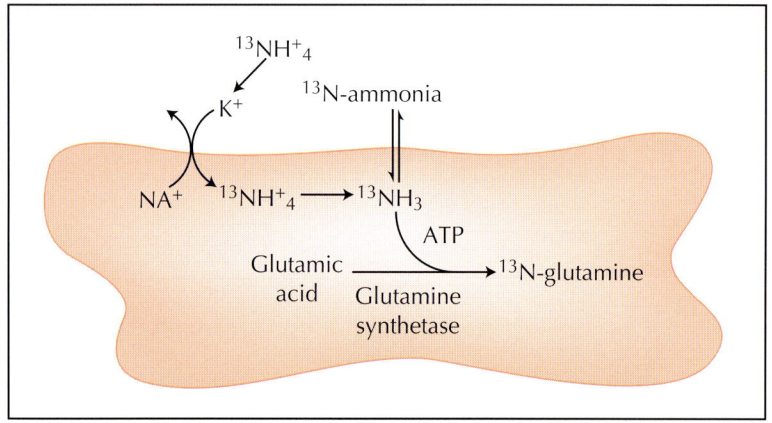

FIGURE 2-31. PET techniques: ^{13}N-ammonia. ^{13}N-ammonia is the extractable perfusion tracer most commonly used with PET. At physiologic pH, ammonia is in its cationic form with a physical half-life of 10 minutes. Myocardial distribution of ammonia is related inversely and nonlinearly to blood flow. Although the exact mechanism of ^{13}N-ammonia transport across the myocardial membrane has not been conclusively established, it has been suggested that ^{13}N-ammonia may cross cell membranes by passive diffusion or as ammonium ion (^{13}NH$^+_4$) by the active sodium-potassium transport mechanism influenced by the concentration gradient across the cell membrane. Once in the myocyte, myocardial retention of ^{13}N-ammonia involves predominantly the conversion of ^{13}N-ammonia and glutamic acid to ^{13}N-labeled glutamine mediated by ATP and glutamine synthetase. Hence, absolute quantification requires two- and three-compartment kinetic models that incorporate both extraction and retention rate constants. Quantification of ammonia is further complicated by the rapid degradation of ammonia, which occurs within 5 minutes after the administration, producing metabolic intermediates such as urea and glutamine that are also extracted by the heart. Experimental studies suggest that myocardial uptake of ammonia reflects absolute blood flows up to 2 to 2.5 mL/g/min and plateaus at flows in the hyperemic range. In the clinical setting, 10 to 20 mCi of ^{13}N-ammonia is administered intravenously.

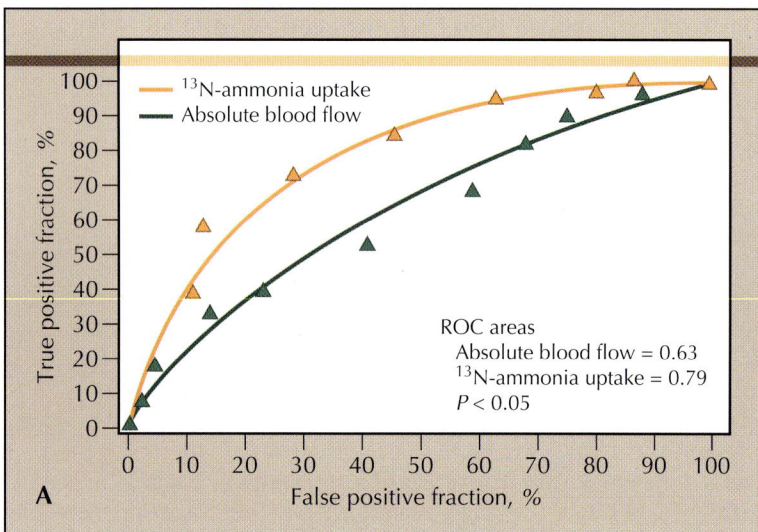

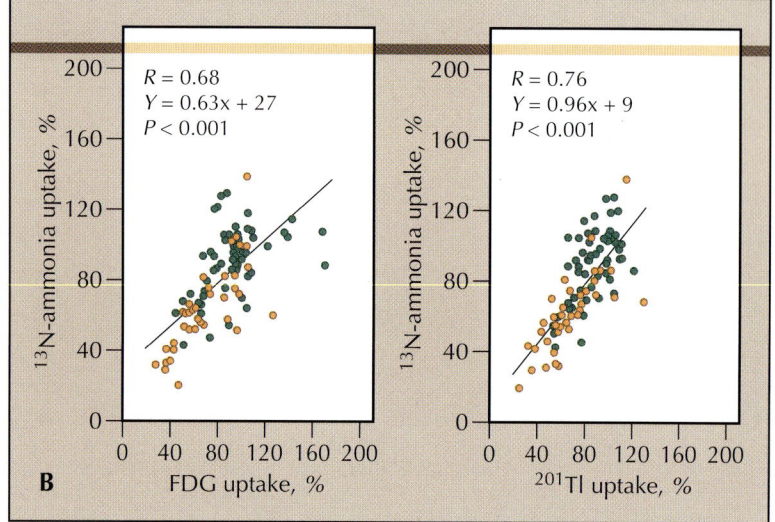

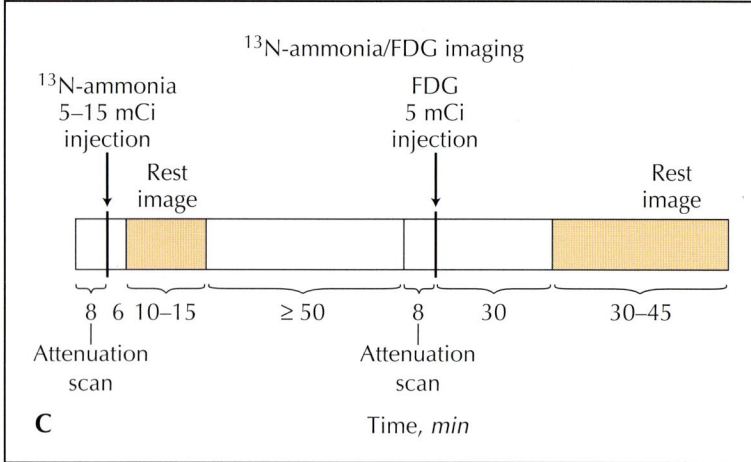

FIGURE 2-32. Mechanism of ^{13}N-ammonia uptake. The interplay between blood flow and metabolism in the extraction and retention of ^{13}N-ammonia is complex. The early extraction phase of freely diffusible ^{13}N-ammonia reflects blood flow while the later, slow turnover phase reflects metabolic trapping of ^{13}N-ammonia. In experimental animals, several investigators have shown that the myocardial extraction and retention of ^{13}N-ammonia are related not only to regional blood flow but also to myocardial oxygenation and metabolism. Under hypoxic or ischemic conditions, the reduction of intracellular ATP to concentrations in the range of the K$_m$ for the enzyme-ATP complex could reduce intracellular ^{13}N-ammonia metabolism by glutamine synthetase. Because the extent of ^{13}N-ammonia metabolism may depend on the ATP state of the myocyte, intracellular levels of ^{13}N-ammonia may reflect cellular viability.

A, In patients with chronic coronary artery disease and left ventricular dysfunction, receiver-operating characteristic (ROC) curves were used to compare the abilities of late ammonia uptake (final 10 to 15 minutes of image acquisition) and absolute blood flow (early extraction phase, approximately 3 minutes after injection) to predict functional improvement of asynergic regions after revascularization. The results show that late ammonia uptake (metabolic trapping) is a significantly better predictor of functional improvement after revascularization when compared to absolute blood flow. **B,** There is a linear relationship between percent late ammonia uptake and [^{18}F]-fluorodeoxyglucose (FDG) uptake (*left*), and ^{201}Tl uptake on redistribution imaging (*right*) in reversible (*green circles*) and irreversible (*orange circles*) asynergic regions after revascularization. **C,** Sequence and timing of ^{13}N-ammonia and FDG PET imaging for assessment of myocardial viability. Thus, beyond ammonia's value as a perfusion tracer, late ammonia images provide important insight regarding cell membrane integrity and myocardial viability. (*Adapted from* Kitsiou *et al.* [31].)

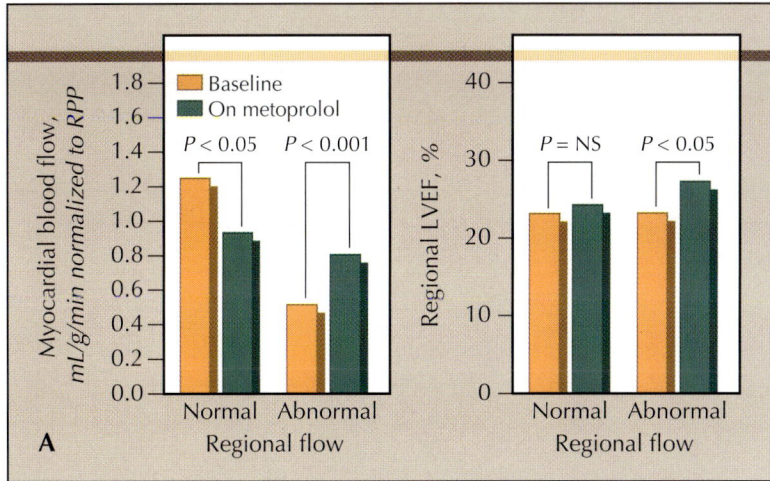
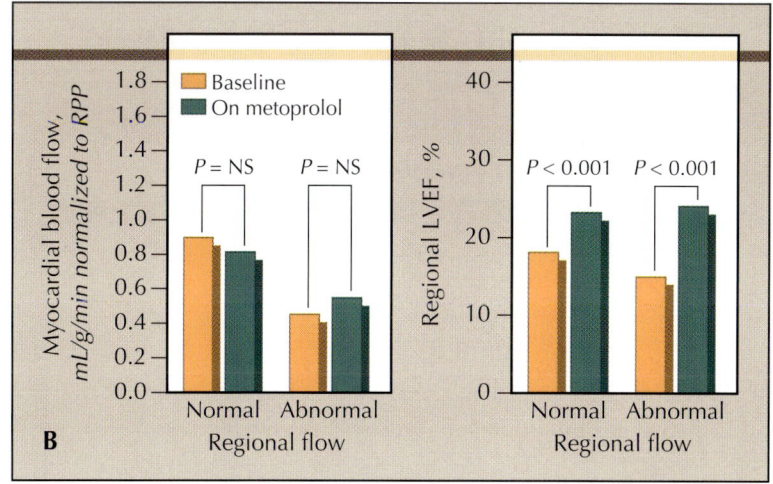

FIGURE 2-33. The effects of 6 months of medical treatment with metoprolol on absolute myocardial blood flow and function in patients with heart failure secondary to ischemic or nonischemic cardiomyopathy. **A,** In patients with ischemic cardiomyopathy, there is favorable redistribution of absolute blood flow (normalized to rate-pressure product [RPP]) from normally perfused myocardium to abnormally perfused myocardium after metoprolol therapy. Increased myocardial blood flow is associated with improvement in regional left ventricular ejection fraction (LVEF) in these abnormally perfused regions of myocardium, while myocardial regions with normal baseline perfusion show no change in regional LVEF. The reduction in blood flow in nonischemic regions by β-blockade most probably reflects the reduction in myocardial oxygen demands induced by the reduction in myocardial contractility and work. On the other hand, the decrease in myocardial oxygen demand of the ischemic area by β-blockade may restore vascular autoregulation and allow the ischemic vasculature to regulate its blood flow. In addition, the lower heart rate achieved with β-blockade results in a decreased number of systolic contractions per minute, allowing more time for diastolic coronary perfusion. By increasing the diastolic coronary perfusion pressure gradient, resistance to flow through the coronary artery narrowing decreases significantly after β-blockade. The final effect of β-blockade in the ischemic region, therefore, is to increase the distal bed vascular resistance and decrease the dynamic severity of coronary artery narrowing. By decreasing myocardial oxygen demand (decrease in heart rate) and increasing myocardial oxygen supply (increased subendocardial blood flow in ischemic myocardium), treatment with metoprolol results in an improvement in oxygen balance of the ischemic myocardium.

B, In patients with nonischemic cardiomyopathy, there is no significant redistribution of absolute myocardial blood flow (normalized to rate-pressure product) from normally perfused myocardium to abnormally perfused myocardium before and after metoprolol therapy. Regional LVEF increased in both normally perfused and abnormally perfused myocardial regions. In patients with ischemic cardiomyopathy, improvement in global left ventricular function during metoprolol therapy may be attributed, in part, to redistribution in absolute myocardial blood flow resulting in increases in regional left ventricular function. However, it appears that other mechanisms of action are key to the improvement in left ventricular function seen in patients with nonischemic cardiomyopathy. NS—not significant. (*Adapted from* Bennett *et al.* [32].)

MYOCARDIAL METABOLISM AND VIABILITY

A. PET TECHNIQUES: ^{11}C-PALMITATE

- Image acquisition to start at 15–20 mCi bolus injection of the tracer and to continue 40–60 min
- Initial uptake and distribution in the myocardium is determined primarily by regional blood flow
- In the cytosol, ^{11}C-palmitate is esterified to ^{11}C-acyl-CoA, which is mediated by thiokinase, an energy-dependent reaction, resulting in trapping of the tracer in the myocardium
- Thereafter, ^{11}C-acyl-CoA either enters the endogenous lipid pool as ^{11}C glycerides and ^{11}C phospholipids or moves via the carnitine shuttle to the mitochondria, where rapid degradation by β-oxidation results in the generation of carbon dioxide

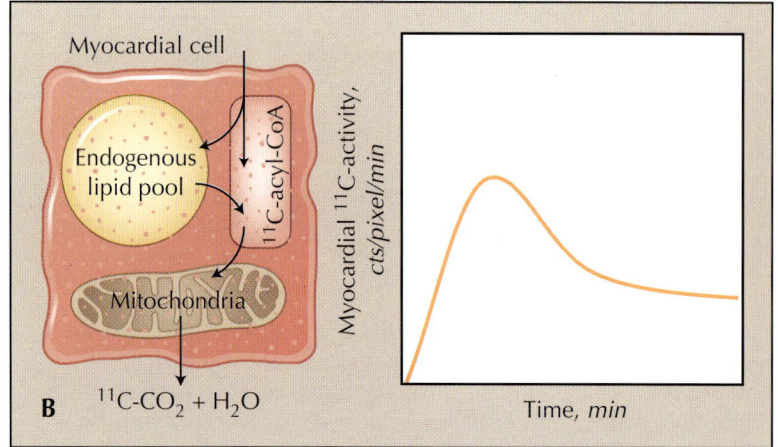

FIGURE 2-34. PET techniques: ^{11}C-palmitate. A, The principle of using a metabolic tracer for myocardial imaging is based on the concept that viable myocytes in hypoperfused and dysfunctional regions are metabolically active, while scarred or fibrotic tissue is metabolically inactive. Under fasting and aerobic conditions, long-chain fatty acids are the preferred fuel in the heart because they supply 65% to 70% of the energy for the working heart, and approximately 15% to 20% of the total energy supply comes from glucose. As such, early studies focused on the characterization of myocardial kinetics of the long-chain fatty acid, ^{11}C-palmitate, using PET. Uptake of ^{11}C-palmitate in the myocardium is dependent on regional perfusion, diffusion across the sarcolemmal membrane, transporter protein, and acceptance in the cytosol by binding to CoA. In normally perfused myocardium, the extraction fraction of ^{11}C-palmitate is 40%. The transporter protein of long-chain fatty acids across myocardial cells has a molecular weight of 40 kD; within the myocyte fatty acids are bound to storage protein with a molecular weight of 12 kD. Once in the cell, metabolic activation of ^{11}C-palmitate occurs by binding to coenzyme A. Depending on demand, about 80% of the extracted ^{11}C-palmitate is activated for transport from the lipid pool into the mitochondria (via the carnitine shuttle) for breakdown by β-oxidation. β-oxidation results in the generation of carbon dioxide, which appears in the venous effluent of the coronary circulation in less than a minute after ^{11}C-acyl-CoA transfer into the mitochondria.

B, External measurement by dynamic PET imaging allows the observation of tracer inflow, peak accumulation, and release of the tracer within a particular region of interest in the myocardium. Fatty acid imaging with radioiodine-labeled fatty acid analogues such as β-methyliodopentadecanoic acid (BMIPP) is also possible using SPECT. (*Panel B adapted from* Feinendegen [33].)

A. PET TECHNIQUES: ^{11}C-ACETATE

Initial tracer uptake provides an indirect estimate of regional myocardial blood flow

In the cytosol, ^{11}C-acetate is converted directly to ^{11}C-acetyl-CoA, and is oxidized by the tricarboxylic acid cycle in the mitochondria to ^{11}C-carbon dioxide and water

Because the washout rate of ^{11}C-acetate from myocardium is directly related to oxidative tricarboxylic acid cycle flux, it is an ideal indicator of myocardial oxidative metabolism

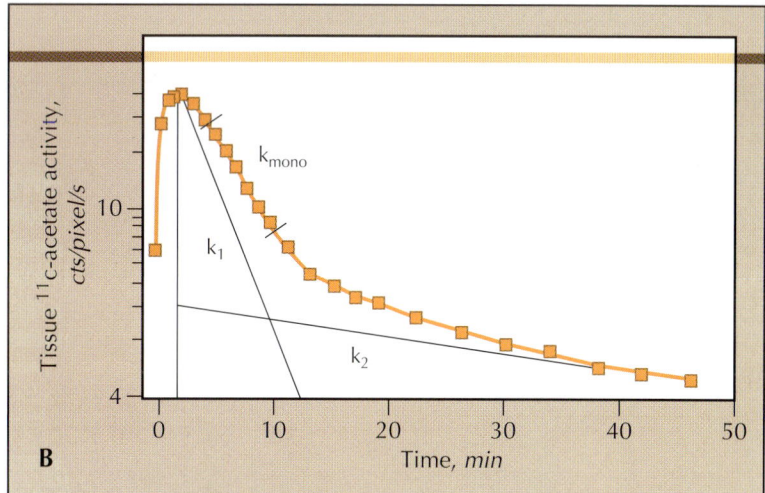

FIGURE 2-35. PET techniques: ^{11}C-acetate. A, ^{11}C-acetate is a short-chain acid that is avidly extracted by the myocardium with a first-pass extraction of 63% at blood flows of 1 mL/g/min and is metabolized predominantly by mitochondrial oxidative metabolism. Once in the cytosol, the tracer is converted to acetyl-CoA by acetyl CoA synthase, and is oxidized by the tricarboxylic acid cycle in the mitochondria to ^{11}C-carbon dioxide and water. Thus, the washout rate of ^{11}C-acetate from myocardium is directly related to oxidative tricarboxylic acid cycle flux. Given the close link between tricarboxylic acid cycle and oxidative phosphorylation, the myocardial turnover and clearance of ^{11}C-acetate in the form of ^{11}C-carbon dioxide may reflect overall oxidative metabolism and provide insight into the mitochondrial function of viable myocardium. Alternative metabolic pathways of ^{11}C-acetate include incorporation into amino acids, ketones, and fatty acids by de novo synthesis or chain elongation. However, these latter pathways are thought to be modest and unlikely to compromise estimation of regional myocardial oxygen consumption per minute.

B, Myocardial ^{11}C-acetate tissue time-activity curve demonstrating biexponential clearance of the tracer from myocardium. Monoexponential fitting of the early portion of the clearance phase yields the slope k_{mono}, while biexponential least-square fitting of the clearance phase yields k_1 and k_2 slopes. The rapid phase of clearance (k_1) represents oxidation of extracted ^{11}C-acetate by the mitochondria to ^{11}C-carbon dioxide, and the slower phase of clearance (k_2) represents incorporation of ^{11}C-acetate into amino acids and other alternate metabolic pathways. In patients with recent myocardial infarction and chronic stable angina, preservation of myocardial oxidative metabolism is shown to predict functional recovery after revascularization [34,35]. When clearance rates of ^{11}C-acetate are within 2 standard deviations of the normal mean, the positive predictive accuracy for recovery of function after revascularization is 84% in patients with recent myocardial infarction and 79% in patients with chronic stable angina. Conversely, when clearance rates of ^{11}C-acetate are more than 2 standard deviations below the normal mean, the negative predictive values are 70% in patients with recent myocardial infarction and 83% in patients with chronic stable angina. (*Panel B adapted from* Schelbert [36].)

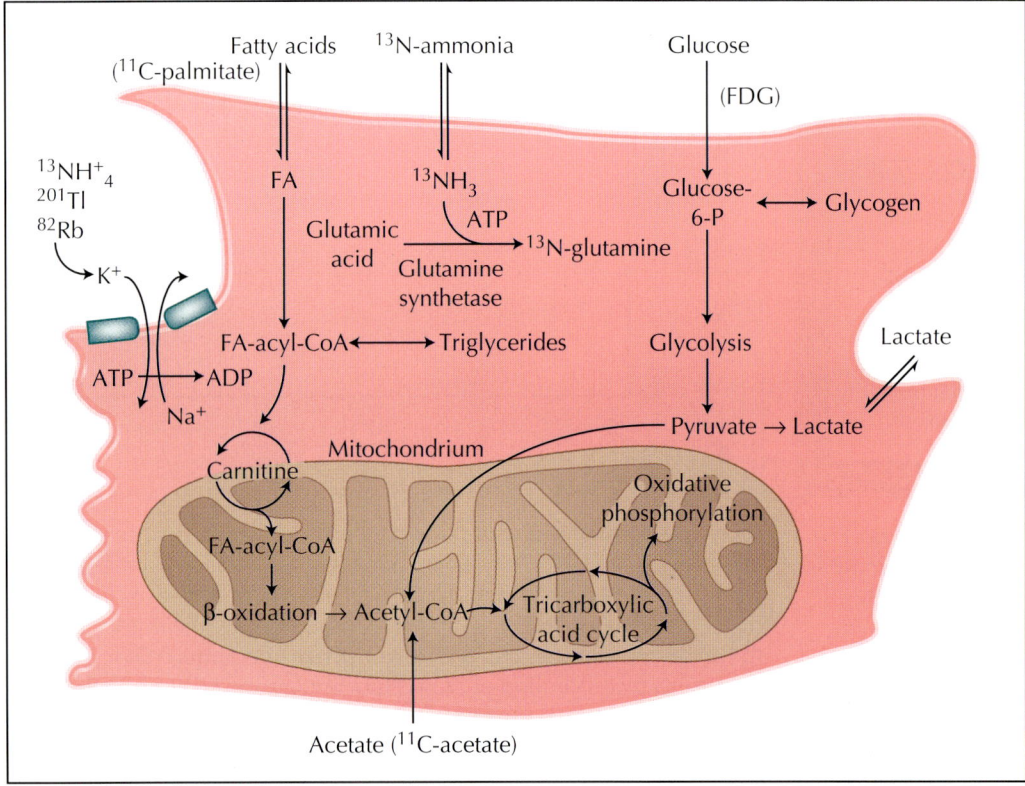

FIGURE 2-36. Major metabolic pathways and regulatory steps of a myocyte. Breakdown of fatty acids in the mitochondria via β-oxidation is exquisitely sensitive to oxygen deprivation. Therefore, in the setting of reduced oxygen supply, the myocytes compensate for the loss of oxidative potential by shifting toward greater utilization of glucose to generate high-energy phosphates. Glycolysis occurs in the cytoplasm under anaerobic conditions and leads to the formation of pyruvate. For every mol of glucose metabolized through glycolysis, 2 mol ATP are generated (anaerobic condition), and 36 mol ATP are generated from pyruvate entering the citric acid cycle in the mitochondria (aerobic oxidative phosphorylation). Because glycolysis can generate ATP under anaerobic conditions, glycolysis becomes an attractive alternate metabolic pathway for ATP generation in hypoperfused myocardium with a limited supply of oxygen. Although the amount of energy produced by glycolysis may be adequate to maintain myocyte viability and preserve the electrochemical gradient across the cell membrane, it may not be sufficient to sustain contractile function. In hibernation, the adaptive response of the myocardium in the setting of prolonged resting hypoperfusion (reduced oxygen supply) is a reduction in myocardial contractile function (reduced oxygen demand), thereby preserving myocardial viability in the absence of clinically evident ischemia. FDG—[^{18}F]-fluorodeoxyglucose. (*Adapted from Dilsizian [37].*)

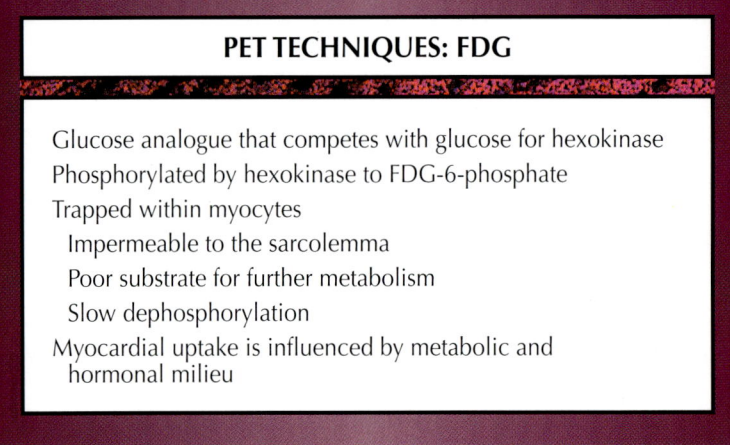

PET TECHNIQUES: FDG

- Glucose analogue that competes with glucose for hexokinase
- Phosphorylated by hexokinase to FDG-6-phosphate
- Trapped within myocytes
  - Impermeable to the sarcolemma
  - Poor substrate for further metabolism
  - Slow dephosphorylation
- Myocardial uptake is influenced by metabolic and hormonal milieu

FIGURE 2-37. PET techniques: [^{18}F]-fluorodeoxyglucose (FDG). FDG is a glucose analogue used to image myocardial glucose utilization with PET. Following intravenous injection of 5 to 10 mCi FDG, FDG rapidly exchanges across the capillary and cellular membranes and is phosphorylated by hexokinase to FDG-6-phosphate. Once phosphorylated, FDG is not metabolized further in the glycolytic pathway, fructose-pentose shunt, or glycogen synthesis. Because the dephosphorylation rate of FDG is slow, essentially it becomes trapped in the myocardium, allowing adequate time to image regional glucose uptake by PET or SPECT. In the fasting and aerobic conditions, fatty acids are the preferred source of myocardial energy production, with glucose accounting for some 15% to 20% of the total energy supply. However, in the fed state, plasma insulin levels increase, glucose metabolism is stimulated, and tissue lipolysis is inhibited, resulting in reduced fatty acid delivery to the myocardium. The combined effects of insulin on these processes and the increased arterial glucose concentration associated with fed state result in preferred glucose utilization by the myocardium.

STANDARDIZATION SCHEMES FOR OPTIMIZING FDG IMAGE QUALITY

INTRAVENOUS BOLUS OF REGULAR INSULIN

- Most common and clinically feasible approach
- Regular insulin is administered according to plasma glucose level and predetermined sliding scale
- Plasma glucose level is assessed every 15 min with administration of additional boluses of insulin, if necessary
- FDG dose is injected once the plasma glucose level is below 140 mg/dL

HYPERINSULINEMIC-EUGLYCEMIC CLAMPING

- Insulin and glucose are infused simultaneously to achieve a stable plasma insulin level of 100 to 120 IU/L and a normal plasma glucose level
- The rate of glucose infusion (20% dextrose solution with potassium chloride) is adjusted intermittently based on measured glucose levels
- Although it provides excellent image quality, the technique is rather tedious and impractical for routine clinical studies

USE OF NICOTINIC ACID DERIVATIVE

- Approximately 2 h before the FDG dose injection, a single dose of nicotinic acid derivative is given orally followed by glucose loading
- FDG image quality is shown comparable to that obtained after the clamp technique in the same patient population

FIGURE 2-38. Standardization schemes for optimizing [^{18}F]-fluorodeoxyglucose (FDG) image quality. Diagnostic quality of FDG imaging is critically dependent on a number of factors, such as hormonal milieu, substrate availability, and regional blood flow. This becomes particularly evident when studying patients with clinical or subclinical diabetes. Most clinical studies are performed after 50 to 75 g glucose loading with oral dextrose approximately 1 to 2 hours before the FDG injection. Although 90% of FDG images are of adequate-to-excellent diagnostic quality in nondiabetic patients, the quality of FDG images after glucose loading is less certain in patients with clinical or subclinical diabetes mellitus. Because the increase in plasma insulin levels after glucose loading may be attenuated in patients with diabetes mellitus, tissue lipolysis is not inhibited, and free fatty acid levels in the plasma remain high. Acquiring good-quality FDG images in diabetics may be challenging. Standardization schemes utilized to optimize FDG image quality include intravenous insulin injections after glucose loading, hyperinsulinemic-euglycemic clamping, and use of nicotinic acid derivative.

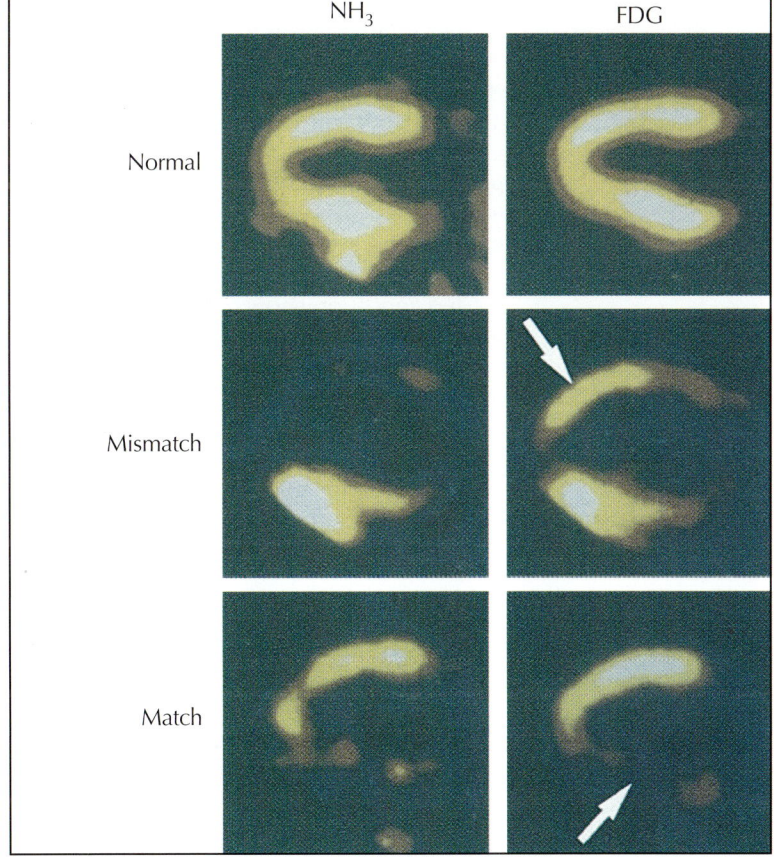

FIGURE 2-39. Patterns of normal, mismatch, and match under glucose-loading. Preserved or increased myocardial glucose utilization in the setting of prolonged hypoperfusion at rest is termed a *mismatch* pattern. On the NH$_3$ images, there is severely reduced blood flow in the anterior and lateral regions that have preserved metabolism on the [^{18}F]-fluorodeoxyglucose (FDG) images (*arrow*) consistent with myocardial viability. Reduced or absent myocardial glucose utilization in hypoperfused myocardial regions is termed a *match* pattern. On the NH$_3$ images, there is severely reduced blood flow in the inferior region that has absent myocardial metabolism on the FDG images (*arrow*) consistent with scarred myocardium. The application of such PET patterns in patients with chronic ischemic left ventricular dysfunction confers high positive and negative predictive accuracies for recovery of regional function after revascularization, with an overall accuracy between 80% and 90% [38]. However, clinically meaningful increases in global left ventricular function after revascularization are best attained if the extent of hibernating and stunned myocardium is 17% to 25% of the left ventricular mass or more [39]. (*Courtesy of* Dr. James Arrighi.)

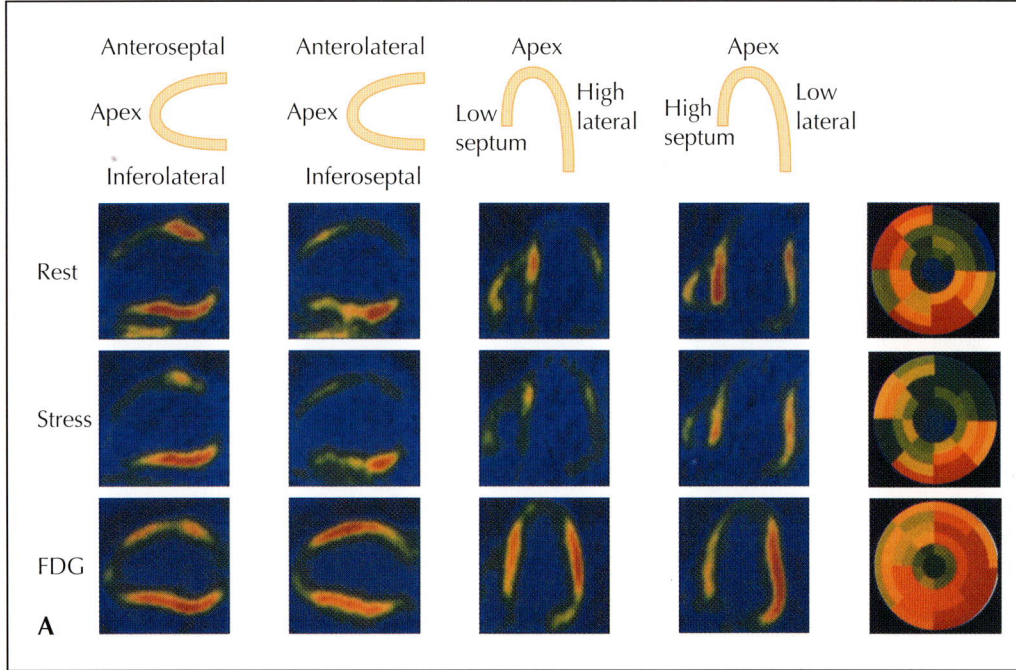

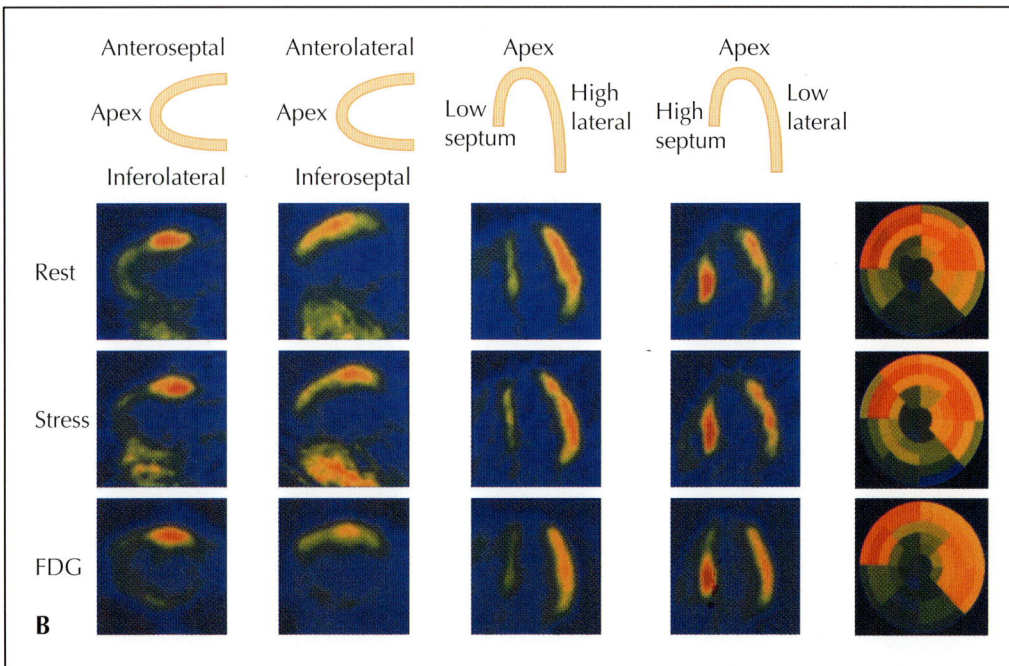

FIGURE 2-40. Examples of PET mismatch and match patterns. Increased [^{18}F]-fluorodeoxyglucose (FDG) uptake in asynergic myocardial regions with reduced blood flow at rest (mismatch pattern) has become a scintigraphic marker of hibernation. **A**, A patient with severely dilated left ventricle, diffuse hypotension, and apical dyskinesis (left ventricular ejection fraction [LVEF], 12%) had severe triple vessel disease. Coronary angiogram revealed 100% occlusion of the proximal left anterior descending coronary artery (LAD), D1, and D2, subtotal occlusion of the proximal right coronary artery (RCA), and 90% OM1 occlusion. In this patient, four long-axis slices (two horizontal long-axis and two vertical long-axis images) encompassing the entire left ventricle along with corresponding bull's-eye images for rest and stress ^{13}N-ammonia and FDG uptake are shown. Rest ^{13}N-ammonia images show irreversible defects in the apical and anterolateral regions with partial reversibility in the anterior and inferoseptal regions. Stress ^{13}N-ammonia images show markedly decreased perfusion in the apical, anterior, anterolateral, and inferoseptal regions. However, FDG images acquired under glucose-loaded conditions show preserved or increased glucose utilization in all abnormally perfused myocardial regions at rest, the scintigraphic hallmark of hibernation. In patients with chronic ischemic left ventricular dysfunction, rest and stress myocardial perfusion images alone may significantly underestimate the presence and extent of hibernating but viable myocardium. **B**, Decreased or absent FDG uptake in asynergic myocardial regions with reduced blood flow at rest (match pattern) represents scarred myocardium. A patient with previous coronary bypass surgery presented with significantly dilated left ventricle, apical dyskinesis, septal and inferior akinesis (LVEF, 36%), and congestive heart failure. Coronary angiogram revealed severe native disease of all three vessels, patent left and right internal mammary grafts to the LAD and RCA, critical stenoses of the OM1 vein graft, and a patent OM2 vein graft. In this patient, rest and stress ^{13}N-ammonia images show irreversible defects in the inferior, apical, and inferoseptal regions. FDG images acquired under glucose-loaded condition show absence of glucose utilization in all abnormally perfused myocardial regions at rest. Such asynergic myocardial regions demonstrating matched reduction in perfusion and metabolism represent scarred myocardium and are unlikely to recover function after revascularization.

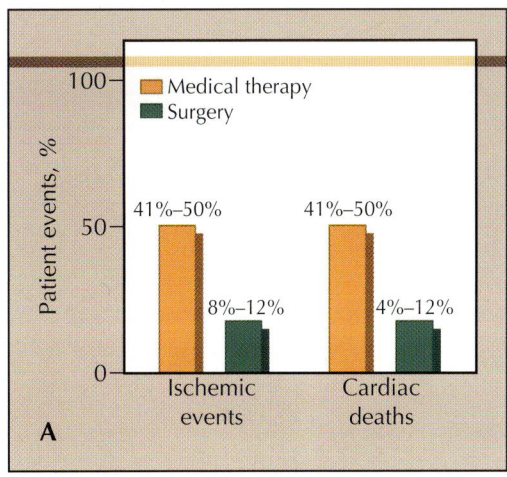 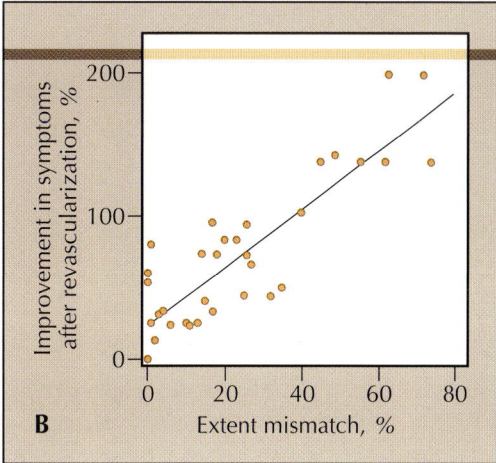 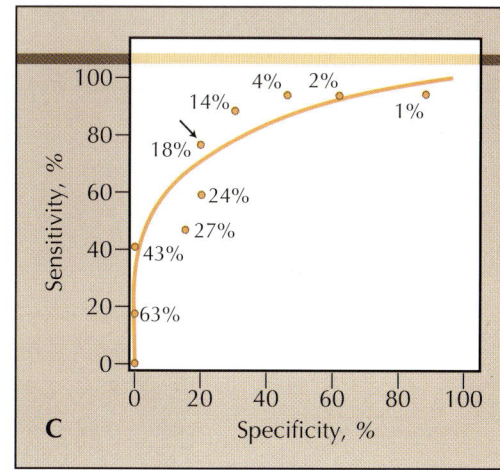

FIGURE 2-41. PET mismatch and prognosis. The prognostic significance of perfusion-metabolism mismatch pattern in ischemic cardiomyopathy has been shown in a number of nonrandomized, retrospective studies with PET [40,41]. **A,** Patients with perfusion-metabolism mismatch pattern who were treated surgically had lower ischemic event rates and fewer deaths when compared with those treated with medical therapy. In contrast, patients with perfusion-metabolism match pattern displayed no such difference in outcomes between surgical and medical management. Moreover, the patients with myocardial viability (mismatch pattern) who underwent revascularization manifested a significant improvement in heart failure symptoms and exercise tolerance [42,43]. **B,** The relation between the anatomic extent of perfusion:metabolism PET mismatch pattern (expressed as percent of the left ventricle) and the change in functional status after revascularization (expressed as percent improvement from baseline) is shown. The scatterplot shows that the greatest improvement in heart failure symptoms occurs in patients with the largest mismatch defects on quantitative analysis of PET images. **C,** Receiver-operating characteristic curve for different anatomic extent of perfusion-metabolism mismatch to predict a change (at least one grade) in functional status after revascularization is shown. When the extent of PET mismatch involves 18% or more of the left ventricular mass, the sensitivity for predicting a change in functional status after revascularization is 76% and the specificity is 78% (area under the fitted curve = 0.82). (*Panel A adapted from* Eitzman *et al.* [40] *and* DiCarli *et al.* [41]; *panels B and C adapted from* DiCarli *et al.* [42].)

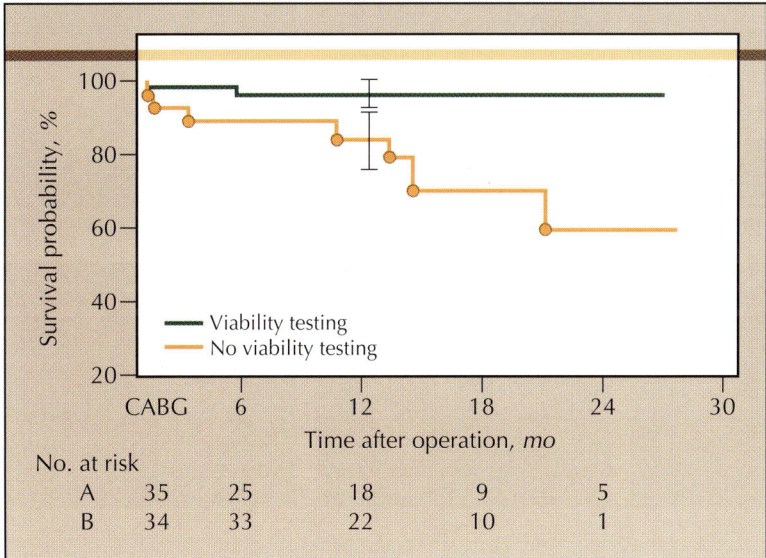

FIGURE 2-42. Assessment of myocardial viability before surgery and clinical outcome. Because patients with chronic ischemic left ventricular dysfunction are at higher risk for perioperative complications associated with coronary artery bypass surgery (CABG), one might question whether assessment of myocardial viability by means of PET before surgery affects clinical outcome with respect to perioperative and postoperative survival. In this retrospective study, the actuarial survival curve, which includes in-hospital mortality after surgery and mortality during follow-up, shows significant different survival between patients who were selected for surgery on the basis of clinical presentation and angiographic data (group A, no viability testing) compared with those who were selected for surgery according to extent of viable myocardium determined by PET (group B, viability testing). One year after surgery, the survival rate of patients with viability testing was 97% ± 3%, while the survival rate of patients with no viability testing was 79% ± 8% ($P < 0.01$). These data suggest that beyond providing prognostic information with regard to recovery of function after revascularization, myocardial viability studies with PET also allow selection of patients who are at low risk for serious perioperative and postoperative complications. (*Adapted from* Haas *et al.* [43].)

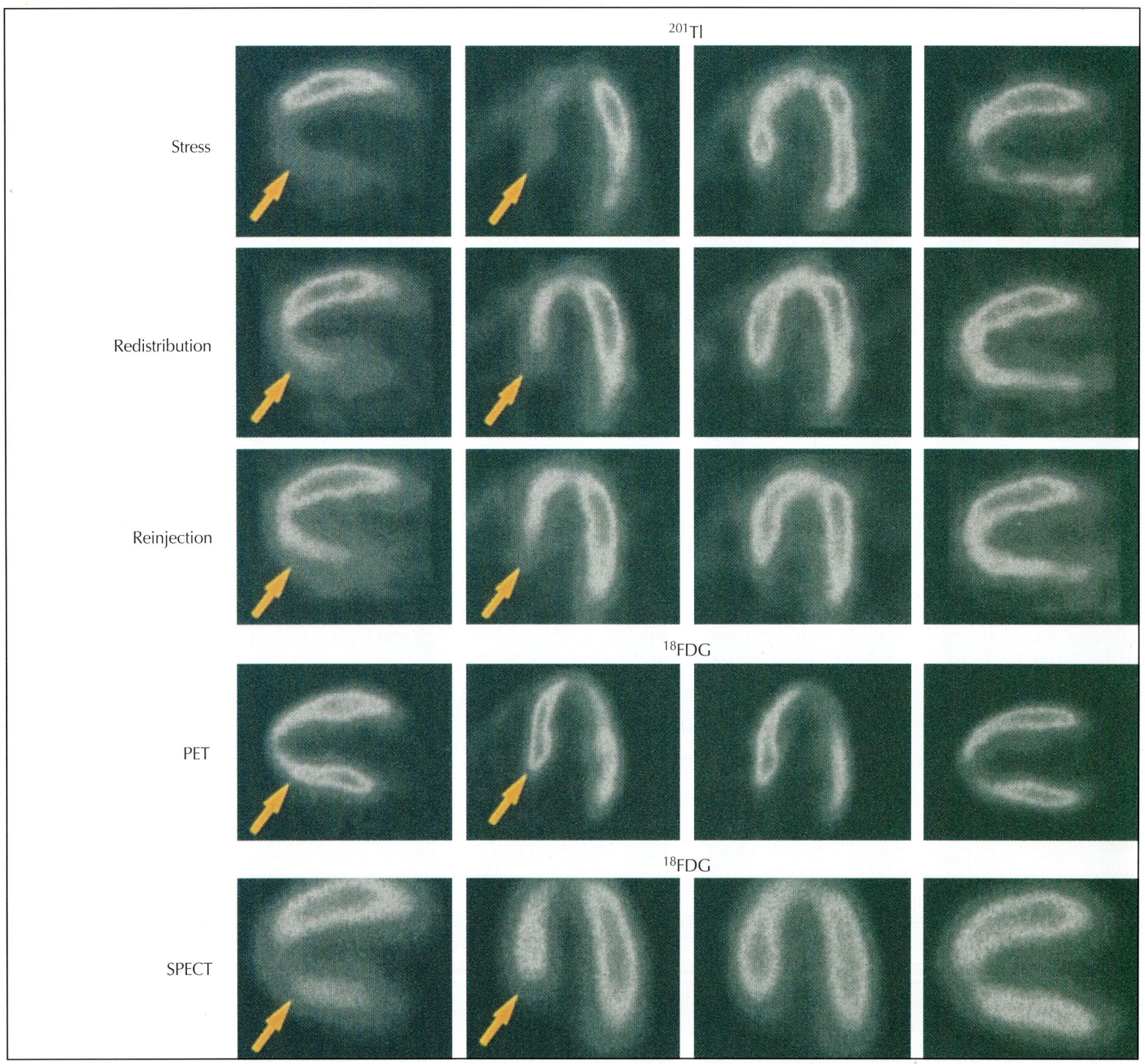

FIGURE 2-43. Recent advances in high-energy collimator design have made imaging the biodistribution of [^{18}F]-fluorodeoxyglucose (FDG) in the heart using SPECT technology a clinical reality. Although positron-emitting radioisotopes emit two 511 keV gamma rays, it is possible to ignore the coincident nature of the two 511 keV photons and image as one would any other single photon–emitting radiotracer using a gamma camera with high energy collimation. An advantage of 511 keV photons over 140 keV photons is that they have less scatter and attenuation in the patient. However, there are limitations to imaging 511 keV photons with SPECT. The collimator must be redesigned (thicker septa), resulting in a lower resolution (typically 15 to 20 mm full-width at half maximum for SPECT versus 6 to 7 mm for PET) and lower sensitivity when compared with PET. They have fewer interactions in the sodium iodide crystal (the substance used in nearly all gamma cameras), resulting in further reduction in sensitivity (which means longer imaging time with SPECT). Of the photons that do interact in the crystal, some will scatter and either leave the crystal or interact within the crystal at another location, resulting in some degradation of spatial resolution. However, despite the technical limitations described, a number of clinical studies have shown a reasonable concordance between cardiac FDG uptake with PET and high-energy collimated SPECT [44]. In the patient example shown, four radial long-axis tomograms are displayed for ^{201}Tl (stress-redistribution-reinjection protocol), FDG PET, and FDG SPECT (applying high-energy collimator). FDG images were obtained under glucose-loaded condition. On the ^{201}Tl images, reversible defects are seen in the apical and inferoseptal regions (*arrows*), representing ischemic but viable myocardium. FDG PET and high-energy collimator SPECT studies show preserved metabolic activity in the apical and inferoseptal regions (viable by FDG), as well as in the remaining myocardial regions with normal ^{201}Tl uptake [37]. (*Courtesy of* Gopal Srinivasan, National Institutes of Health, Bethesda, MD.)

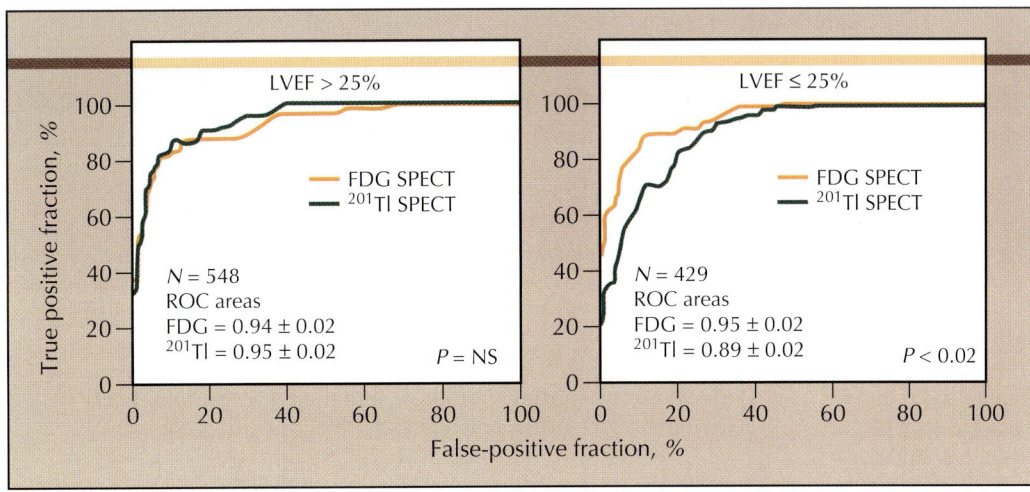

FIGURE 2-44. In patients with chronic coronary artery disease, differences between high-energy collimator SPECT and PET technologies and [^{18}F]-fluorodeoxyglucose (FDG) and ^{201}Tl tracers are examined for their ability to differentiate viable from nonviable myocardium. Plots of receiver-operating characteristic (ROC) curves for ^{201}Tl and FDG SPECT to predict myocardial viability as defined by 60% FDG PET threshold value for patients with left ventricular ejection fraction (LVEF) above 25% (*left*) and for patients with LVEF 25% or less (*right*) are shown. Area under the ROC curve for FDG SPECT and ^{201}Tl SPECT are displayed for each panel. ^{201}Tl tends to underestimate myocardial viability in patients with LVEF 25% or less, but not in patients with LVEF above 25%. Of the severe asynergic regions, 73% of discordant regions between ^{201}Tl and FDG PET were located in the inferior segment, compared with only 27% of regions with concordance between ^{201}Tl and FDG PET ($P < 0.001$). (*Adapted from* Srinivasan *et al.* [44]).

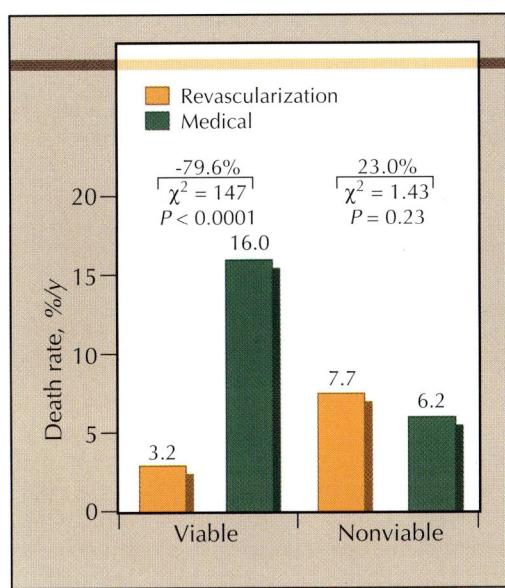

FIGURE 2-45. Prognostic implications of myocardial viability testing in patients with coronary artery disease and left ventricular dysfunction. Data from meta-analysis of 3088 patients (mean left ventricular ejection fraction, 32%, followed for 25 ± 10 months) demonstrates that in patients with preserved myocardial viability, the annual mortality rate was significantly lower in those who were treated with revascularization (3.2%) compared with those treated with medical therapy alone (16%). This represents a 79.6% decrease in annual mortality for patients with viability treated with revascularization ($P < 0.0001$). Moreover, there was a direct relationship between severity of left ventricular dysfunction and magnitude of benefit from revascularization among patients with myocardial viability ($P < 0.001$). In contrast, among patients without evidence of viable myocardium, there was no incremental benefit of revascularization over medical therapy. These data, along with other papers presented in this chapter, support the role of myocardial viability testing for the management of patients with chronic left ventricular dysfunction and in guiding therapeutic decisions for revascularization. (*Adapted from* Allman *et al.* [45].)

References

1. Gibson RS, Watson DD, Craddock GB, *et al.*: Predication of cardiac events after uncomplicated myocardial infarction: A prospective study comparing predischarge exercise thallium-201 scintigraphy and coronary angiography. *Circulation* 1983, 68:321–336.

2. Kiat H, Berman DS, Maddahi J, *et al.*: Late reversibility of tomographic myocardial thallium-201 defects: An accurate marker of myocardial viability. *J Am Coll Cardiol* 1988, 12:1456–1463.

3. Cloninger KG, DePuey EG, Garcia EV, *et al.*: Incomplete redistribution in delayed thallium-201 single photon emission computed tomographic (SPECT) images: An overestimation of myocardial scarring. *J Am Coll Cardiol* 1988, 12:955–963.

4. Dilsizian V: Thallium-201 scintigraphy: experience of two decades. In *Myocardial Viability: A Clinical and Scientific Treatise*. Edited by Dilsizian V. Armonk, New York: Futura; 2000:265–313.

5. Dilsizian V, Rocco TP, Freedman NM, *et al.*: Enhanced detection of ischemic but viable myocardium by the reinjection of thallium after stress-redistribution imaging. *N Engl J Med* 1990, 323:141–146.

6. Zimmermann R, Mall G, Rauch B, *et al.*: Residual Tl-201 activity in irreversible defects as a marker of myocardial viability: clinico-pathological study. *Circulation* 1995, 91:1016–1021.

7. Kayden DS, Sigal S, Soufer R, *et al.*: Thallium-201 for assessment of myocardial viability: Quantitative comparison of 24-hour redistribution imaging with imaging after reinjection at rest. *J Am Coll Cardiol* 1991, 18:1480–1486.

8. Shirani J, Alaeddini J, Pick R, Dilsizian V: Variations in collagen content of asynergic left ventricular segments in explanted hearts of men with ischemic cardiomyopathy. *Am J Cardiol* 2002, 89:865–869.

9. Shirani J, Lee J, Quigg RJ, *et al.*: Relation of thallium uptake to morphologic features of chronic ischemic heart disease: evidence for myocardial remodeling in non-infarct myocardium. *J Am Coll Cardiol* 2001, 38:84–90.

10. Kitsiou AN, Srinivasan G, Quyyumi AA, *et al.*: Stress-induced reversible and mild-to-moderate irreversible thallium defects: Are they equally accurate for predicting recovery of regional left ventricular function after revascularization? *Circulation* 1998, 98:501–508.

11. Petretta M, Cuocolo A, Bonaduce D, *et al.*: Prognostic value of thallium reinjection after stress-redistribution imaging in patients with previous myocardial infarction and left ventricular dysfunction. *J Nucl Med* 1997, 38:195–200.

12. Arrighi JA, Dilsizian V: Identification of viable, nonfunctioning myocardium. In *Cardiac Intensive Care*. Edited by Brown DL. Philadelphia: W.B. Saunders; 1998:307–327.

13. Gioia G, Milan E, Giubbini R, *et al.*: Prognostic value of tomographic rest-redistribution thallium-201 imaging in medically treated patients with coronary artery disease and left ventricular dysfunction. *J Nucl Cardiol* 1996, 3:150–156.

14. Gioia G, Powers J, Heo J, Iskandrian AS: Prognostic value of rest-redistribution tomographic thallium-201 imaging in ischemic cardiomyopathy. *Am J Cardiol* 1995, 75:759–762.

15. Pagley PR, Beller GA, Watson DD, *et al.*: Improved outcome after coronary artery bypass surgery in patients with ischemic cardiomyopathy and residual myocardial viability. *Circulation* 1997, 95:793–800.

16. Meleca MJ, McGoron AJ, Gerson MC, *et al.*: Flow versus uptake comparisons of thallium-201 with technetium-99m perfusion tracers in a canine model of myocardial ischemia. *J Nucl Med* 1997, 38:1847–1856.

17. Piwnica-Worms D, Chiu ML, Kronauge JF, *et al.*: Divergent kinetics of 201Tl and 99mTc-SESTAMIBI in cultured chick ventricular myocytes during ATP depletion. *Circulation* 1992, 85:1531–1541.

18. Narahara KA, Vilaneuva-Meyer J, Thompson CJ, *et al.*: Comparison of thallium-201 and technetium-99m hexakis 2-methoxyisobutyl isonitrile single-photon emission computed tomography for estimating the extent of myocardial ischemia and infarction in coronary artery disease. *Am J Cardiol* 1990, 66:1438–1444.

19. Leon AR, Eisner RL, Martin SE, *et al.*: Comparison of single-photon emission computed tomographic (SPECT) myocardial perfusion imaging with thallium-201 and technetium-99m sestamibi in dogs. *J Am Coll Cardiol* 1992, 20:1612–1625.

20. Li QS, Solot G, Frank TL, *et al.*: Myocardial redistribution of technetium-99m-methoxyisobutyl isonitrile (sestamibi). *J Nucl Med* 1990, 31:1069–1076.

21. Dilsizian V, Arrighi JA, Diodati JG, *et al.*: Myocardial viability in patients with chronic coronary artery disease: comparison of ^{99m}Tc-sestamibi with thallium reinjection and ^{18}F-fluorodeoxyglucose. *Circulation* 1994, 89:578–587.

22. Franceschi M, Guimond J, Zimmerman RE, *et al.*: Myocardial clearance of Tc-99m hexakis-2-methoxy-2-methylpropyl isonitrile (MIBI) in patients with coronary artery disease. *Clin Nucl Med* 1990, 15:307–312.

23. Bisi G, Sciagra R, Santoro GM, *et al.*: Technetium-99m-sestamibi imaging with nitrate infusion to detect viable hibernating myocardium and predict postrevascularization recovery. *J Nucl Med* 1995, 36:1994–2000.

24. Mehry Y, Latour JG, Arsenault A, Rousseau G: Effect of coronary reperfusion on technetium-99m methoxyisobutylisonitrile uptake by viable and necrotic myocardium in the dog. *Eur J Nucl Med* 1992, 19:503–510.

25. Udelson JE, Coleman PS, Metherall JA, *et al.*: Predicting recovery of severe regional ventricular dysfunction: comparison of resting scintigraphy with ^{201}Tl and ^{99m}Tc-sestamibi. *Circulation* 1994, 89:2552–2561.

26. Delbeke D, Videlefsky S, Patton JA, *et al.*: Rest myocardial perfusion/metabolism Imaging using simultaneous dual-isotope acquisition SPECT with technetium-99m-MIBI/fluorine-18-FDG. *J Nucl Med* 1995, 36:2110–2119.

27. Gould KL, Yoshida K, Hess MJ, *et al.*: Myocardial metabolism of fluorodeoxyglucose compared to cell membrane integrity for the potassium analogue rubidium-82 for assessing infarct size in man by PET. *J Nucl Med* 1991, 32:1–9.

28. Iida H, Rhodes CG, de Silva R, *et al.*: Myocardial tissue fraction: Correction of partial volume effects and measure of tissue viability. *J Nucl Med* 1991, 32:2169–2175.

29. Bergmann SR, Herrero P, Markham J, *et al.*: Noninvasive quantitation of myocardial blood flow in human subjects with oxygen-15-labeled water and positron emission tomography. *J Am Coll Cardiol* 1989, 14:639–652.

30. Yamamoto Y, de Silva R, Rhodes CG, *et al.*: A new strategy for the assessment of viable myocardium and regional myocardial blood flow using 15O-water and dynamic positron emission tomography. *Circulation* 1992, 86:167–178.

31. Kitsiou AN, Bacharach SL, Bartlett ML, *et al.*: ^{13}N-ammonia myocardial blood flow and uptake: Relation to functional outcome of asynergic regions after revascularization. *J Am Coll Cardiol* 1999, 33:678–686.

32. Bennett SK, Smith MF, Gottlieb SS, *et al.*: Effect of metoprolol on absolute myocardial blood flow in patients with heart failure secondary to ischemic or non-ischemic cardiomyopathy. *Am J Cardiol* 2002, 89:1431–1434.

33. Feinendegen LE: Myocardial imaging of lipid metabolism with labeled fatty acids. In *Myocardial Viability: A Clinical and Scientific Treatise*. Edited by Dilsizian V. Armonk, New York: Futura; 2000:349–389.

34. Gropler RJ, Siegel BA, Sampathkumaran K, *et al.*: Dependence of recovery of contractile function on maintenance of oxidative metabolism after myocardial infarction. *J Am Coll Cardiol* 1992, 19:989–997.

35. Gropler RJ, Geltman EM, Sampathkumaran K, *et al.*: Functional recovery after coronary revascularization for chronic coronary artery disease is dependent on maintenance of oxidative metabolism. *J Am Coll Cardiol* 1992, 20:569–577.

36. Schelbert HR: Principles of positron emission tomography. In *Marcus Cardiac Imaging: A Companion to Braunwald's Heart Disease*, edn 2. Edited by Skorton DJ, Schelbert HR, Wolf GL, Brundage BH. Philadelphia: W.B. Saunders; 1996:1063–1092.

37. Dilsizian V: Perspectives on the study of human myocardium: viability. In *Myocardial Viability: A Clinical and Scientific Treatise*. Edited by Dilsizian V. Armonk, New York: Futura; 2000:3–22.

38. Tillisch JH, Brunken R, Marshall R, *et al.*: Reversibility of cardiac wall-motion abnormalities predicted by positron tomography. *N Engl J Med* 1986; 314:884–888.

39. Dilsizian V, Arrighi JA: Myocardial viability in chronic coronary artery disease: perfusion, metabolism and contractile reserve. In *Cardiac Nuclear Medicine*, edn 3. Edited by Gerson MC. New York: McGraw-Hill; 1996:143–191.

40. Eitzman D, Al-Aouar Z, Kanter HL, *et al.*: Clinical outcome of patients with advanced coronary artery disease after viability studies with positron emission tomography. *J Am Coll Cardiol* 1992, 20:559–565.

41. DiCarli MF, Davidson M, Little R, *et al.*: Value of metabolic imaging with positron emission tomography for evaluating prognosis in patients with coronary artery disease and left ventricular dysfunction. *Am J Cardiol* 1994, 73:527–533.

42. DiCarli MF, Asgarzadie F, Schelbert HR, *et al.*: Quantitative relation between myocardial viability and improvement in heart failure symptoms after revascularization in patients with ischemic cardiomyopathy. *Circulation* 1995, 92:3436–3444.

43. Haas F, Haehnel CJ, Picker W, *et al.*: Preoperative positron emission tomography viability assessment and perioperative and postoperative risk in patients with advanced ischemic heart disease. *J Am Coll Cardiol* 1997, 30:1693–1700.

44. Srinivasan G, Kitsiou AN, Bacharach SL, *et al.*: ^{18}F-fluorodeoxyglucose single photon emission computed tomography: Can it replace PET and thallium SPECT for the assessment of myocardial viability? *Circulation* 1998, 97:843–850.

45. Allman KC, Shaw LJ, Hachamovitch R, Udelson JE: Myocardial viability testing and impact of revascularization on prognosis in patients with coronary artery disease and left ventricular dysfunction: a meta-analysis. *J Am Coll Cardiol* 2002, 39:1151–1158.

CHAPTER 3

PHARMACOLOGIC STRESSORS IN CORONARY ARTERY DISEASE

D. Douglas Miller

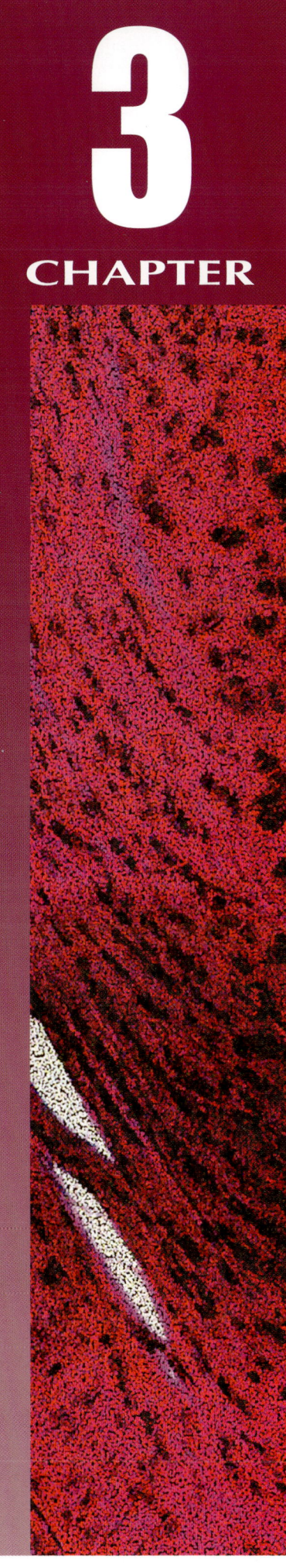

The use of pharmacologic agents to stress patients who are unsuitable for maximal exercise stress has evolved into an essential clinical tool for the diagnosis of coronary artery disease (CAD) and for noninvasive cardiac risk assessment. The initial administration of a drug to create differential coronary hyperemia (using oral then intravenous dipyridamole), as an adjunct to planar ^{201}Tl myocardial perfusion imaging for the diagnosis of CAD in stable patients, has been extended to include the following: use with single photon and positron nuclear tomography, 2-D echocardiography, and MRI; use with ^{99m}Tc-labeled myocardial radiotracers (sestamibi, tetrofosmin, etc.); Food and Drug Administration-approved indication for the definition of the risk of future cardiac events (ie, prognosis); development of short-acting, highly specific hyperemic agents (adenosine and its analogues); use of catecholamine infusion in patients with contraindications to hyperemic agents (dobutamine, arbutamine); protocols combining drug stress with submaximal exercise stress (isometric or dynamic); and safe use early after uncomplicated acute coronary syndromes (unstable angina, myocardial infarction).

The progressive, evidence-based evolution in drug stress pharmacology and related imaging protocols provides strong evidence for the safety and utility of this testing modality in clinical medicine. This widespread acceptance into the clinical practice of cardiovascular specialists and referring physicians has been reinforced by expert consensus as reflected in practice guidelines. Based on the strength of evidence in the medical literature, American College of Physicians/American College of Cardiology/American Heart Association practice guidelines [1] feature and recommend the use of drug stress imaging in a wide range of clinical settings. It is estimated that up to 40% of all current stress imaging studies are performed in combination with pharmacologic stressors, with more than 50% of these procedures being performed in elderly patients [2].

The target populations who benefit most from the incremental diagnostic and prognostic value of drug stress imaging are those at higher risk of severe CAD and related serious cardiac events due to their comorbid conditions (ie, generalized vascular disease) and/or poor functional capacity, which renders them unable to perform the preferred stress modality, maximal dynamic exercise stress.

Triaging patients for further cardiac evaluation based on clinical risk predictors and the type of surgical procedure is now recommended and widely practiced. Pharmacologic stress myocardial perfusion imaging is an excellent adjunctive method for identifying high- and low-risk patients from within an intermediate clinical risk pool. The stress imaging results with each of the available pharmacologic stressors are qualitatively similar for discriminating low- and high-risk groups for postoperative cardiac events, although the reported clinical experience to date with adenosine and dobutamine is somewhat limited. With the routine use of electrocardiograph-gated SPECT imaging, the left ventricular ejection fraction can also be obtained, adding further prognostic value to the perfusion data. Patients with more extensive stress-induced myocardial hypoperfusion or ischemia are at highest risk, and are best evaluated with coronary angiography with the goal of preoperative revascularization based on the current published guidelines. Although the American College of Cardiology/American Heart Association Task Force guidelines have not been prospectively validated, several small studies support these expert, evidence-based recommendations [1].

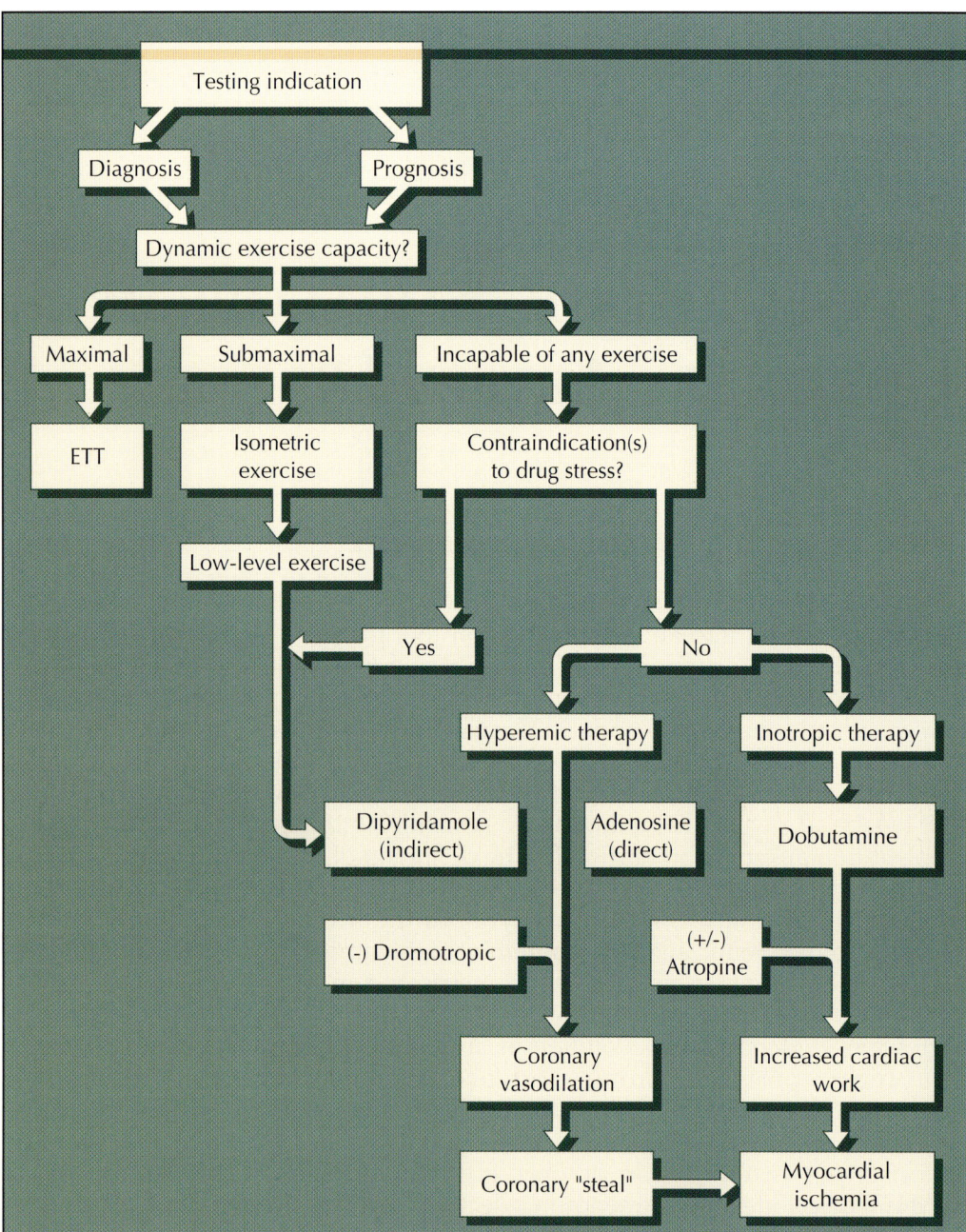

FIGURE 3-1. Patient protocol selection algorithm. The decision analysis for pharmacologic stress imaging illustrates the clinical issues that should be addressed: whether the patient can perform dynamic exercise, whether there are contraindications for drug stress, the type of drug stress (*ie*, hyperemic or inotropic), and the resulting physiologic and pathophysiologic endpoints. ETT—exercise treadmill testing.

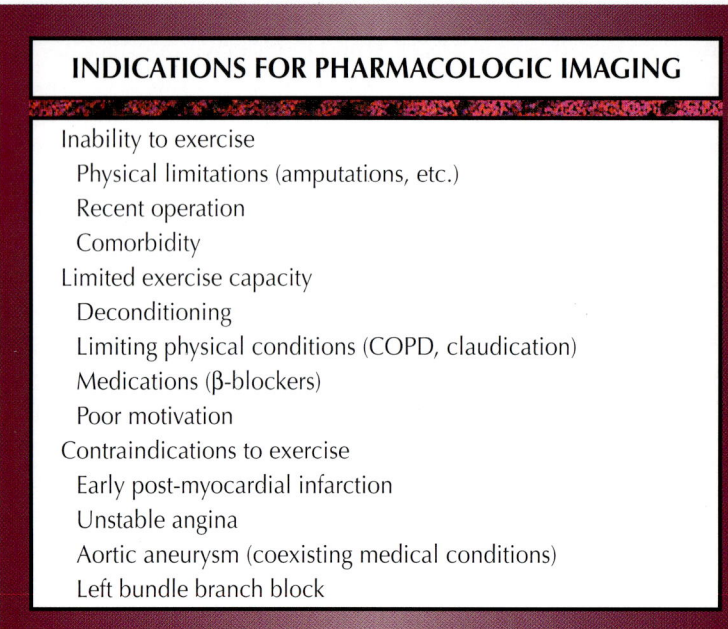

FIGURE 3-2. Indications for pharmacologic stress imaging. These indications include inability to exercise, limited exercise capacity, and relative or absolute contraindications to exercise. While exercise remains the preferred modality of stress testing in the majority of cases, a significant number of patients cannot complete a maximum stress test. Some patient populations are well suited for vasodilator stress imaging, such as patients with aortic stenosis, where excellent diagnostic accuracy and safety have been shown [3]. Patients with electrocardiographic left bundle branch block (LBBB) have a high false-positive rate with exercise or dobutamine stress testing due to abnormal patterns of septal perfusion and contradiction [4,5]. The diagnostic accuracy in patients with LBBB is 86% to 90% with adenosine or dipyridamole, compared to 50% or less with exercise perfusion imaging. Supplemental exercise is not advised for patients with LBBB. COPD—chronic obstructive pulmonary disease.

PHARMACOLOGIC STRESS TESTING CHARACTERISTICS*

	DIAGNOSIS	PROGNOSIS
Primary endpoint	Disease detection (CAD)	Risk stratification
Pretest variables	Disease probability (clinical)	Clinical risk index
	Exercise capacity	Preceding events
		Exercise capacity
		Anticipated future stress (ie, surgery)
Test performance characteristics	Sensitivity	Positive predictive value
	Specificity (or normalcy)	Negative predictive value
	Diagnostic accuracy	
Post-test variables	Disease probability	Incremental value (versus clinical assessment, other tests)
Sources of bias	Patient selection (test indication)	Follow-up (duration, lost patients)
	Verification (referral for coronary angiography)	Censoring (after events, interventions)
		Event type (hard, soft, both)
		Event frequency (adequate endpoints)

*In patients with known or suspected CAD.

FIGURE 3-3. Pharmacologic stress testing characteristics. Pharmacologic stress testing is useful for the diagnosis of coronary artery disease (CAD) and for defining the likelihood of future cardiac events. While both diagnostic and prognostic information can be derived from the same testing procedure, it is important to identify the primary indication for testing prior to performing the procedure. It is also important that this primary question (or endpoint) be addressed in the report generated from the drug stress study. The other variables are considered important in clinical research designed to evaluate the efficacy, effectiveness, and validity of pharmacologic stress imaging for diagnosis and prognosis.

OPTIONS FOR NONEXERCISE STRESS TESTING

- Cold pressor test
- Atrial pacing
  - Transthoracic
  - Intravenous
  - Transesophageal
- Pharmacologic stress
  - Vasodilator stress
    - Dipyridamole
    - IV adenosine
  - Inotropic/anatropic/chronotropic
    - IV dobutamine

FIGURE 3-4. Options for nonexercise stress testing. These options include less frequently used techniques such as cold pressor testing and atrial pacing, and more commonly used pharmacologic stress with vasodilators or inotropic agents. General contraindications for pharmacologic stress testing include hypersensitivity to the particular stress agent or its antidote, testing within 24 hours of an acute coronary syndrome, and uncompensated congestive heart failure. Dipyridamole and adenosine are contraindicated for patients with hypotension, bronchospasm, and advanced atrioventricular block; dobutamine is contraindicated for patients with hypertension, high-grade ventricular ectopy, uncontrolled atrial fibrillation/flutter, left ventricular outflow tract obstruction, and expanding aortic aneurysm. Published data support the safety of adenosine or dipyridamole in patients with lung disease in the absence of wheezing, and if peak flow rates on spirometry are normal before testing [6,7]. IV—intravenous.

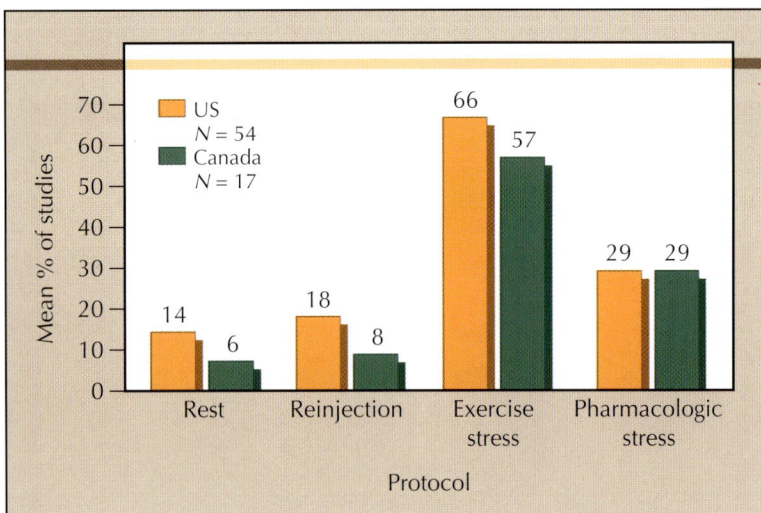

FIGURE 3-5. Myocardial perfusion imaging protocols used in the United States and Canada. Pharmacologic stress testing is performed in approximately 29% of all studies in both countries [2].

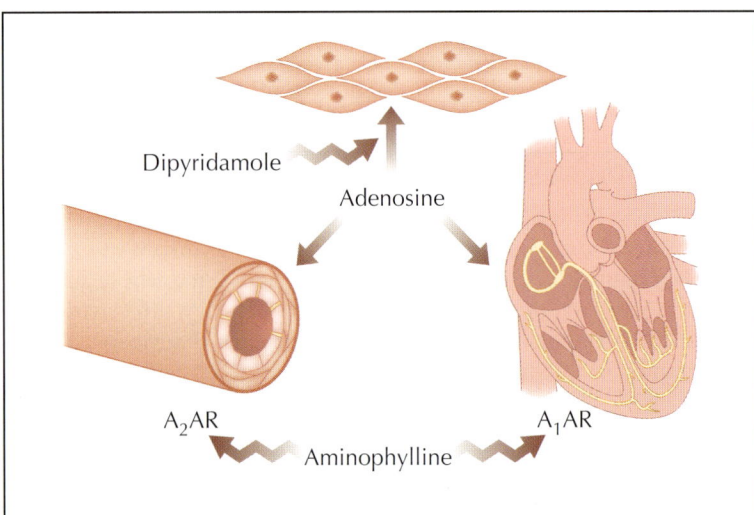

FIGURE 3-6. The direct and indirect action of adenosine and dipyridamole on vascular smooth muscle cells (A_2 receptors [A_2AR]) and on cardiac conduction cells (A_1 receptors [A_1AR]). The "antidote" that reverses the effects of dipyridamole or adenosine is aminophylline. Patient preparation for pharmacologic stress testing is similar to that for 12 to 24 hours for exercise stress, although all methylxanthines must be withheld before adenosine or dipyridamole testing [8]. β-Blockers should be withheld for 24 hours before dobutamine stress testing. With vasodilator SPECT imaging, the increased splanchnic activity mandates a delay in image acquisition for 30 to 60 minutes following the injection of a ^{99m}Tc agent [9,10].

Adenosine is a small, heterocyclic, endogenous compound produced by the endothelial cell. It activates A_2 receptors, causing vasodilatation via the production of adenyl cyclase and the subsequent local increase in cylic AMP. Theophylline and other methylxanthines, including caffeine, are competitive antagonists of adenosine, blocking their effects at the A_2 receptor. Adenosine enters endothelial and red blood cells by a facilitated transport mechanism. Intracellular adenosine is then deaminated or converted to other inactive metabolites. Selective A_2 receptor agonists, such as MRI-0470, CVT-3146, ATL-146e, and CGS-21680, induce coronary hyperemia with less systemic vasodilation and fewer side effects, including chest pain and atrioventricular block [11,12]. Stress testing with intravenous adenine triphosphate has also been successful.

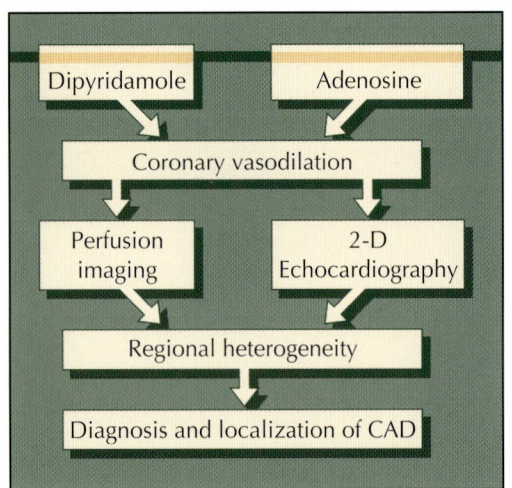

FIGURE 3-7. The effects of hyperemic stress with dipyridamole or adenosine on coronary vasodilation, establishing flow heterogeneity (usually in the absence of ischemia), leading to the diagnosis and localization of coronary artery disease (CAD). Adenosine and dipyridamole reduce coronary vascular resistance and increase blood flow three- to fivefold, to near maximal levels. Myocardial ischemia is not a prerequisite for the detection of obstructive CAD, because poststenotic flow disparities may be imaged in the setting of critical stenoses. Synthetic catecholamines such as dobutamine increase myocardial oxygen consumption by increasing heart rate and inotropy, thereby reproducing some of the physiology of exercise.

CHARACTERISTICS OF METHODS OF STRESS TESTING

	EXERCISE	DOBUTAMINE	DIPYRIDAMOLE	ADENOSINE
CBF increase	2–3X	2X	3–4X	3–5X
Ischemia provocation	Frequent	Common	Rare	Uncommon
Onset of effect	3–5 min	2–4 min	4–6 min	1–2 min
Duration after stopping	2–5 min	4–6 min	10–30 min	0.5–1 min
AV block occurrence	No	No	Rare	Common (transient)
Ventricular ectopy	Uncommon	Common	Rare	Rare

FIGURE 3-8. Characteristics of stress testing with regard to responses from exercise, dobutamine, dipyridamole, and adenosine. AV—atrioventricular; CBF—coronary blood flow.

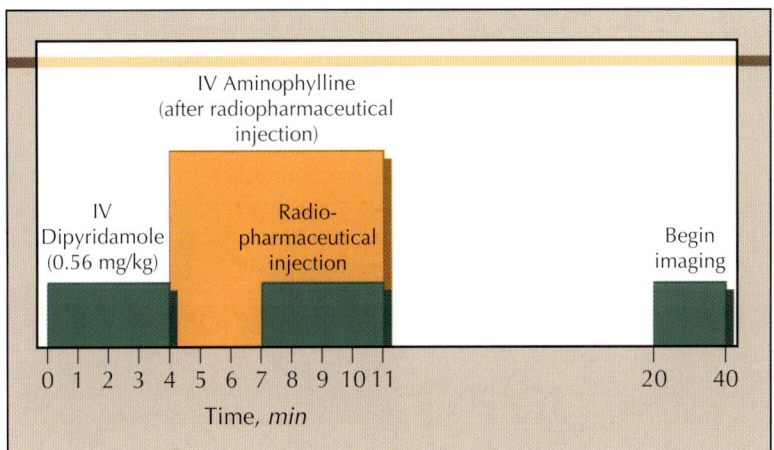

FIGURE 3-9. Intravenous dipyridamole myocardial perfusion imaging protocol. This timeline indicates that optimal injection of the radiopharmaceutical agent should occur 3 to 4 minutes after the completion of dipyridamole infusion. ^{99m}Tc-agent imaging is usually started 20 to 40 minutes thereafter. Aminophylline should be administered only after radiopharmaceutical injection. Dipyridamole, a purine base, acts indirectly by blocking transport of endogenous adenosine into cells, thereby increasing the local levels of adenosine to interact with the A_2 receptor. This agent is administered intravenously (IV) at a dose of 140 µg/kg/min for 6 minutes by an infusion pump or slow drip/push. The half-life of dipyridamole is 20 to 30 minutes.

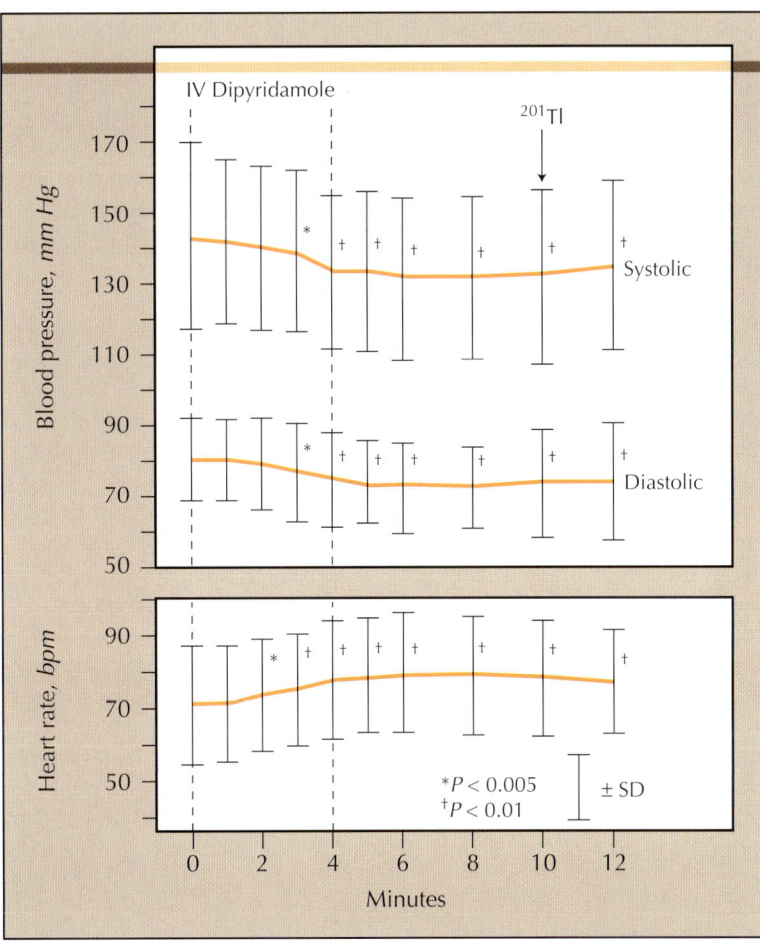

FIGURE 3-10. Hemodynamic responses to intravenous (IV) dipyridamole. The response usually entails a slight (10%–15%) decrease in blood pressure with compensatory (reflex) tachycardia. (*Adapted from* Homma *et al.* [11].)

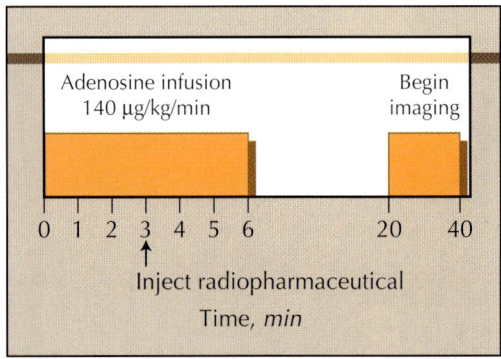

FIGURE 3-11. Adenosine infusion protocol. This timeline indicates that optimal injection of the radiopharmaceutical should occur at approximately 3 to 4 minutes after the onset of continuous pump infusion. The peak hyperemic effect is established by 3 minutes. ^{99m}Tc-agent imaging is started 20 to 40 minutes thereafter. Adenosine is administered in a dose of 140 µg/kg/min over 6 minutes, although protocols using infusion times of 3 to 4 minutes have been successful. Adenosine is administered by an infusion pump through a small caliber tube to avoid sudden bolus administration.

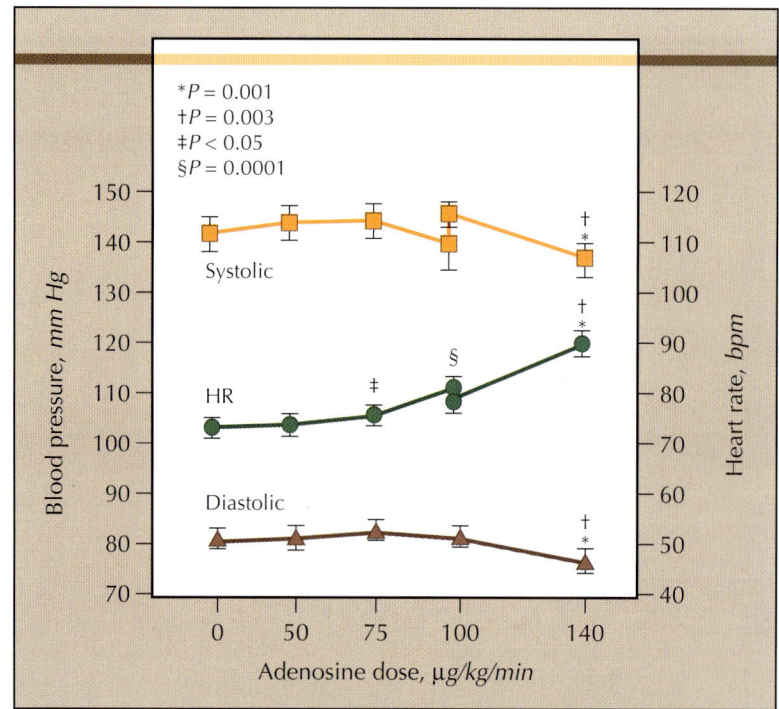

FIGURE 3-12. Peripheral hemodynamic responses to adenosine. Blood pressure decreases by 10% to 15% in a dose-dependent fashion during infusion, with compensatory (reflex) tachycardia. BPM—beats per minute; HR—heart rate. (*Adapted from* Verani *et al.* [12].)

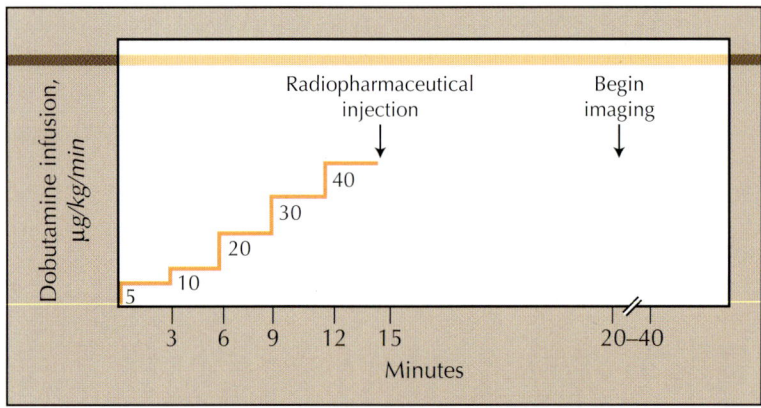

FIGURE 3-13. Intravenous (IV) dobutamine infusion protocol. Incremental doses of dobutamine are given at 3-minute intervals to a maximum of 50 µg/kg/min over 15 to 20 minutes. Radiopharmaceutical injection is performed at the peak of drug effect (measured by cardiac double product), with imaging initiated 20 to 40 minutes thereafter. Dobutamine, a synthetic catecholamine, produces a predominantly β-adrenergic effect, causing increased inotropy and relatively small changes in blood pressure. Atropine can be safely added to increase heart rate and to help reach the target heart rate in most patients. Side effects include frequent supraventricular and ventricular ectopy; ventricular tachycardia occurs in only 4% of patients [13]. These arrhythmias are successfully treated with termination of the infusion and the occasional use of an IV β-blocker (esmolol or metoprolol). Radiopharmaceutical (IV) injection should occur at the peak heart rate that should be maintained for at least one additional minute [14]. No deaths or myocardial infarctions attributable to dobutamine have occurred.

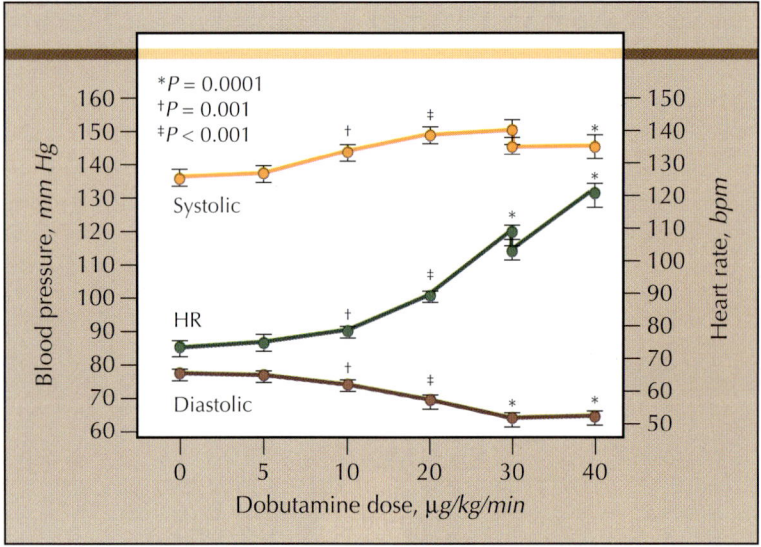

FIGURE 3-14. Peripheral hemodynamic responses to dobutamine. The responses entail a predictable increase in systolic blood pressure, widening of the pulse pressure, and a chronotropic impact on heart rate (HR), which may be augmented by atropine (0.4–0.6 mg intravenous bolus). ST segment alterations are predictive of significant coronary disease with exercise, but there is controversy regarding the diagnostic value of ST depression with pharmacologic stress testing [15]. ST depression is predictive of both scintigraphic evidence of myocardial ischemia and more severe coronary artery disease. Electrocardiographic changes are more common with dobutamine than with vasodilators, perhaps due to the increased cardiac workload (demand) [8]. With adenosine and dipyridamole, ST depression reflects coronary "steal," as collateral vessels are usually associated with adenosine- or dipyridamole-induced ST depression [16]. BPM—beats per minute. (*Adapted from* Hays *et al.* [14].)

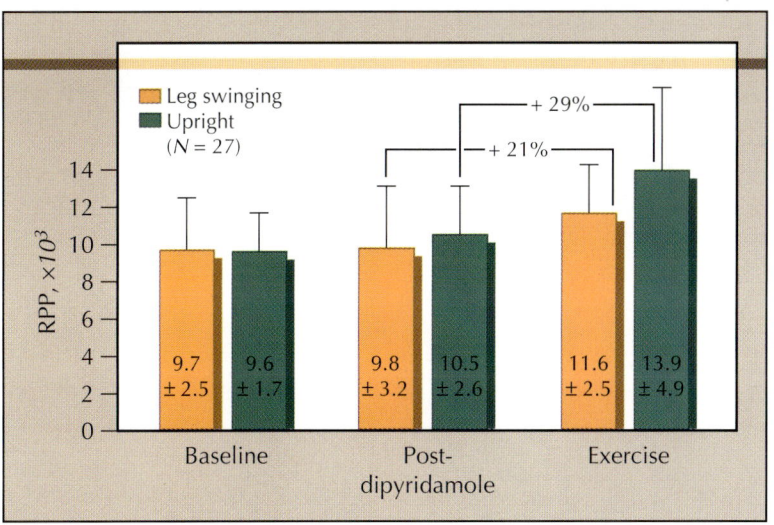

FIGURE 3-15. Impact of adjunctive leg swinging and upright submaximal treadmill walking on cardiac rate-pressure product (RPP) in patients receiving a dipyridamole infusion prior to exercise. Significant increases in RPP are observed with the addition of exercise following dipyridamole infusion in 27 patients, usually associated with fewer drug side effects and less gut tracer uptake on images. The use of low-level exercise has been shown to reduce subdiaphragmatic hepatic activity and improve target-to-background ratios for both adenosine and dipyridamole [17,18]. Additionally, adjunctive exercise reduces the occurrence and severity of noncardiac side effects, as well as the incidence of atrioventricular block. By enhancing cardiac work, it may also increase ischemia detection.

REPORTED SIDE EFFECTS OF INTRAVENOUS ADENOSINE AND DIPYRIDAMOLE IMAGING

	ADENOSINE, %	DIPYRIDAMOLE, %
Noncardiac		
Flushing	36.5	3.4
Dyspnea	35.2	2.6
Chest pain	34.6	19.7
Gastrointestinal distress	14.6	5.6
Headache	14.2	12.2
Dizziness	8.5	11.8
Cardiorespiratory		
AV block	7.6	0
ST-T wave changes	5.7	7.5
Arrhythmia	3.3	5.2*
Hypotension	1.8	4.6
Bronchospasm	0.1	0.15
Myocardial infarction	0.0001	0.05
Death	0†	0.05

*Ventricular arrhythmias.
†One subsequent death reported. All data are reported as percent of patients.

FIGURE 3-16. Side effect comparison between intravenous adenosine and dipyridamole imaging in multicenter studies for both noncardiac and cardiorespiratory events [7]. Adenosine side effects are common, predominantly flushing, nonspecific chest pain, dyspnea, headache, and nausea. Chest pain is not necessarily associated with the presence of coronary artery disease, because adenosine also stimulates the nociceptors. Caution is advised in patients with severe asthma or chronic obstructive pulmonary disease due to the direct bronchoconstrictive effect that may be precipitated by adenosine. First- and second-degree heart block occurs in up to 10% of patients, but is generally well tolerated and brief [19,20]. The safety of dipyridamole stress testing is well-documented [21,22]. The incidence of serious adverse events (death, myocardial infarction or cerebrovascular accident) was less than 0.02% in a series of more than 73,000 patients. Side effects are similar to adenosine; although less frequent, atrioventricular (AV) block is uncommon. Adverse effects generally last longer with dipyridamole, and more often require treatment. In a direct comparison, dipyridamole and adenosine had similar diagnostic accuracy, with a myocardial segmental concordance of 87% [23]. Adenosine provokes slightly more frequent myocardial ischemia during infusion. (*Adapted from* Miller and Labovitz [7].)

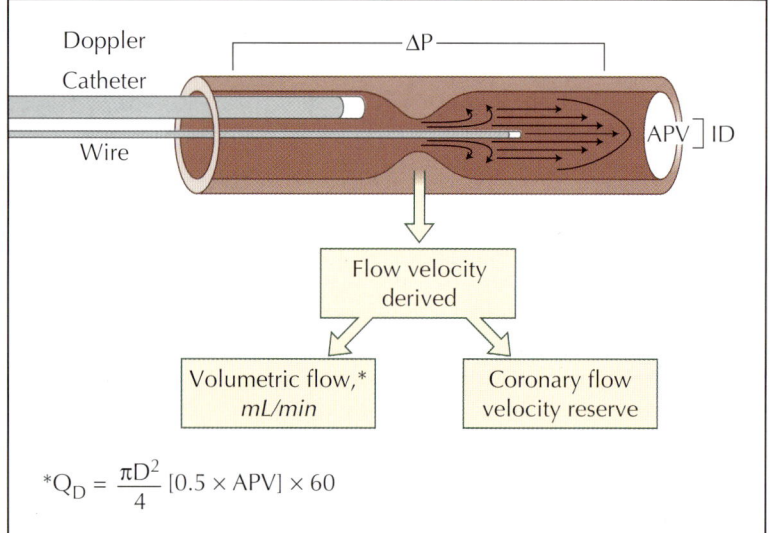

FIGURE 3-17. Schematic illustration of a Doppler flow wire crossing a coronary stenosis for measurement of average peak velocity (or pressure drop using a pressure wire). Flow velocity can be used to derive volumometric flow or coronary flow velocity reserve, which normally increases twofold or greater under the effects of hyperemic drug stress. This physiologic catheterization laboratory technique has been correlated with SPECT and PET imaging. APV—average peak velocity; ΔP—pressure drop.

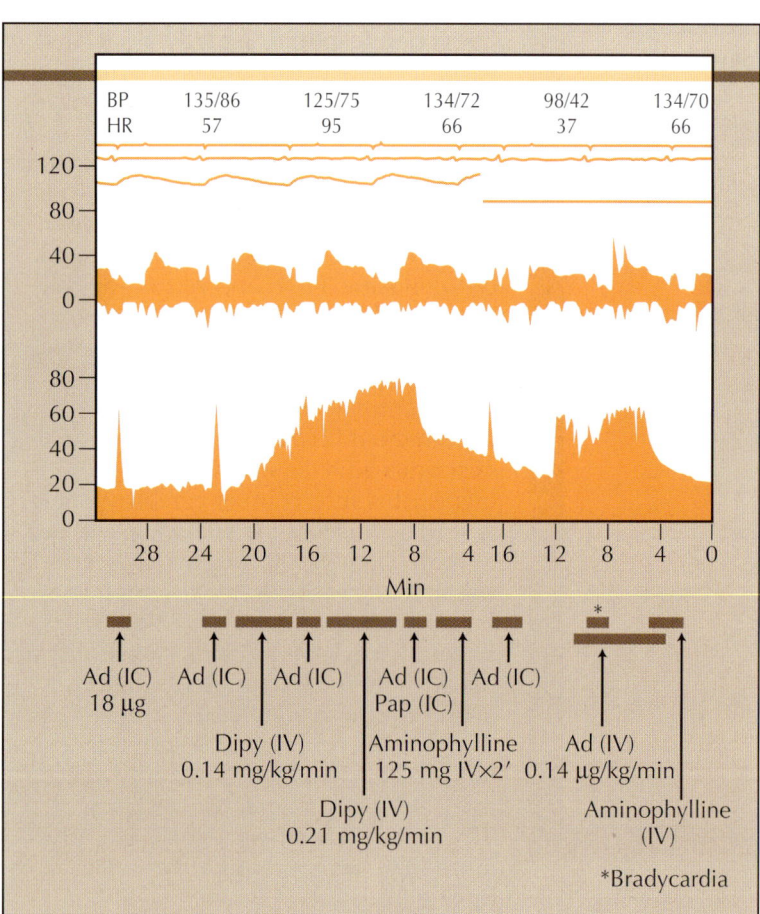

FIGURE 3-18. Typical continuous coronary Doppler flow wire tracing in a patient receiving a series of hyperemic agents, including intracoronary (IC) adenosine (Ad), intravenous (IV) dipyridamole (Dipy), IV Ad, and IC papaverine (Pap). Intracoronary drug boluses create a flow spike of immediate coronary hyperemia. IV dipyridamole creates a gradual increase in coronary flow velocity, which can gradually and serially be reversed by boluses of aminophylline. Peripheral blood pressure (BP) and heart rate (HR) are also recorded. Because the half-life of exogenous IV Ad is less than 2 seconds, hemodynamic changes and side effects usually resolve in less than one minute. Therefore, drug reversal treatment is rarely indicated, as effects subside with termination of the infusion. Aminophylline, a competitive antagonist (50–250 mg by IV push), reverses the effects of dipyridamole. Patients with lung disease are at increased risk for bronchoconstriction; vasodilator stress testing is contraindicated if active wheezing or respiratory failure is present. In patients with chronic obstructive pulmonary disease, routine reversal with IV aminophylline (50–250 mg IV push) may be appropriate.

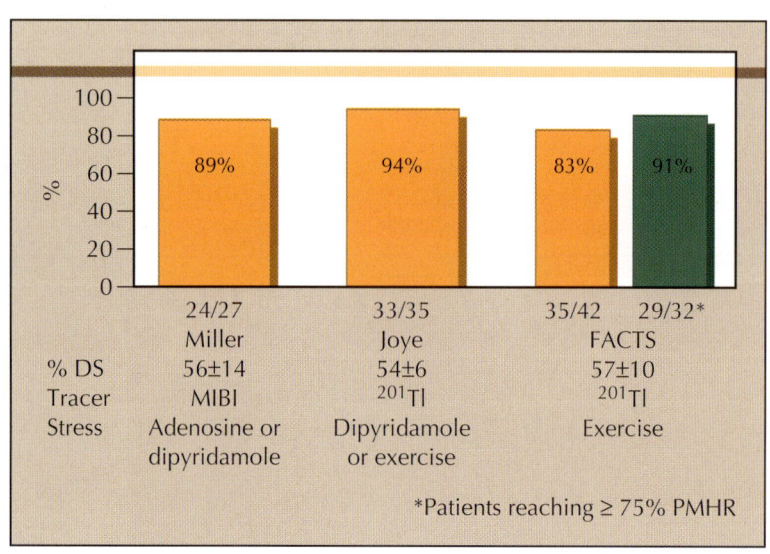

FIGURE 3-19. Comparison of coronary flow velocity reserve with SPECT myocardial perfusion imaging results in three studies. The overall segmental correlation between these two physiologic measurements of coronary stenosis severity is high, ranging from 83% to 94%. This relationship is preserved regardless of the type of tracer or stress used. DS—diameter stenosis; MIBI—sestamibi; PMHR—predicted maximum heart rate. (*Data from* Miller *et al.* [24], Joye *et al.* [25], and Heller *et al.* [26].)

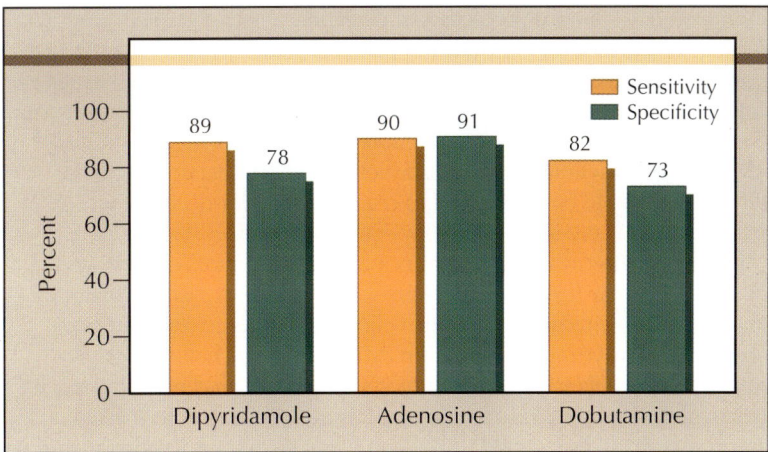

FIGURE 3-20. Cumulative test accuracy data from multiple studies of pharmacologic stress imaging using dipyridamole, adenosine, or dobutamine in combination with myocardial perfusion SPECT. Average sensitivity ranges from 82% to 90%, and specificity ranges from 73% to 91%. Drug stress provides comparable diagnostic value to exercise for the detection of coronary artery disease as well as superior accuracy to submaximal exercise testing. The diagnostic accuracy of drug stress imaging is high, irrespective of age or gender. Transient left ventricular cavity dilation or increased lung ^{201}Tl activity are markers of more severe or extensive coronary disease; these markers of disease burden also portend an increased risk for cardiac events. Adenosine, dipyridamole, and dobutamine have each been successfully employed in conjunction with all available myocardial perfusion tracers (^{201}Tl, ^{99m}Tc-sestamibi, ^{99m}Tc-tetrofosmin) [8]. Diagnostic accuracy may be slightly reduced with certain protocol combinations, such as dobutamine–^{99m}Tc-sestamibi [9] and dipyridamole–^{99m}Tc-tetrofosmin [10].

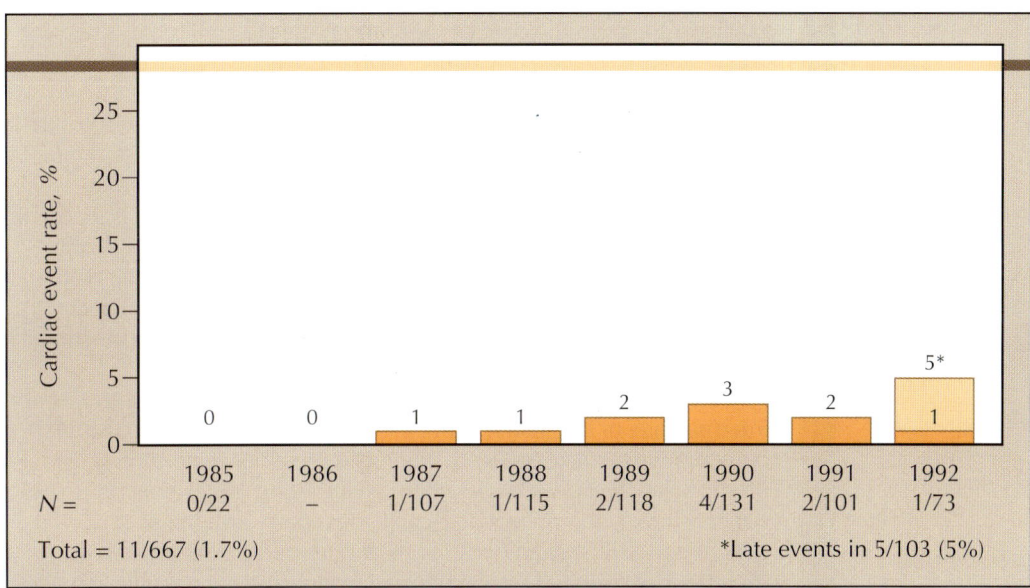

FIGURE 3-21. Prognostic value of preoperative peripheral vascular disease (PVD) assessment using dipyridamole–^{201}Tl imaging. In serial studies reported between 1985 and 1992 in patients with a normal scan, the cardiac event (death or myocardial infarction) rate ranges from 0 to 3% [27,28]. The overall average heart event rate in patients with PVD with a normal scan is 1.7%. Data regarding the excellent prognostic value of adenosine, dipyridamole, or dobutamine is widely reported [29]. Data have also demonstrated excellent risk stratification in patients who present with medically stabilized unstable angina [30], following an uncomplicated acute myocardial infarction [31–33], and for preoperative assessment in patients before vascular surgery or organ transplantation [34,35].

CARDIAC RISK STRATIFICATION*
FOR NONCARDIAC SURGICAL PROCEDURES

HIGH (CARDIAC RISK OFTEN > 5%)

Emergency major operations, particularly in the elderly
Aortic and other major vascular surgery
Peripheral vascular surgery
Anticipated prolonged surgical procedures associated with large fluid shifts and/or blood loss

INTERMEDIATE (CARDIAC RISK GENERALLY < 5%)

Carotid endarterectomy
Head and neck surgery
Intraperitoneal and intrathoracic surgery
Orthopedic surgery
Prostate surgery

LOW (CARDIAC RISK GENERALLY < 1%)

Endoscopic procedures
Superficial procedures
Cataract surgery
Breast surgery

*Combined incidence of cardiac death and nonfatal myocardial infarction.
†Patients do not generally require further preoperative cardiac testing.

FIGURE 3-22. The clinical role of cardiac imaging in evaluating patients prior to noncardiac surgery has been steadily expanding since 1985 [29,36], because both the number of procedures performed each year and the age and complexity of patients referred for surgery has increased. A careful history and physical examination are mandatory to assess whether pre-existing medical conditions exist, and to determine the likelihood of occult underlying cardiovascular disease [37–40]. The decision to perform surgery and the associated cardiovascular risk must also be placed in context of the urgency and type of the procedure to be performed. This is particularly true for vascular surgery [41–50], where there is a high (30%–50%) prevalence of underlying coronary artery disease. In other procedures associated with large fluid shifts and/or blood loss that can lead to hemodynamic instability, event risk is also high. In emergency surgery for a life-threatening condition when preoperative risk stratification is not possible, perioperative medical management and careful monitoring for cardiac complications is essential [51]. In patients referred for less urgent or elective procedures, complete risk evaluation can be based on clinical variables and the results of noninvasive testing. Comparisons of stress imaging data to left ventricular function assessments, at rest or with stress, have also been performed [52–55]. (*Adapted from* Eagle *et al.* [1].)

CLINICAL PREDICTORS OF PERIOPERATIVE EVENTS

MAJOR

Unstable coronary syndromes
  Recent MI* with evidence of important ischemic risks by clinical symptoms or noninvasive study
  Unstable or severe† angina (Canadian class III or IV)
Decompensated congestive heart failure
Significant arrhythmias
  High-grade AV block
  Symptomatic ventricular arrhythmias in the presence of underlying heart disease
  Supraventricular arrhythmias with uncontrolled ventricular rate
Severe valvular disease

INTERMEDIATE

Mild angina pectoris (Canadian class I or II)
Prior MI by history of pathologic Q waves
Compensated or prior congestive heart failure
Diabetes mellitus

MINOR

Advanced age
Abnormal ECG (LV hypertrophy, LBBB, ST-T abnormalities)
Rhythm other than sinus (*eg*, atrial fibrillation)
Low functional capacity (*eg*, inability to climb one flight of stairs with a bag of groceries)
History of stroke
Uncontrolled systemic hypertension

*Recent is defined as more than 7 days but less than or equal to 30 days.
†May include stable angina in unusually sedentary patients.

FIGURE 3-23. Clinical predictors of perioperative events. The American College of Cardiology/American Heart Association (ACC/AHA) Task Force has published and updated practice guidelines for perioperative cardiovascular evaluation prior to noncardiac surgery [1]. These recommendations embody expert and evidence-based considerations, and identify specific clinical markers, patient functional capacity, and the type of surgery to be performed as crucial factors for deciding which patients need more intensive preoperative evaluation.

The major, intermediate, and minor clinical predictors of increased perioperative cardiovascular risk are summarized. A medical history and physical examination can elicit clinical risk predictors including angina, prior myocardial infarction (MI), congestive heart failure, arrhythmias, diabetes, peripheral vascular disease, and prior coronary revascularization procedures. Asymptomatic patients with known coronary artery disease who have had coronary revascularization within the past 5 years require no further evaluation. Surgery can also proceed in patients with coronary artery disease when the results of a recent cardiac catheterization or stress test reflect clinical stability.

In patients who have any of the recognized major clinical predictors of risk, a full cardiac work-up is warranted prior to surgery. The appropriate assessment would include coronary angiography, echocardiography to assess left ventricular (LV) ejection function and valvular abnormalities, or noninvasive stress imaging to detect myocardial ischemia. In the intermediate-risk category, the functional capacity of the patient and the type of surgical procedure determine whether further testing is indicated. Cardiac testing is necessary in intermediate-risk patients with a functional capacity of fewer than 4 METs (metabolic equivalents of the task) and those with moderate or excellent functional capacity who are undergoing a high-risk surgical procedure.

Patients with good functional capacity who are undergoing an intermediate- or low-risk surgical procedure do not generally require preoperative cardiac testing. In patients with minor or no clinical risk predictors, surgery can be performed without further evaluation unless patients have poor functional capacity or surgery is high risk.

Although functional capacity is an important determinant of risk, exercise stress testing (with or without imaging) is not possible in many patients who require further preoperative evaluation. Elderly or obese patients, those with prior MI, congestive heart failure, or pulmonary disease, and patients referred for peripheral vascular, orthopedic, and neurologic procedures may not be able to exercise adequately. In this setting, pharmacologic stress myocardial perfusion imaging is the preferred method of preoperative screening. AV—atrioventricular; LBBB—left bundle branch block. (*Adapted from* Eagle *et al.* [1].)

DIPYRIDAMOLE–^{201}Tl IMAGING FOR PREOPERATIVE ASSESSMENT OF CARDIAC RISK

STUDY	N	PATIENTS WITH ISCHEMIA BY ^{201}TL–RD, N (%)	MI/DEATH, N (%)	PERIOPERATIVE EVENTS	
				RD SCAN POSITIVE PREDICTIVE VALUE, % (N)	NORMAL SCAN NEGATIVE PREDICTIVE VALUE, % (N)
VASCULAR SURGERY					
Boucher et al. [36]	48	16 (33)	3 (6)	19 (3/160)	100 (32/32)
Cutler and Leppo [50]	116	54 (47)	11 (10)	20 (11/54)	100 (60/60)
Fletcher et al. [56]	67	15 (22)	3 (4)	20 (3/15)	100 (56/56)
Sachs et al. [57]	46	14 (31)	2 (4)	14 (2/14)	100 (24/24)
Eagle et al. [38]	200	82 (41)	15 (8)	16 (13/82)	98 (61/62)
McEnroe et al. [53]	95	34 (36)	7 (7)	9 (3/34)	96 (44/46)
Younis et al. [58]	111	40 (36)	8 (7)	15 (6/40)	100 (51/51)
Mangano et al. [51]	60	22 (37)	3 (5)	5 (1/22)	95 (19/20)
Strawn and Guernsey [59]	68	NA	4 (6)	NA	100 (21/21)
Watters et al. [55]	26	15 (58)	3 (12)	20 (3/15)	100 (11/11)
Hendel et al. [41]	327	167 (51)	28 (9)	14 (23/167)	99 (97/98)
Lette et al. [46]	355	161 (45)	30 (8)	17 (28/161)	99 (160/162)
Madsen et al. [40]	65	45 (69)	5 (8)	11 (5/45)	100 (20/20)
Brown and Rowen [27]	231	77 (33)	12 (5)	13 (10/77)	99 (120/121)
Kresowik et al. [43]	170	67 (39)	5 (3)	4 (3/67)	98 (64/65)
Baron et al. [52]	457	160 (35)	22 (5)	4 (7/160)	96 (195/203)*
Bry et al. [48]	237	110 (46)	17 (7)	11 (12/110)	100 (97/97)
Total	2679	107 (41)	178 (6.6)	12 (33/1079)	99 (1132/1149)
NONVASCULAR SURGERY					
Camp et al. [34]	40	9 (23)	6 (15)	67 (6/9)	100 (23/23)
Iqbal et al. [35]	31	11 (41)	3 (11)	27 (3/11)	100 (20/20)
Coley et al. [49]	100	36 (36)	4 (4)	8 (3/36)	98 (63/64)
Shaw et al. [60]	60	28 (47)	6 (10)	21 (6/28)	100 (19/19)
Takase et al. [54]	53	15 (28)	6 (11)	27 (4/15)	100 (32/32)
Younis et al. [61]	161	50 (31)	15 (9)	18 (9/50)	98 (87/89)
Total	445	149 (33)	40 (9)	21 (31/149)	99 (244/247)

*Nonfatal MI only.
†Studies utilizing pharmacologic and/or exercise ^{201}Tl testing.
All studies except those by Coley et al. [49] acquired patient information prospectively. Only in reports by Mangano et al. [51] and Baron et al. [52] were scan results blinded from attending physicians.
Patients with fixed defects were omitted from calculation of positive and negative predictive value.

FIGURE 3-24. Dipyridamole–^{201}Tl imaging for preoperative assessment of cardiac risk. Dipyridamole–^{201}Tl myocardial scintigraphy has been used extensively as a noninvasive approach to assess perioperative cardiac risk in patients prior to vascular and nonvascular surgery [55,56,58,59,61,62]. Dipyridamole–^{99m}Tc-sestamibi scintigraphy for preoperative risk stratification has also been evaluated [63,64]. Patients with a normal ^{201}Tl or sestamibi myocardial perfusion study are at very low likelihood for peri- or postoperative cardiac events. Events (including death and nonfatal myocardial infarction [MI]) occur in approximately 20% of patients with scintigraphic evidence of ischemia. Patients with fixed perfusion defects are at lower risk for perioperative cardiac events, but their long-term prognosis is similar to that in patients with chronic coronary artery disease with myocardial ischemia. Although drug-induced myocardial hypoperfusion or ischemia predicts a high risk for cardiac events, approximately 80% of patients survive the surgical procedure without complications (ie, low positive predictive value). Risk stratification may be improved by identifying not only the presence but also the extent of myocardial ischemia. Patients with multiple ischemic defects in several vascular beds are at higher risk than those with a single ischemic segment. Quantitative SPECT imaging permits the determination of the percent and location of ischemic myocardium.

Continued on next page

FIGURE 3-24. *(Continued)* Of 231 patients undergoing noncardiac surgery who had dipyridamole studies with 1 month of operation [27], the number of segments with ^{201}Tl redistribution (RD) was the best predictor of perioperative cardiac death or nonfatal MI ($P = 0.0001$), although a history of diabetes mellitus was also predictive in this study ($P = 0.006$). When dipyridamole perfusion scintigraphy was performed in 66 consecutive patients undergoing predominantly vascular surgeries, only 9% of patients with a "small" ischemic defect had a cardiac event compared with 80% of patients with more extensive ischemia. Levinson *et al.* [47] reported a significantly higher cardiac event rate in patients with ^{201}Tl redistribution in four or more segments (38%) compared with those with less extensive ischemia (12%).

The optimal approach for identifying risk in surgical candidates should integrate clinical and imaging variables. In 200 patients undergoing major vascular surgery [37], clinical and imaging parameters were evaluated to optimize risk stratification in patient subsets. Logistic regression analysis identified five clinical predictors of cardiac event risk: electrocardiographic Q waves; ventricular ectopic activity; diabetes; age over 70 years; and a history of angina. The presence of ^{201}Tl redistribution was also found to be a significant risk predictor. In the 64 patients who had no clinical predictors, only 3.1% had ischemic events, with no deaths. Most of these patients also had no scintigraphic evidence of ischemia, and therefore would have been classified as low risk by imaging. Conversely, 50% of patients with more than three clinical risk factors had cardiac events, and scintigraphic ischemia involving multiple vascular territories was frequent in this subgroup. The majority of patients had one or two clinical variables (68%); of these, 15.5% had a postoperative event, defining a large group at intermediate clinical risk. Without dipyridamole–^{201}Tl redistribution, 3.2% had a subsequent cardiac event compared with 30% with defect redistribution.

Among younger patients without a prior cardiovascular history, clinical criteria can effectively define a low-risk group, and stress imaging is generally not warranted [1]. In patients with multiple cardiac risk factors, imaging is useful as a guide to coronary revascularization prior to surgery. In heterogeneous clinical populations with variable risk, drug stress perfusion imaging is valuable for defining patients most likely to have cardiac events based on the presence and extent of myocardial ischemia.

Despite the increased use of adenosine and dobutamine as pharmacologic stressors [28,29,42,60,62,65], less data are available for these agents in preoperative risk stratification than for dipyridamole. When adenosine–^{201}Tl tomography was used as a preoperative screening test in patients referred for vascular orthopedic or general surgery, patients with defect redistribution had a 25% event rate, whereas no events occurred in patients without myocardial ischemia [60].

Adenosine–^{201}Tl tomography, when performed in 106 patients undergoing vascular surgery, was abnormal in 54% of patients, of whom 82% demonstrated defect ischemia [42]. Eleven percent of the patients with scintigraphic ischemia had an event, but none of the patients without ischemia had an event. By quantitative analysis, the size of the total and reversible perfusion defects was larger in patients with events compared with those without perfusion defects.

In 126 patients awaiting vascular surgery, dobutamine was administered in doses up to 20 µg/kg/min, with atropine given to 47 patients to further increase heart rate [62]. Sixty-seven percent had either a normal ^{201}Tl SPECT or only a fixed defect, with cardiac event rates of 1.8% and 11%, respectively. In the 42 patients who demonstrated ^{201}Tl defect redistribution, 15 operations were canceled, 9 underwent coronary revascularization, and 18 proceeded with their vascular procedures. Nine of the 18 patients who did not undergo revascularization with scintigraphic ischemia (50%) had a postoperative cardiac event.

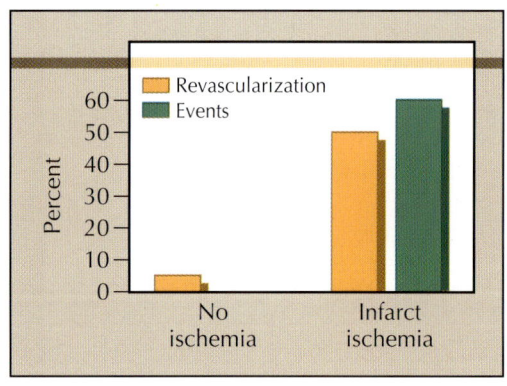

FIGURE 3-25. Predictive accuracy of early post-myocardial infarction imaging with dipyridamole-^{201}Tl. The presence of infarct zone ischemia is predictive of a higher rate of coronary revascularization and other cardiac events. In the absence of ischemia, revascularization and cardiac events are very low. Imaging in this multicenter study was safely performed 2 to 4 days following uncomplicated myocardial infarction (MI). Pharmacologic testing is useful for identifying both early and late risk for cardiac events. For example, data demonstrate that early (2 to 4 days) dipyridamole sestamibi perfusion imaging after an uncomplicated MI is a safe and powerful predictor of future cardiac death and recurrent MI [28], and offers incremental prognostic value to that of submaximal exercise testing. (*Adapted from* Brown *et al.* [66].)

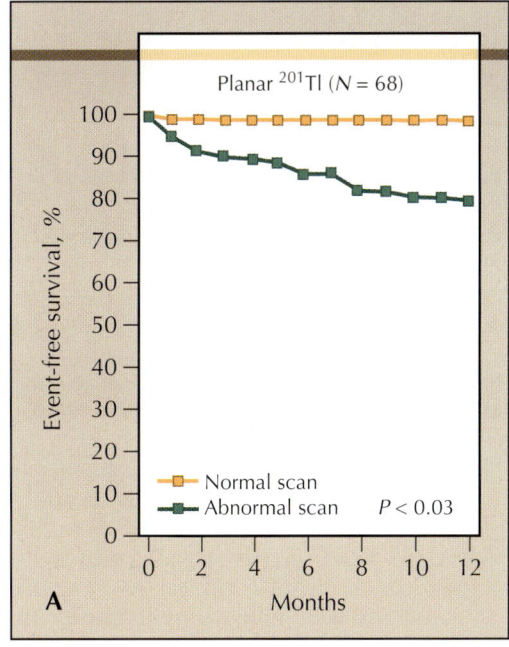
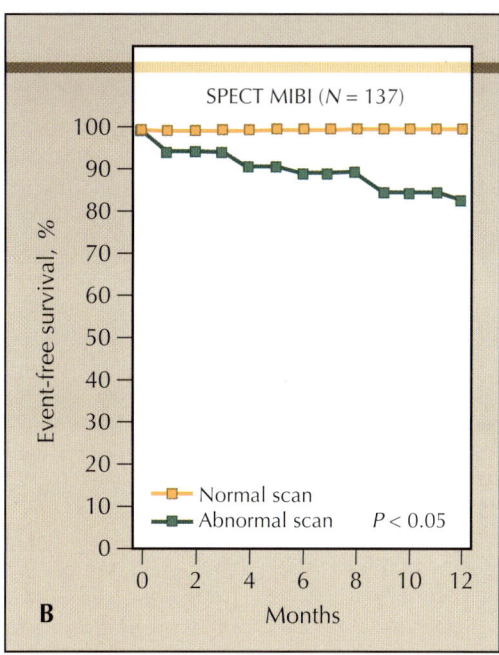

FIGURE 3-26. Prognostic value of predischarge dipyridamole stress myocardial imaging for predicting cardiac death or myocardial infarction (MI), in combination with (**A**) planar ^{201}Tl ($N = 68$) or (**B**) SPECT sestamibi (MIBI) ($N = 137$), in patients with a medically stabilized recent ischemic event (MI or unstable angina). Both techniques identify a low-risk subset with a normal scan and few cardiac events over 1 year following the acute ischemic event. The event rate in patients with an abnormal scan is significantly higher, regardless of the imaging technique. In patients with unstable angina, the very low mortality rate associated with a normal scan supports a conservative medical management approach [32,53]. (*Panel A adapted from* Younis *et al.* [67]; *panel B adapted from* Miller *et al.* [33].)

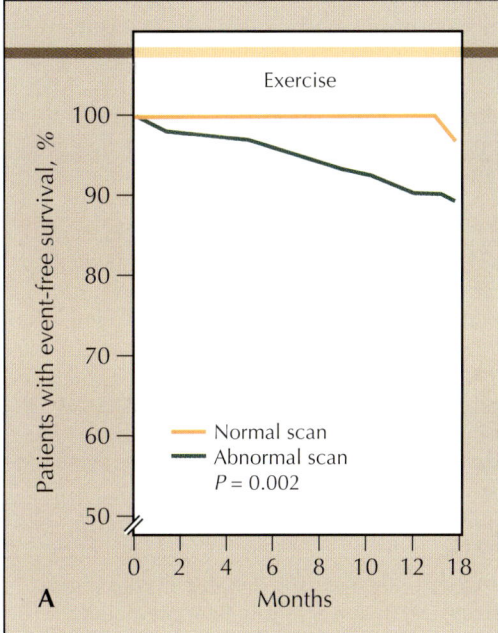
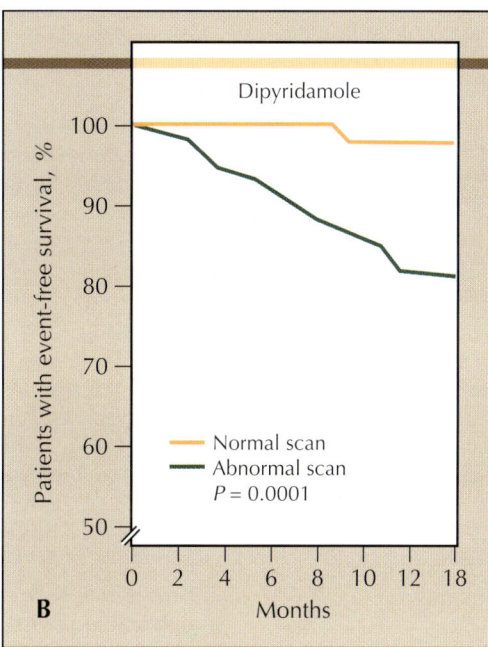

FIGURE 3-27. Prognostic value of ^{99m}Tc-sestamibi imaging in patients with stable chest pain, comparing exercise testing (**A**) with dipyridamole testing (**B**) in similar populations. A normal scan is associated with a low 18-month cardiac event rate and good cardiac event-free survival, regardless of the stress approach utilized. Significantly higher cardiac event rates and poorer cardiac event-free survival occur in the presence of an abnormal scan in stable chest pain patients [68,69]. (*Panel A adapted from* Stratmann *et al.* [68]; *panel B adapted from* Stratmann *et al.* [70].)

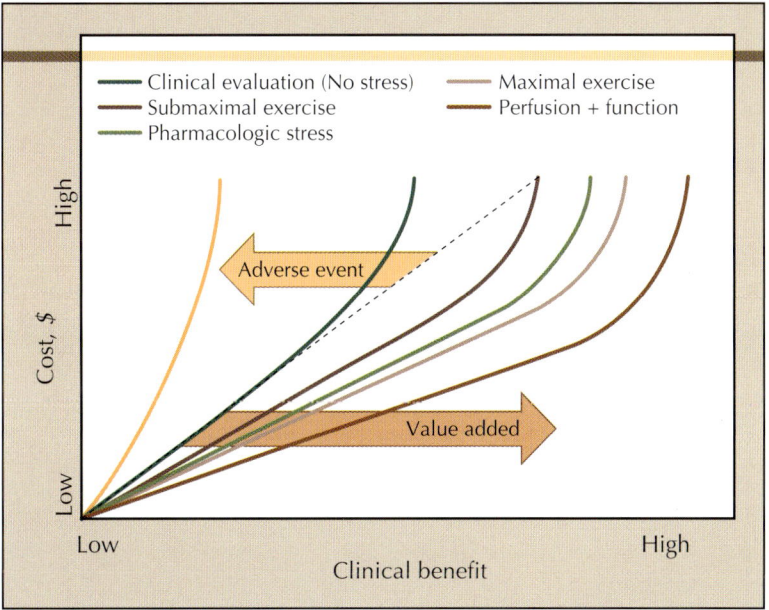

FIGURE 3-28. Relationship between cost and clinical benefit (incremental diagnostic or prognostic data derived) for various stress imaging techniques to evaluate coronary artery disease. Value is added to a baseline level of clinical benefit (incremental value in proportion to incremental cost) when submaximal exercise, pharmacologic stress, maximal exercise, and perfusion plus function imaging are utilized. An adverse event during testing can reduce the clinical benefit and significantly accelerate the incremental cost of patient care [71].

REFERENCES

1. Eagle KA, Brundage BH, Chaitman BR, *et al.*: Report of the American College of Cardiology/American Heart Association Task Force on Practice Guidelines (Committee on Perioperative Cardiovascular Evaluation for Noncardiac Surgery). *J Am Coll Cardiol* 1996, 27:910–948.

2. Miller DD, Keiss M, Freeman M, Taillefer R: Northern exposure: nuclear cardiology in the Canadian Health System. *J Nucl Cardiol* 1995, 2:53–61.

3. Samuels B, Kiat H, Friedman JD, Berman DS: Adenosine pharmacologic stress myocardial perfusion tomographic imaging in patients with significant aortic stenosis. Diagnostic efficacy and comparison of clinical, hemodynamic and electrocardiographic variables with 100 age-matched control subjects. *J Am Coll Cardiol* 1995, 25:99–106.

4. O'Keefe JH Jr, Bateman TM, Barnhart CS: Adenosine thallium-201 is superior to exercise thallium-201 for detecting coronary artery disease in patients with left bundle branch block. *J Am Coll Cardiol* 1993, 21:1332–1338.

5. Wagdy HM, Hodge D, Christian TF, *et al.*: Prognostic value of vasodilator perfusion imaging in patients with left bundle-branch block. *Circulation* 1998, 97:1563–1570.

6. Shaffer J, Simbartl L, Render ML, *et al.*: Patients with stable chronic obstructive pulmonary disease can safely undergo intravenous dipyridamole thallium-201 imaging. *Am Heart J* 1998, 36:307–313.

7. Miller DD, Labovitz AJ: Dipyridamole and adenosine vasodilator stress for myocardial imaging: vive la difference! *J Am Coll Cardiol* 1994, 23:390–392.

8. Pennell DJ, Ell PJ: Whole-body imaging of thallium-201 after six different stress regimens. *J Nucl Med* 1994, 35:425–428.

9. Wu JC, Yuyn JJ, Heller EN, *et al.*: Limitations of dobutamine for enhancing flow heterogeneity in the presence of single coronary artery stenosis: implications for technetium-99m-sestamibi imaging. *J Nucl Med* 1998, 39:417–425.

10. Levine MG, Ahlberg A, Mann A, *et al.*: Comparison of exercise, dipyridamole, adenosine, and dobutamine stress with the use of Tc-99m tetrofosmin tomographic imaging. *J Nucl Cardiol* 1999, 6:389–396.

11. Homma S, Gilliland Y, Guiney TE, *et al.*: Safety of intravenous dipyridamole for stress testing with thallium imaging. *Am J Cardiol* 1987, 59:152–154.

12. Verani MS, Mahmarian JJ, Hixson JB, *et al.*: Diagnosis of coronary artery disease by controlled coronary vasodilation with adenosine and thallium-201 scintigraphy in patients unable to exercise. *Circulation* 1990, 82:80–87.

13. Elhendy A, Valkema R, van Domburg RT, *et al.*: Safety of dobutamine-atropine stress myocardial perfusion scintigraphy. *J Nucl Med* 1998, 39:1662–1669.

14. Hays JT, Mahmarian JJ, Cochran AJ, Verani MS: Dobutamine thallium-201 tomography for evaluating patients with suspected coronary artery disease unable to undergo exercise or vasodilatory pharmacologic stress testing. *J Am Coll Cardiol* 1993, 21:1583–1590.

15. Marshall ES, Raichlen JS, Tighe DA, *et al.*: ST-segment depression during adenosine infusion as a predictor of myocardial ischemia. *Am Heart J* 1994, 127:305–311.

16. Nishimura S, Mahmarian JJ, Boyce TM, Verani MS: Equivalence between adenosine and exercise thallium-201 myocardial tomography: a multicenter, prospective, crossover trial. *J Am Coll Cardiol* 1992, 20:265–275.

17. Samady H, Wackers FJ, Joska TM, *et al.*: Pharmacologic stress perfusion imaging with adenosine: role of simultaneous low-level treadmill exercise. *J Am Coll Cardiol* 2002, 9:188–196.

18. Jamil G, Ahlberg A, Elliott MD, *et al.*: Impact of limited treadmill exercise on adenosine Tc-99m sestamibi single-photon emission computed tomographic myocardial perfusion imaging in coronary artery disease. *Am J Cardiol* 1999, 84:400–403.

19. Alkoutami GS, Reeves WC, Movahed A: The safety of adenosine pharmacologic stress testing in patients with first-degree atrioventricular block in the presence and absence of atrioventricular blocking medications. *J Nucl Cardiol* 1999, 6:495–497.

20. Cerqueira MD, Verani MS, Schwaiger M, *et al.*: Safety profile of adenosine stress perfusion imaging: results from the Adenoscan Multicenter Trial Registry. *J Am Coll Cardiol* 1994, 23:384–389.

21. Lette J, Waters D, Bernier H, *et al.*: Preoperative and long-term cardiac risk assessment: predictive value of 23 clinical descriptors, 7 multivariate scoring systems, and quantitative dipyridamole imaging in 360 patients. *Ann Surg* 1992, 216:192–204.

22. Ranhosky A, Kempthorne-Rawson J: The safety of intravenous dipyridamole thallium myocardial perfusion imaging. Intravenous Dipyridamole Thallium Imaging Study Group. *Circulation* 1990, 81:1205–1209.

23. Taillefer R, Amyot R, Turpin S, *et al.*: Comparison between dipyridamole and adenosine as pharmacologic coronary vasodilators in detection of coronary artery disease with thallium 201 imaging. *J Nucl Cardiol* 1996, 3:204–211.

24. Miller DD, Donohue TJ, Younis LT, *et al.*: Correlation of pharmacological 99mTc-sestamibi myocardial perfusion imaging with poststenotic coronary flow reserve in patients with angiographically intermediate coronary artery stenoses. *Circulation* 1994, 89:2150–2160.

25. Joye JD, Schulman DS, Lasorda D, *et al.*: Intracoronary Doppler guide wire versus stress single-photon emission computed tomographic thallium-201 imaging in assessment of intermediate coronary stenoses. *J Am Coll Cardiol* 1994, 24:940–947.

26. Heller LI, Popma J, Cates C, *et al.*: Functional assessment of stenosis in the cath lab: a comparison of Doppler and Tl-201 imaging. *J Interv Cardiol* 1995, 7:23A.

27. Brown KA, Rowen M: Extent of jeopardized viable myocardium determined by myocardial perfusion imaging best predicts perioperative cardiac events in patients undergoing noncardiac surgery. *J Am Coll Cardiol* 1993, 21:325–330.

28. Hachamovitch R, Berman DS, Kiat H, *et al.*: Incremental prognostic value of adenosine stress myocardial perfusion single-photon emission computed tomography and impact on subsequent management in patients with or suspect of having myocardial ischemia. *Am J Cardiol* 1997, 80:426–433.

29. Shaw LJ, Eagle KA, Gersh BJ, Miller DD: Meta-analysis of intravenous dipyridamole-thallium-201 imaging (1985 to 1994) and dobutamine echocardiography (1991 to 1994) for risk stratification before vascular surgery. *J Am Coll Cardiol* 1996, 27:787–798.

30. Stratmann HG, Tamesis BR, Younis LT, *et al.*: Prognostic value of predischarge dipyridamole technetium 99m sestamibi myocardial tomography in medically treated patients with unstable angina. *Am Heart J* 1995, 130:734–740.

31. Brown KA, Heller GV, Landin RS, *et al.*: Early dipyridamole Tc-99m sestamibi single photon emission computed tomographic imaging 2 to 4 days after acute myocardial infarction predicts in-hospital and postdischarge cardiac events: comparison with submaximal exercise. *Circulation* 1999, 100:2060–2066.

32. Mahmarian JJ, Mahmarian AC, Marks GF, et al.: Role of adenosine thallium-201 tomography for defining long-term risk in patients after acute myocardial infarction. *J Am Coll Cardiol* 1995, 25:1333–1340.

33. Miller DD, Stratmann HG, Shaw LJ, et al.: Dipyridamole technetium 99m sestamibi myocardial tomography as an independent predictor of cardiac event-free survival after acute ischemic events. *J Nucl Cardiol* 1994, 1:72–82.

34. Camp AD, Garvin PJ, Hoff J, et al.: Prognostic value of intravenous dipyridamole thallium imaging in patients with diabetes mellitus considered for renal transplantation. *Am J Cardiol* 1990, 65:1459–1463.

35. Iqbal A, Gibbons RJ, McGoon MD, et al.: Noninvasive assessment of cardiac risk in insulin-dependent diabetic patients being evaluated for pancreatic transplantation using thallium-201 myocardial perfusion scintigraphy. *Transplant Proc* 1991, 23(pt 2):1690–1691.

36. Boucher CA, Brewster DC, Darling RC, et al.: Determination of cardiac risk by dipyridamole-thallium imaging before peripheral vascular surgery. *N Engl J Med* 1985, 312:389–394.

37. Eagle KA, Singer DE, Brewster DC, et al.: Dipyridamole-thallium scanning in patients undergoing vascular surgery: optimizing preoperative evaluation of cardiac risk. *JAMA* 1987, 257:2185–2189.

38. Eagle KA, Coley CM, Newell JB, et al.: Combining clinical and thallium data optimizes preoperative assessment of cardiac risk before major vascular surgery. *Ann Intern Med* 1989, 110:859–866.

39. Lette J, Waters D, Bernier H, et al.: Preoperative and long-term cardiac risk assessment: predictive value of 23 clinical descriptors, 7 multivariate scoring systems, and quantitative dipyridamole imaging in 360 patients. *Ann Surg* 1992, 216:192–204.

40. Madsen PV, Vissing M, Munck O, Kelbaek H: A comparison of dipyridamole thallium 201 scintigraphy and clinical examination in the determination of cardiac risk before arterial reconstruction. *Angiology* 1992, 43:306–311.

41. Hendel RC, Whitfield SS, Villegas BJ, et al.: Prediction of late cardiac events by dipyridamole thallium imaging in patients undergoing elective vascular surgery. *Am J Cardiol* 1992, 70:1243–1249.

42. Koutelou MG, Asimacopoulos PJ, Mahmarian JJ, et al.: Preoperative risk stratification by adenosine thallium-201 single-photon emission computed tomography in patients undergoing vascular surgery. *J Nucl Cardiol* 1995, 2:389–394.

43. Kresowik TF, Bower TR, Garner SA, et al.: Dipyridamole thallium imaging in patients being considered for vascular procedures. *Arch Surg* 1993, 128:299–302.

44. Lane SE, Lewis SM, Pippin JJ, et al.: Predictive value of quantitative dipyridamole-thallium scintigraphy in assessing cardiovascular risk after vascular surgery in diabetes mellitus. *Am J Cardiol* 1989, 64:1275–1279.

45. Leppo JA, Plaja J, Gionet M, et al.: Noninvasive evaluation of cardiac risk before elective vascular surgery. *J Am Coll Cardiol* 1987, 9:269–276.

46. Lette J, Walters D, Cerino M, et al.: Preoperative coronary artery disease risk stratification based on dipyridamole imaging and a simple three-step, three-segment model for patients undergoing noncardiac vascular surgery or major general surgery. *Am J Cardiol* 1992, 69:1553–1558.

47. Levinson JR, Boucher CA, Coley CM, et al.: Usefulness of semiquantitative analysis of dipyridamole-thallium-201 redistribution for improving risk stratification before vascular surgery. *Am J Cardiol* 1990, 66:406–410.

48. Bry JD, Belkin M, O'Donnell TF Jr, et al.: An assessment of the positive predictive value and cost-effectiveness of dipyridamole myocardial scintigraphy in patients undergoing vascular surgery. *J Vasc Surg* 1994, 19:112–121.

49. Coley CM, Field TS, Abraham SA, et al.: Usefulness of dipyridamole-thallium scanning for preoperative evaluation of cardiac risk for nonvascular surgery. *Am J Cardiol* 1992, 69:1280–1285.

50. Cutler BS, Leppo JA: Dipyridamole thallium-201 scintigraphy to detect coronary artery disease before abdominal aortic surgery. *J Vasc Surg* 1987, 5:91–100.

51. Mangano DT, London MJ, Tubau JF, et al.: Dipyridamole thallium-201 scintigraphy as a preoperative screening test: a reexamination of its predictive potential. Study of Perioperative Ischemia Research Group. *Circulation* 1991, 84:493–502.

52. Baron JF, Mundler O, Bertrand M, et al.: Dipyridamole-thallium scintigraphy and gated radionuclide angiography to assess cardiac risk before abdominal aortic surgery. *N Engl J Med* 1994, 330:663–669.

53. McEnroe CS, O'Donnell RF Jr, Yeager A, et al.: Comparison of ejection fraction and Goldman risk factor analysis of dipyridamole-thallium-201 studies in the evaluation of cardiac morbidity after aortic aneurysm surgery. *J Vasc Surg* 1990, 11:497–504.

54. Takase B, Younis LT, Byers SL, et al.: Comparative prognostic value of clinical risk indexes, resting two-dimensional echocardiography, and dipyridamole stress thallium-201 myocardial imaging for perioperative cardiac events in major nonvascular surgery patients. *Am Heart J* 1993, 126:1099–1106.

55. Watters TA, Botvinick EH, Dae MW, et al.: Comparison of the findings on preoperative dipyridamole perfusion scintigraphy and intraoperative transesophageal echocardiography: implications regarding the identification of myocardium at ischemic risk. *J Am Coll Cardiol* 1991, 18:93–100.

56. Fletcher JP, Antico JF, Gruenewald S, et al.: Dipyridamole-thallium scan for screening of coronary artery disease prior to vascular surgery. *J Cardiovasc Surg (Torino)* 1988, 29:666–669.

57. Sachs RN, Tellier P, Larmignat P, et al.: Assessment by dipyridamole-thallium-201 myocardial scintigraphy of coronary risk before peripheral vascular surgery. *Surgery* 1988, 103:584–587.

58. Younis LT, Aguirre F, Byers SL, et al.: Perioperative and long-term prognostic value of intravenous dipyridamole thallium scintigraphy in patients with peripheral vascular disease. *Am Heart J* 1990, 119:1287–1292.

59. Strawn DJ, Guernsey JM: Dipyridamole thallium scanning in the evaluation of coronary artery disease in elective abdominal aortic surgery. *Arch Surg* 1991, 126:880–884.

60. Shaw LJ, Miller DD, Kong BA, et al.: Determination of perioperative cardiac risk by adenosine thallium-201 myocardial imaging. *Am J Heart J* 1992, 124:861–869.

61. Younis LT, Stratmann HG, Takase B, et al.: Preoperative clinical assessment and dipyridamole thallium-201 scintigraphy for prediction and prevention of cardiac events in patients having major noncardiovascular surgery and known or suspected coronary artery disease. *Am J Cardiol* 1994, 74:311–317.

62. Elliott BM, Robison JG, Zellner JL, et al.: Dobutamine-thallium-201 imaging: Assessing cardiac risks associated with vascular surgery. *Circulation* 1991; 84(suppl III):III54–III60.

63. Stratmann HG, Younis LT, Wittry MD, et al.: Dipyridamole technetium-99m sestamibi myocardial tomography for preoperative cardiac risk stratification before major or minor nonvascular surgery. *Am Heart J* 1996, 132:536–541.

64. Amanullah AM, Berman DS, Erel J, *et al.*: Incremental prognostic value of adenosine myocardial perfusion single-photon emission computed tomography in women with suspected coronary artery disease. *Am J Cardiol* 1998, 15:725–730.

65. Stratmann HG, Younis LT, Wittry MD, *et al.*: Dipyridamole technetium-99m sestamibi myocardial tomography in patients evaluated for elective vascular surgery: Prognostic value for perioperative and late cardiac events. *Am Heart J* 1996, 131:923–929.

66. Brown KA, O'Meara J, Chambers CE, Plante DA: Ability of dipyridamole-thallium-201 imaging one to four days after acute myocardial infarction to predict in-hospital and late recurrent myocardial ischemic events. *Am J Cardiol* 1990, 65:160–167.

67. Younis LT, Byers S, Shaw L, *et al.*: Prognostic value of intravenous dipyridamole thallium scintigraphy after an acute myocardial ischemic event. *Am J Cardiol* 1989, 64:161–166.

68. Stratmann HG, Williams GA, Wittry MD, *et al.*: Exercise technetium-99m sestamibi tomography for cardiac risk stratification of patients with stable chest pain. *Circulation* 1994, 89:615–622.

69. Younis LT, Stratmann H, Takase BR, *et al.*: Preoperative clinical assessment and dipyridamole thallium-201 scintigraphy for the prediction of prevention of cardiac events in major non–cardiovascular surgery patients. *Am J Cardiol* 1994, 74:311–317.

70. Stratmann HG, Tamesis BR, Younis LT, *et al.*: Prognostic value of dipyridamole technetium-99m sestamibi myocardial tomography in patients with stable chest pain who are unable to exercise. *Am J Cardiol* 1994, 73:647–652.

71. Miller DD: Cost efficacy of diagnostic and management strategies. Paper presented at the 2nd International Conference of Nuclear Cardiology; April 25, 1995; Cannes, France.

CHAPTER 4

SPECT DETECTION OF CORONARY ARTERY DISEASE

Frans J. Th. Wackers

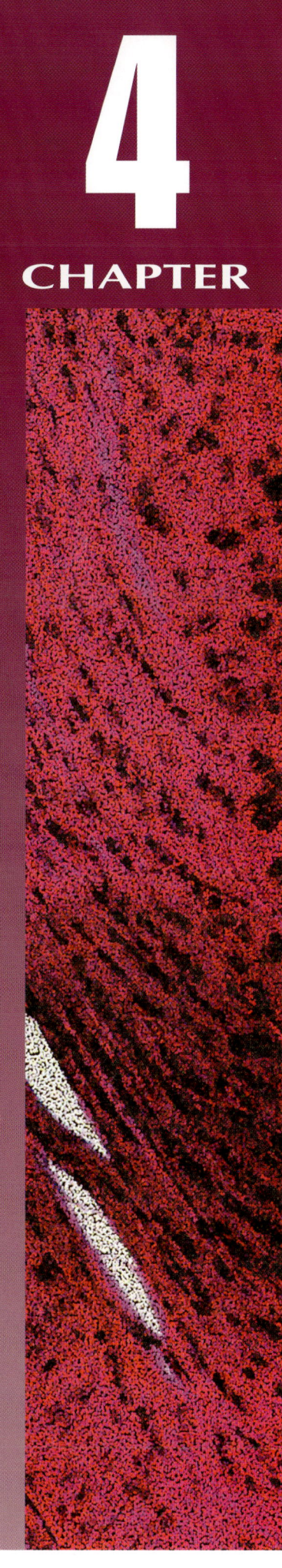

Radionuclide myocardial perfusion imaging, with either physical or pharmacologic stress, is one of the main pillars of the diagnostic work-up of patients with symptoms suspicious for coronary artery disease. The basic concepts of exercise myocardial perfusion imaging were developed in the early 1970s, using ^{43}K and rectilinear nuclear scanning equipment. When ^{201}Tl became commercially available in the mid-1970s and planar imaging with Anger-type gamma cameras provided consistently good quality images, the clinical use of radionuclide myocardial perfusion imaging rapidly gained clinical acceptance. The principles of pharmacologic vasodilation with dipyridamole as an alternate mode of stress were developed in the early 1980s. This made it possible to test patients who could not exercise and who previously could not be evaluated adequately.

The main purpose of stress testing initially was the noninvasive detection of angiographically significant coronary artery disease. Subsequently, it became clear that stress myocardial perfusion images provided not only *diagnostic* information but also powerful *prognostic* and *risk-stratifying* information. Quantification of images was allowed for reproducible determination of the degree and extent of myocardial perfusion abnormalities. Imaging and computer technology improved considerably from the mid-1980s to the late 1990s. Single-head planar projection imaging was gradually replaced by tomographic imaging with multiple detector heads. This resulted in improved detection of coronary artery disease, in particular in various coronary artery territories. ^{201}Tl was the only available imaging agent for more than 15 years. New ^{99m}Tc-labeled myocardial perfusion imaging agents were developed and approved for clinical use in the early 1990s. This was an important stimulus for the further clinical acceptance and spread of radionuclide myocardial perfusion imaging. Using ^{99m}Tc-labeled agents, *eg*, sestamibi and tetrofosmin, excellent- to good-quality SPECT imaging became standard. Importantly, the ^{99m}Tc-labeled agents also allowed for ECG-gated acquisition and simultaneous assessment of myocardial perfusion and function.

Why not perform cardiac catheterization and coronary angiography in all patients suspected of having coronary artery disease? The contrast coronary angiogram displays the anatomic extent of epicardial coronary artery disease, the severity of luminal narrowing, and the number of diseased vessels. Stress radionuclide myocardial perfusion imaging, on the other hand, displays the downstream functional consequences of epicardial coronary artery disease in the myocardium. It also may visualize the regional effects of microvascular endothelial dysfunction and impairment of regional coronary flow reserve.

One can expect to see continued improvements in equipment and radiotracers over time. The development and validation of attenuation correction devices will be extremely important for the further advancement of clinical myocardial perfusion imaging. Once soft tissue attenuation can be corrected for, the absolute uptake of radiopharmaceutical in the myocardium and consequently absolute myocardial blood flow will be quantifiable. This will improve the early detection of disease in various coronary artery territories. Although the available radiotracers have an excellent record of clinical usefulness, none of them are ideal for imaging under all circumstances in all patients. New radiopharmaceuticals, *eg*, ^{99m}Tc-NOET, with different imaging characteristics, are currently being evaluated in clinical testing and may become available in the near future. This chapter presents characteristics of routinely used radiotracers, the principles of imaging, and the interpretation and diagnostic value of clinical radionuclide myocardial perfusion imaging.

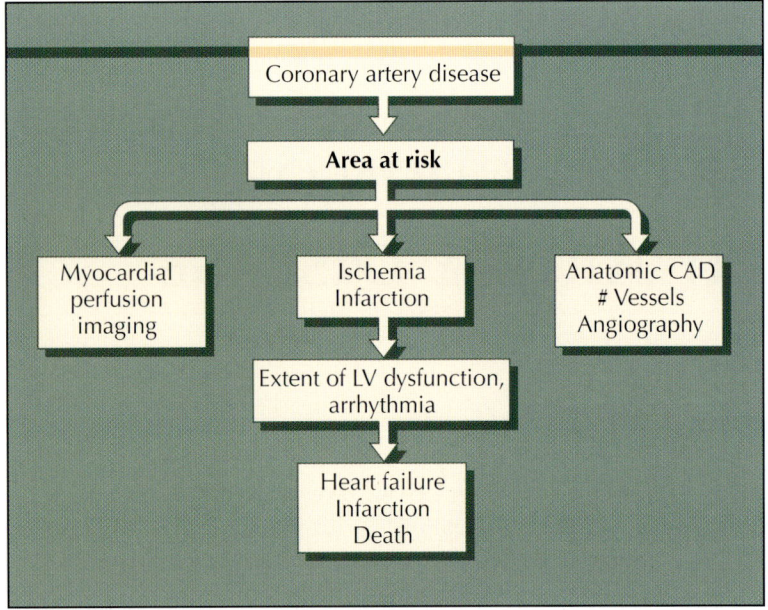

FIGURE 4-1. Clinical morbidity of coronary artery disease. The clinical morbidity of coronary artery disease (CAD) is the result of myocardial ischemia and infarction. The ultimate clinical outcome, *ie*, heart failure, myocardial infarction, and death, is determined by the extent of damage caused by obstructive CAD. The extent of myocardial damage can be predicted by the magnitude of the area at risk. The area at risk can be assessed either by stress myocardial perfusion imaging, which visualizes the regional distribution of myocardial blood flow, or coronary angiography, which visualizes the anatomic extent of CAD. LV—left ventricular.

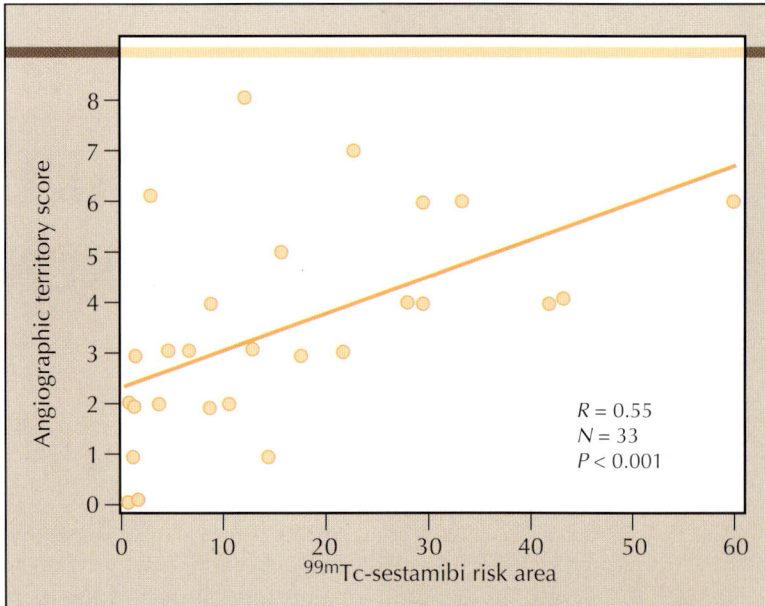

FIGURE 4-2. Angiographic territory score and ^{99m}Tc-sestamibi risk area. Although it is generally assumed that the extent of the myocardial area at risk for ischemia or infarction can be estimated from the conventional contrast coronary angiogram, this may not always be true. In patients with totally occluded coronary arteries who experience acute myocardial infarction, prior studies have shown that ^{99m}Tc-sestamibi perfusion defects accurately quantify the extent of myocardial infarction [1,2]. However, this relation is not as strong in patients with coronary artery disease who are not experiencing acute myocardial infarction. In patients undergoing single-vessel coronary artery angioplasty, when ^{99m}Tc-sestamibi was injected at the time of angioplasty balloon inflation, the estimated myocardial area at risk with ^{99m}Tc-sestamibi correlated weakly with angiographic risk scoring. Thus, in an individual patient, it would be very difficult to predict the myocardial area at risk from coronary angiography alone. (*Adapted from* Haronian *et al.* [3].)

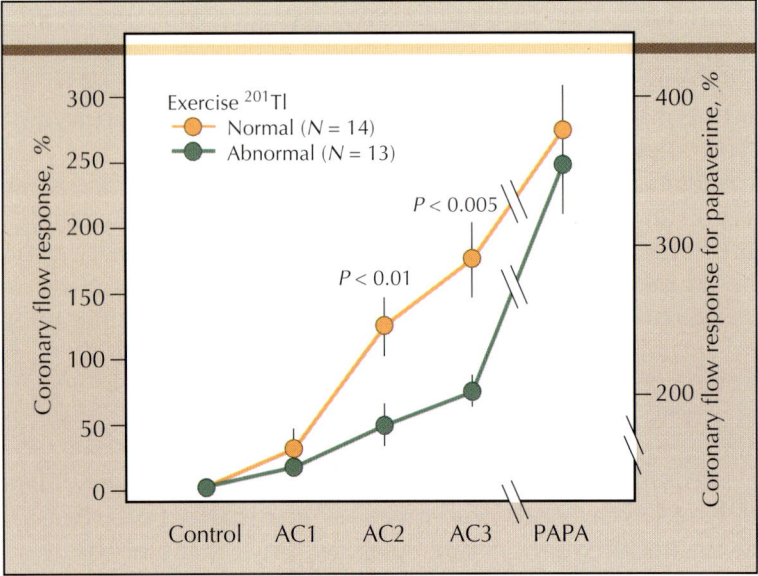

FIGURE 4-3. Normal coronary angiography. Lack of epicardial coronary artery disease does not necessarily mean absence of coronary artery disease. The response of coronary blood flow to increasing doses of intracoronary acetylcholine (AC) and papaverine (PAPA) is shown in patients with normal coronary angiograms and normal exercise thallium images, and in patients with normal coronary angiograms and abnormal thallium images (presumably false-positive). In patients with true-negative thallium images, the dose-related increase of coronary blood flow to acetylcholine is normal. In contrast, in patients with false-positive thallium images, dose-related increase of coronary blood flow to acetylcholine is blunted. Because the blood flow response to acetylcholine is endothelium-dependent, these data suggest that the "false-positive" thallium images in fact are true positives, and that regional microvascular endothelial dysfunction is detected in the absence of epicardial coronary artery disease. Both groups respond with similar normal blood flow increases to administration of papaverine, which increases blood flow by smooth muscle relaxation. These data suggest that myocardial perfusion studies examine the entire coronary tree, from epicardial coronary arteries to small myocardial vessels, including endothelial function, and not exclusively epicardial coronary artery patency. (*Adapted from* Zeiher *et al.* [4].)

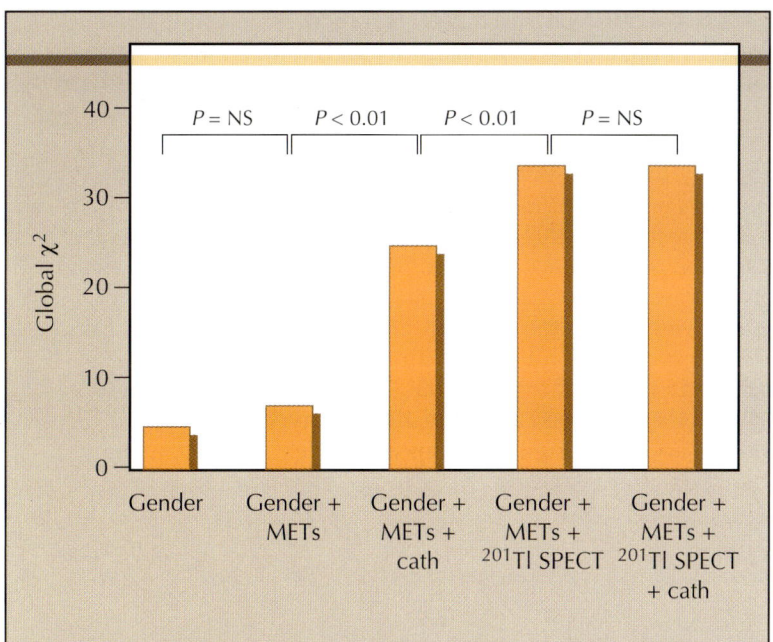

FIGURE 4-4. Incremental prognostic value of stress myocardial perfusion imaging over readily available clinical parameters and coronary angiography. The statistical power of variables for predicting cardiac events is measured as the global χ^2. In patients who underwent exercise radionuclide SPECT imaging and coronary angiography, clinical variables such as gender and the total metabolic equivalents (METs) performed on treadmill exercise demonstrated modest predictive power for cardiac events. If information from the coronary angiogram (single vessel versus multivessel disease) was added to these clinical variables, the power to predict events increased significantly. If the information obtained from ^{201}Tl SPECT perfusion imaging (low risk versus high risk) instead of coronary angiography was added to the clinical variables of gender and METs, the statistical power for predicting cardiac events was greater. Moreover, coronary angiography provided no further predictive power when added to the information from SPECT imaging. These data have been confirmed by subsequent studies. Stress myocardial perfusion imaging provides unique and powerful prognostic information that exceeds that of the coronary angiogram. Cath—catheterization; NS—not significant. (*Adapted from* Iskandrian et al. [5].)

CLINICAL IMAGING

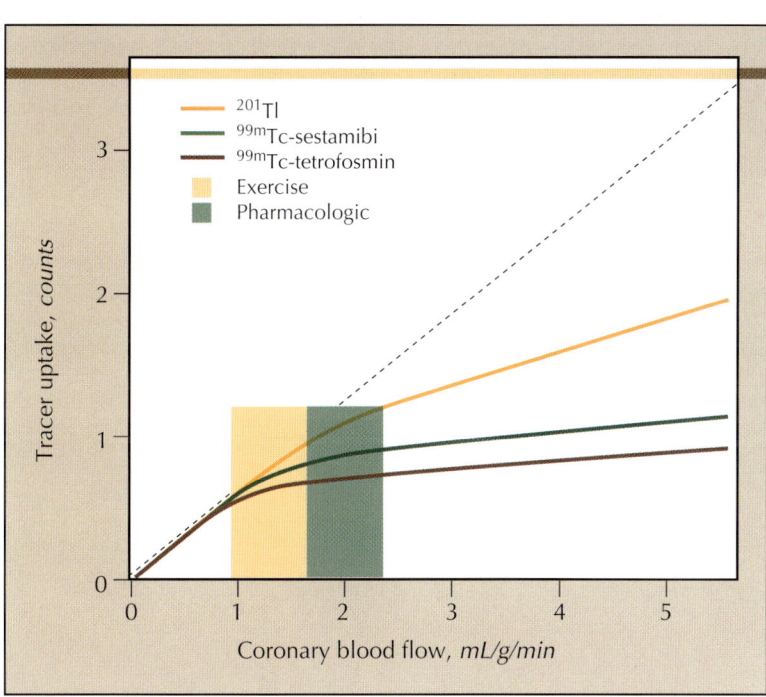

FIGURE 4-5. Radionuclide myocardial perfusion imaging. Two classes of radiotracers are used for stress myocardial perfusion SPECT imaging: ^{201}Tl, used since the mid 1970s, and ^{99m}Tc-labeled perfusion tracers, used since the early 1990s. These two classes of radiotracers have different physical half-lives, energy of photons emitted, and dosage allowances. ^{201}Tl is a radioisotopic potassium analogue with a relatively long half-life of 78 hours. The isotope emits low-energy photons predominantly at 80 keV and 10% at 160 keV. Because of the long half-life of thallium, only a low dose of 2.5–4.0 mCi can be administered to patients. ^{99m}Tc has a short half-life of 6 hours and emits photons with a medium energy at 140 keV. Because of its shorter half-life, a higher dose of ^{99m}Tc (15–30 mCi) can be administered. If both radioisotopes are used for clinical imaging, a protocol commonly referred to as the "dual isotope protocol," thallium should be given first because of its lower energy. Both ^{201}Tl and ^{99m}Tc-labeled perfusion tracers distribute within the myocardium proportional to regional blood flow.

^{201}Tl is a potassium analogue that enters the myocytes by an active process using the Na-K ATPase pump. In contrast, both ^{99m}Tc-sestamibi and ^{99m}Tc-tetrofosmin pass across the sarcolemmal and mitochondrial cell membranes by passive diffusion, and are retained within the mitochondria because of a large negative transmembrane potential. The first-pass extraction of ^{201}Tl and ^{99m}Tc-labeled perfusion tracers, which ultimately determines the regional uptake relative to regional myocardial blood, differ as well. While the extraction fraction of ^{201}Tl is high at 85%, the extraction fraction of ^{99m}Tc-sestamibi is only 60%, and that of ^{99m}Tc-tetrofosmin is approximately 54%. The extraction fraction is determined experimentally in a Langendorf preparation and represents the extraction during one single pass. In patients, many recirculations occur, and during every passage through the heart radiotracer is extracted. Similar to the potassium ion, ^{201}Tl is subject to continuous exchange across the Na-K ATPase pump, whereas ^{99m}Tc-sestamibi and ^{99m}Tc-tetrofosmin remain essentially fixed within the myocytes. The higher extraction fraction of ^{201}Tl is offset by the relatively rapid washout from the cells, whereas the lower extraction fraction of ^{99m}Tc-sestamibi and ^{99m}Tc-tetrofosmin is compensated for by the stable fixation within the myocytes. This schematic illustrates radiotracer uptake and regional myocardial blood flow. An ideal myocardial perfusion tracer would be expected to show a perfect linear relationship (line of identity, *dotted line*) to myocardial blood flow over a wide range of flow rates in mL/g/min. This is not the case for either ^{201}Tl or ^{99m}Tc-labeled sestamibi and tetrofosmin. Under resting conditions, myocardial blood flow is approximately 1 mL/g/min. During physical exercise, myocardial blood flow may increase to 2 mL/g/min, whereas with pharmacologic vasodilation (adenosine or dipyridamole), flow may exceed 2 mL/g/min. All three radiotracers demonstrate "roll-off" at high flow levels, *ie*, the relationship between tracer uptake and flow deviates more and more from the line of identity. Although this is true for ^{201}Tl, it is particularly marked for ^{99m}Tc-sestamibi and ^{99m}Tc-tetrofosmin. The practical implication of this is that at higher flow levels, relative myocardial uptake of these radiotracers may underestimate regional myocardial blood flow deficits. Clinical studies have shown that this "roll-off" phenomenon does not significantly affect the detection of significant (> 80%) coronary artery stenoses. However, mild coronary artery stenoses (50%–70%) may go undetected, especially with ^{99m}Tc-sestamibi and ^{99m}Tc-tetrofosmin.

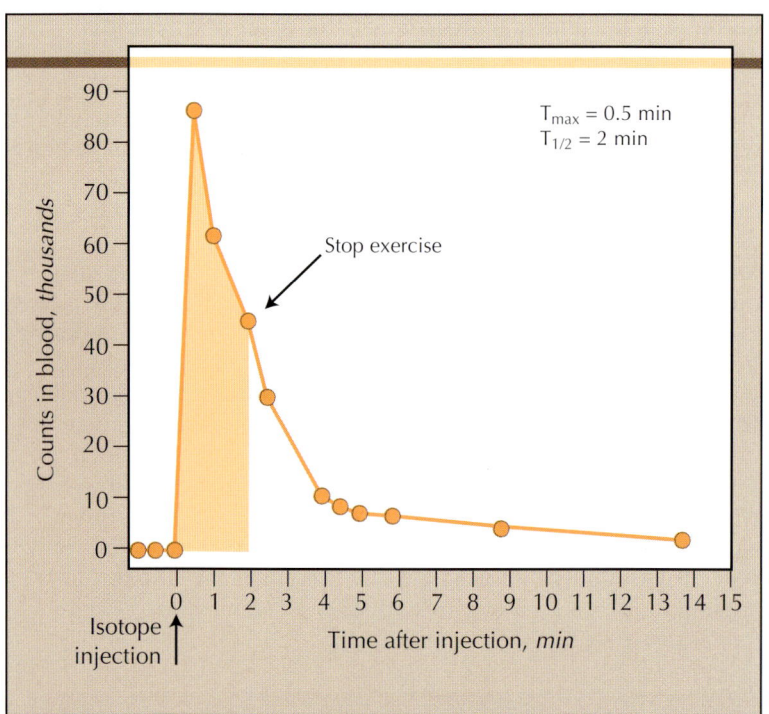

FIGURE 4-6. Radiotracer blood clearance. Once a radiotracer is injected at peak stress, it is rapidly accumulated in the heart in proportion to regional myocardial blood flow. All clinically used radiotracers clear rapidly from the blood in 5 to 7 minutes after injection. Because ^{201}Tl is cleared more rapidly from the blood than ^{99m}Tc-sestamibi or ^{99m}Tc-tetrofosmin, the patient should be encouraged to continue exercising for approximately 1 minute after injection of ^{201}Tl at peak exercise, and for 2 minutes after injection of ^{99m}Tc-sestamibi or ^{99m}Tc-tetrofosmin at peak exercise. In the case of ^{99m}Tc-sestamibi and ^{99m}Tc-tetrofosmin, if the patient is allowed to stop too early, *eg*, 1 minute after radiotracer injection during exercise, a substantial amount of the injected dose is still recirculating. This important point is not widely recognized. If exercise is stopped too early, further myocardial uptake occurs under resting conditions and the extent of ischemia may be underestimated.

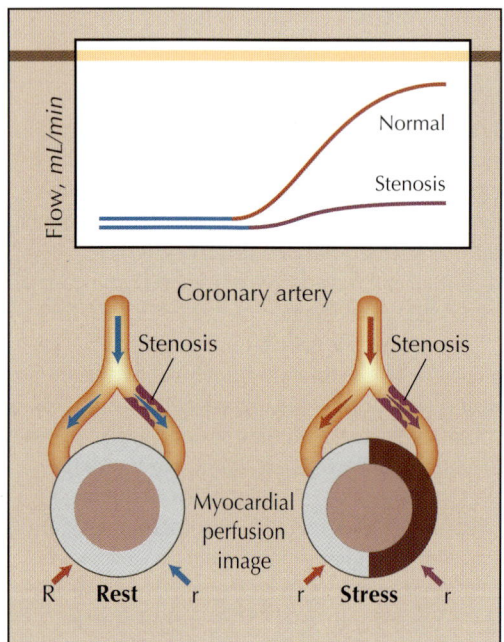

FIGURE 4-7. Pathophysiology underlying radionuclide myocardial perfusion imaging. Coronary blood flow in each of the coronary artery branches at rest and during stress is shown in the graph. At rest, regional myocardial blood flow is similar in both coronary artery branches. When a myocardial perfusion radiotracer is injected at rest, myocardial uptake of radiotracer is homogeneous, and consequently the short-axis image is normal. During stress, coronary blood flow increases 2.0 to 2.5 times in the normal branch, but not to the same extent in the stenotic branch, resulting in heterogeneous distribution of regional myocardial blood flow. This heterogeneity of blood flow can be visualized with ^{201}Tl, ^{99m}Tc-sestamibi, or ^{99m}Tc-tetrofosmin as an area with relatively decreased myocardial accumulation, *ie*, an image with a myocardial perfusion defect (*bottom, right*). Anatomic delineation of a normal (left branch) and an abnormal (right branch) coronary artery is shown. R—normal resistance; r—low resistance.

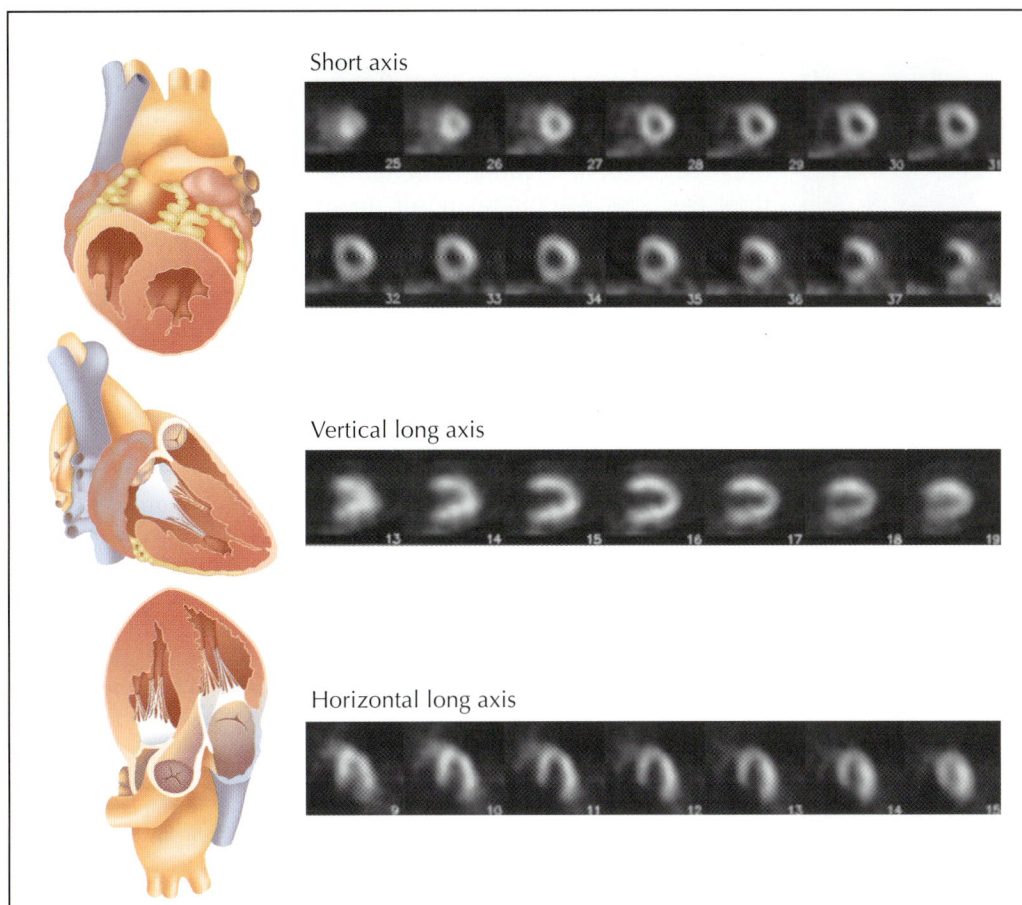

FIGURE 4-8. Normal exercise SPECT myocardial perfusion images. The display of SPECT myocardial perfusion imaging is standardized. The short-axis slices are presented from apex to base, the vertical long-axis slices are displayed from septum to lateral wall, and the horizontal long-axis slices are displayed from inferior to anterior. The radiotracer uptake is homogeneous in each of the slices.

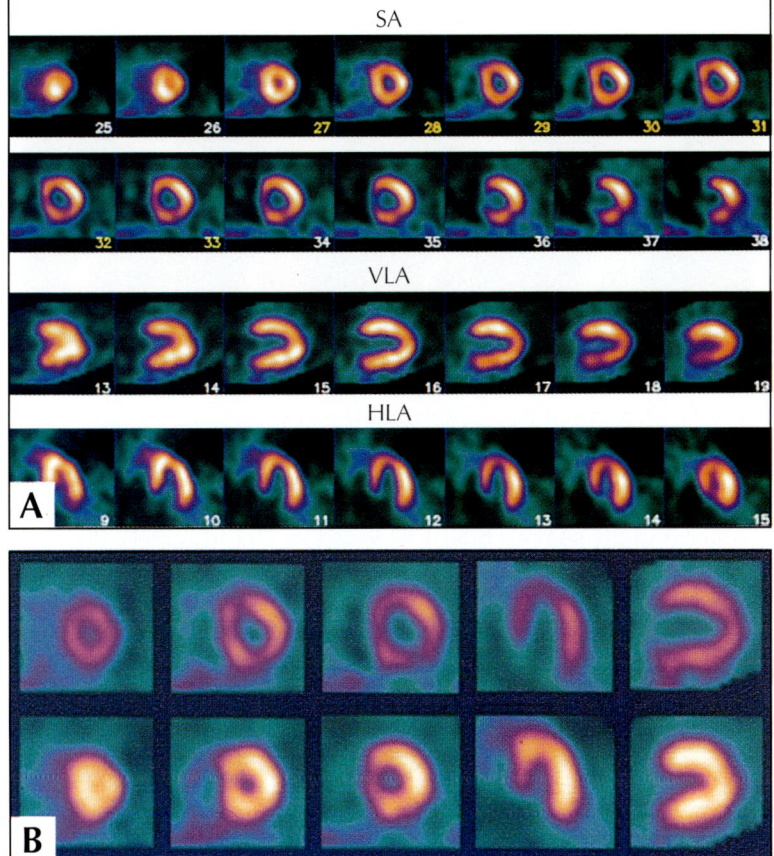

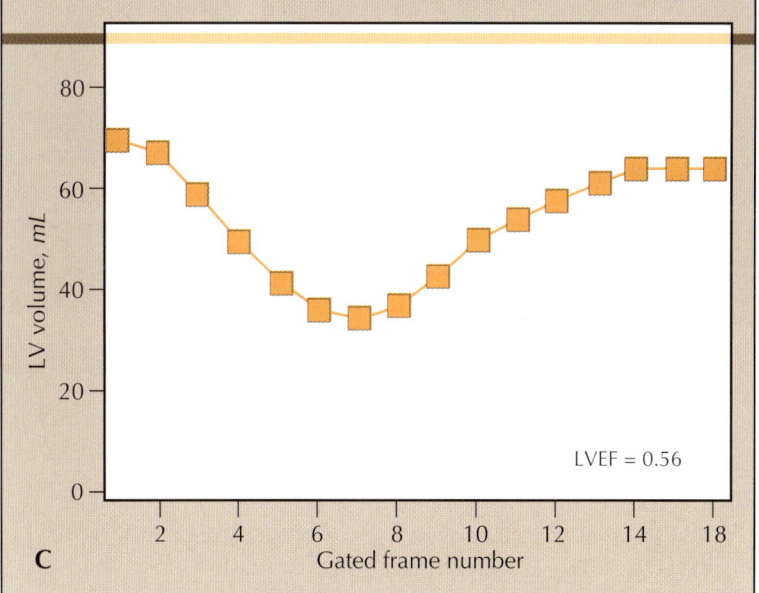

FIGURE 4-9. Example of normal gated SPECT images. **A**, Color normal exercise SPECT myocardial perfusion images from Figure 4-10. **B**, Normal ECG-gated SPECT. The acquisition of the images in *panel A* was performed with ECG gating. The end-diastolic (ED) and end-systolic (ES) images are shown. Regional thickening of the left ventricular wall can be appreciated by a change in color from dark purple to yellow and white. These images demonstrate uniformly normal contraction of the left ventricle (LV). **C**, Left ventricular ejection fraction (LVEF) is 56%. HLA—horizontal long axis; SA—short axis; VLA—vertical long axis.

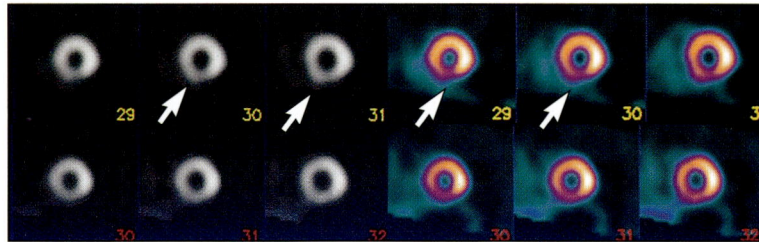

FIGURE 4-10. Diaphragmatic attenuation. Normal variation of radiotracer uptake on exercise SPECT myocardial perfusion images.

Stress (*top row*) and rest (*bottom row*) short-axis slices are displayed. The *arrows* point toward areas with slightly decreased uptake in the inferior wall due to inferior attenuation; this represents a normal variation. Several corrective measures can be attempted to either correct or recognize this artifact. The patient can be re-imaged in a different position, *eg*, prone or in right-side decubitus position. In these positions, diaphragmatic attenuation is diminished and improved uptake can be noted. If the inferior defect is fixed (*ie*, both at stress and at rest), normal inferior wall motion is suggestive of attenuation artifact. Finally, the only method to truly deal with attenuation artifacts is to apply attenuation compensation devices.

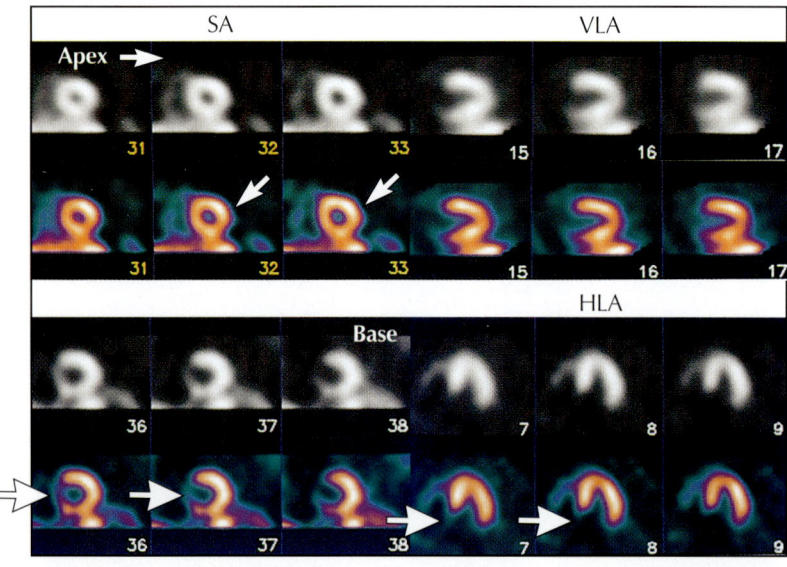

FIGURE 4-11. Normal variations of SPECT images. Normal SPECT images frequently show areas of mildly reduced radiotracer uptake that represent normal variations. Although normal images appear to have homogeneous radiotracer uptake, on closer inspection and on enhancement by color display, one can note that there may be slight inhomogeneities. These inhomogeneities may be due to tissue attenuation or may be a normal variation of cardiac anatomy. On normal short-axis (SA) SPECT images, the high lateral wall is usually the area with maximal radiotracer uptake (*small arrows*) and the anterior wall, septum, and inferior wall consequently appear to have slightly less uptake. This is a normal variation. At the base of the heart, a septal defect is present in most basal SA slices (*large arrows*). This is the membranous septum that contains no myocardium. The horizontal long-axis (HLA) slices are useful for determining whether there is a normal membranous septum, which usually involves less than a third of the basal septum, or a true septal myocardial perfusion defect that usually involves more than a third of the septum extending toward the apex. VLA—vertical long axis.

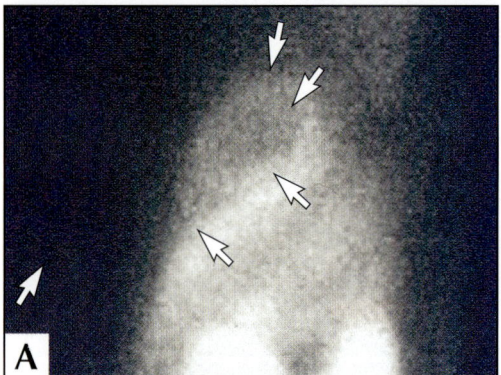
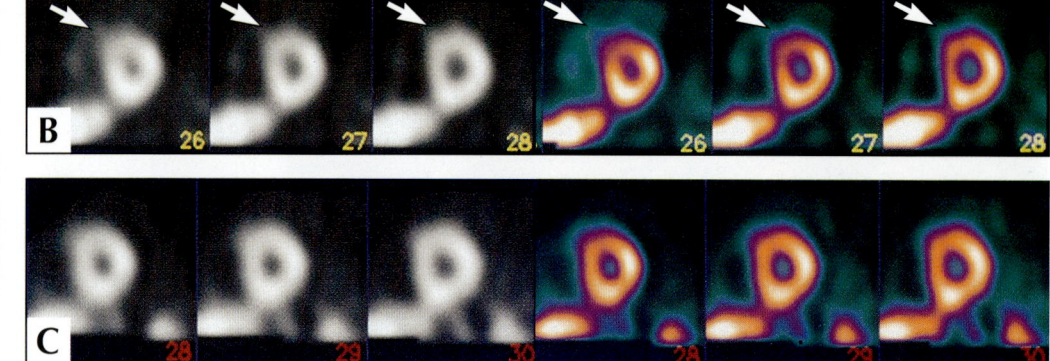

FIGURE 4-12. Breast attenuation. Breast attenuation artifacts used to be a serious interpretive problem on planar imaging. Fortunately, with SPECT imaging, breast attenuation is less of a problem, although it still occurs. Breast attenuation can be recognized on the rotating planar projection images as a shadow moving over the heart in certain projections, usually from left anterior oblique projections to the left lateral projections. **A**, The planar left lateral image shows marked attenuation of cardiac radiotracer uptake of the anterior wall. The contour of the breast is marked with *arrows*. **B**, The short-axis SPECT images show mild anterior wall defects (*arrows*). **C**, When SPECT imaging was repeated and the breast moved by the use of taping, the anterior wall appears normal.

ECG-gated images are often helpful in recognizing breast artifacts. When the attenuation artifact is present on both the stress and rest images (fixed defect), normal wall motion and thickening on movie display strongly suggest breast attenuation. Unfortunately, the breast may not always be in exactly the same position on the stress and rest images, and a reversible defect may be mimicked. Usually the cine display of the rotating images may then be helpful for recognizing the difference in position of the breast. The only definitive solution in dealing with attenuation artifacts is accurate attenuation correction.

Image Interpretation and Quantification

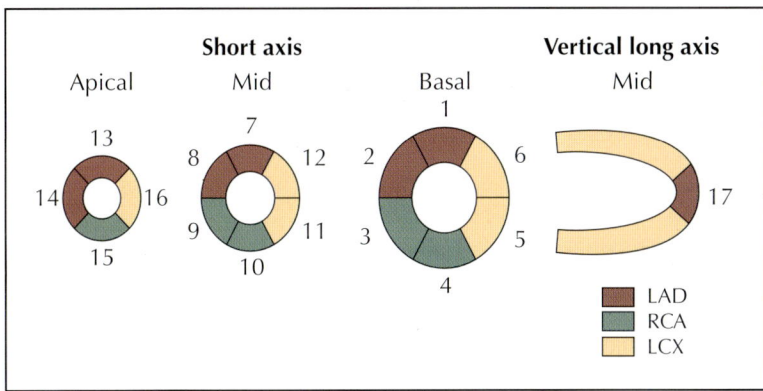

FIGURE 4-13. Coronary artery territories. Although the anatomy of coronary arteries may vary substantially in individual patients, the location of myocardial perfusion abnormalities on SPECT imaging allows for a general prediction of which coronary artery is likely to be diseased. The diagram shown represents the standardized assignment of coronary artery territories of the left anterior descending coronary artery (LAD), the right coronary artery (RCA), and the left circumflex coronary artery (LCX). The prediction of disease in the LAD is often quite accurate. The prediction of disease in the RCA and LCX is often less accurate because of substantial variation in extent of myocardial territories supplied by these arteries. (*Adapted from* Port [6].)

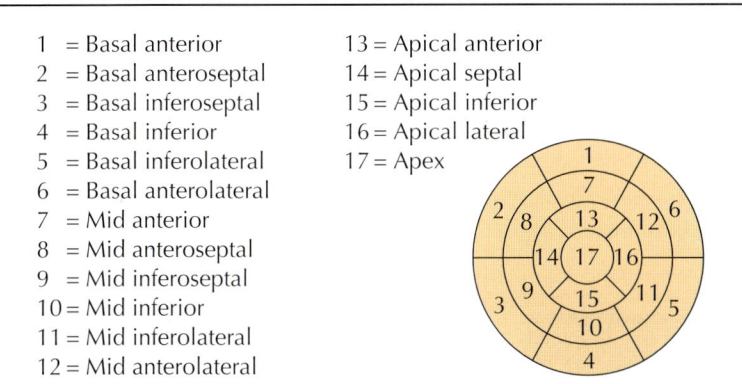

FIGURE 4-14. Standard nomenclature and segmentation commonly used for SPECT myocardial perfusion imaging. The 17-segment model is preferred, although a 20-segment model is acceptable as well. The standard nomenclature divides the short-axis slices of the left ventricle in three major portions: apical, midventricular, and basal. The apex is a separate portion, which is analyzed from a vertical long-axis slice. The midventricular and basal short-axis slices are each divided into six segments, whereas the apical short-axis slices are divided into four segments. The apex on the vertical long-axis slice represents one more segment. In the 20-segment model, the apex is divided into two segments and the apical short-axis slices are divided into six segments. Since the latter model leads to overrepresentation of the apex, the 17-segment model is preferred. Standardization of analysis of images is important in order to communicate effectively the results of SPECT myocardial perfusion imaging [7]. (*Adapted from* Port [6].)

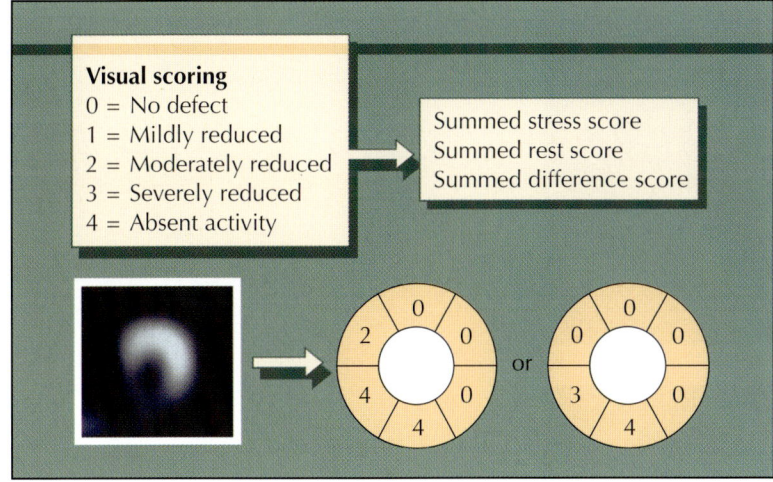

FIGURE 4-15. Visual scoring. SPECT myocardial perfusion images are interpreted by expressing the extent and severity of the myocardial perfusion abnormality using segmentation and visual scoring. The observer divides the image in his mind into segments according to the segmentation model described in Figure 4-14. A well-accepted visual scoring method (0–4) is shown. This methodology is obviously subjective, and therefore may lack reproducibility. As shown, the same abnormality can be described as involving three segments or two segments. In addition, the visual scoring may vary slightly and result in a defect score of 10 or 7. Nevertheless, this scoring method, using summed stress scores, summed rest scores, or summed difference scores, has been used successfully for evaluation of the prognostic value of SPECT myocardial perfusion imaging in the literature [8].

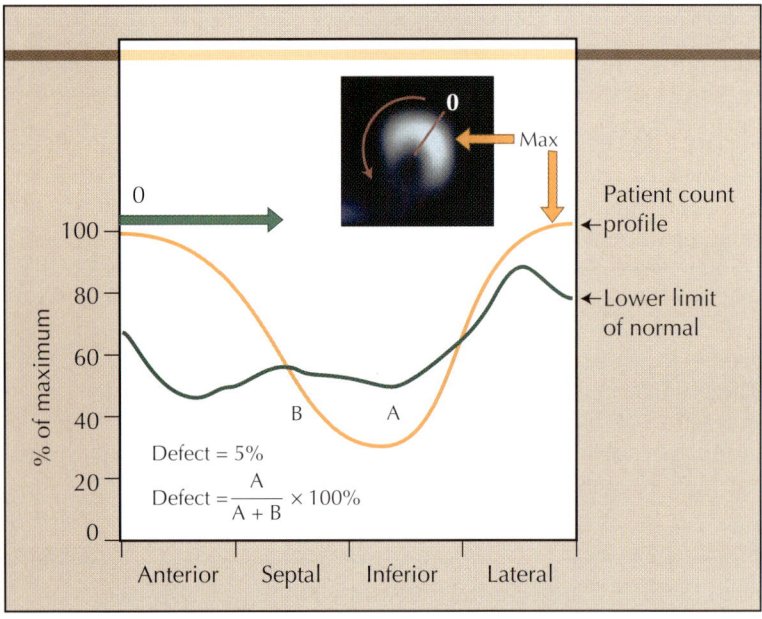

applied to a short-axis SPECT image with an inferoseptal myocardial perfusion defect is shown. Maximal (Max) count density is in the high lateral wall (*orange arrows*); this location is designated the value of 100%. The patient's count profile displays the distribution of counts in the SPECT slice relative to maximal counts counterclockwise, starting at 0, from anterior to septal, to inferior, to lateral wall. The trough of the *orange curve* represents lowest counts, which corresponds to the inferoseptal defect. The *green curve* displays the lower limit of normal count distribution (mean –2 SD) derived from a group of subjects with a low likelihood of coronary artery disease. The inferoseptal myocardial perfusion defect is the area between the curves (*A*). This area, which integrates the extent and severity of the defect, can be quantified as a percentage of the total area of the slice. Obviously, one does not know what the patient's circumferential profile would have been had the image been normal. However, the image would have looked normal if all portions of the circumferential profile were above the lower limit of normal curve. The presumed normal curve in this patient therefore would involve at least both portions of the orange curve above the lower limit of normal curve and the portion of the green curve where the defect is. If the area under the orange curve is labeled *B* and the defect as *A*, the minimal potentially visualized area of normal myocardium would include (*A* + *B*). The defect *A* therefore can be quantified as percent of normal myocardium: *A* divided by *A* + *B* × 100%. In the example shown, the defect is 5% of the potentially visualized normal myocardium in this slice.

FIGURE 4-16. Quantification of perfusion defect. Radionuclide images are intrinsically digital images. Shades of gray or color reflect the number of photons that reached the gamma camera at a certain location. True quantification of images, therefore, is feasible [9,10]. The methodology of quantification using circumferential profiles

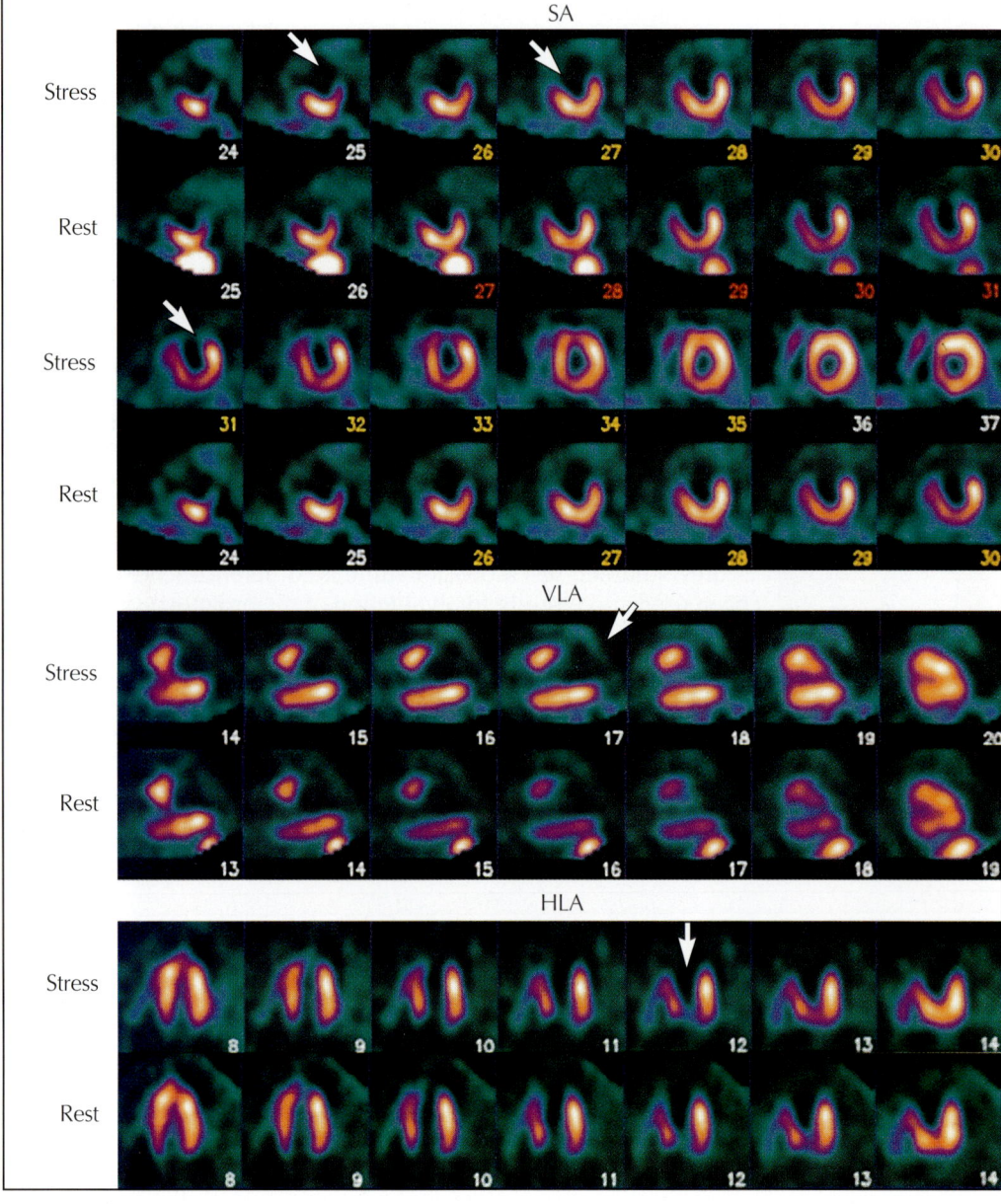

FIGURE 4-17. Example of a patient with a large, fixed (irreversible) myocardial perfusion defect. Both on the stress and rest images, large, severely reduced, anteroseptal and apical defects are evident (*arrows*). HLA—horizontal long axis; SA—short axis; VLA—vertical long axis.

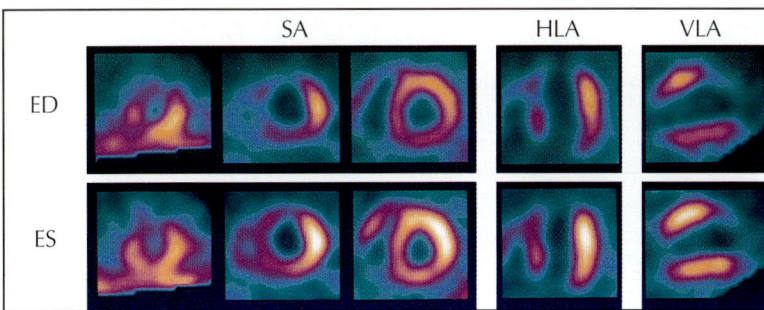

FIGURE 4-18. ECG-gated SPECT. The acquisition of the images in Figure 4-17 was performed with ECG gating. The end-diastolic (ED) and end-systolic (ES) images are shown. Regional thickening of the left ventricular wall can be appreciated as a change in color from dark purple to yellow and white. On these images, there is no appreciable change in color from ED to ES in the region with the anteroseptal defect, indicating severe regional dysfunction in the area of infarction. The left ventricular ejection fraction was 25%. HLA—horizontal long axis; SA—short axis; VLA—vertical long axis.

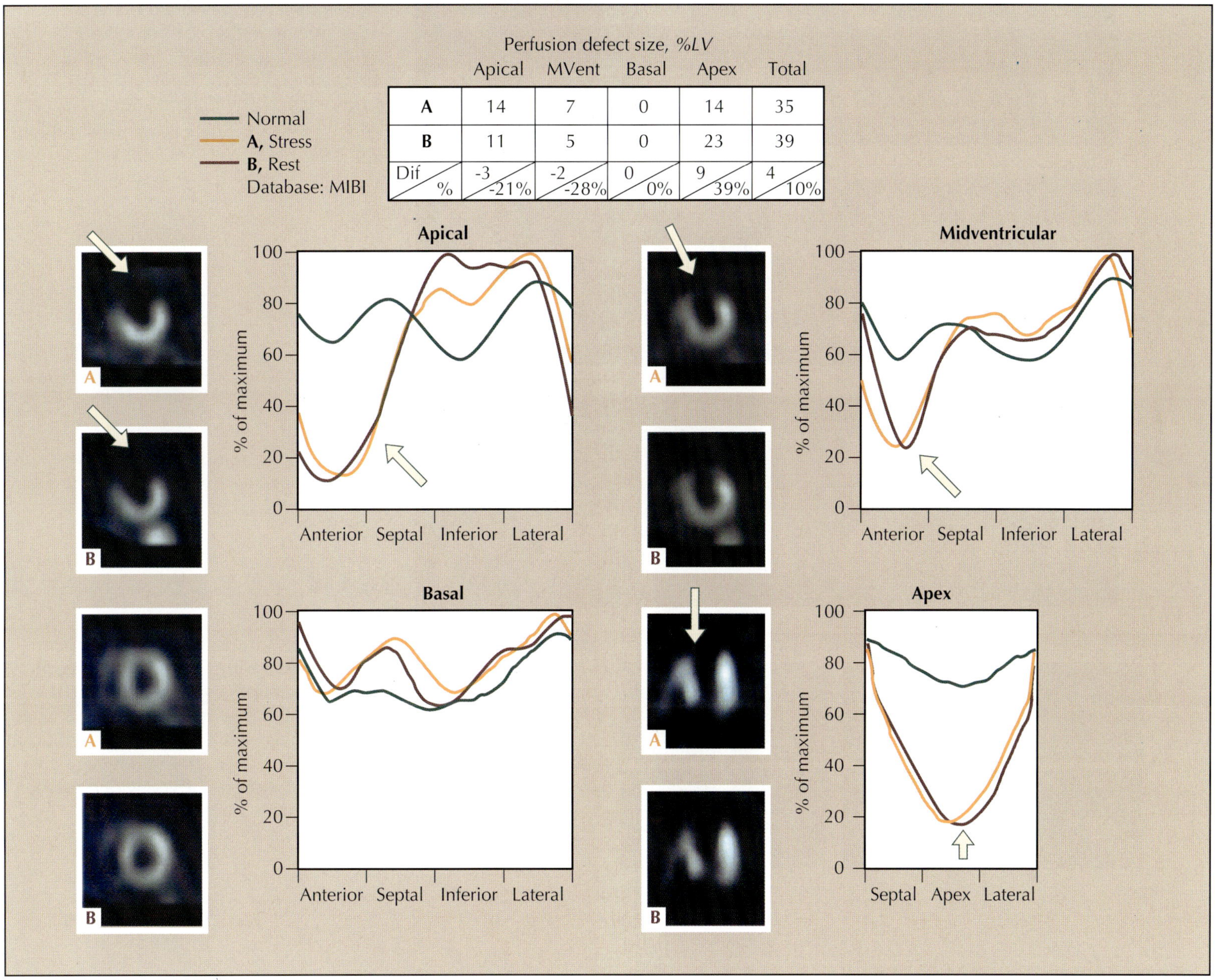

	Apical	MVent	Basal	Apex	Total
A	14	7	0	14	35
B	11	5	0	23	39
Dif	-3	-2	0	9	4
%	-21%	-28%	0%	39%	10%

Perfusion defect size, %LV

— Normal
— A, Stress
— B, Rest
Database: MIBI

FIGURE 4-19. Quantification of myocardial perfusion SPECT images from the patient in Figure 4-18 with fixed anteroseptal and apical defect. The stress curves are below the lower limit of normal in anteroseptal and lateral walls in the apical and midventricular (MVent) short-axis slices. There is no defect in the basal slices. There is a large defect in the apex, as shown in the horizontal long-axis slice. Note that the stress and rest curves are virtually identical, indicating a fixed myocardial perfusion abnormality, or scar, without ischemia. Results of computer quantification are shown in the table. The total stress defect size is large and involves 35% of the left ventricle (LV). The rest defect is quantified as 39%, which is not significantly different from the stress defect. The reproducibility of quantification of defect size is within 3% variation. MIBI—^{99m}Tc-sestamibi.

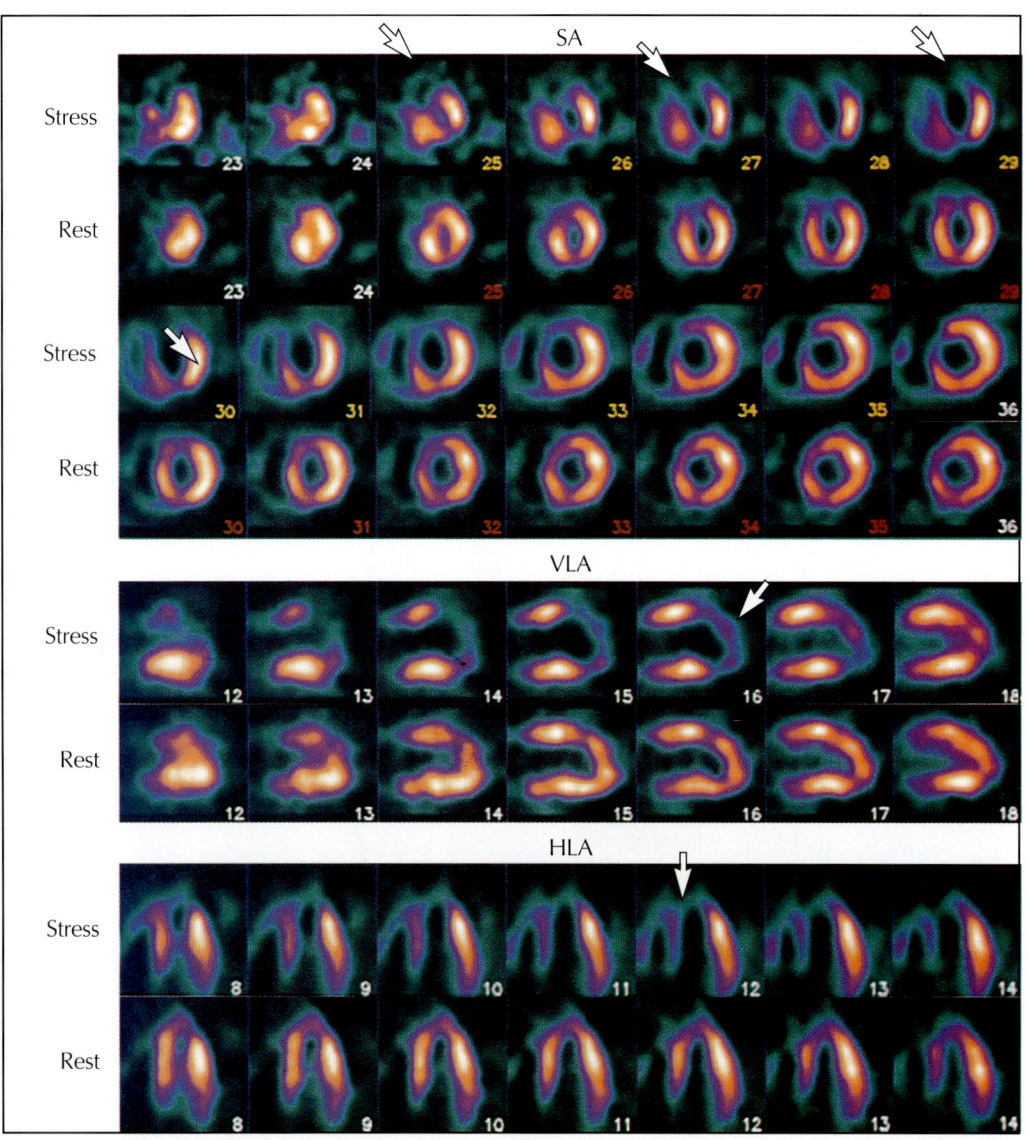

FIGURE 4-20. Example of a patient with a large, reversible myocardial perfusion defect. There are large, severely reduced, anteroseptal and apical defects (*arrows*) suggestive of myocardial ischemia evident on both stress and rest images. In addition, there is mild transient ischemic cavity dilation of the left ventricle on the stress images compared with the rest images. The rest images are almost normal, except for a small residual defect in the anterior wall on the apical short-axis (SA) slices. These images are typical for a large reversible stress-induced myocardial perfusion defect. The transient left ventricular cavity dilation suggests severe ischemia during stress. HLA—horizontal long axis; VLA—vertical long axis.

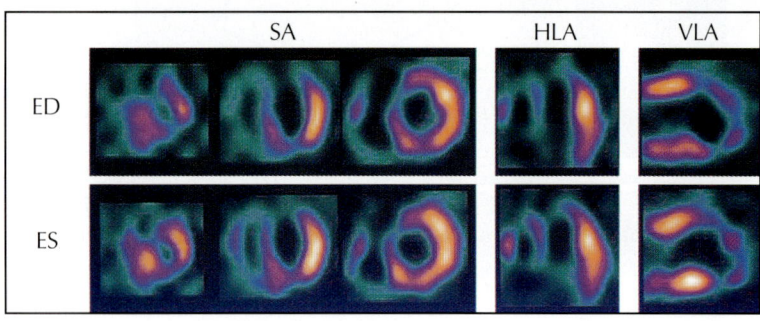

FIGURE 4-21. ECG-gated SPECT. The acquisition of the images in Figure 4-20 was performed with ECG gating. The post-stress end-diastolic (ED) and end-systolic (ES) images are shown. Regional thickening of the left ventricular wall can be appreciated as a change in color from dark purple to yellow and white. There is no significant change in color in the area of the defect, indicating severe regional dysfunction. Global left ventricular function is severely depressed with a calculated left ventricular ejection fraction of 35%. HLA—horizontal long axis; SA—short axis; VLA—vertical long axis.

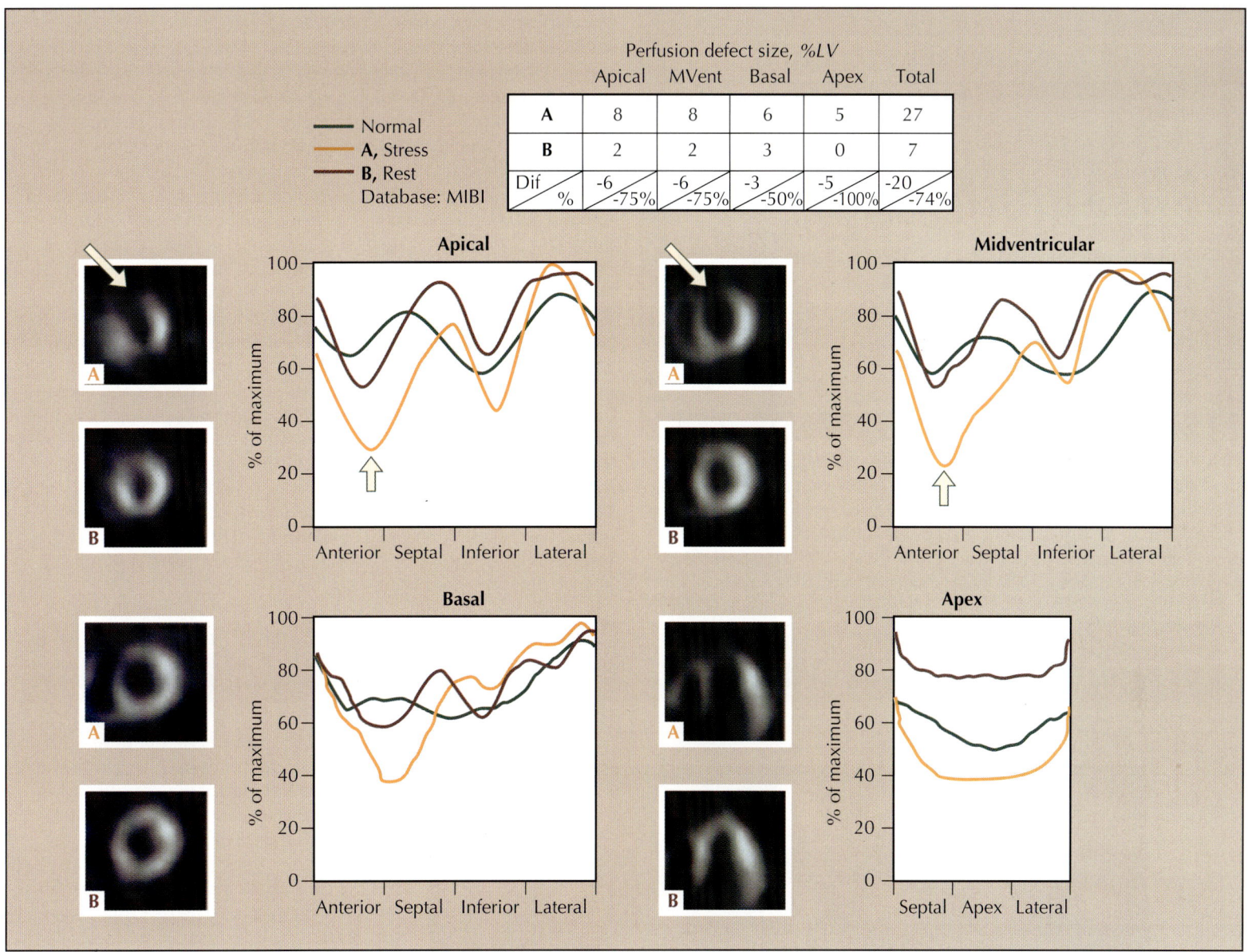

FIGURE 4-22. Quantification of myocardial perfusion SPECT results from a patient with a reversible anteroseptal and apical defect. The stress curves are below the lower limit of normal in anteroseptal walls in the apical, midventricular (MVent), and basal short-axis slices. In the apical short-axis slices, there is also a small inferior defect due to a wrap-around anteroapical defect. There is also a defect in the apex visible in the horizontal long-axis slice. The rest circumferential profiles are largely within the normal range, except for small residual anterior wall defects. The results of computer quantification are shown in the table. The total stress defect size is large and involves 27% of the left ventricle. The rest defect is quantified as 7%, which is significantly less than the stress defect. The ischemic burden is large and involves 20% of the left ventricle (LV). MIBI—^{99m}Tc-sestamibi.

HIGH- AND LOW-RISK SPECT IMAGES

<u>HIGH-RISK</u>

Large perfusion defect on stress imaging
Multiple coronary artery territories
Large reversibility
Increased lung uptake
Transient LV dilation

<u>LOW-RISK</u>

Normal stress images
Small stress defect
Small reversibility

FIGURE 4-23. High- and low-risk SPECT images. SPECT images should not be interpreted as either normal or abnormal. The prognosis of a patient is related to the degree of myocardial perfusion abnormality. Quantification or semiquantification provides that important prognostic information. High-risk SPECT images are characterized by large perfusion defects on the stress images that involve multiple coronary artery territories (if two or more coronary territories are involved, the study should be considered to indicate high risk for the patient). Large stress-induced reversible defects represent extensive myocardial ischemia, which may be associated with increased lung uptake, transient ischemic left ventricular (LV) cavity dilation, and transient increased right ventricular myocardial visualization.

One of the strongest features of stress myocardial perfusion SPECT imaging is its ability to identify low-risk patients. Patients with unequivocal normal exercise or pharmacologic stress myocardial perfusion SPECT images exhibit less than a 1% future cardiac event rate, the same as the general population. For those undergoing an exercise study, this presumes that the patient achieved greater than 85% predicted maximum heart rate for a man or woman of their age. Similarly, presuming that adequate exercise was performed, patients with small myocardial perfusion defects on stress and small regions of defect reversibility have low risk for future cardiac events. These patients should be treated aggressively with medical therapy because of the presence of coronary artery disease. It is important to emphasize that stress myocardial perfusion SPECT images should always be interpreted in conjunction with clinical and electrocardiographic data. For example, a rare patient may have a markedly abnormal exercise portion of the test but normal or near-normal SPECT images. It is the responsibility of the nuclear cardiologist to determine the significance of such disparate data.

CARDIOMYOPATHY

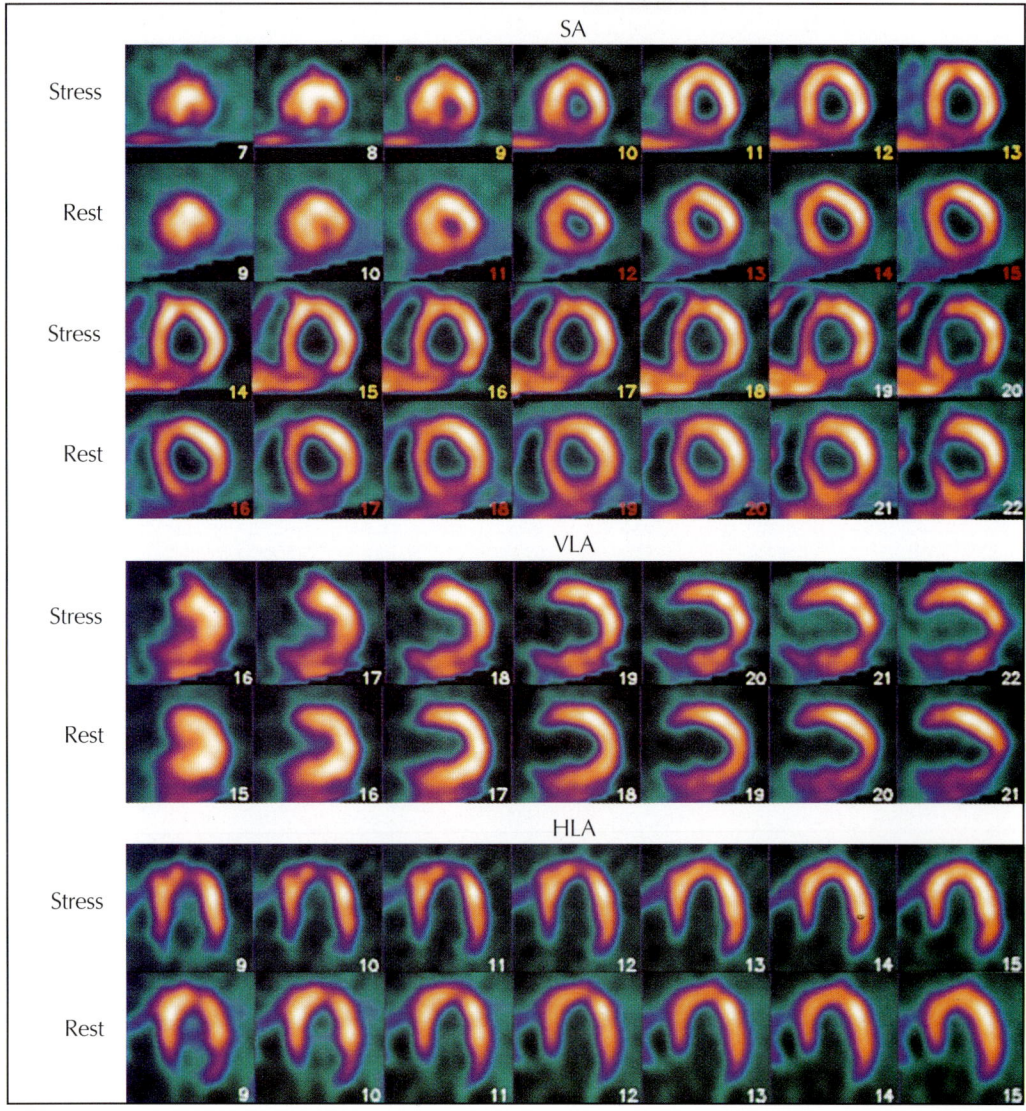

FIGURE 4-24. Example of a patient with nonischemic cardiomyopathy. On the stress images, the left ventricular cavity size is dilated without associated myocardial perfusion defect. The mild decrease in uptake in the inferior wall on the short-axis (SA) SPECT slices most likely represents inferior attenuation. The rest images are similar to the stress images without evidence of myocardial ischemia or infarction. HLA—horizontal long axis; VLA—vertical long axis.

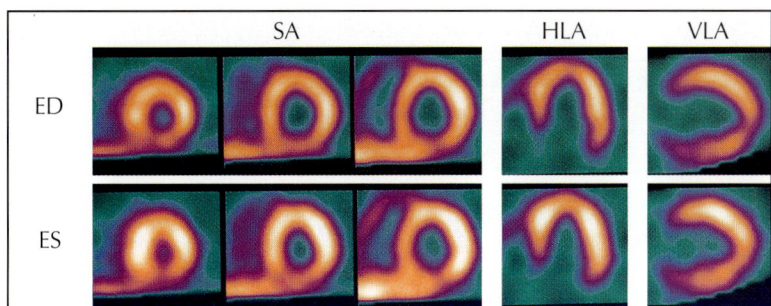

FIGURE 4-25. ECG-gated SPECT in a patient with cardiomyopathy. The acquisition of the images in Figures 4-24 and 4-26 was performed with ECG gating. The post-stress end-diastolic (ED) and end-systolic (ES) images are shown. Regional thickening of the left ventricular wall can be appreciated by a change in color from dark purple to yellow and white. The left ventricle of this patient with nonischemic cardiomyopathy is enlarged, and there is no significant change in myocardial color from ED to ES, indicating diffuse hypokinesis. Global left ventricular function is severely depressed with a calculated left ventricular ejection fraction of 32%. HLA—horizontal long axis; SA—short axis; VLA—vertical long axis.

Perfusion defect size, %LV

	Apical	MVent	Basal	Apex	Total
A	0	0	0	0	0
B	0	0	0	0	0
Dif / %	0 / 0%	0 / 0%	0 / 0%	0 / 0%	0 / 0%

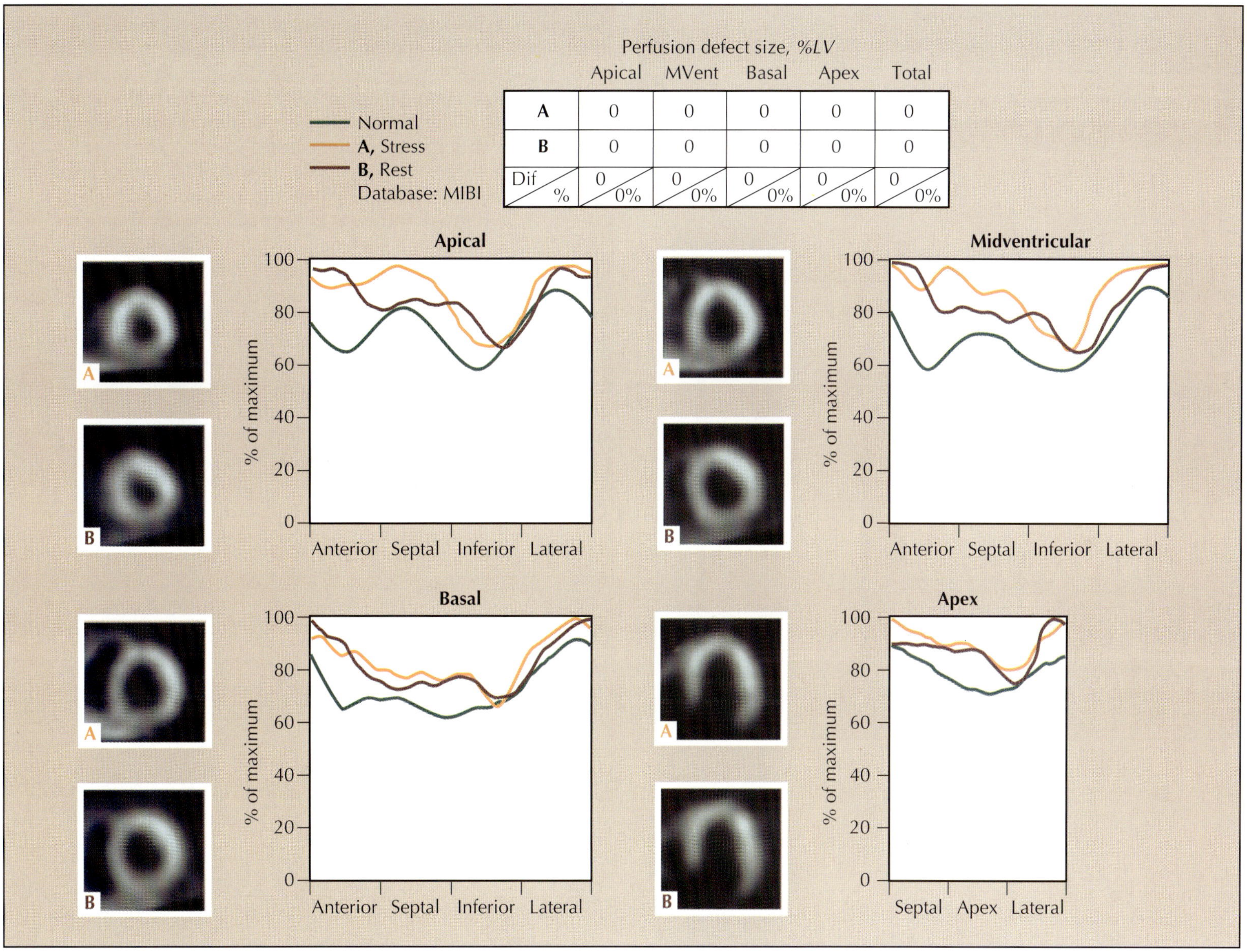

FIGURE 4-26. Quantification of myocardial perfusion SPECT results from a patient with nonischemic cardiomyopathy. Stress and rest curves are above the lower limit of normal, indicating that there are no myocardial perfusion defects. Accordingly, the quantification table shows zeros. LV—left ventricle; MIBI—^{99m}Tc-sestamibi; MVent—midventricular.

Clinical Indications for SPECT Imaging and Diagnostic Yield

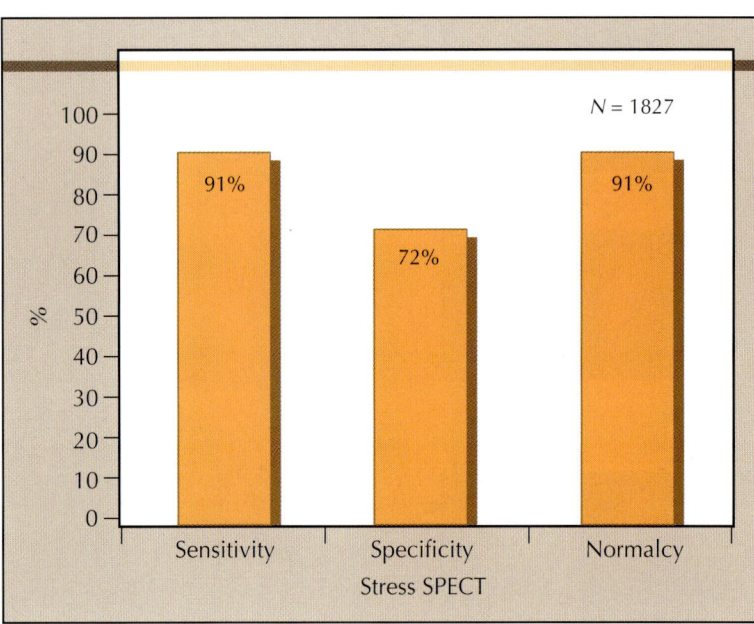

CLINICAL INDICATIONS FOR MYOCARDIAL PERFUSION IMAGING

- Detection of coronary artery disease
- Evaluation of known coronary artery disease
- Risk stratification
- Preoperative evaluation

FIGURE 4-27. Clinical indications for myocardial perfusion imaging. The clinical indications for stress-rest myocardial perfusion SPECT imaging are well established [11]. Most patients are referred because of chest pain symptoms and suspected coronary artery disease. However, patients with known coronary artery disease are referred as well. In these patients, the purpose of testing may be to evaluate the effect of therapy or to determine the cause of changes in symptom patterns. In addition, many patients are referred for risk stratification after acute myocardial infarction. Stress-rest SPECT imaging plays an important role in the preoperative evaluation of patients who are scheduled to undergo major noncardiac surgery. The most important and useful clinical application of SPECT myocardial perfusion imaging is to stratify patients into low- and high-risk categories, and thus contribute to the management of patients.

FIGURE 4-28. Detection of angiographic coronary artery disease with radiotracers. Extensive literature exists on the diagnostic yield of stress SPECT myocardial perfusion imaging [12–23]. Among 1827 patients referred for evaluation of chest discomfort (pooled data from 12 studies performed between 1989 and 1999), the overall sensitivity of myocardial perfusion SPECT for the detection of angiographic coronary artery disease was 91%, the specificity was 72%, and the normalcy rate (in subjects with low likelihood for coronary artery disease who did not undergo coronary angiography) was 91%.

References

1. Boucher CA, Wackers FJ, Zaret BL, Mena IG: Technetium-99m sestamibi myocardial imaging at rest for assessment of myocardial infarction and first-pass ejection fraction. *Am J Cardiol* 1992, 9(1):22–27.

2. Gibbons RJ, Miller TD, Christian TF: Infarct size measured by single photon emission computed tomographic imaging with (99m)Tc-sestamibi: A measure of the efficacy of therapy in acute myocardial infarction. *Circulation* 2000, 101(1):101–108.

3. Haronian H, Remetz MS, Sinusas AJ, *et al.*: Myocardial risk area defined by technetium-99m-sestamibi imaging during percutaneous transluminal coronary angioplasty: comparison to coronary angiography. *J Am Coll Cardiol* 1993, 22:1033–1043.

4. Zeiher AM, Krause T, Schächinger V, *et al.*: Impaired endothelium-dependent vasodilation of coronary resistance vessels is associated with exercise-induced myocardial ischemia. *Circulation* 1995, 91:2345–2352.

5. Iskandrian AS, Chae SC, Heo J, *et al.*: Independent and incremental prognostic value of exercise single-photon emission computed tomographic (SPECT) thallium imaging in coronary artery disease. *J Am Coll Cardiol* 1993, 22:665–670.

6. Port SC: Imaging guidelines for nuclear cardiology procedures: Part 2. *J Nucl Cardiol* 1999, 6:G49–G84.

7. Cerqueira MD, Weissman NJ, Dilsizian V, *et al.*: Standardized myocardial segmentation and nomenclature for tomographic imaging of the heart. *Circulation* 2002, 105:539–542.

8. Hachamovitch R, Berman DS, Shaw LJ, *et al.*: Incremental prognostic value of myocardial perfusion single photon emission computed tomography for the prediction of cardiac death. *Circulation* 1998, 97:535–543.

9. Liu YH, Sinusas AJ, Deman P, *et al.*: Quantification of SPECT myocardial perfusion images: Methodology and validation of the Yale-CQ method. *J Nucl Cardiol* 1999, 6:190–203.

10. Wackers FJTh: The clinical importance of quantification of stress-rest SPECT radionuclide myocardial perfusion images. *ACC Curr J Rev* 1999, 8:65–70.

11. Ritchie JL, Bateman TM, Bonow RO, *et al.*: Guidelines for the clinical use of cardiac radionuclide imaging: a report of the American College of Cardiology/American Heart Association Task Force on assessment of diagnostic and therapeutic procedures (Committee on Radionuclide Imaging). *J Am Coll Cardiol* 1995, 25:521–547; *J Nucl Cardiol* 1995, 2:172–192.

12. Maddahi J, Van Train K, Prigent F, *et al.*: Quantitative single photon emission computed thallium-201 tomography for detection and localization of coronary artery disease: optimization and prospective validation of a new technique. *J Am Coll Cardiol* 1989, 14:1689.

13. Fintel DJ, Links JM, Brinker JA, *et al.*: Improved diagnostic performance of exercise thallium-201 single photon emission computed tomography over planar imaging in the diagnosis of coronary artery disease: A receiver operating characteristic analysis. *J Am Coll Cardiol* 1989, 13:600, 1989.

14. Iskandrian AS, Heo J, Kong B, *et al.*: Effect of exercise level on the ability of thallium-201 tomographic imaging in detecting coronary artery disease: analysis of 461 patients. *J Am Coll Cardiol* 1989, 14:1477.

15. Go RT, Marwick TH, MacIntyre WJ, *et al.*: A prospective comparison of rubidium-82 PET and thallium-201 SPECT myocardial perfusion imaging utilizing a single dipyridamole stress in the diagnosis of coronary artery disease. *J Nucl Med* 1990, 31:1899.

16. Mahmarian JJ, Boyce, Goldberg RK, *et al.*: Quantitative exercise thallium-201 single photon emission computed tomography for the enhanced diagnosis of ischemic heart disease. *J Am Coll Cardiol* 1990, 15:318.

17. van Train KF, Maddahi J, Berman DS, *et al.*: Quantitative analysis of tomographic stress thallium-201 myocardial scintigrams: A multicenter trial. *J Nucl Med* 1990, 31:1168.

18. Kiat H, Maddahi J, Roy L, *et al.*: Comparison of technetium 99m methoxy isobutyl isonitrile and thallium-201 for evaluation of coronary artery disease by planar and tomographic methods. *Am Heart J* 1989, 117:111.

19. Iskandrian AS, Heo J, Long B, *et al.*: Use of technetium-99m isonitrile (RP-30A) in assessing left ventricular perfusion and function at rest and during exercise in coronary artery disease, and comparison with coronary arteriography and exercise thallium-201 SPECT imaging. *Am J Cardiol* 1989, 64:270.

20. Kahn JK, McGhie I, Akers MS, *et al.*: Quantitative rotational tomography ^{201}Tl and ^{99m}Tc 2-methoxly-isobutyl-isonitrile. *Circulation* 1989, 79:1282.

21. Solot G, Hermans J, Merlo P, *et al.*: Correlation of 99Tcm-sestamibi SPECT with coronary angiography in general hospital practice. *Nucl Med Commun* 1993, 14:23.

22. Van Train KF, Garcia EV, Maddahi J, *et al.*: Multicenter trial validation for quantitative analysis of same-day rest-stress technetium-99m-sestamibi myocardial tomograms. *J Nucl Med* 1994, 35:609.

23. Azzarelli S, Galassi AR, Foti R, *et al.*: Accuracy of 99m-tetrofosmin myocardial tomography in the evaluation of coronary artery disease. *J Nucl Cardiol* 1999, 6:183.

CHAPTER 5

PET Quantitation of Myocardial Blood Flow

Heinrich R. Schelbert and Maria Angela Oxilia-Estigarribia

Positron-emission tomography affords the noninvasive measurement of regional myocardial blood flow in units of milliliters of blood per minute per gram myocardium. With this capability, PET expands the diagnostic possibilities of more traditional nuclear medicine approaches for explaining the human heart's function and for identifying abnormalities in cardiovascular disease. More conventional nuclear medicine approaches, *eg*, SPECT, delineate the relative distribution of myocardial blood flow at rest or during physical or pharmacologically induced stress. While accurately identifying flow-limiting coronary stenoses, their location, and extent, such evaluations of the relative distribution of myocardial blood flow have remained incomplete for two reasons. First, myocardial regions with the highest radiotracer uptake are defined as normal on the images when, in fact, they may be subtended by diseased coronary arteries. Second, evaluating only the relative distribution of myocardial blood flow may fail to uncover balanced coronary artery stenosis or identify coronary artery disease still without flow-limiting stenosis. The flow tracer may distribute homogeneously throughout the left ventricular myocardium, while myocardial blood flow in absolute units may be abnormal. It is now widely accepted that the majority of acute coronary events originate in coronary vessels without significant angiographic stenosis. Therefore, identification of such preclinical disease could prove clinically important. Recognition of early coronary disease could prove clinically relevant because coronary risk factor modification may significantly diminish cardiac risk. Findings through quantitative measurements of myocardial blood flow might thus identify individuals at risk or provide a strong rationale for therapeutic interventions and, at the same time, provide a means for monitoring their efficacy.

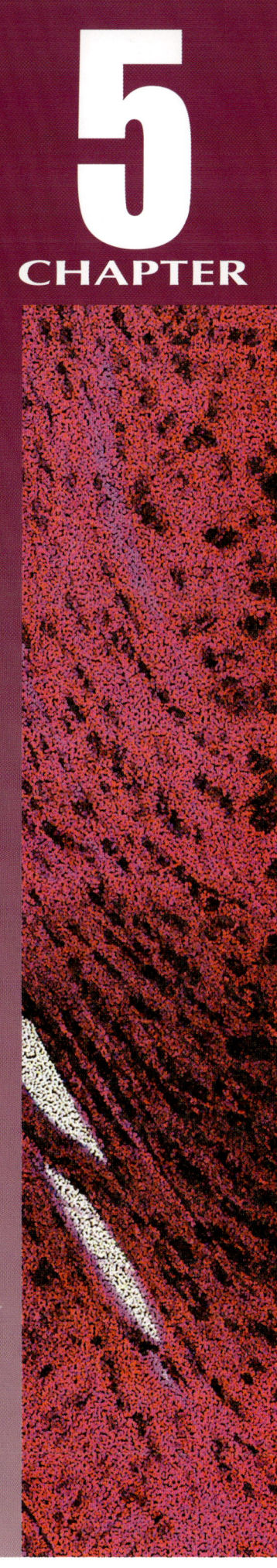

Methodology

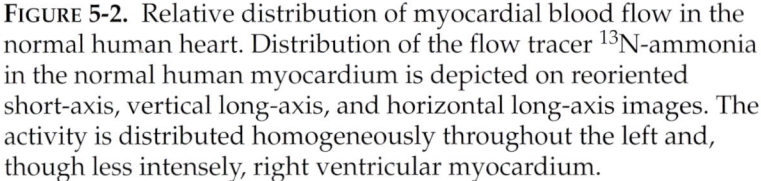

FIGURE 5-1. Positron-emitting tracers of myocardial blood flow. Several positron-emitting tracers of myocardial blood flow are available. Their ultra-short physical half-life allows serial measurements at time intervals ranging from 8 to 50 minutes. Retention of these positron-emitting flow tracers follows myocardial blood flow, generally in a curvilinear fashion. In the low-flow range, myocardial tracer concentrations rise steeply with increases in myocardial blood flow, while flow increases in the hyperemic flow range are associated with progressively smaller increments in flow tracer concentrations. Tracer compartment models describe the kinetics of the radiotracer in blood and tissue relative to myocardial blood flow and correct for the flow-dependent, nonlinear tracer uptake in the myocardium. Measurements of myocardial blood flow are performed through intravenous administration of the flow tracer, acquisition of serial images or dynamic imaging of the tracer transit through the central circulation and accumulation of the tracer in the myocardium, determination of the arterial tracer input function and the myocardial tissue response from regions of interest assigned to the left ventricular blood pool and the left ventricular myocardium, and, finally, fitting of the resulting time-activity curves with the tracer compartment model.

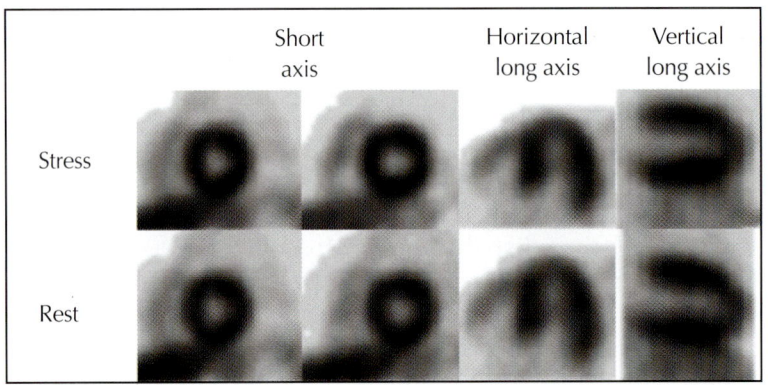

FIGURE 5-2. Relative distribution of myocardial blood flow in the normal human heart. Distribution of the flow tracer ^{13}N-ammonia in the normal human myocardium is depicted on reoriented short-axis, vertical long-axis, and horizontal long-axis images. The activity is distributed homogeneously throughout the left and, though less intensely, right ventricular myocardium.

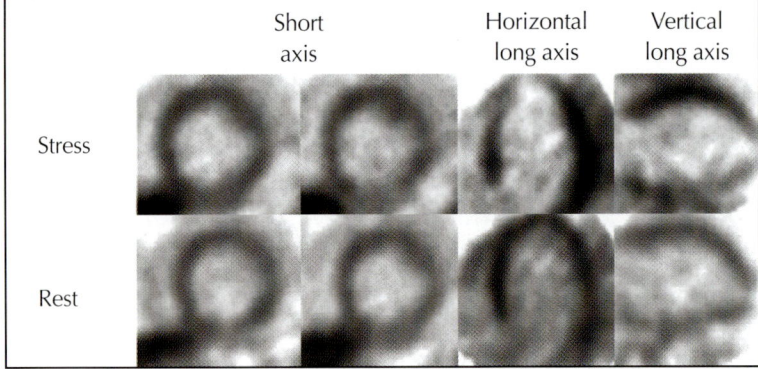

FIGURE 5-3. Relative distribution of myocardial blood flow in a patient with coronary artery disease. Distribution of the flow tracer ^{13}N-ammonia in the myocardium is depicted on reoriented short-axis, vertical long-axis, and horizontal long-axis images. The diminished tracer concentrations in the anterior and the anteroseptal wall and the anterior septum of the left ventricular myocardium reflect a flow defect resulting from an 85% diameter stenosis of the left anterior descending coronary artery. Relative myocardial perfusion appears best preserved in the lateral wall. However, a 50% diameter stenosis of the left circumflex coronary artery remains unidentified on the perfusion images.

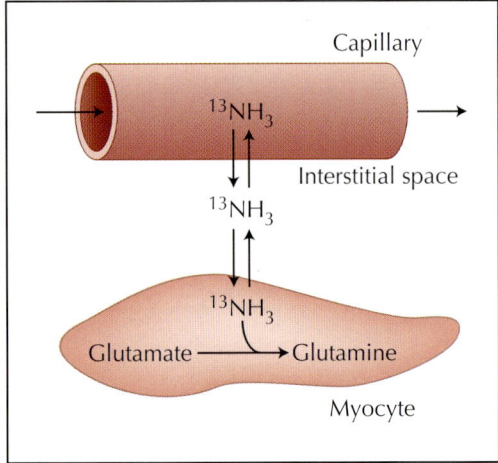

FIGURE 5-4. Myocardial tissue kinetics of the flow tracer ^{13}N-ammonia. Injected intravenously in minute, true-tracer quantities, ^{13}N-ammonia (^{13}NH$_3$) rapidly exchanges across the capillary wall, transits through the interstitial spaces, and reaches the myocardial cell. A fraction of tracer then diffuses back from tissue into blood while another fraction becomes metabolically trapped and retained in the myocardium through the α-ketoglutarate-to-glutamate and the glutamate-to-glutamine reactions [1]. Over the 10- to 20-minute duration of serial image acquisition required for flow measurements, myocardial ^{13}N-ammonia concentrations remain constant without loss of the ^{13}N-labeled glutamine from the myocardium.

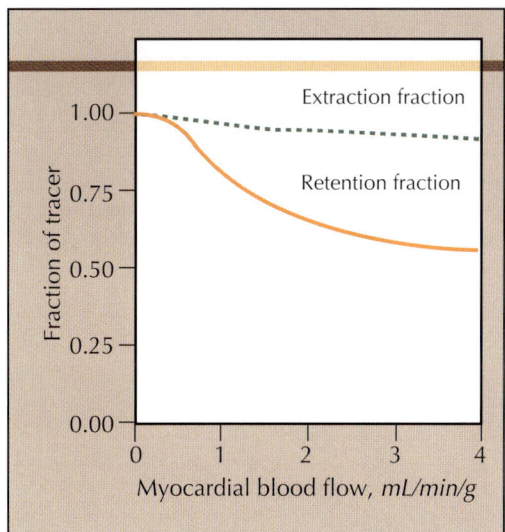

FIGURE 5-5. First-pass extraction and retention fractions of flow tracers. The first-pass extraction fraction, defined as the fraction of tracer that crosses the capillary membrane during the first transit through the coronary circulation, approaches unity for ^{13}N-ammonia and does not significantly decline with higher flow velocities [1]. Back diffusion of tracer from tissue to blood increases with higher flows, however, so that an increasingly smaller fraction becomes available for metabolic trapping and the first-pass retention fraction progressively declines with higher coronary flows.

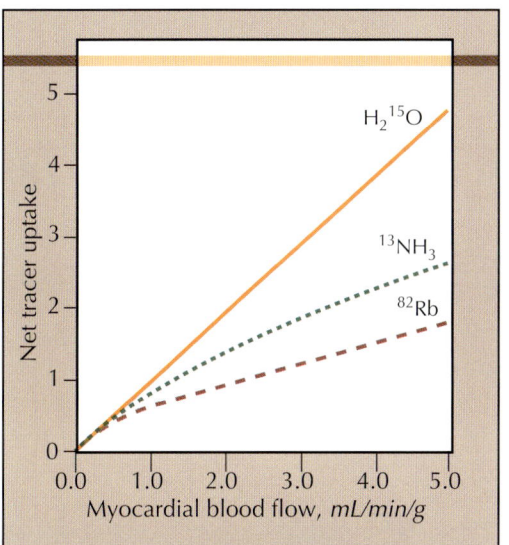

FIGURE 5-6. Net myocardial tracer uptake and myocardial blood flow. The net myocardial uptake of a tracer is the product of the first-pass retention fraction of the tracer and of myocardial blood flow, *eg*, the amount of tracer delivered to the myocardium. Because the first-pass extraction fraction for ^{15}O-water ($H_2{}^{15}O$) approaches 1 and is independent of blood flow, its net uptake increases linearly with myocardial blood flow. In contrast, the net uptake of ^{13}N-ammonia ($^{13}NH_3$) and rubidium-82 (^{82}Rb) increases nonlinearly with higher flows. For the same flow, the net uptake of $^{13}NH_3$ is higher than that of ^{82}Rb because of its higher first-pass extraction fraction.

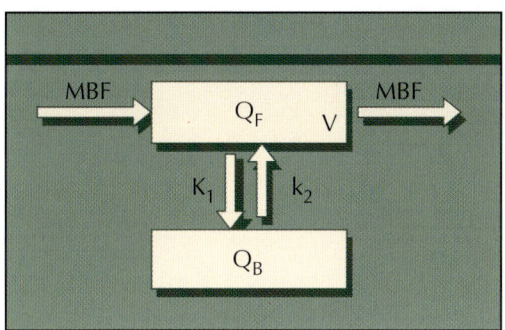

FIGURE 5-7. Tracer compartment model. Tracer compartment models are fundamental for establishing operational equations that permit estimates of myocardial blood flow (MBF). The tracer kinetic model, shown here for the flow tracer ^{13}N-ammonia, describes quantitatively the exchange of tracer between blood and tissue and within tissue in terms of functional compartments of different sizes or volumes of distribution (V) of that tracer [2,3]. The amount of radiotracer Q_F present at any time after tracer injection in freely diffusible form is shown in the *upper box*, the first compartment. Because the first-pass extraction fraction of ^{13}N-ammonia approaches unity, freely diffusible tracer present in blood, interstitium, and the cell is "lumped" into a single functional compartment. The metabolically trapped tracer activity (Q_B) is described in the *bottom box*, the second compartment. Forward and reverse (back diffusion) tracer exchange between the two functional compartments is described by first-order rate constants, or k_1 and k_2. The product of the forward rate constant k_1 and the concentration (or mass) of ^{13}N-ammonia then describes the mass flux of ^{13}N-ammonia from blood into tissue (K_1).

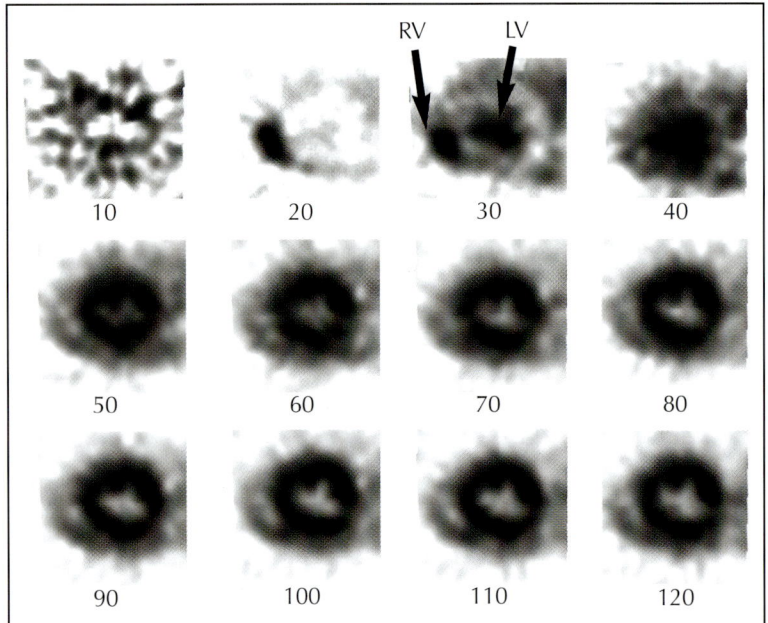

Figure 5-8. Transit of a ^{13}N-ammonia bolus through the central circulation. The serially acquired 10-second short-axis images illustrate the transit of the intravenous radiotracer bolus through the central circulation. The early images depict the tracer activity predominantly in the right heart, followed by dispersion of the tracer bolus into both lungs, return into the left ventricular (LV) cavity, and subsequent clearance of tracer activity from arterial blood into the myocardium. The late static image depicts the tracer activity retained in the LV myocardium after the radiotracer largely has disappeared from the blood. RV—right ventricle.

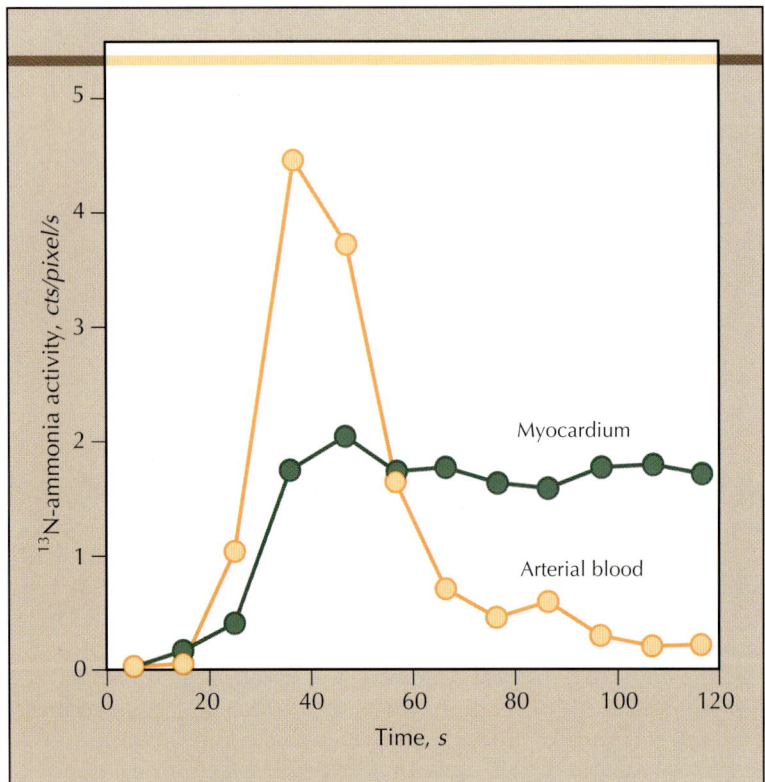

Figure 5-9. Arterial radiotracer input function and myocardial tissue response. From regions of interest assigned to the left ventricular blood pool and the left ventricular myocardium on the serially acquired images, time-activity curves are derived that describe the changes in radiotracer activity in arterial blood and in myocardium as a function of time. Through fitting of the time-activity curves with the operational equation formulated from the tracer kinetic model, estimates of myocardial blood flow in units of milliliters of blood per minute per gram myocardium are obtained.

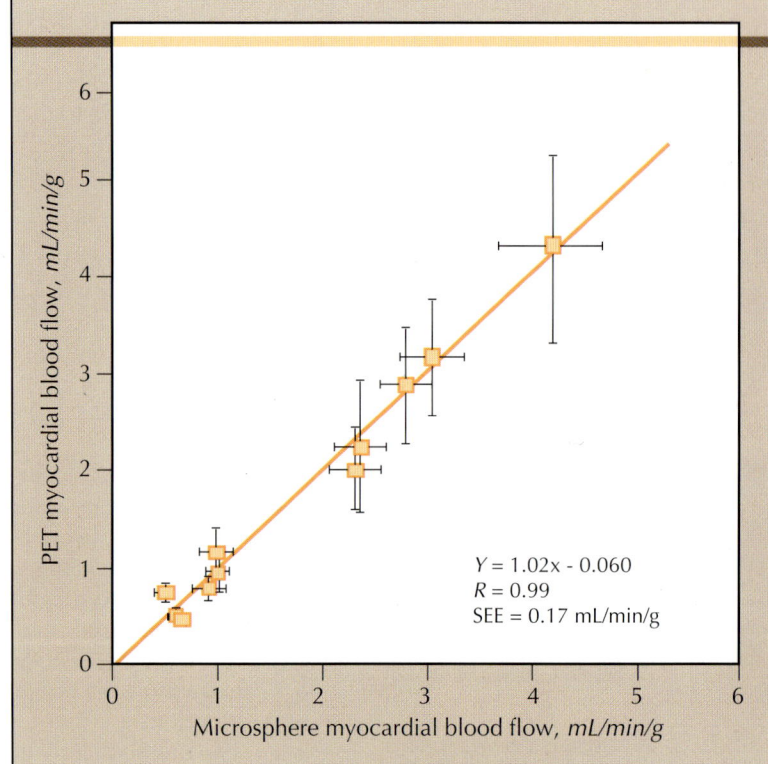

Figure 5-10. Validation of PET-based measurements of myocardial blood flow. Comparison of myocardial blood flows measured simultaneously with intravenous ^{13}N-ammonia and PET and with radiolabeled microspheres injected into the left ventricular cavity and postmortem tissue counting in dog experiments is shown [3]. The error bars indicate the standard deviations of the segmental blood flow relative to the mean left ventricular myocardial blood flow. SEE—standard error of the estimate.

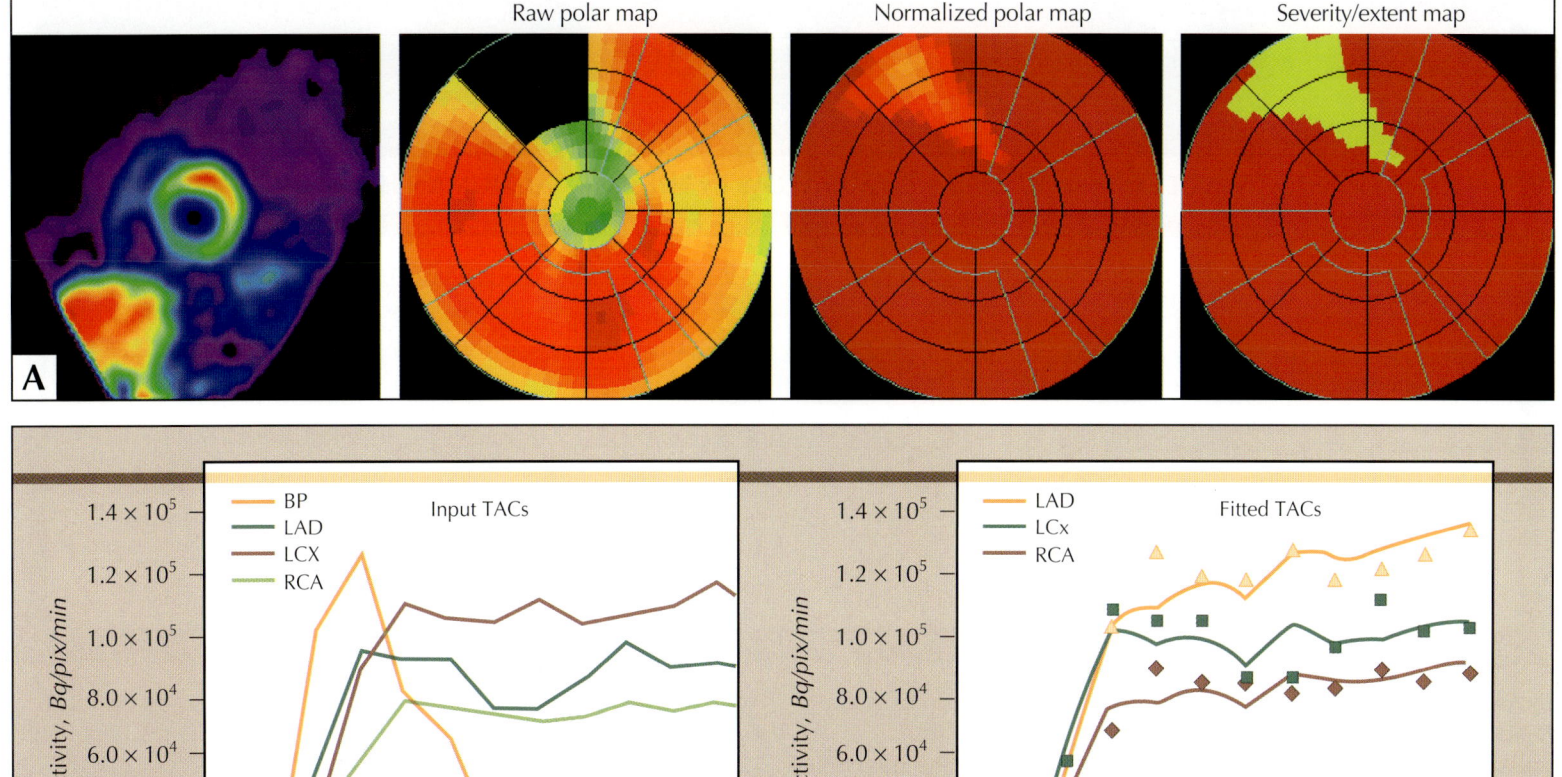

FIGURE 5-11. Polar map approach for estimating regional myocardial blood flow. Software algorithms facilitate determinations of myocardial blood flow. **A,** The last of the serially acquired transaxial images is reoriented into short-axis slices (*left*). The images are assembled into a polar map of the relative distribution of the flow tracer in the left ventricular myocardium. Regions of interest are assigned to the territories of the three coronary arteries (left anterior descending coronary artery [LAD], left circumflex coronary artery [LCX], and right coronary arteries [RCA]) and to the center of the left ventricular cavity (BP). The reorientation parameters are then applied to the serially acquired images. The regions of interest are copied to the serial polar maps. **B,** Time-activity curves (TAC) for each coronary artery territory are fitted with the tracer compartment model so that estimates of regional myocardial blood flows are obtained. In this example, flow is estimated for a region of interest corresponding to a stress-induced flow defect in the territory of the LAD and the entire LCX and RCA territories.

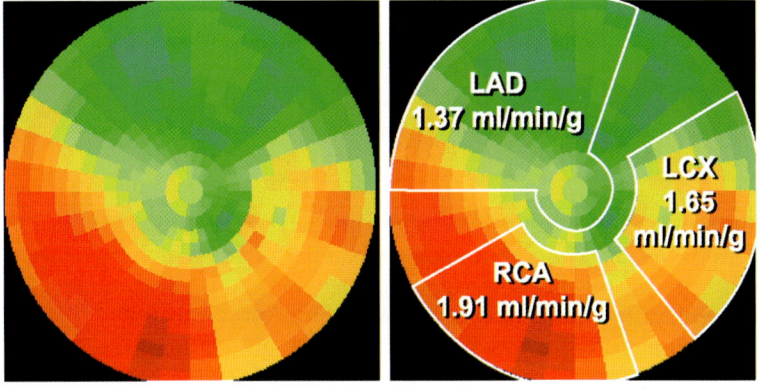

FIGURE 5-12. Polar map of myocardial tracer activity concentrations in a patient with coronary artery disease. The stress myocardial perfusion polar map depicts a flow defect in the territory of the left anterior descending coronary artery (LAD) and the left circumflex coronary artery (LCX) (*green, light yellow*). Myocardial blood flow during adenosine hyperemia in the LAD is 1.37 mL/min/g, in the LCX territory 1.65 mL/min/g, and 1.91 mL/min/g in the RCA territory. The myocardial flow reserve and the apparently "normal" RCA territory is only 2.2 and thus diminished when compared to flow reserves in normal volunteers.

Findings in the Normal Heart

VALUES OF MYOCARDIAL BLOOD FLOW IN THE NORMAL HUMAN HEART

STUDY	N	AGE, y	METHOD	REST MBF, ML/G/MIN	STRESS MBF, ML/G/MIN	FLOW RESERVE
Bergmann et al. [4]	11	25.5	$H_2{}^{15}O$	0.90 ± 0.22	3.55 ± 1.15	4.1 ± 1.2
Araujo et al. [5]	11	26 ± 7	$H_2{}^{15}O$	0.84 ± 0.09	3.52 ± 1.12	4.2 ± 1.3
Pitkänen et al. [6]	20	31 ± 8	$H_2{}^{15}O$	0.83 ± 0.13	4.49 ± 1.27	5.4 ± 1.5
Yokoyama et al. [7]	13	56 ± 7	$H_2{}^{15}O$	0.80 ± 0.39	2.92 ± 1.66	3.7 ± 1.4
Kaufmann et al. [8]	21	45 ± 8	$H_2{}^{15}O$	0.89 ± 0.15	3.51 ± 0.45	NR
Tadamura et al. [9]	20	23 ± 3	$H_2{}^{15}O$	0.67 ± 0.16	4.33 ± 1.23	NR
Hutchins et al. [10]	7	24 ± 4	$^{13}NH_3$	0.88 ± 0.17	4.17 ± 1.12	4.8 ± 1.3
Chan et al. [11]	20	35 ± 16	$^{13}NH_3$	1.10 ± 0.20	4.3 ± 1.3	4.0 ± 1.3
Czernin et al. [12]	18	31 ± 9	$^{13}NH_3$	0.76 ± 0.25	3.0 ± 0.8	4.1 ± 0.9

FIGURE 5-13. Values of myocardial blood flow in the normal human heart. Estimates of myocardial blood flow (MBF) in healthy volunteers at rest and during pharmacologically induced hyperemia and myocardial flow reserves as reported in several investigations (method, measurement of MBF with ^{15}O-water [$H_2{}^{15}O$] or ^{13}N-ammonia [$^{13}NH_3$]) are shown. Although generally of similar magnitude, considerable interindividual variations are observed for both rest and hyperemic MBF. MBF at rest largely depends on oxygen demand and, thus, on cardiac work, estimated by the rate pressure product. Adenosine- or dipyridamole-stimulated hyperemic MBF represents the total integrated coronary vasodilator capacity as a function of vascular smooth muscle relaxation and of the flow-dependent, endothelium-mediated dilation of the resistance and the conductance vessels. Hyperemic flows further depend on the coronary driving pressure, on extravascular myocardial resistive forces, and on neurohumoral factors. NR—not reported.

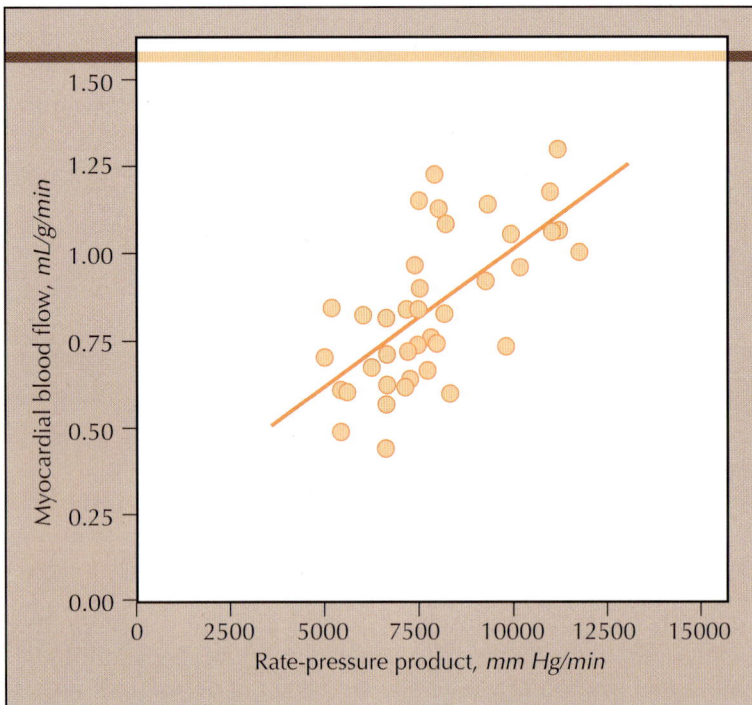

FIGURE 5-14. Dependency of myocardial blood flow at rest on cardiac work. In the normal myocardium, blood flows at rest correlate with cardiac work estimated by the rate-pressure product [12]. Such dependency of blood flows as determined with PET is consistent with findings through invasive techniques. It has prompted laboratories to normalize myocardial blood flows at rest to the rate-pressure product as a readily available index of cardiac work at the time of the blood flow measurement.

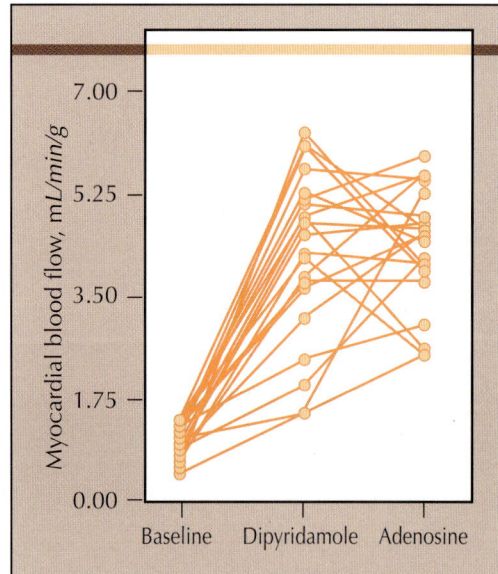

FIGURE 5-15. Pharmacologic stress and myocardial hyperemia. Direct vascular smooth muscle relaxants like adenosine (140 µg/kg/min) or dipyridamole (0.56 mg/kg infused intravenously over 4 minutes) are used to induce myocardial hyperemia in 20 healthy men. Both agents induce comparable hyperemic myocardial blood flows [11]. The mean group values are virtually identical for both hyperemic agents. However, individual responses vary greatly between the two vasodilator agents and, further, between individuals. Similar individual variations in the hyperemic flow response to adenosine or papaverine have been observed with independent invasive techniques, *eg*, intracoronary flow velocity probes [13].

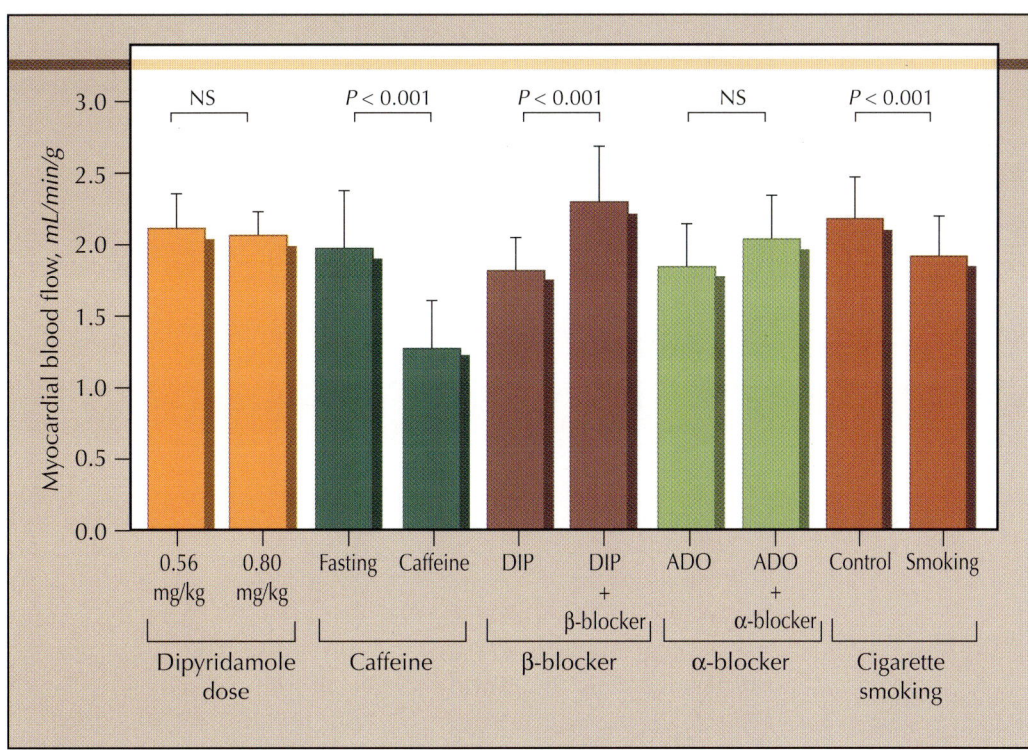

FIGURE 5-16. Determinants of pharmacologically induced hyperemia. Possible factors that might account for the interindividual variations in the response of myocardial blood flow to adenosine (ADO)- or dipyridamole (DIP)-stimulated vasodilation have been explored in several investigations. As depicted by the bars on the left, standard dose dipyridamole infusion (0.56 mg/kg) produces a maximum flow response; higher doses of dipyridamole (0.80 mg/kg) did not produce higher flows [14]. Caffeine significantly reduces the hyperemic flow response; dipyridamole flows were 35% lower after caffeine intake as compared to those after abstention from caffeine for 24 hours [15]. Indeed, the degree of attenuation of hyperemic blood flows correlates inversely with plasma caffeine concentrations. Adenosine- or dipyridamole-stimulated hyperemia further is augmented by administration of β-adrenergic blockers but not by α-adrenergic receptor blockers [16,17]. $α_2$-Adrenoreceptor stimulation with intravenous dobutamine raises myocardial blood flow in a dose-dependent manner and in proportion to cardiac work as defined again by the rate-pressure product [18,19]. Co-injection of atropine was found to augment dobutamine-induced hyperemia by as much as 36%, so that hyperemic myocardial blood flows exceeded those observed in the same study after dipyridamole [9]. Cigarette smoking during dipyridamole-induced hyperemia significantly reduced the level of hyperemic blood flows, most likely due to α-adrenergically mediated vasoconstriction [20].

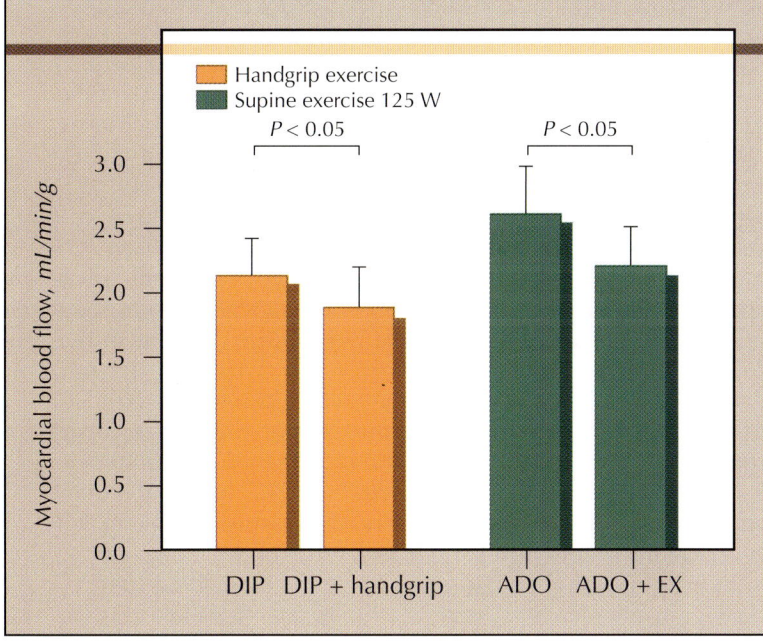

FIGURE 5-17. Coronary driving pressure and hyperemic myocardial blood flow. Increases in coronary perfusion pressures induced by either sustained handgrip or supine bicycle exercise (EX) lowered dipyridamole (DIP)-stimulated blood flows [14,21]. With handgrip, systolic arterial blood pressure rose from 123 ± 8 mm Hg to 147 ± 10 mm Hg and during supine exercise from 125 ± 17 mm Hg to 186 ± 24 mm Hg. Though unexpected, the decline in blood flow most likely resulted from an increase in extravascular resistive forces ascribed to higher systolic blood pressures and increased heart rates associated with physical exercise. ADO—adenosine.

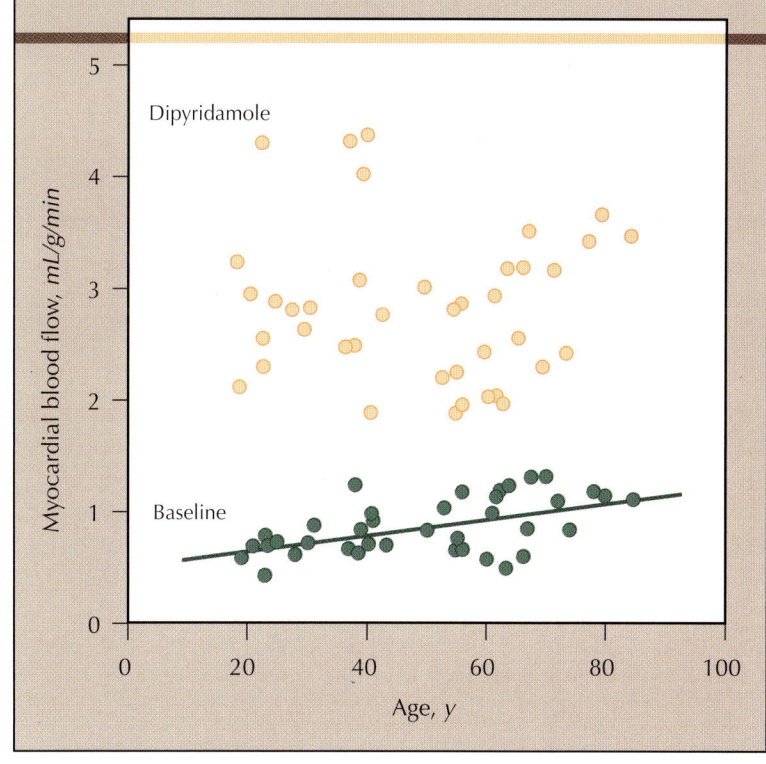

FIGURE 5-18. Age, myocardial blood flow, and myocardial flow reserve. Myocardial blood flows both at rest (*green circles*) and during dipyridamole-stimulated hyperemia (*orange circles*) are plotted as a function of age [12]. Myocardial blood flows at rest progressively increase with age. In this study, cardiac work as defined by the rate-pressure product similarly increased with age so that the age-dependency of myocardial blood flow appears most likely explained by an age-dependent increase in cardiac work. However, dipyridamole-stimulated hyperemic blood flows were independent of age in this study.

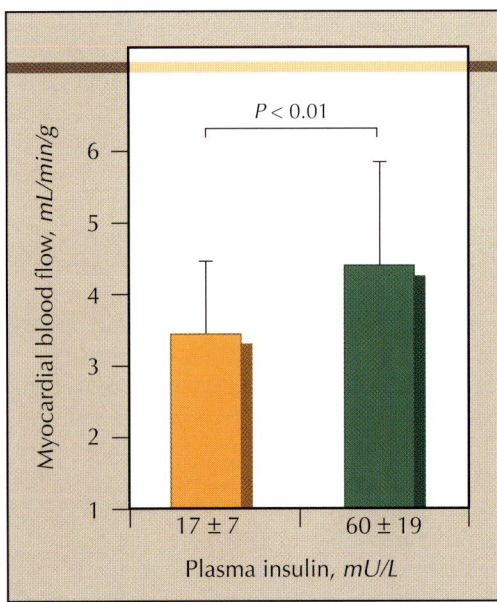

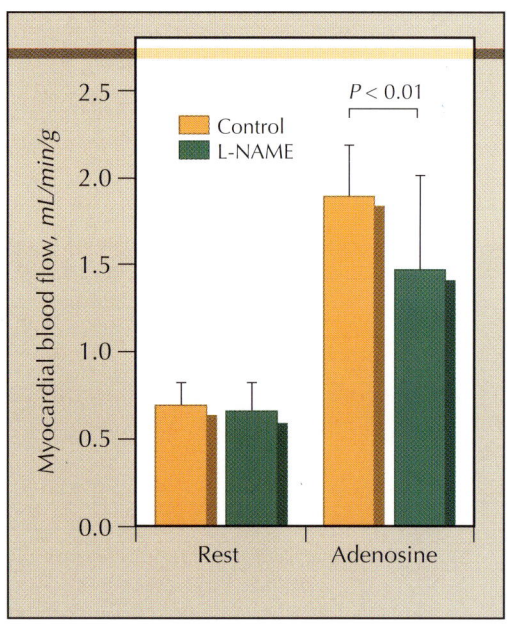

FIGURE 5-19. Insulin and pharmacologically induced hyperemic myocardial blood flows. Myocardial blood flow during pharmacologic vasodilation also depends on plasma insulin concentrations. In 16 healthy patients, myocardial blood flow during standard dose adenosine infusion was significantly lower than during the euglycemic-hyperinsulinemic clamp, which raised plasma insulin concentrations from 17 ± 7 to 60 ± 19 mU/L while plasma glucose levels remained essentially unchanged [22]. The effect of insulin on hyperemic myocardial blood flow appears to be dose-dependent, as indicated in another study in healthy men with supraphysiologic insulin plasma concentrations [23].

FIGURE 5-20. Inhibition of nitric oxide synthase and myocardial blood flow at rest and during adenosine-stimulated hyperemia. Intravenous administration of N^G-nitro-L-arginine methyl ester (L-NAME), an inhibitor of the nitric oxide synthase, in 12 healthy patients caused modest increases in mean arterial blood pressure and a decrease in heart rate but did not significantly change myocardial blood flow at rest [17]. In contrast, adenosine-stimulated hyperemic myocardial blood flows were 21% lower after L-NAME administration than at the time of the placebo study, implicating the coronary endothelium as a modulator of hyperemic myocardial blood flows.

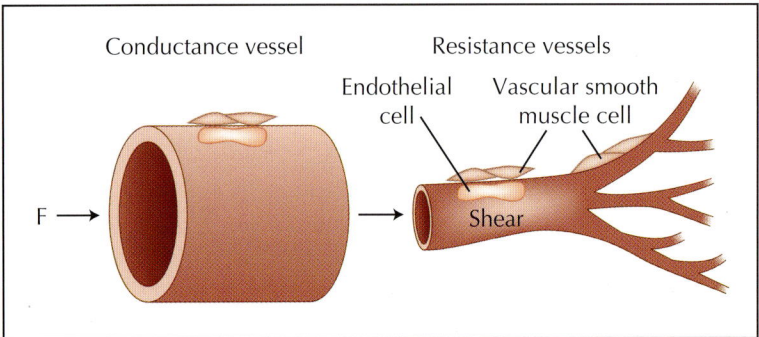

FIGURE 5-21. Schematic representation of coronary circulation. The coronary circulation has been viewed as a two-compartment system consisting of the large epicardial conductance and resistance vessels. In normal coronary circulation, the intraluminal pressure in the conductance vessels equals that in the aortic root (or the coronary driving pressure), but steeply declines within the resistance vessels to values moderately higher than those in the right atrium, so that a pressure gradient between the coronary circulation and the right atrium is maintained. Direct vascular smooth muscle dilation as affected through adenosine or dipyridamole lowers the resistance to flow. Acceleration of coronary flow (F) prompts a flow-dependent, endothelium-mediated additional dilation of the resistance vessels but also an approximately 15% to 25% flow-dependent increase in the diameter of the conductance vessels. This flow-dependent dilation of the conductance vessels offsets an increase in resistance to higher flow velocities. The total adenosine- or dipyridamole-stimulated hyperemic flows therefore reflect the total integrated vasodilator capacity of the coronary circulation. Factors that modify hyperemic myocardial blood flow in the normal heart include gender and age, cardiac work, the coronary driving pressure, heart rate, left ventricular diastolic and systolic pressures, effects of insulin, norepinephrine and epinephrine, and nitric oxide bioactivity.

Myocardial Blood Flow in Cardiovascular Disease

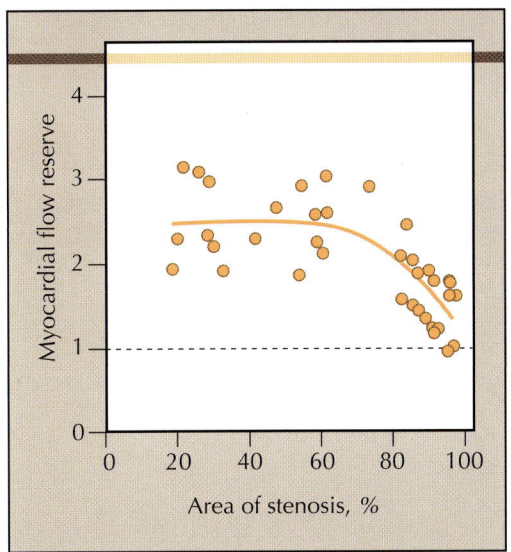

Figure 5-22. Angiographic coronary stenoses and myocardial blood flow. Comparison between stenosis severity defined as percent cross-sectional area reduction on quantitative angiography and the myocardial flow reserve as examined in 18 patients with coronary artery disease through measurements of regional myocardial blood flow at rest and during dipyridamole-stimulated hyperemia [24]. The curvilinear correlation is similar to the one observed in chronically instrumented dogs with idealized coronary stenosis [25].

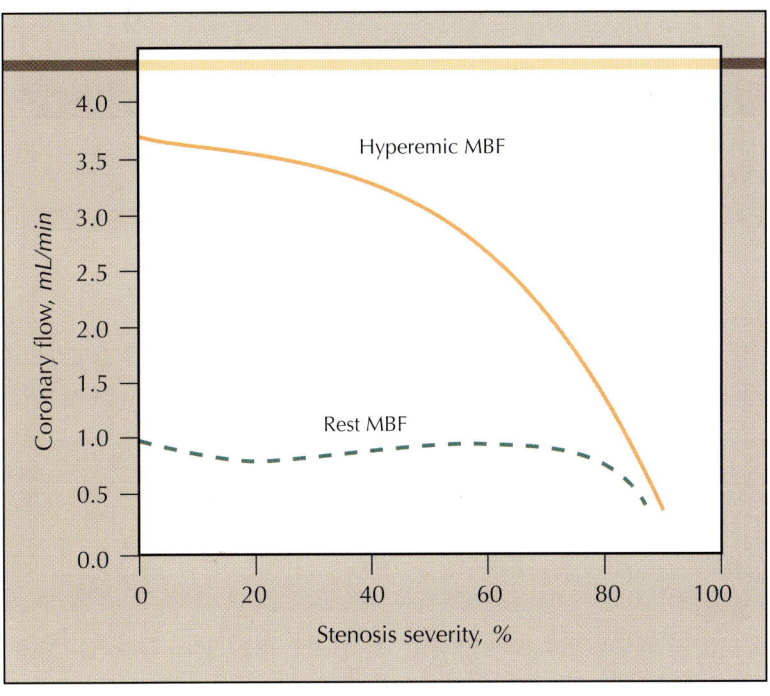

Figure 5-23. Classic correlation between severity of coronary stenoses and coronary blood flow velocities in dogs. Coronary blood flow was measured at rest and during contrast-induced hyperemia with Doppler flow velocity probes while stenosis severity was determined by quantitative angiography [25]. The findings in human coronary artery disease as shown in Figure 5-22 confirm the coronary flow–coronary stenosis relationship as established in experimental animals. Additional clinical studies with PET in patients have reported similar reductions in hyperemic blood in stenosis-dependent myocardium, but fail to find a similar curvilinear correlation [26,27]. This is most likely because this relationship was observed only for myocardium without collateral blood flow or without prior myocardial infarction and only after vessels with stenosis in series were excluded. MBF—myocardial blood flow.

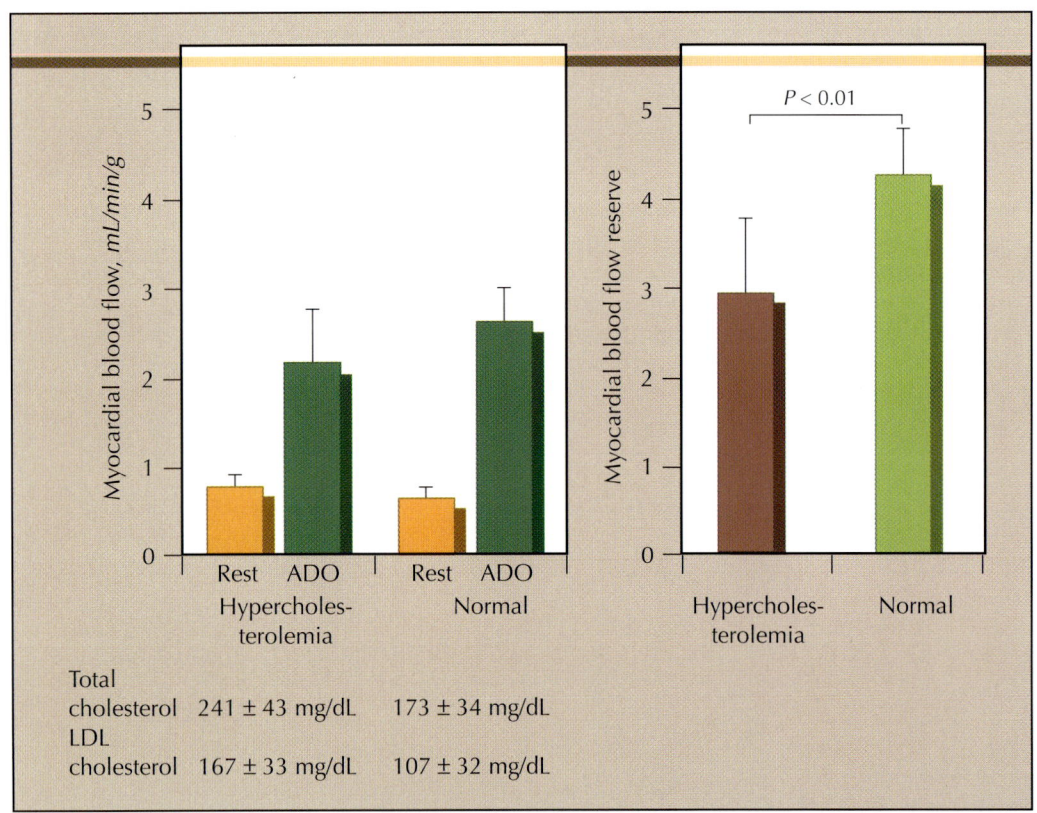

FIGURE 5-24. Diminished hyperemic blood flows in patients with coronary risk factors. In 16 middle-aged men (49.0 ± 0.5 years of age) with elevated plasma cholesterol levels but without clinical evidence of coronary artery disease, myocardial blood flow at rest was similar to that in an age-matched group of normals without coronary risk factors. However, during adenosine (ADO)-induced hyperemia, myocardial flows tended to be lower in the at-risk group than in the control group. Importantly, the myocardial flow reserve was significantly lower in the at-risk patients than in the normal control group [28]. LDL—low-density lipoprotein

REDUCED VASODILATOR CAPACITY IN PATIENTS WITH RISK FACTORS BUT WITHOUT ANGIOGRAPHIC CORONARY ARTERY DISEASE

| | | PATIENTS | | | CONTROLS | | | |
| | | MBF, mL/min/g | | | MBF, mL/min/g | | | |
STUDY	N	REST	STRESS	N	REST	STRESS	DIFFERENTIAL, %	P VALUE
Dayanikli et al. [28]	16	0.76 ± 0.19	2.18 ± 0.56	11	0.66 ± 0.09	2.84 ± 0.39	−17	< 0.001
Pitkänen et al. [6]	15	0.92 ± 0.24	3.19 ± 1.59	20	0.83 ± 0.13	4.49 ± 1.27	−29	< 0.01
Yokoyama et al. [29]	11	0.70 ± 0.21	2.10 ± 0.71	11	0.75 ± 0.35	3.22 ± 1.64	−35	< 0.01
	11	0.81 ± 0.31	1.29 ± 0.19				−60	< 0.01
Pitkänen et al. [30]	21	0.79 ± 0.19	3.54 ± 1.59	21	0.88 ± 0.20	4.54 ± 1.17	−22	< 0.025

FIGURE 5-25. Reduced vasodilator capacity in patients with risk factors but without angiographic coronary artery disease. Rest and hyperemic myocardial blood flow (MBF) in patients without coronary artery disease but with coronary risk factors was studied by four investigators [6,28–30].

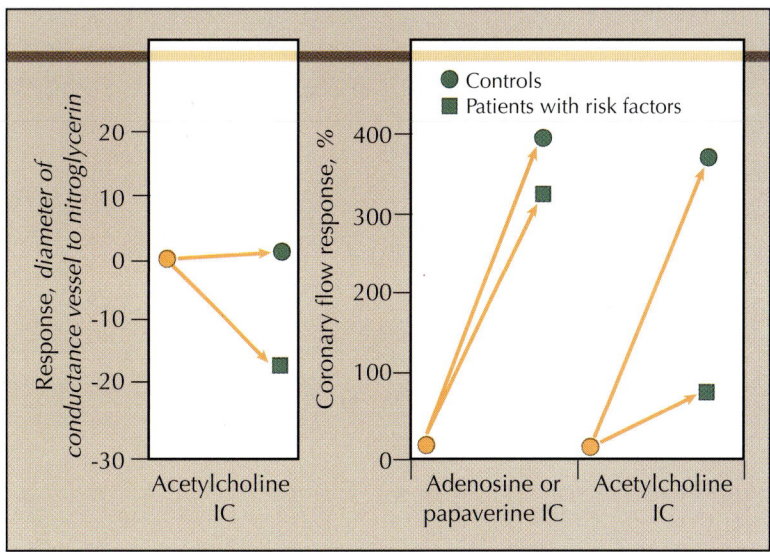

FIGURE 5-26. Coronary risk factors and coronary vasomotor function. The findings made with PET-based noninvasive measurements of myocardial blood flow appear consistent with those obtained through invasive techniques in patients with coronary risk factors but without angiographically significant coronary artery disease. These studies employed quantitative coronary angiography, intracoronary Doppler flow velocity probes, and intracoronary administration of vascular smooth muscle dilators (*eg*, adenosine or papaverine) and acetylcholine for testing endothelial function. In response to nitroglycerin, the conductance vessels dilated or remained unchanged in control patients but constricted in at-risk patients. Responses of coronary blood flow to direct vascular smooth muscle relaxation were fully preserved in patients with risk factors because flow increased as it did in the control group. However, intracoronary acetylcholine stimulation produced markedly attenuated increases in coronary flow velocities, indicating the presence of endothelial dysfunction associated with coronary risk factors [31].

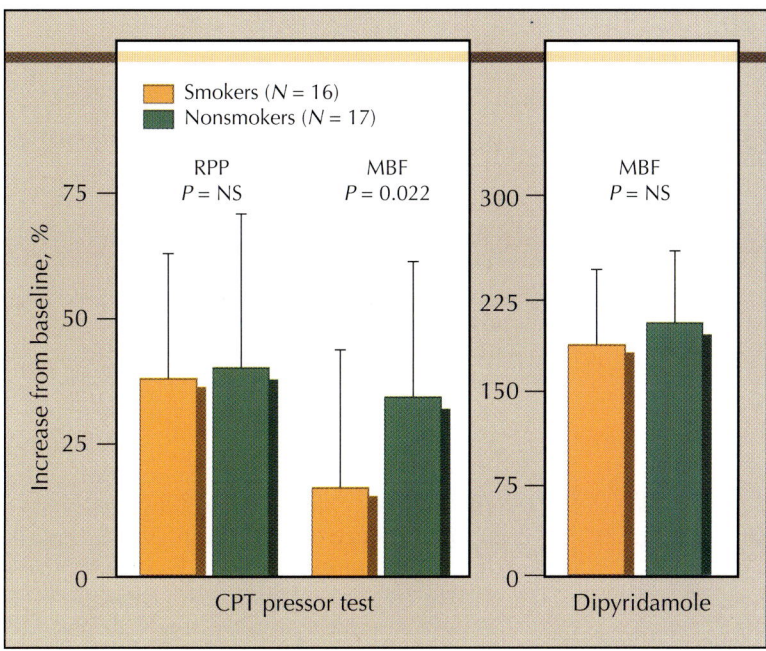

FIGURE 5-27. Coronary vasomotion in long-term smokers. In long-term smokers without clinical evidence of cardiovascular disease, myocardial blood flow (MBF) both at rest and during dipyridamole-induced hyperemia was similar to that in an age-matched control group of nonsmokers and thus was considered normal. Because of known adverse effects of nicotine and smoking byproducts on the endothelium, the response of MBF to cold pressor testing (CPT) as a means for more selectively examining or evaluating endothelial function was measured [32]. CPT promptly raised heart rate and systolic blood pressure, and the rate-pressure product (RPP) increased by approximately 40% to 50%. In the age-matched group of nonsmokers, MBF rose in proportion to the increase in cardiac work but did not in long-term smokers despite a normal increase in the RPP. NS—not significant.

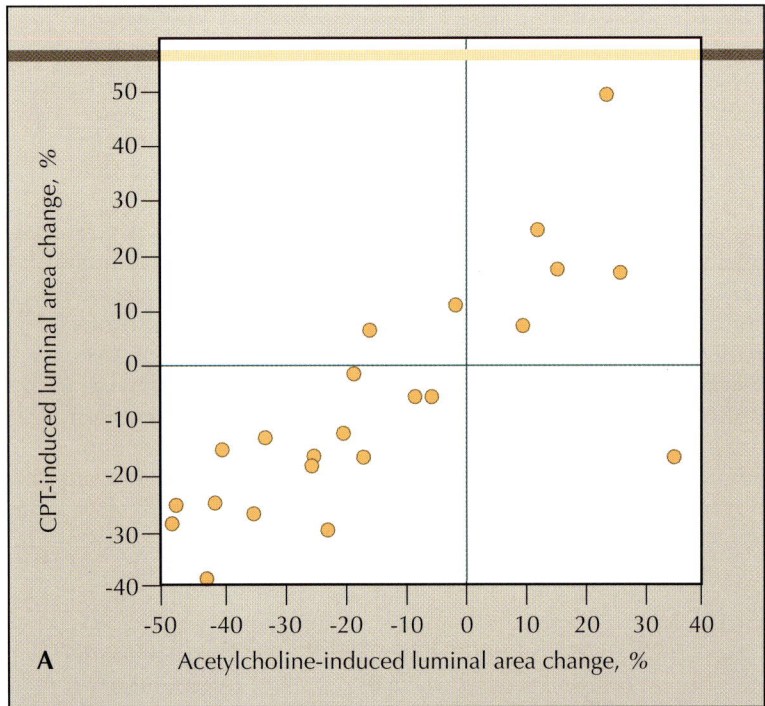
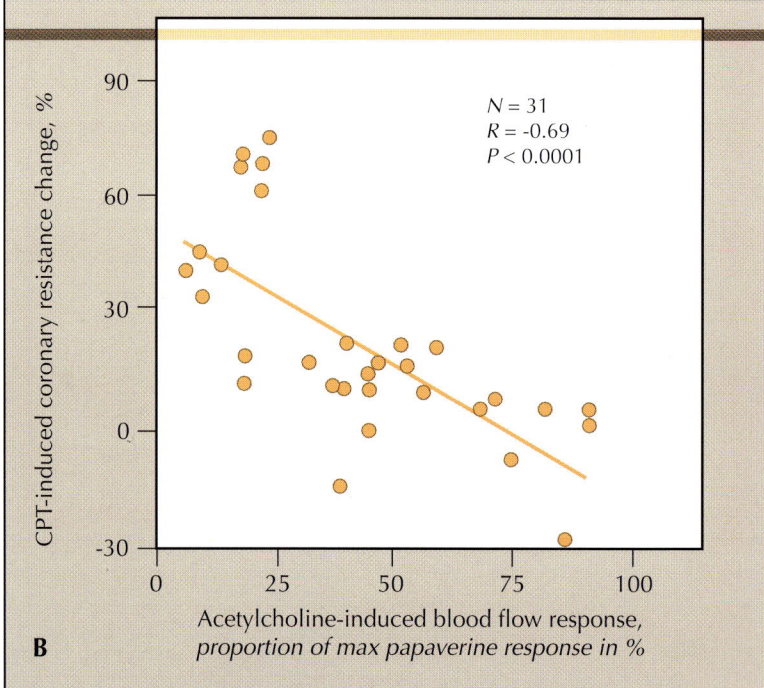
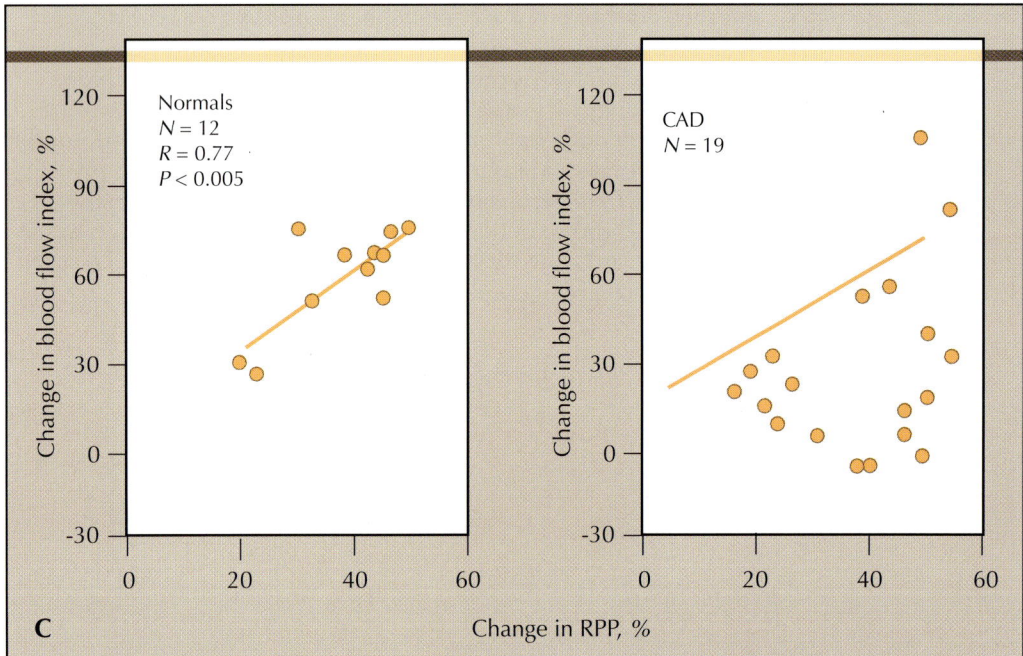

Figure 5-28. Flow responses to cold pressor testing (CPT) as a measure of endothelial function. The adrenergically mediated response of the coronary circulation to cold parallels several features linked directly to stimulation of the coronary endothelium as determined through invasive measurements. **A**, Increases in coronary flow associated with exposure to cold in the normal circulation lead to a flow-dependent dilation of the coronary conductance vessels. In abnormal states, the flow-dependent dilation is diminished or absent or paradoxical vasoconstriction may occur. These changes and their magnitude correlate directly with those evoked by intracoronary injection of acetylcholine or the flow-dependent, nitric oxide–mediated dilation of the conduit vessel in response to injections of papaverine or adenosine into the distal coronary circulation [33]. **B**, Acetylcholine stimulation raises flow in the normal coronary circulation, while flow responses in the presence of risk factors are diminished or even absent. Flow responses elicited by cold correlate with those in response to intracoronary acetylcholine stimulation [34–37]. **C**, Directly measured coronary flows increase in the normal coronary circulation in direct proportion to the increase in the rate-pressure product (RPP). In abnormal states, however, the responses in coronary blood flow to cold no longer correspond to changes in RPP; flow may increase only modestly, remain unchanged, or even decline in response to cold (*right panel*). *Continued on next page*

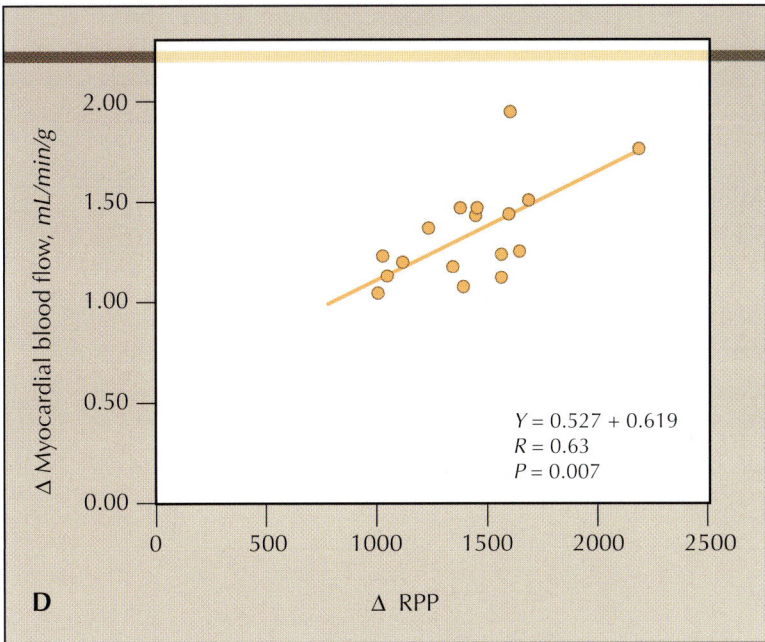

FIGURE 5-28. *(Continued)* **D**, Measurements of myocardial blood flow with PET in healthy patients reveal a similar increase in flow that again is proportionate to the cold-induced increase in the RPP. CAD—coronary artery disease.

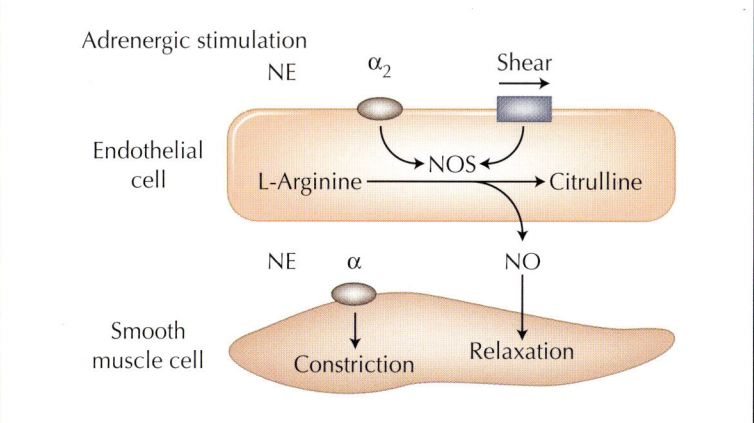

FIGURE 5-29. Cold pressor test. Coronary flow responses to cold depend on the close interaction between the endothelium and the vascular smooth muscle cell. Release of norepinephrine (NE) from adrenergic neuron terminals in response to adrenergic stimulation leads to predominantly α_2-adrenoreceptor–mediated vascular smooth muscle constriction. The increase in heart rate and blood pressure associated with cold-induced adrenergic stimulation is associated with an increase in coronary flow velocity, which in turn increases the shear stress-mediated greater availability of nitric oxide and, consequently, vascular smooth muscle relaxation. Norepinephrine-mediated stimulation of α-adrenoreceptors of the endothelium causes release of nitric oxide. Both shear stress and adrenergically mediated nitric oxide released from the endothelial cell oppose the vascular smooth muscle constriction. If the endothelium is dysfunctional, release of the vasodilating nitric oxide is diminished or even absent, so the vasoconstrictor effect of norepinephrine on the vascular smooth muscle cell prevails and coronary and myocardial blood flow do not increase or may even decline. NOS—nitric oxide synthase.

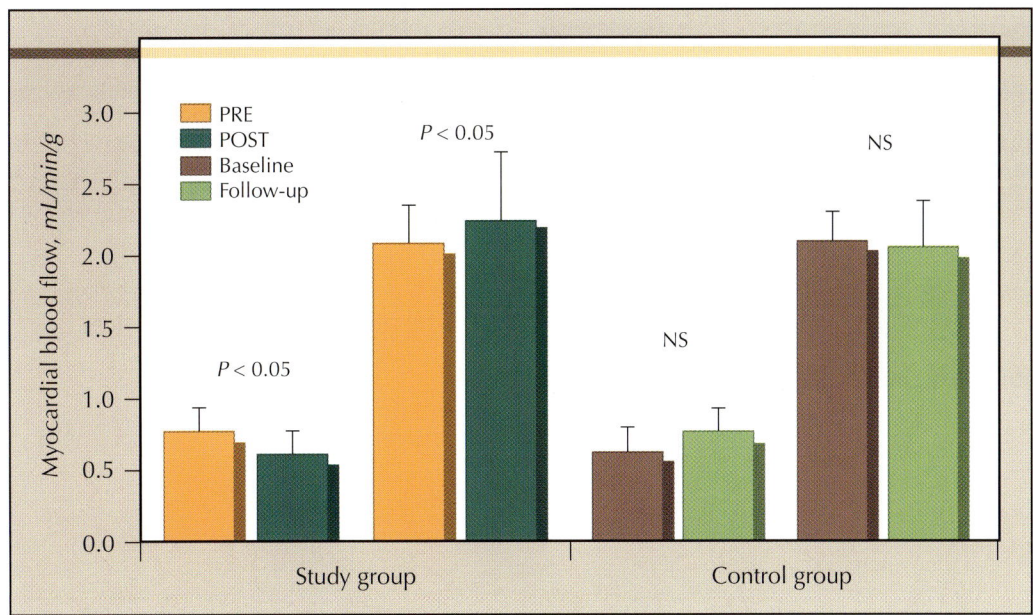

FIGURE 5-30. Cardiovascular conditioning and myocardial blood flow. Cardiovascular conditioning with six weeks of regular physical exercise, weight loss, and low cholesterol diet significantly improves myocardial flow reserve [38]. Myocardial blood flow at rest decreased moderately but significantly from baseline (PRE) to treatment (POST) in the study group of 13 patients but not in an age-matched control group. This most likely resulted from a decrease in the rate-pressure product that at follow-up was significantly lower than at baseline. Furthermore, dipyridamole-stimulated hyperemic myocardial blood flows increased significantly by an average of 9% from baseline to follow-up possibly because of lower systolic pressures and heart rates or lower plasma cholesterol levels or, alternatively, an improvement in the total vasodilator capacity.

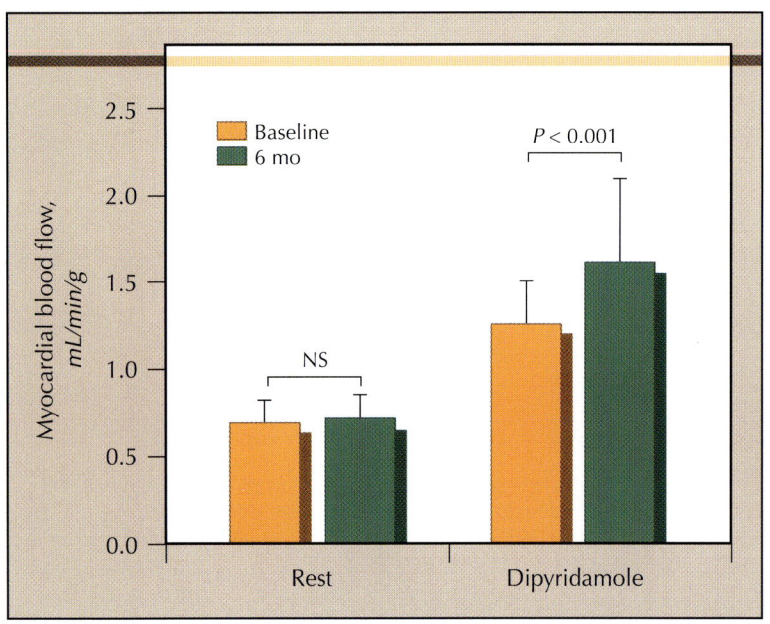

FIGURE 5-31. HMG CoA–reductase inhibitors and myocardial blood flow. In 23 hypercholesteremic patients with angiographically normal or minimally diseased coronary arteries, treatment with simvastatin for 6 months significantly lowered total and low-density lipid cholesterol levels (by 30% and 42%, respectively) while high-density lipid cholesterol increased [39]. At baseline, myocardial blood flow was normal at rest but markedly diminished during dipyridamole-induced hyperemia. After treatment, myocardial blood flow at rest was unchanged but hyperemic blood flows had increased by an average of 31%, so that the myocardial flow reserve approached near-normal values (from 2.2 ± 0.6 to 2.64 ± 0.06; $P < 0.01$). NS—not significant.

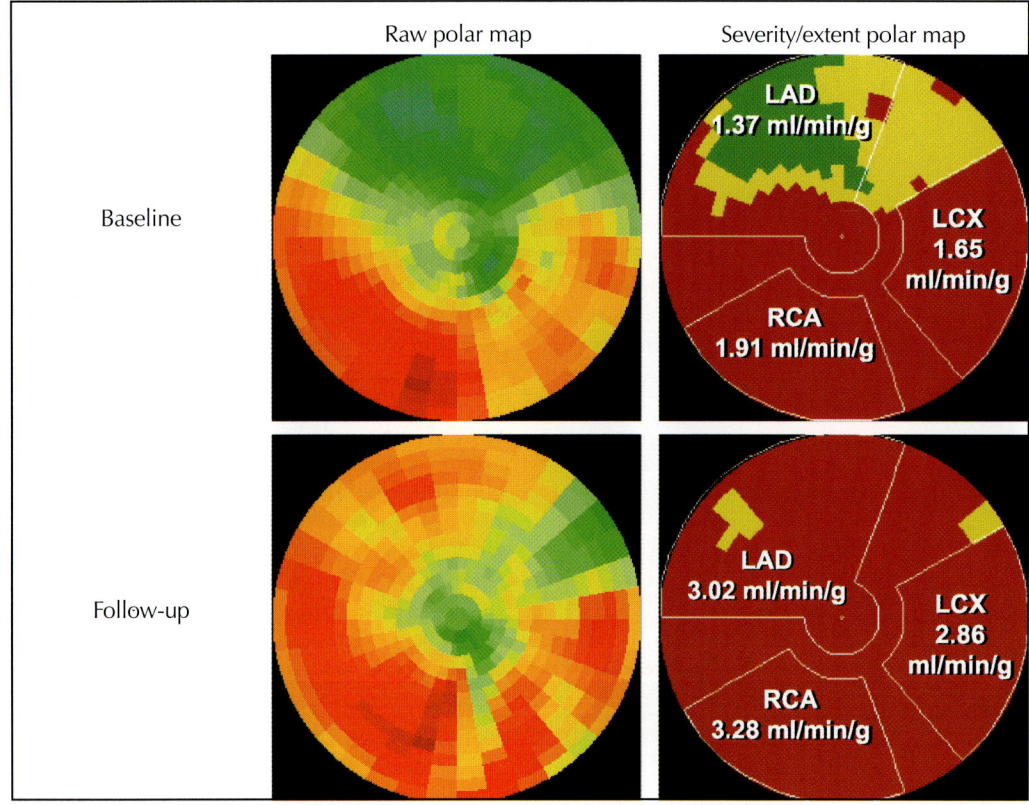

FIGURE 5-32. HMG CoA–reductase inhibitors and regional myocardial blood flow. Polar maps of the distribution of myocardial blood flow during adenosine-stimulated hyperemia in a patient with coronary artery disease at baseline and after 1 year of treatment with pravastatin. The extent of the stress-induced defect declined from 51% of the left anterior descending coronary artery (LAD) territory to only 3%. Myocardial blood flow in each of the three coronary artery territories increased and normalized in the region with a prior stress-induced defect. Only measurements of myocardial blood flow but not the evaluation of the relative distribution of the radiotracer uptake in the myocardium demonstrate the improvement in the flow reserve in remote or normal-appearing myocardium. LCX—left circumflex coronary artery; RCA—right coronary artery.

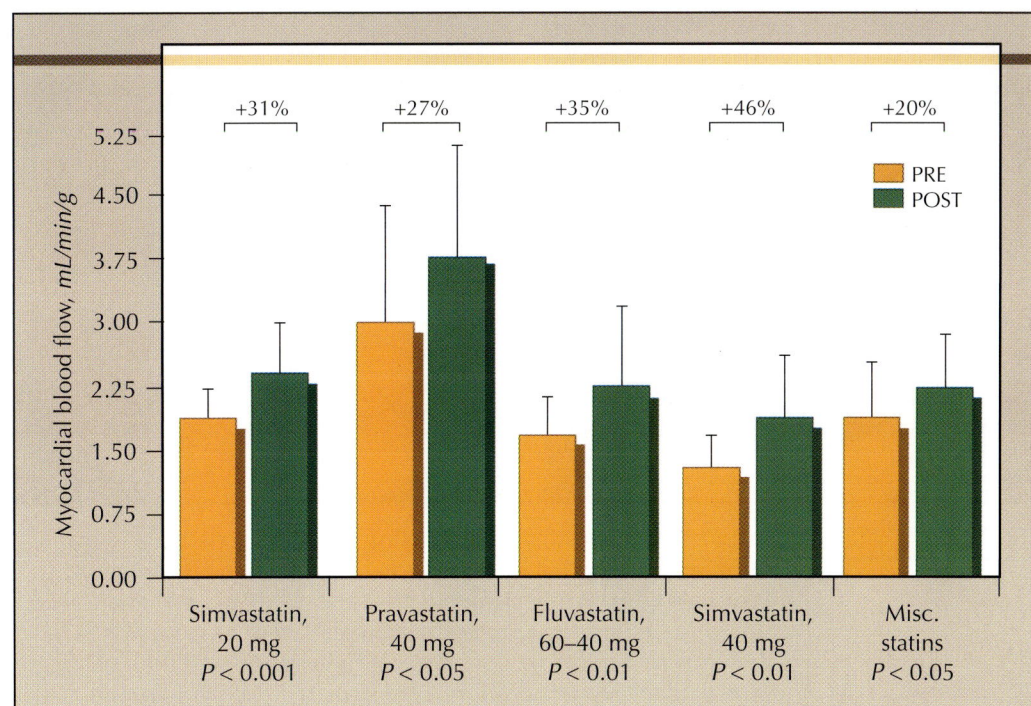

FIGURE 5-33. HMG CoA–reductase inhibitor treatment and myocardial blood flows in hypercholesteremia patients. Effects of HMG CoA–reductase inhibitor treatment on myocardial blood flow during dipyridamole- or adenosine-induced hyperemia in patients with and without coronary artery disease. Hyperemic myocardial blood flows after treatment (POST) are compared to those at baseline (PRE) for each study. The percent improvement in hyperemic myocardial blood flows in each study is indicated by the numbers above the columns [39–44]. The specific agent used in each of these studies and the daily dose are indicated below each pair of bars.

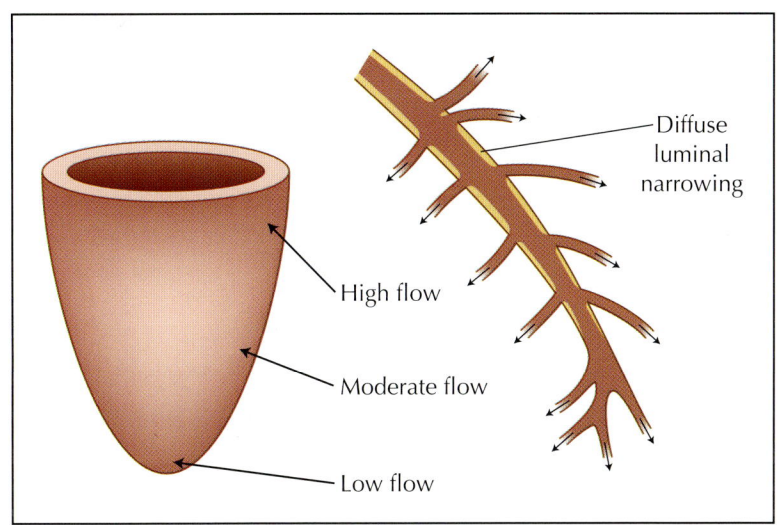

FIGURE 5-34. Diffuse coronary artery luminal narrowing and myocardial blood flow. Diffuse luminal narrowing of the epicardial conduit vessels can cause a longitudinal base to apex myocardial perfusion gradient [45,46]. Because resistance to flow through the conduit vessel relates according to the Hagen-Poiseuille equation to the 4th power of the radius, the intracoronary pressure may decline progressively along the epicardial vessels from proximal to distal so that the perfusion pressure significantly declines in myocardium in the distal distribution of the coronary arteries. Such longitudinal perfusion can be especially prominent during hyperemic blood flows when resistance to coronary flow is especially high and accentuated if the conduit vessel does not dilate. (*Adapted from* Gould *et al.* [46].)

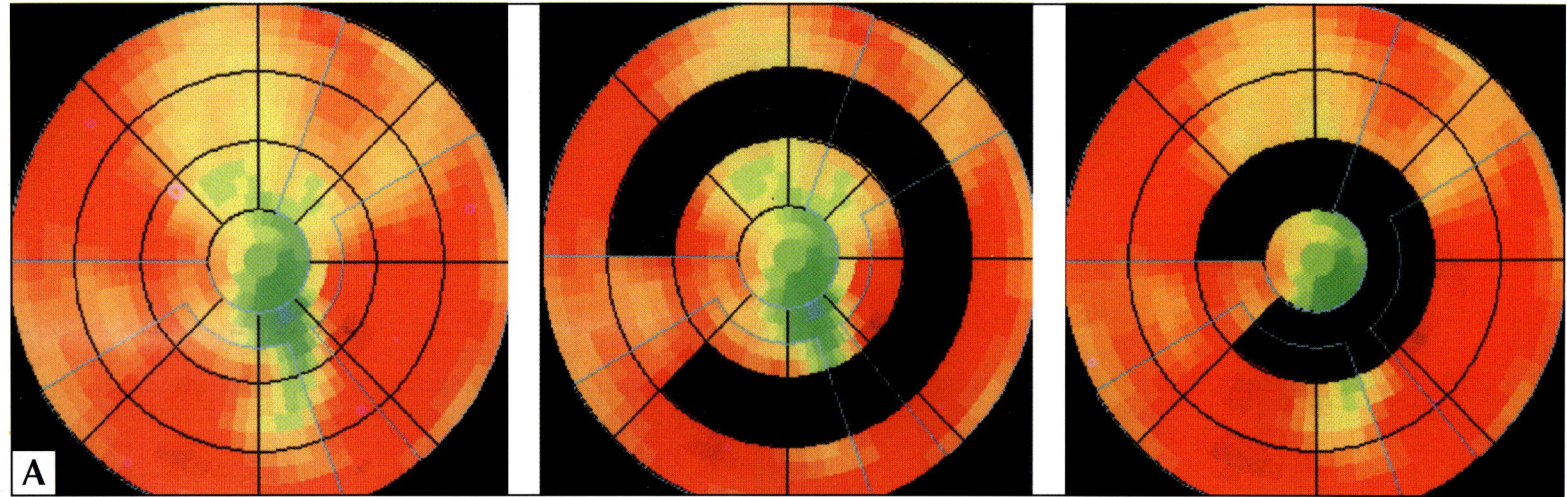

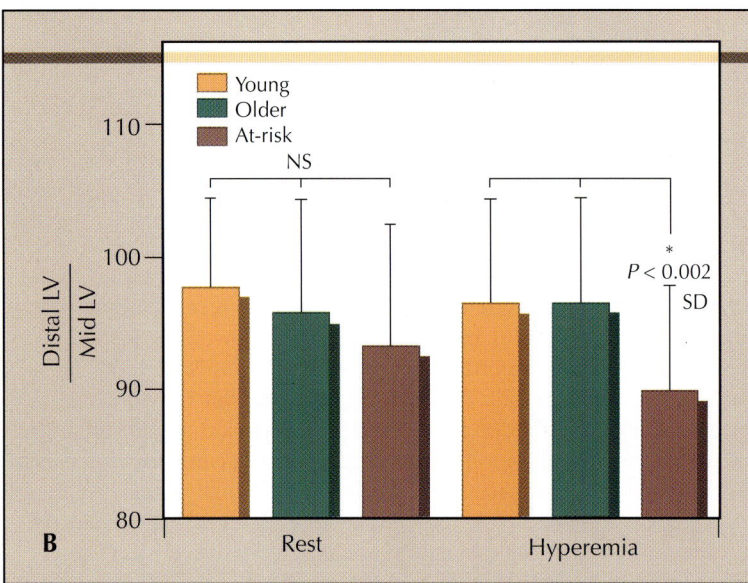

FIGURE 5-35. Base to apex perfusion gradient in patients with coronary risk factors. **A**, Myocardial blood flow was measured at rest and during dipyridamole hyperemia in the mid and apical circumference of the left ventricle, as shown on polar maps [47]. **B**, Ratios of myocardial blood flow in the apical and mid left ventricular (LV) circumference are depicted. No statistically diminished ratios are observed in either of the three study groups at rest. However, during hyperemia, the ratio is significantly reduced in the at-risk group as compared with the age-matched and young healthy patients. This diminished ratio reflects the longitudinal perfusion gradient, *ie*, a proximal to distal decline in the coronary perfusion pressure during hyperemia. Infracoronary pressure measurements have confirmed the existence of such a longitudinal pressure gradient, which most likely represents a functional or structural alteration of the coronary circulation [45]. NS—not significant.

ACKNOWLEDGMENTS

The authors wish to thank Diane Martin and Luke Deltredici for preparing the illustrations and Rita Rubins for her assistance in preparing this manuscript. This work was supported in part by the Director of the Office of Energy Research, Office of Health and Environmental Research, Washington, DC, and in part by Research Grant #HL 33177, National Institutes of Health, Bethesda, MD.

References

1. Schelbert HR, Phelps ME, Huang SC, et al.: N-13 ammonia as an indicator of myocardial blood flow. *Circulation* 1981, 63:1259–1272.

2. Krivokapich J, Smith GT, Huang SC, et al.: 13N ammonia myocardial imaging at rest and with exercise in normal volunteers. Quantification of absolute myocardial perfusion with dynamic positron emission tomography. *Circulation* 1989, 80:1328–1337.

3. Kuhle WG, Porenta G, Huang SC, et al.: Quantification of regional myocardial blood flow using 13N-ammonia and reoriented dynamic positron emission tomographic imaging. *Circulation* 1992, 86:1004–1017.

4. Bergmann SR, Herrero P, Markham J, et al.: Noninvasive quantitation of myocardial blood flow in human subjects with oxygen-15-labeled water and positron emission tomography. *J Am Coll Cardiol* 1989, 14:639–652.

5. Araujo L, Lammertsma A, Rhodes C, et al.: Noninvasive quantification of regional myocardial blood flow in coronary artery disease with oxygen-15-labeled carbon dioxide inhalation and positron emission tomography. *Circulation* 1991, 83:875–885.

6. Pitkänen OP, Raitakari OT, Niinikoski H, et al.: Coronary flow reserve is impaired in young men with familial hypercholesterolemia. *J Am Coll Cardiol* 1996, 28:1705–1711.

7. Yokoyama I, Ohtake T, Momomura S, et al.: Altered myocardial vasodilatation in patients with hypertriglyceridemia in anatomically normal coronary arteries. *Arterioscler Thromb Vasc Biol* 1998, 18:294–299.

8. Kaufmann PA, Gnecchi-Ruscone T, Yap JT, et al.: Assessment of the reproducibility of baseline and hyperemic myocardial blood flow measurements with 15O-labeled water and PET. *J Nucl Med* 1999, 40:1848–1856.

9. Tadamura E, Iida H, Matsumoto K, et al.: Comparison of myocardial blood flow during dobutamine-atropine infusion with that after dipyridamole administration in normal men. *J Am Coll Cardiol* 2001, 37:130–136.

10. Hutchins GD, Schwaiger M, Rosenspire KC, et al.: Noninvasive quantification of regional blood flow in the human heart using N-13 ammonia and dynamic positron emission tomographic imaging. *J Am Coll Cardiol* 1990, 15:1032–1042.

11. Chan SY, Brunken RC, Czernin J, et al.: Comparison of maximal myocardial blood flow during adenosine infusion with that of intravenous dipyridamole in normal men. *J Am Coll Cardiol* 1992, 20:979–985.

12. Czernin J, Müller P, Chan S, et al.: Influence of age and hemodynamics on myocardial blood flow and flow reserve. *Circulation* 1993, 88:62–69.

13. Wilson R, Laughlin D, Ackell P: Transluminal subselective measurement of coronary artery blood flow velocity and vasodilator reserve in man. *Circulation* 1985, 72:82–89.

14. Czernin J, Auerbach M, Sun KT, et al.: Effects of modified pharmacologic stress approaches on hyperemic myocardial blood flow. *J Nucl Med* 1995, 36:575–580.

15. Böttcher M, Czernin J, Sun KT, et al.: Effect of caffeine on myocardial blood flow at rest and during pharmacological vasodilation. *J Nucl Med* 1995, 36:2016–2021.

16. Böttcher M, Czernin J, Sun K, et al.: Effect of beta 1 adrenergic receptor blockade on myocardial blood flow and vasodilatory capacity. *J Nucl Med* 1997, 38:442–446.

17. Buus NH, Böttcher M, Hermansen F, et al.: Influence of nitric oxide synthase and adrenergic inhibition on adenosine-induced myocardial hyperemia. *Circulation* 2001, 104:2305–2310.

18. Krivokapich J, Czernin J, Schelbert HR: Dobutamine positron emission tomography: absolute quantitation of rest and dobutamine myocardial blood flow and correlation with cardiac work and percent diameter stenosis in patients with and without coronary artery disease. *J Am Coll Cardiol* 1996, 28:565–572.

19. Krivokapich J, Huang SC, Schelbert HR: Assessment of the effects of dobutamine on myocardial blood flow and oxidative metabolism in normal human subjects using nitrogen-13 ammonia and carbon-11 acetate. *Am J Cardiol* 1993, 71:1351–1356.

20. Czernin J, Sun K, Brunken R, et al.: Effect of acute and long-term smoking on myocardial blood flow and flow reserve. *Circulation* 1995, 91:2891–2897.

21. Müller P, Czernin J, Choi Y, et al.: Effect of exercise supplementation during adenosine infusion on hyperemic blood flow and flow reserve. *Am Heart J* 1994, 128:52–60.

22. Laine H, Nuutila P, Luotolahti M, et al.: Insulin-induced increment of coronary flow reserve is not abolished by dexamethasone in healthy young men. *J Am Coll Cardiol* 2000, 35:419A.

23. Sundell J, Nuutila P, Laine H, et al.: Dose-dependent vasodilating effects of insulin on adenosine-stimulated myocardial blood flow. *Diabetes* 2002, 51:1125–1130.

24. Di Carli M, Czernin J, Hoh CK, et al.: Relation among stenosis severity, myocardial blood flow, and flow reserve in patients with coronary artery disease. *Circulation* 1995, 91:1944–1951.

25. Gould KL, Lipscomb K, Hamilton GW: Physiologic basis for assessing critical coronary stenosis. Instantaneous flow response and regional distribution during coronary hyperemia as measures of coronary flow reserve. *Am J Cardiol* 1974, 33:87–94.

26. Beanlands RS, Muzik O, Melon P, et al.: Noninvasive quantification of regional myocardial flow reserve in patients with coronary atherosclerosis using nitrogen-13 ammonia positron emission tomography. Determination of extent of altered vascular reactivity. *J Am Coll Cardiol* 1995, 26:1465–1475.

27. Uren NG, Melin JA, De Bruyne B, et al.: Relation between myocardial blood flow and the severity of coronary-artery stenosis. *N Engl J Med* 1994, 330:1782–1788.

28. Dayanikli F, Grambow D, Muzik O, et al.: Early detection of abnormal coronary flow reserve in asymptomatic men at high risk for coronary artery disease using positron emission tomography. *Circulation* 1994, 90:808–817.

29. Yokoyama I, Ohtake T, Momomura S, et al.: Reduced coronary flow reserve in hypercholesterolemic patients without overt coronary stenosis. *Circulation* 1996, 94:3232–3238.

30. Pitkänen OP, Nuutila P, Raitakari OT, et al.: Coronary flow reserve in young men with familial combined hyperlipidemia. *Circulation* 1999, 99:1678–1684.

31. Reddy KG, Nair RN, Sheehan HM, Hodgson JM: Evidence that selective endothelial dysfunction may occur in the absence of angiographic or ultrasound atherosclerosis in patients with risk factors for atherosclerosis. *J Am Coll Cardiol* 1994, 23:833–843.

32. Campisi R, Czernin J, Schöder H, et al.: Effects of long-term smoking on myocardial blood flow, coronary vasomotion, and vasodilator capacity. *Circulation* 1998, 98:119–125.

33. Zeiher AM: Endothelial modulation of coronary vasomotor tone in humans. Effects of atherosclerosis and risk factors for coronary artery disease. *Arzneimittelforschung* 1994, 44:439–442.

34. Zeiher AM, Drexler H: Coronary hemodynamic determinants of epicardial artery vasomotor responses during sympathetic stimulation in humans. *Basic Res Cardiol* 1991, 86:203–213.

35. Zeiher AM, Drexler H, Wollschlaeger H, *et al.*: Coronary vasomotion in response to sympathetic stimulation in humans: importance of the functional integrity of the endothelium. *J Am Coll Cardiol* 1989, 14:1181–1190.

36. Zeiher AM, Drexler H, Wollschlager H, Just H: Endothelial dysfunction of the coronary microvasculature is associated with coronary blood flow regulation in patients with early atherosclerosis. *Circulation* 1991, 84:1984–1992.

37. Zeiher AM, Drexler H, Wollschlager H, Just H: Modulation of coronary vasomotor tone in humans. Progressive endothelial dysfunction with different early stages of coronary atherosclerosis. *Circulation* 1991, 83:391–401.

38. Czernin J, Barnard RJ, Sun KT, *et al.*: Effect of short-term cardiovascular conditioning and low-fat diet on myocardial blood flow and flow reserve. *Circulation* 1995, 92:197–204.

39. Baller D, Notohamiprodjo G, Gleichmann U, *et al.*: Improvement in coronary flow reserve determined by positron emission tomography after 6 months of cholesterol-lowering therapy in patients with early stages of coronary atherosclerosis. *Circulation* 1999, 99:2871–2875.

40. Guethlin M, Kasel AM, Coppenrath K, *et al.*: Delayed response of myocardial flow reserve to lipid-lowering therapy with fluvastatin. *Circulation* 1999, 99:475–481.

41. Huggins GS, Pasternak RC, Alpert NM, *et al.*: Effects of short-term treatment of hyperlipidemia on coronary vasodilator function and myocardial perfusion in regions having substantial impairment of baseline dilator reserve. *Circulation* 1998, 98:1291–1296.

42. Janatuinen T, Laaksonen R, Vesalainen R, *et al.*: Effect of lipid-lowering therapy with pravastatin on myocardial blood flow in young mildly hypercholesterolemic adults. *J Cardiovasc Pharmacol* 2001, 38:561–568.

43. Yokoyama I, Momomura S, Ohtake T, *et al.*: Improvement of impaired myocardial vasodilatation due to diffuse coronary atherosclerosis in hypercholesterolemics after lipid-lowering therapy. *Circulation* 1999, 100:117–122.

44. Yokoyama I, Yonekura K, Inoue Y, *et al.*: Long-term effect of simvastatin on the improvement of impaired myocardial flow reserve in patients with familial hypercholesterolemia without gender variance. *J Nucl Cardiol* 2001, 8:445–451.

45. De Bruyne B, Hersbach F, Pijls NH, *et al.*: Abnormal epicardial coronary resistance in patients with diffuse atherosclerosis but "normal" coronary angiography. *Circulation* 2001, 104:2401–2406.

46. Gould KL, Nakagawa Y, Nakagawa K, *et al.*: Frequency and clinical implications of fluid dynamically significant diffuse coronary artery disease manifest as graded, longitudinal, base-to-apex myocardial perfusion abnormalities by noninvasive positron emission tomography. *Circulation* 2000, 101:1931–1939.

47. Hernandez-Pampaloni M, Keng FY, Kudo T, *et al.*: Abnormal longitudinal, base-to-apex myocardial perfusion gradient by quantitative blood flow measurements in patients with coronary risk factors. *Circulation* 2001, 104:527–532.

CHAPTER 6

RISK STRATIFICATION AND PATIENT MANAGEMENT

Daniel S. Berman, Rory Hachamovitch, and Guido Germano

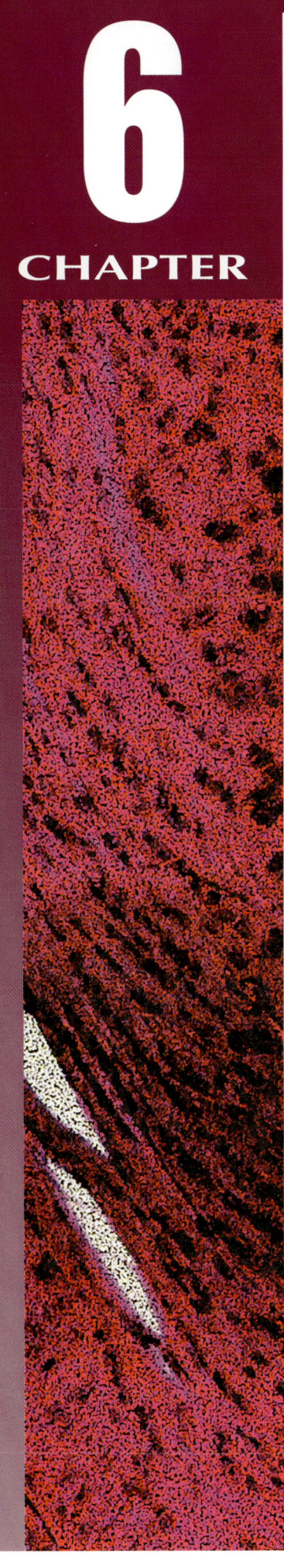

Since the early 1970s, a number of noninvasive testing modalities have become widely available in clinical cardiology. Today, state-of-the-art nuclear cardiology allows for the precise measurement of both myocardial function and relative regional perfusion at rest and under stress, providing accurate risk assessment in a variety of patient subsets. This chapter deals with stress myocardial perfusion SPECT, which currently accounts for approximately 95% of the procedures performed in this field.

The main use of nuclear cardiology studies for guiding management decisions is determining which patients with suspected or known coronary artery disease (CAD) require catheterization with consideration of revascularization. In patients who have chest pain symptoms that, despite medical therapy, affect their well being, nuclear cardiology studies play a limited role, chiefly being useful for identifying the culprit coronary lesion and determining which vessel or vessels might be most appropriate for revascularization. Because revascularization has been shown to relieve anginal symptoms in patients with CAD, it would not be cost effective to use myocardial perfusion SPECT to study all patients. On the other hand, if revascularization is being considered for purposes of improving prognosis, myocardial perfusion SPECT can be helpful in determining whether the patient's risk is high enough to warrant revascularization.

The most rapidly growing area of application of myocardial perfusion SPECT is risk stratification, based on increased acceptance of this new paradigm in patient management. A risk-based approach to patients with suspected CAD appears better suited to the modern environment of cost containment and dramatic improvements in medical therapy than the approach focusing on simple diagnosis, in which all patients with suspected disease undergo coronary angiography and then are frequently revascularized based on coronary anatomic findings. With the risk-based approach, the focus is not on predicting who has anatomic CAD, but on identifying and separating patients at risk, versus not at risk, for cardiac death.

The basic concept in the use of nuclear tests for risk stratification is that they are best applied to patients with an intermediate risk of a subsequent cardiac event, analogous to the optimal diagnostic application of nuclear testing of patients with an intermediate likelihood of having CAD. For prognostic testing, patients known to be at high risk or low risk would not be appropriate patients for cost-effective risk stratification, since they are already risk stratified. In chronic CAD, it has been suggested that a greater than 3% per year mortality rate can be used to identify patients with minimal symptoms whose mortality rate can be improved by coronary artery bypass grafting [1]. For purposes of risk assessment, it has been proposed that low risk is defined as a less than 1% cardiac mortality rate per year, high risk as a greater than 3% cardiac mortality rate per year, and intermediate risk as between 1% to 3% cardiac mortality rate per year [2]. Because the mortality risk associated with either coronary artery bypass grafting or angioplasty is greater than 1% [3], mildly symptomatic patients with a less than 1% mortality rate would not be candidates for revascularization to improve survival, and would be appropriately classified by this rate as having a low risk of death. Note that for diagnostic testing, nuclear imaging would be most appropriate in patients with an intermediate likelihood of CAD [2]; for risk stratification, this appropriateness extends to the groups of patients with a high likelihood of CAD. Thus, the risk stratification application in patients with suspected CAD considerably extends the group of appropriate patients for nuclear stress testing.

The basis for the power of nuclear testing for risk stratification is found in the fact that the major determinants of prognosis in CAD can be assessed by measurements of stress-induced perfusion or function. These measurements include the amount of infarcted myocardium, the amount of jeopardized myocardium (supplied by vessels with hemodynamically significant stenosis), and the degree of jeopardy (tightness of the individual coronary stenosis). An additional important factor in prognostic assessment is the stability (or instability) of the CAD process. This last consideration may help explain what appears to be a clinical paradox: nuclear tests, which in general are expected to be positive only in the presence of hemodynamically significant stenosis, are associated with a very low risk of either cardiac death or nonfatal myocardial infarction (MI) when results are normal. In contrast, it has been observed that most MIs occur in regions with premyocardial infarction coronary plaques causing less than 50% stenosis [4,5]. It has been postulated that this paradox may be explained by the different response to stress of mild stenosis associated with stable and unstable plaque. For example, it has been shown that mild coronary narrowings associated with unstable plaque manifest a vasoconstrictive response to acetylcholine stimulation due to abnormal endothelial function, whereas stable, mild coronary lesions respond to acetylcholine with vasodilation [6]. It is possible that factors released during exercise or vasodilator stress may be similar to acetylcholine in terms of stimulation of a differential endothelial response in stable and unstable plaque. Thus, beyond the ability to define anatomic stenosis, nuclear tests (by virtue of their assessment of physiology) would be able to discern abnormalities of endothelial function associated with high risk, even in the absence of significant stenosis.

Recent evidence in large patient cohorts has revealed that factors estimating the extent of left ventricular dysfunction (left ventricular ejection fraction, extent of infarcted myocardium, transient ischemic dilation of the left ventricle, and increased lung uptake) are excellent predictors of cardiac mortality. In contrast, measurements of inducible ischemia are better predictors of the development of acute ischemic syndromes. These include exertional symptoms and electrocardiographic changes, as well as the extent of perfusion defect reversibility and new ventricular dyssynergy. Several reports have shown that nuclear testing yields incremental prognostic value over clinical information with respect to cardiac death, or the combination of cardiac death and nonfatal MI as isolated endpoints. By understanding how clinical information and nuclear test markers can be used to estimate varying outcomes, it is now possible to tailor therapeutic decision-making for an individual patient based upon the combination of clinical factors and nuclear scan results. For example, a patient with severe perfusion abnormalities on their stress image may have a five- to tenfold higher likelihood of cardiac death compared with a patient with a normal myocardial perfusion SPECT. If the defects are stress-induced (reversible), therapies known to improve survival might be chosen in order to result in an optimized outcome for that patient.

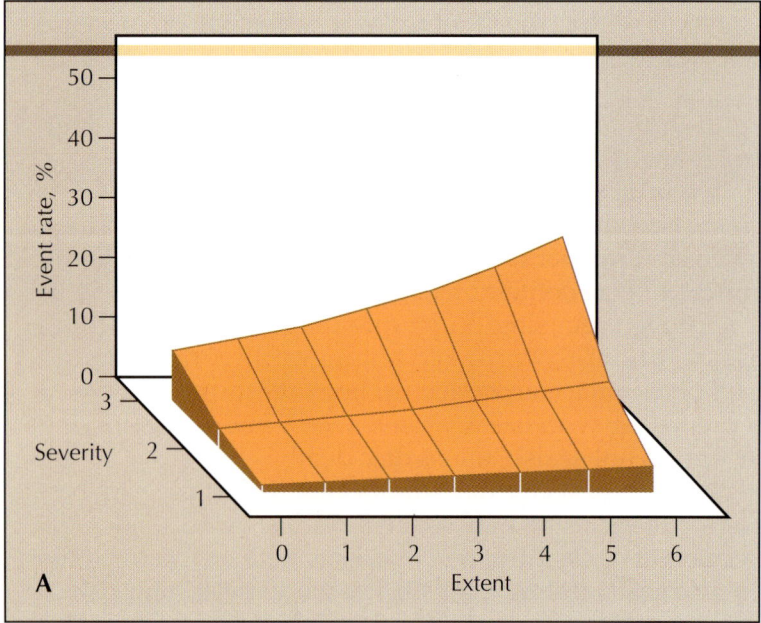

FIGURE 6-1. Extent and severity of reversible myocardial hypoperfusion as independent variables in predicting subsequent cardiac events in patients with suspected coronary artery disease (CAD). Ladenheim *et al.* [7] assessed 1689 patients with suspected CAD but without prior myocardial infarction (MI) or revascularization. All of the patients were followed for 1 year following planar ^{201}Tl myocardial perfusion scintigraphy; 74 patients had coronary events including 12 cardiac deaths, 29 nonfatal myocardial infarctions, and 42 referrals for bypass surgery more than 60 days after testing (late revascularization, shown to be an accurate marker of clinical worsening). Stepwise logistic regression identified only three independent predictors of events: the number of regions with reversible defects (an index of the extent of hypoperfusion), the magnitude of hypoperfusion (an index of the severity of hypoperfusion), and the achieved heart rate (an index of exercise performance). **A,** The 1414 patients who were able to exercise to at least 85% of maximal predicted heart rate (average 99%).

Continued on next page

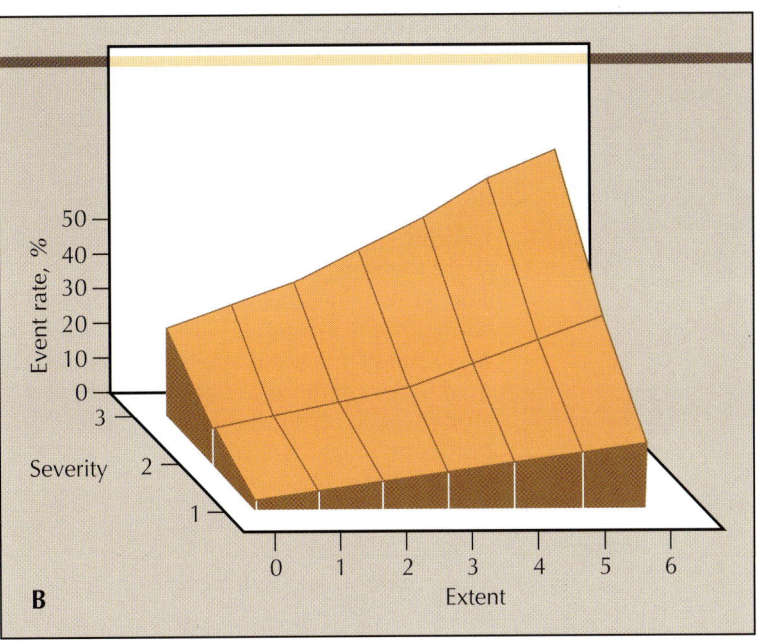

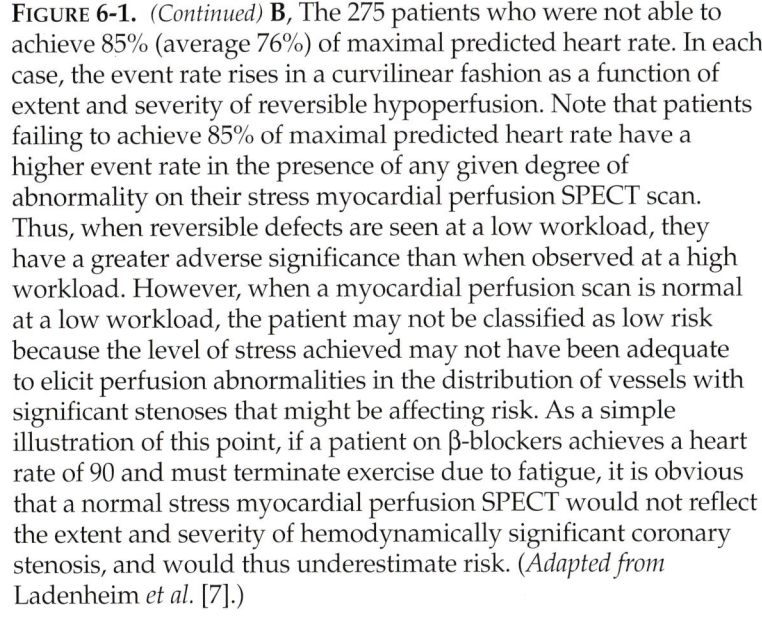

FIGURE 6-1. *(Continued)* **B**, The 275 patients who were not able to achieve 85% (average 76%) of maximal predicted heart rate. In each case, the event rate rises in a curvilinear fashion as a function of extent and severity of reversible hypoperfusion. Note that patients failing to achieve 85% of maximal predicted heart rate have a higher event rate in the presence of any given degree of abnormality on their stress myocardial perfusion SPECT scan. Thus, when reversible defects are seen at a low workload, they have a greater adverse significance than when observed at a high workload. However, when a myocardial perfusion scan is normal at a low workload, the patient may not be classified as low risk because the level of stress achieved may not have been adequate to elicit perfusion abnormalities in the distribution of vessels with significant stenoses that might be affecting risk. As a simple illustration of this point, if a patient on β-blockers achieves a heart rate of 90 and must terminate exercise due to fatigue, it is obvious that a normal stress myocardial perfusion SPECT would not reflect the extent and severity of hemodynamically significant coronary stenosis, and would thus underestimate risk. *(Adapted from* Ladenheim *et al.* [7].)

FIGURE 6-2. Definition of scintigraphic indices. Scoring perfusion defects in each individual segment is useful in deriving summed perfusion parameters, which incorporate the global extent and severity of perfusion abnormality [10]. The summed stress score (SSS) reflects the extent and severity of perfusion defects at stress, and is affected by prior myocardial infarction as well as by stress-induced ischemia. The summed rest score (SRS) reflects the amount of infarcted or hibernating myocardium. The summed difference score (SDS) is a measure of the extent and severity of stress-induced ischemia. These global perfusion parameters can be considered the perfusion analogs of left ventricular ejection fraction, the most commonly employed global ventricular function parameter. By incorporating the extent and severity of perfusion defects, these global parameters allow assessment of the variables shown in Figure 6-1 to be incrementally important in assessing risk from perfusion scintigraphy. *(Adapted from* Berman *et al.* [8].)

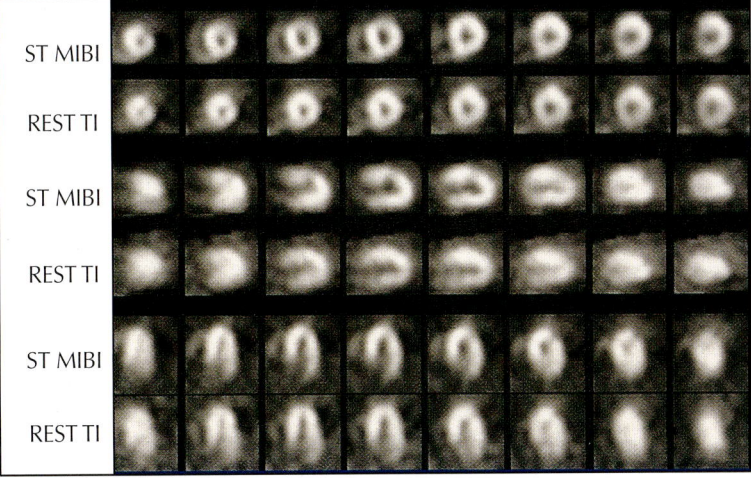

FIGURE 6-3. Example of a patient with a small stress perfusion defect resulting in a mildly abnormal summed stress score. The patient is a 69-year-old man with atypical angina whose only risk factor for coronary disease was hypercholesterolemia. The patient exercised for 7 minutes, 20 seconds to a heart rate of 139 (92% of maximal predicted) and had a normal blood pressure response. He developed minimal chest discomfort during stress, which was considered equivocal for an ischemic response. The electrocardiographic response to stress was normal. Exercise stress ^{99m}Tc-sestamibi (ST MIBI) and rest ^{201}Tl (REST Tl) images are interlaced in the alternate rows, which show short-axis images (*top two rows*), vertical long-axis images (*middle two rows*), and horizontal long-axis images (*bottom two rows*). The images reveal a small defect in the distal anterior left ventricular wall with sparing of the interventricular septum and the apex. This pattern is classic for the territory of the mid to distal portion of diagonal branch of the left anterior descending coronary artery. The summed stress score is 7.

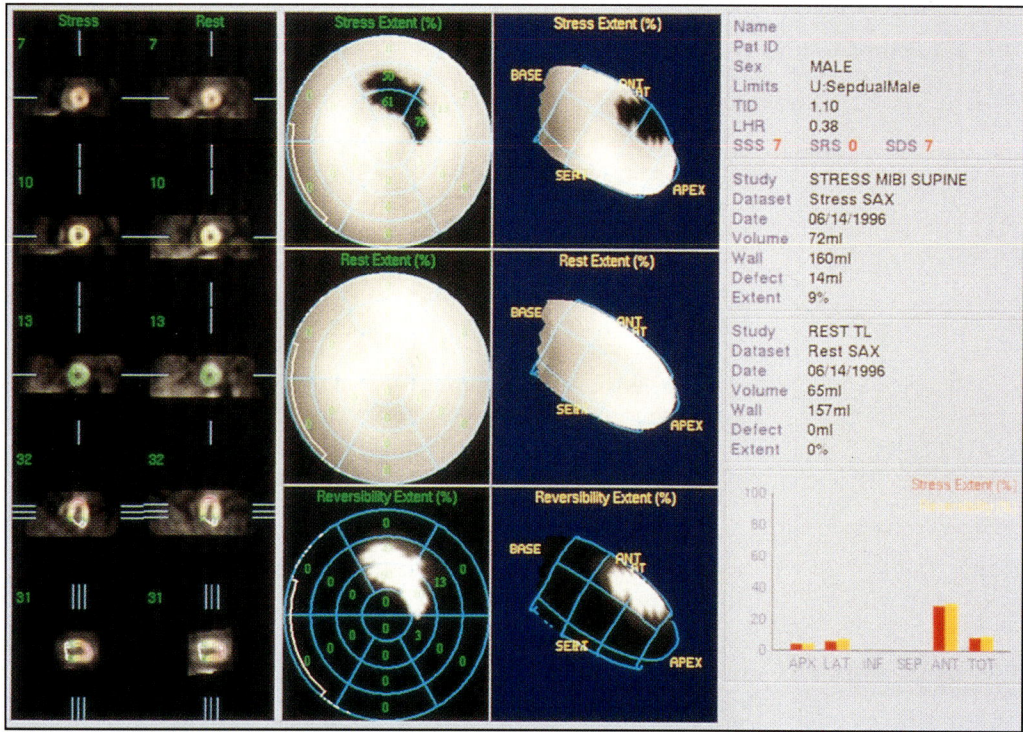

FIGURE 6-4. Quantitative perfusion SPECT analysis of the patient in Figure 6-3 indicating the presence of a small perfusion defect in the diagonal coronary territory. The summed stress score (SSS) attributed to the images in Figure 6-3 is illustrated in the upper right corner. The SSS of 7 indicates a mild abnormality. The quantitative perfusion defect extent is 9%. The typical diagonal territory location is shown in the 2-D (*middle panel*) and 3-D (*right panel*) images at stress with a normal quantitative pattern at rest. This patient's study would be borderline based on perfusion alone with respect to the need for subsequent catheterization.

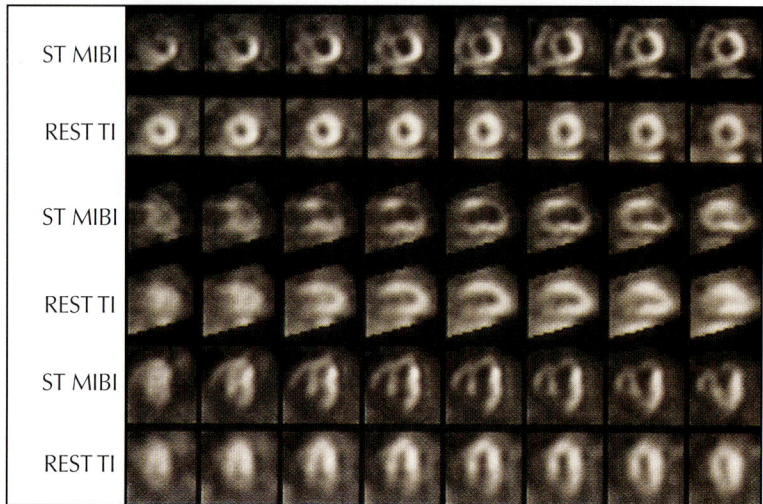

FIGURE 6-5. Example of a patient with a severe and extensive stress-induced perfusion defect. A 69-year-old man with atypical chest pain who had hypertension and diabetes as risk factors as well as left ventricular hypertrophy on resting ECG exercised for 5 minutes to a heart rate of 139 (87% of maximal predicted). The patient did develop chest discomfort and had an ischemic ECG response to stress. There was no exercise hypotension. Exercise stress ^{99m}Tc-sestamibi (ST MIBI) and rest ^{201}Tl (REST Tl) images are interlaced in the alternate rows, which show short-axis images (*top two rows*), vertical long-axis images (*middle two rows*), and horizontal long-axis images (*bottom two rows*). The REST Tl/ST MIBI dual isotope myocardial perfusion SPECT images reveal a severe perfusion defect throughout the distribution of the left anterior descending coronary artery. The summed stress score is very high at 31, the summed rest score is low at 3, and the summed difference score is 28. Severe and extensive ischemia is confirmed by evidence of transient ischemic dilation of the left ventricle, measured at 1.43 [9].

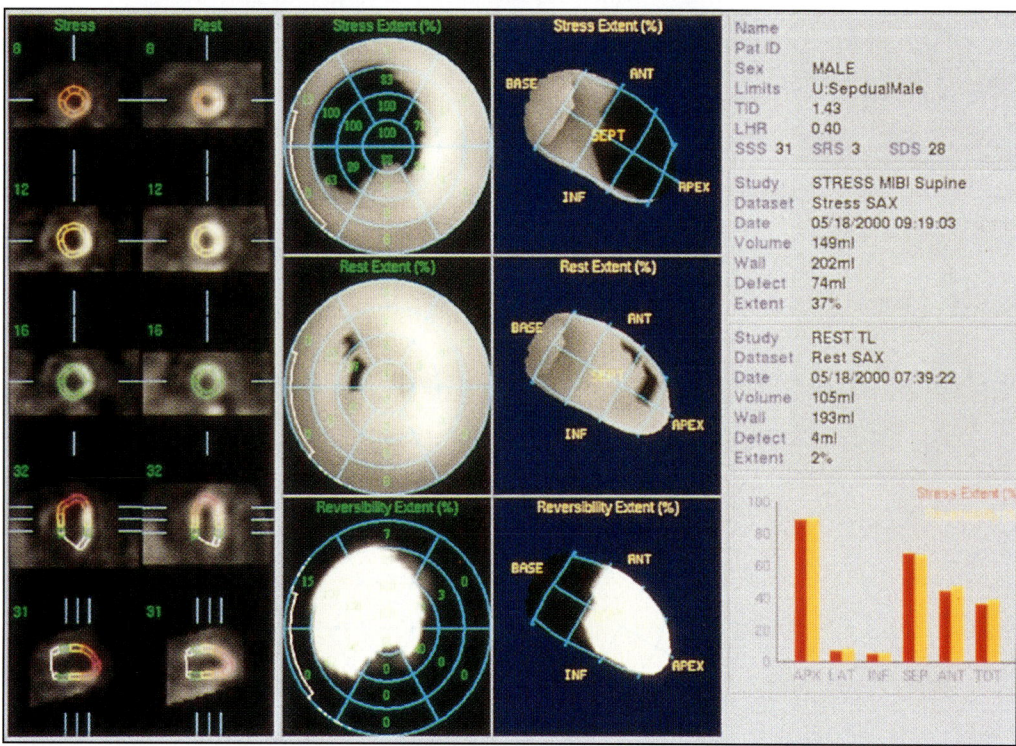

FIGURE 6-6. Quantitative perfusion SPECT analysis of the patient in Figure 6-5. This study revealed that 37% of the left ventricle is abnormal after stress, corresponding to the entire left anterior descending coronary artery (LAD) territory. The resting perfusion defect extent is measured as 2%. Note that the 37% abnormality is very close to the 40%, generally considered the proportion of the myocardium supplied by the LAD. Thus, the findings are predictive of a proximal stenosis of the LAD, and the severity of the perfusion defect allows the interpreter to state that the proximal LAD is likely to have a critical stenosis (> 90%) [10,11]. At catheterization, the patient was found to have a 100% proximal stenosis of the LAD, a 60% circumflex lesion, and a 50% to 60% mid right coronary artery stenosis.

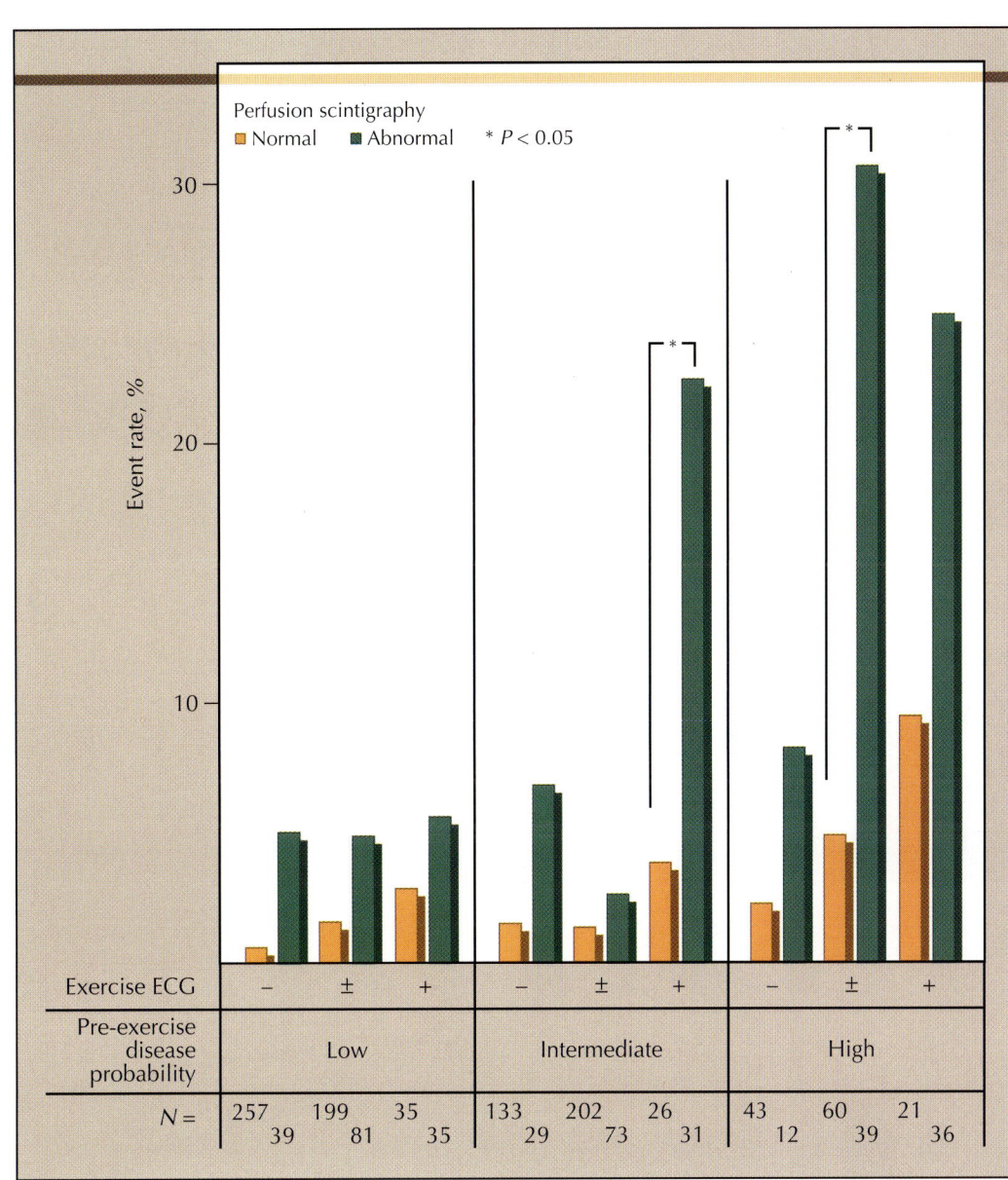

Figure 6-7. Incremental prognostic value of myocardial perfusion scintigraphy in a large series of patients without known coronary artery disease (CAD). Patients were categorized by their pre-exercise probability of CAD, by their response to stress testing, and then by their response on planar myocardial perfusion scintigraphy [12]. In the nine categories illustrated, an abnormal ^{201}Tl scan was associated with a higher risk than a normal scan. However, marked differences in event rates were noted only in categories in patients with an intermediate likelihood of CAD and an abnormal stress test response, and patients with a high likelihood of CAD. Until the time of this study, the use of ^{201}Tl imaging was confined predominantly to patients with an intermediate likelihood of having CAD, because prior research had shown that testing with nuclear studies in this patient population was highly effective for diagnostic purposes. The results of this study demonstrated that for prognostic purposes, patients with a high likelihood of CAD either before or after treadmill ECG are the patients in whom the greatest incremental benefit of myocardial perfusion scintigraphy is noted. (*Adapted from* Ladenheim *et al.* [12].)

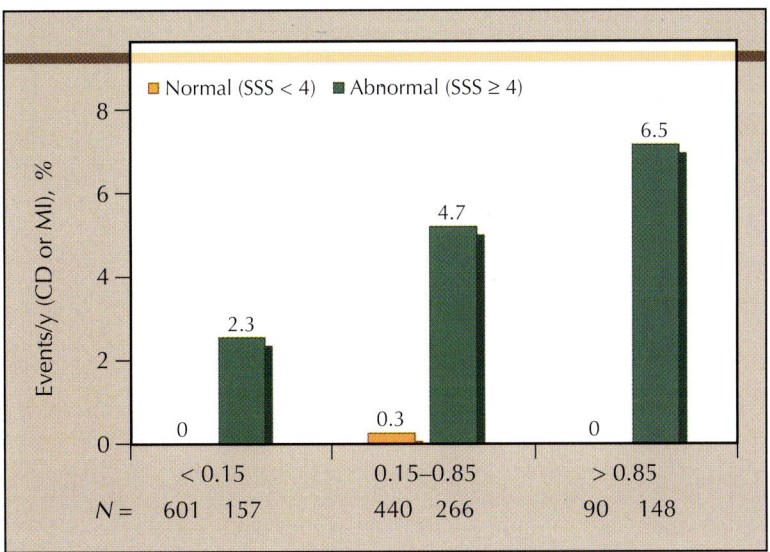

Figure 6-8. Incremental prognostic value of stress sestamibi SPECT over prescan likelihood of coronary artery disease (CAD). Similar to the experience using ^{201}Tl in a study of 1702 patients undergoing ^{99m}Tc-sestamibi imaging, a normal ^{99m}Tc-sestamibi scan was associated with a very low (0.2%) likelihood of cardiac death (CD) or myocardial infarction (MI) over a 20-month period. The figure illustrates the rate of CD or nonfatal MI throughout the follow-up period as a function of SPECT results and prescan likelihood of CAD (low likelihood, < 0.15; intermediate likelihood, 0.15–0.85; high likelihood, > 0.85). These results demonstrate that myocardial perfusion SPECT could be used for prognostic purposes throughout the range of likelihood of CAD. SSS—summed stress score. (*Adapted from* Berman *et al.* [13].)

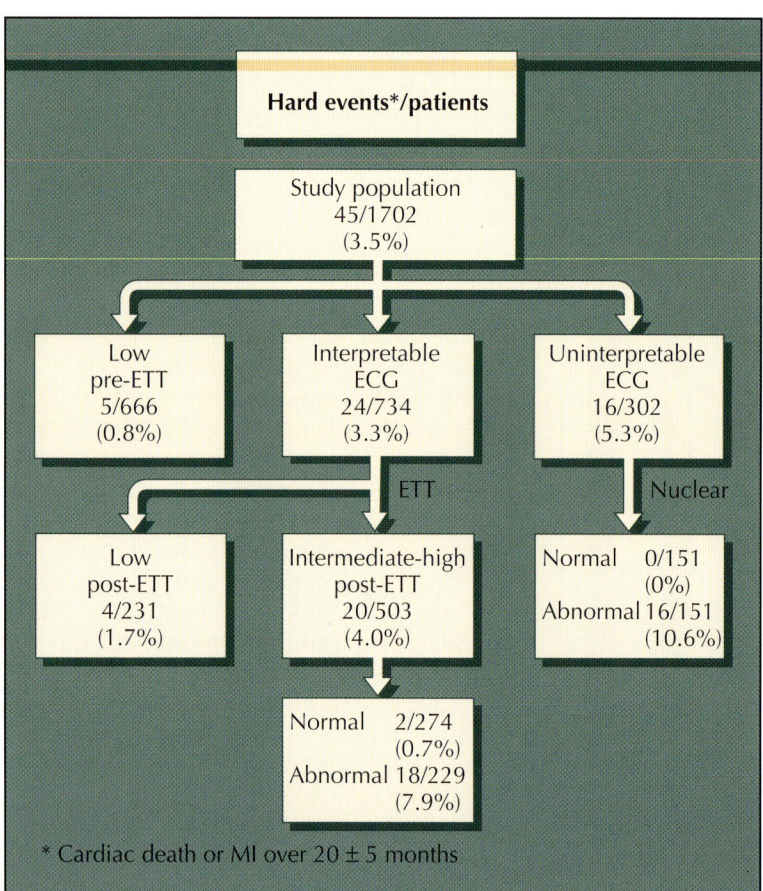

FIGURE 6-9. Optimized strategy for risk stratification of patients using myocardial perfusion SPECT. This flow chart is very similar to the current recommendations of the guidelines committees of the American Heart Association and the American College of Cardiology [2]. Patients with a low likelihood of coronary artery disease (CAD) before treadmill testing (low pre-ETT) do not need further study for prognostic purposes. Of the remaining patients, those with an uninterpretable ECG can skip exercise testing and go straight to stress myocardial perfusion SPECT, which stratifies the patients into very low-risk and very high-risk groups. In the patients in whom the exercise ECG can be interpreted, a subgroup can be considered to have a low risk following stress testing based on a low post-stress ECG likelihood of CAD (low post-ETT [< 15%]). In the remaining patients, an intermediate risk of hard events is present (intermediate–high post-ETT [≥ 15%]). Excellent risk stratification is then provided by nuclear testing into very low-risk and very high-risk groups. (*Adapted from* Berman *et al.* [13].)

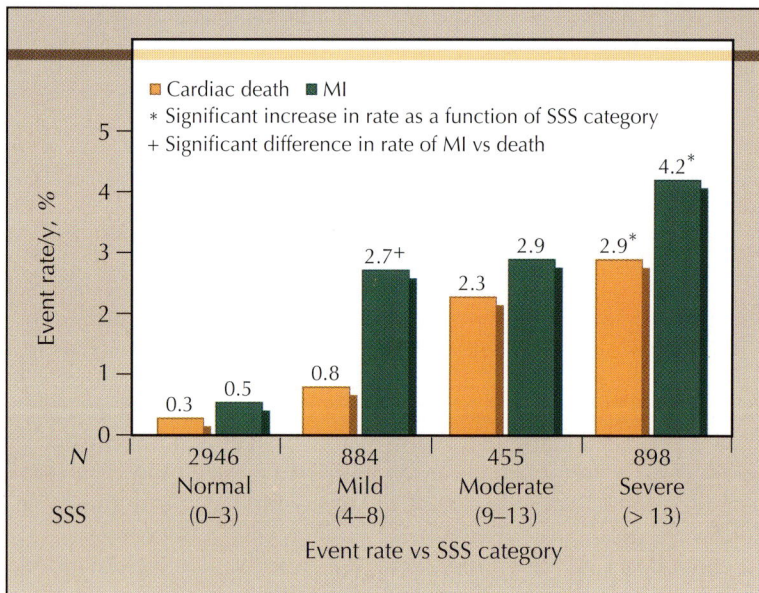

FIGURE 6-10. Prediction of myocardial infarction (MI) versus cardiac death by myocardial perfusion SPECT. The extent of abnormality of the myocardial perfusion SPECT provides important additional information regarding risk. The annualized cardiac death and MI rates of a large group of patients undergoing stress myocardial perfusion SPECT is shown. The extent of stress perfusion defect as measured by the summed stress score (SSS) is plotted horizontally. The progressive increase in the cardiac death rate as a function of the SSS is shown. The rate of nonfatal MI is low when the scans are normal but increases abruptly even when mild myocardial perfusion in defect is noted. (*Adapted from* Hachamovitch *et al.* [14].)

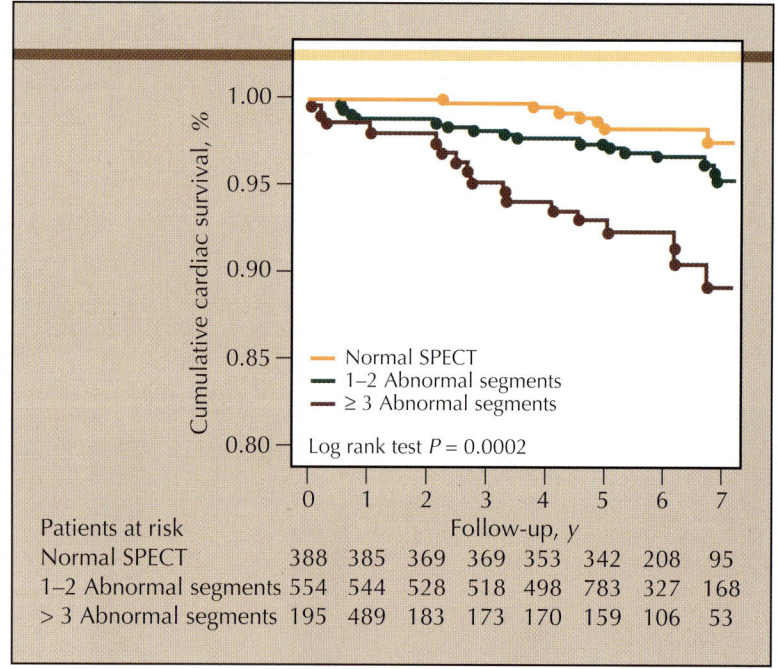

FIGURE 6-11. Long-term prognostic value of ^{201}Tl SPECT. Vanzetto *et al.* [15] reported the results of a large series of patients who were followed for long-term cardiac events. In the presence of a normal ^{201}Tl SPECT study, the event-free survival was excellent. A progressive worsening of event-free survival was noted as a function of the number of abnormal segments on stress myocardial perfusion SPECT studies. (*Adapted from* Vanzetto *et al.* [15].)

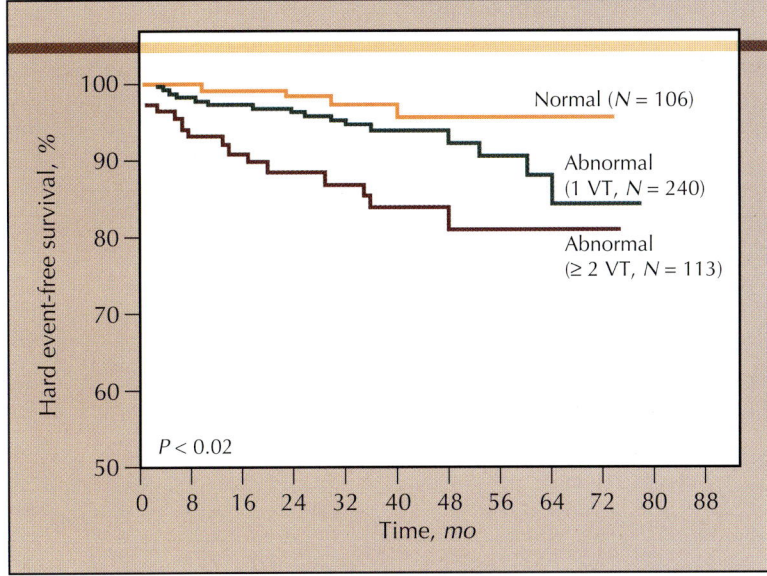

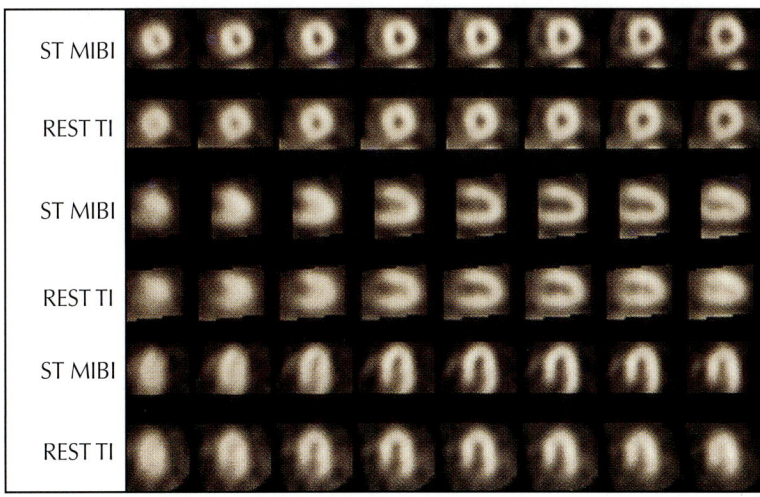

FIGURE 6-12. Hard event-free survival in patients with normal and abnormal ^{99m}Tc-tetrofosmin SPECT scans from a series of 459 patients. Similar to the results of the previously illustrated studies, the normal tetrofosmin SPECT study was associated with an excellent hard event-free survival, while the patients with abnormal tetrofosmin SPECT studies had lower hard event-free survival in proportion to the extent of abnormality observed. Although the greatest amount of prognostic information is available in the literature regarding the use of ^{99m}Tc-sestamibi, there is also extensive prognostic literature based on ^{201}Tl SPECT. Recent studies have demonstrated excellent prognostic stratification with ^{99m}Tc-tetrofosmin. VT—vascular territories. (*Adapted from* Galassi *et al.* [16].)

FIGURE 6-13. Stress myocardial perfusion SPECT in a patient with a high likelihood of coronary artery disease. The patient, a 71-year-old woman, had chronic, mild typical angina pectoris and a history of hypertension. Because she was unable to exercise, she underwent an adenosine stress test with normal clinical and electrocardiographic responses. Exercise stress ^{99m}Tc-sestamibi (ST MIBI) and rest ^{201}Tl (REST Tl) images are interlaced in the alternate rows, which show short-axis images (*top two rows*), vertical long-axis images (*middle two rows*), and horizontal long-axis images (*bottom two rows*). The myocardial perfusion SPECT images are entirely normal. With this result, the patient was treated medically. Six years following the initial stress imaging study, the patient remained free from cardiac catheterization and free from cardiac events.

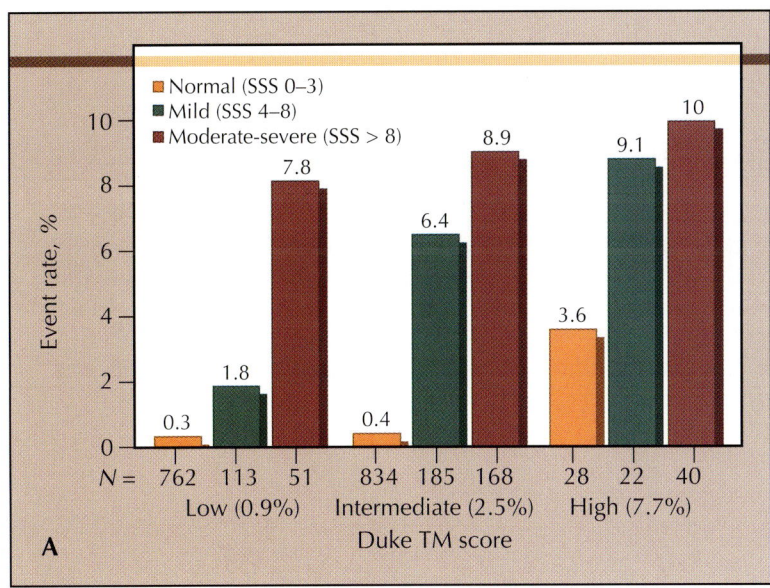

FIGURE 6-14. Hard event rate as a function of summed stress score (SSS) and Duke University treadmill score (TM). In patients with interpretable stress ECGs, it has been demonstrated that the Duke TM score can separate patients into groups with low, intermediate, and high risk of cardiac events. Thus, current guidelines suggest beginning with a stress ECG in these patients [2]. However, nuclear testing is useful in the patients with intermediate- or high-risk Duke TM scores. **A,** Stress myocardial perfusion SPECT studies further risk-stratify patients within each of these Duke TM score categories [17]. All patients examined had no known coronary artery disease (patients with prior catheterization, myocardial infarction [MI], or revascularization were excluded). The hard event (cardiac death or MI) rate as a function of the Duke treadmill score category and the nuclear scan results (SSS) are illustrated. The normal, mild, and severe SSS categories are based on the subgroups of SSS abnormality described in Figure 6-2. Due to small patient numbers, for purposes of this study those patients with moderate to severe SSS were categorized as severe. Overall, patients with a low-risk Duke TM score had such a low rate of cardiac events that it would not be cost effective to study them for prognostic purposes. Additionally, since patients with a high-risk Duke TM score usually undergo catheterization, these patients are generally not sent for further nuclear testing. However, 55% of the population had the intermediate risk Duke TM score with a cardiac event rate of 2.5%. Thus, myocardial perfusion SPECT provided excellent stratification of these patients with respect to risk of hard event [17].

Continued on next page

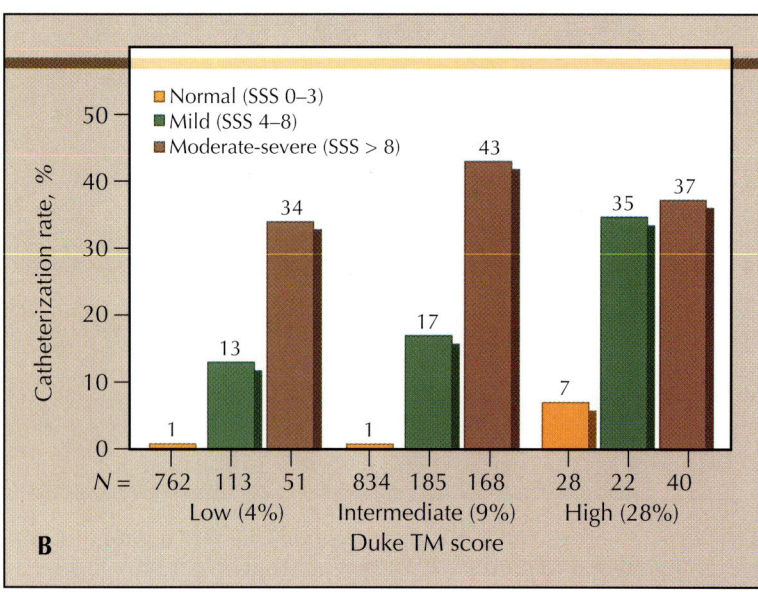

FIGURE 6-14. *(Continued)* B, Catheterization rate as a function of SSS and the Duke TM score. The catheterization rates are seen to follow the event rates in *panel A*. Note that of the patients in the intermediate Duke TM score group, only 1% of the patients found to have a normal myocardial perfusion SPECT study underwent subsequent early catheterization. Similarly, in the patients in the high Duke TM score group, only 7% of the patients found to have a normal myocardial perfusion SPECT study underwent subsequent early catheterization. (*Adapted from* Hachamovitch et al. [17].)

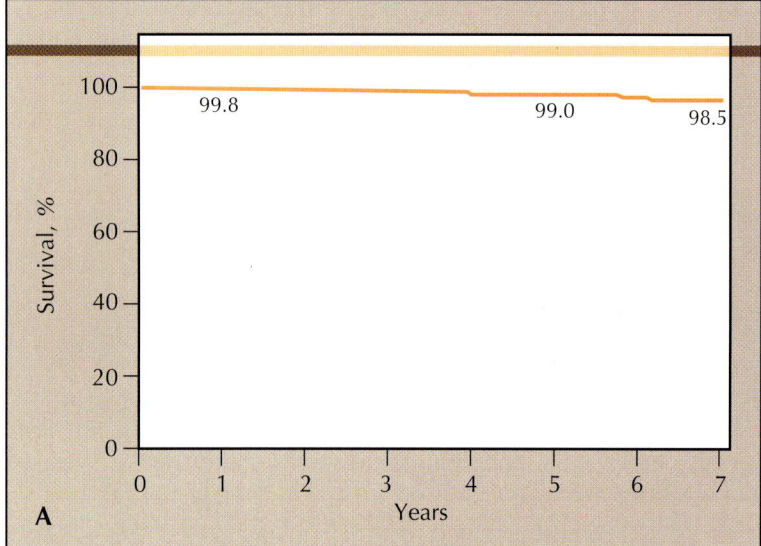

FIGURE 6-15. A, Long-term outcome of 4649 patients from four institutions with an intermediate risk exercise electrocardiogram based on the Duke treadmill score and no or minimal stress myocardial perfusion defects. The mortality rate is extremely low for patients with no stress myocardial perfusion defect. B, The cumulative incidence of coronary angiography in patients with an intermediate risk Duke treadmill score and no stress myocardial perfusion defect. Note that the clinicians involved in the decision-making process seldom chose to perform cardiac catheterization in these patients. The findings of this study add strength to the concept that stress myocardial perfusion SPECT is highly effective in the clinical decision-making applied to the management of patients with intermediate risk Duke treadmill scores. (*Adapted from* Gibbons et al. [18].)

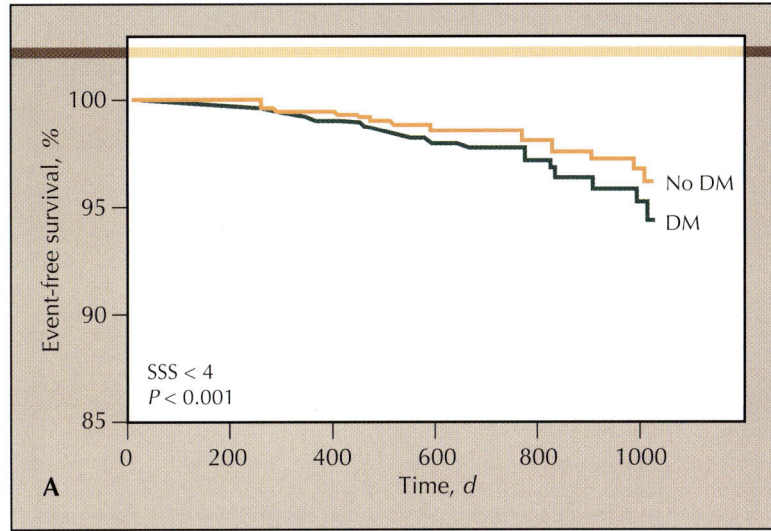
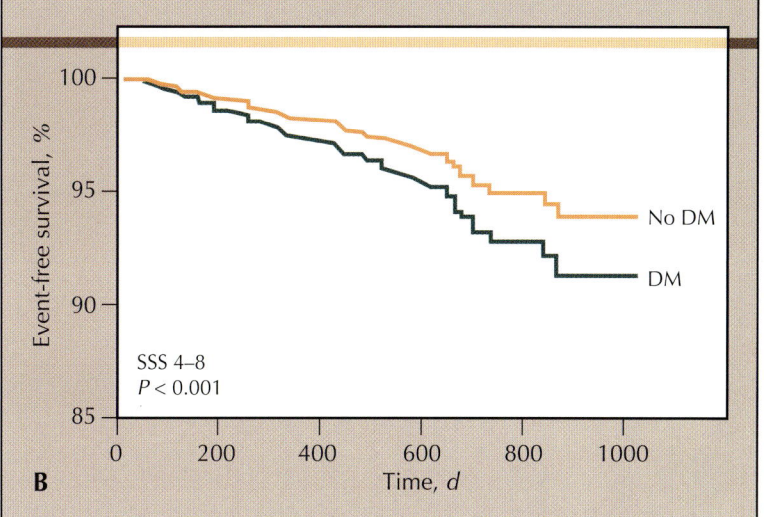
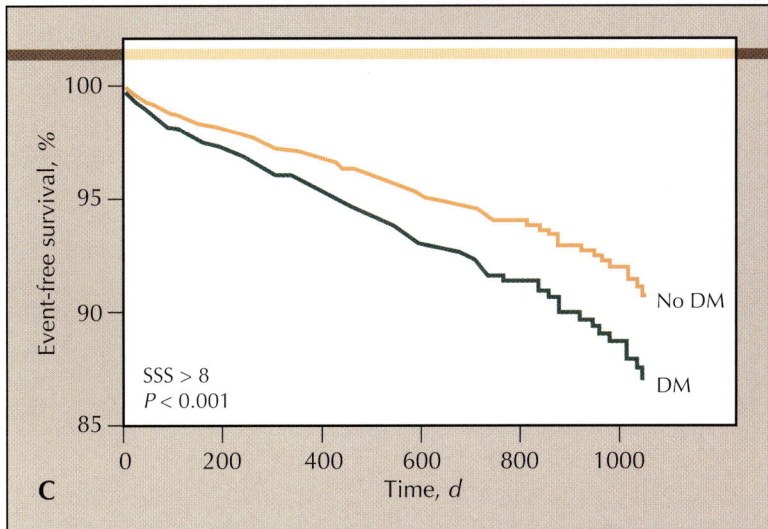

FIGURE 6-16. Prognostic value of summed stress scores in sestamibi SPECT in diabetic patients. Risk stratification using myocardial perfusion SPECT has been proven effective in a variety of patient subgroups, most importantly among diabetic patients. This figure illustrates the hard cardiac event-free survival rate in diabetic patients (DM) and patients without diabetes (no DM) categorized by the summed stress scores (SSS) as **A**, normal (SSS < 4), **B**, mildly abnormal (SSS 4–8), and **C**, moderately to severely abnormal (SSS > 8). The study was composed of 1271 patients with diabetes and 5862 patients without diabetes who underwent dual isotope myocardial perfusion SPECT. After risk adjustment for prescan likelihood of coronary artery disease, inability to exercise (requiring pharmacologic stress), history of coronary artery disease, and SSS, the patients with diabetes had a lower event-free survival in each of the SSS categories than the patients without diabetes. Given this result, a diabetic patient with only mildly abnormal myocardial perfusion scan results might be considered for cardiac catheterization in the presence of minimal symptoms, whereas in general, patients with only mildly abnormal scans might be considered appropriate for aggressive medical management without catheterization [2,14]. Similar results were obtained in a smaller diabetic population from a multicenter registry [19]. (*Adapted from* Kang *et al.* [20].)

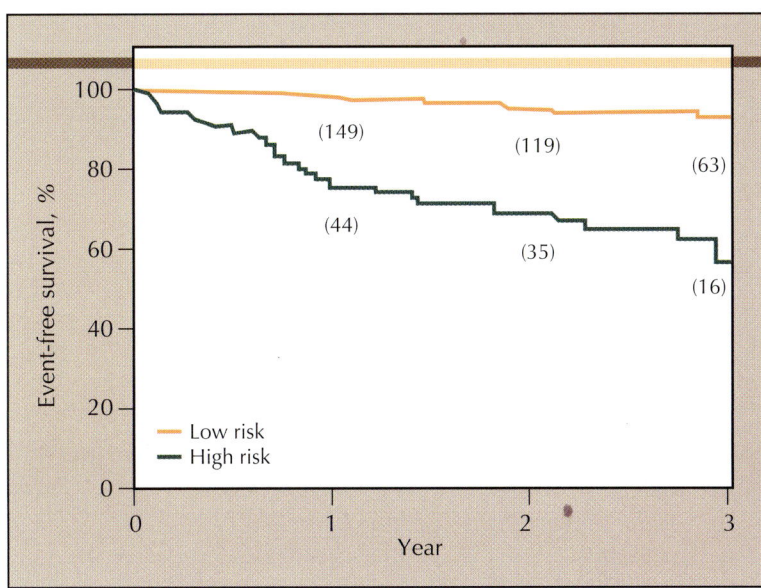

FIGURE 6-17. Prognostic value of vasodilator SPECT in left bundle branch block (LBBB). When patients with LBBB are considered for testing, vasodilator SPECT is the preferred form of stress in order to avoid the frequent stress-induced septal perfusion defect associated with high heart rates during exercise. This figure illustrates the effectiveness of vasodilator myocardial perfusion SPECT for risk stratification of patients with LBBB. In a relatively large group of patients with LBBB undergoing vasodilator ^{201}Tl SPECT, survival free of cardiac death, myocardial infarction, or cardiac transplantation is significantly higher among patients with low-risk myocardial perfusion scans compared with those with high-risk myocardial perfusion scans. (*Adapted from* Wagdy *et al.* [21].)

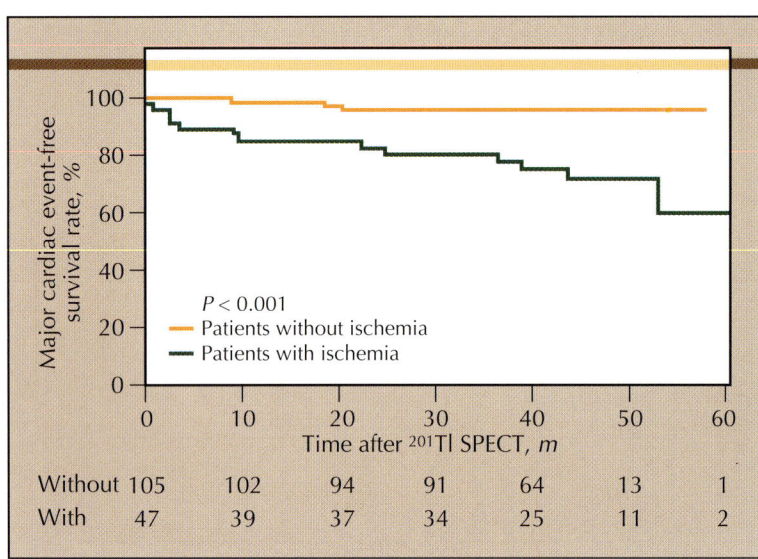

FIGURE 6-18. Long-term prognostic value of ^{201}Tl myocardial perfusion SPECT after coronary stenting. Myocardial perfusion SPECT has been demonstrated to be useful in risk stratification following percutaneous coronary intervention. In patients without ischemia on myocardial perfusion SPECT, the likelihood of a major cardiac event is very low and clearly distinct from the event-free survival rate of patients demonstrating myocardial ischemia following stenting. (*Adapted from* Cottin *et al.* [22].)

NUCLEAR CARDIOLOGY FOR RISK STRATIFICATION IN CHRONIC CORONARY ARTERY DISEASE

Specific patient subsets
- Women
- Elderly
- Diabetic
- LBBB, LVH
- Intermediate Duke treadmill score
- After coronary angiography
- After MI
- After PCI, CABG

FIGURE 6-19. Nuclear cardiology for risk stratification in chronic coronary artery disease. Nuclear cardiology has been shown to be effective for risk stratification in several relevant clinical subsets. Several randomized trials in progress should provide a higher level of evidence for this risk stratification application. Among these trials are COURAGE (Clinical Outcomes Utilizing Revascularization and Aggressive Drug Evaluation), BARI 2D (Bypass Angioplasty Revascularization Investigation 2 Diabetes), INSPIRE (Intravascular Ultrasound Study of Predictor of Restenosis), and DIAD (Detection of Ischemia in Asymptomatic Diabetics). CABG—coronary artery bypass grafting; LBBB—left bundle branch block; LVH—left ventricular hypertrophy; MI—myocardial infarction; PCI—percutaneous coronary intervention. (*Adapted from* Gibbons *et al.* [2].)

MYOCARDIAL PERFUSION SPECT DATA ON RISK STRATIFICATION

- Early revascularization and/or aggressive medical therapy leads to loss of prognostic information in highest risk patients
- Recent technical advances not included
  - Quantitative lung uptake
  - Transient ischemic dilation
  - Gated SPECT
    - Ejection fraction
    - Regional wall motion/thickening
    - Absolute LV volume

FIGURE 6-20. Myocardial perfusion SPECT data on risk stratification. Myocardial perfusion SPECT data for risk stratification may underestimate the strength of the modality. LV—left ventricle.

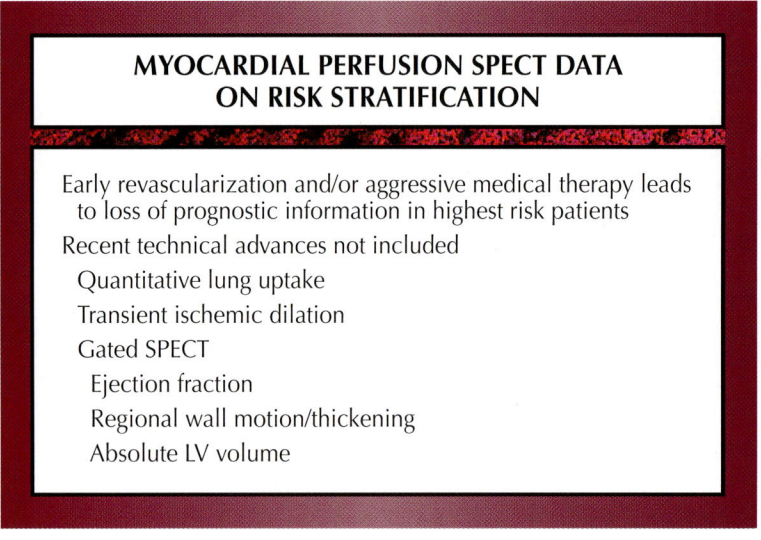

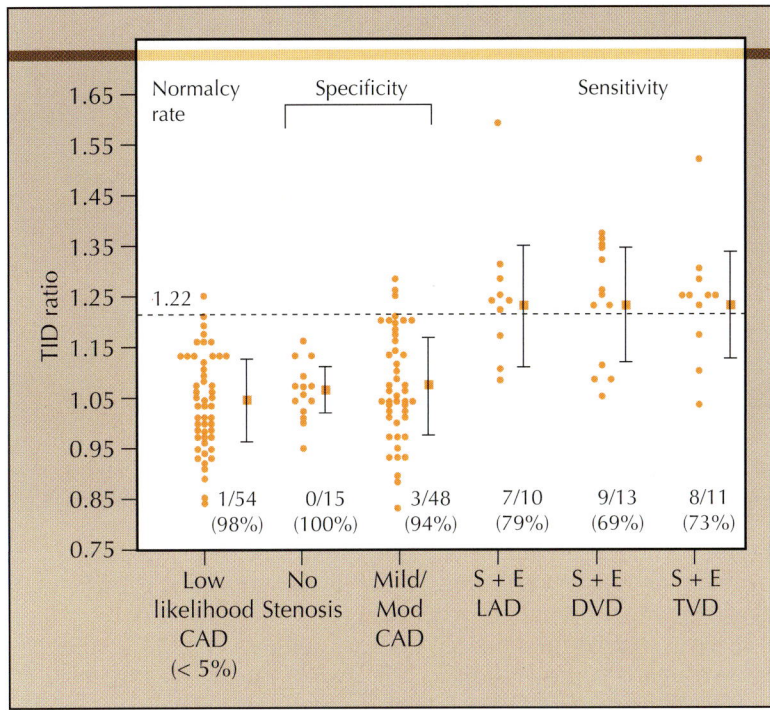

FIGURE 6-21. Relationship between transient ischemic dilation and the presence and extent of angiographic coronary artery disease. For purposes of risk stratification, it is reasonable to consider patients with severe (> 90% stenosis) and extensive (S + E) coronary artery disease (CAD) to be at high risk. The findings provide the basis for the statement that on myocardial perfusion SPECT, the finding of transient ischemic dilation (TID) is usually associated with a greater than 90% stenosis of either the proximal left anterior descending coronary artery (LAD) or the multiple vessels. Thus, consideration of the presence of TID will augment the prognostic value of myocardial perfusion SPECT over the information provided by indices such as summed stress score and summed difference score. DVD—double vessel disease; TVD—triple vessel disease. (*Adapted from* Mazzanti *et al.* [9].)

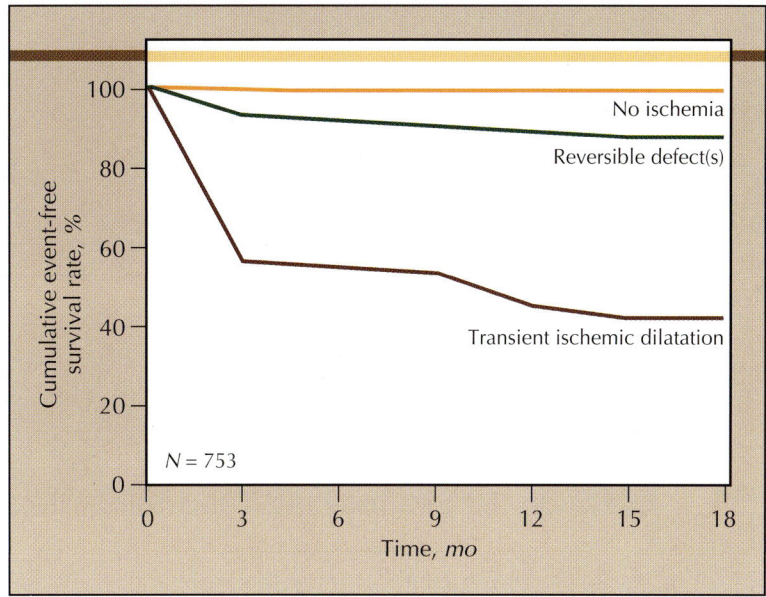

FIGURE 6-22. Long-term risk stratification with dipyridamole planar ^{201}Tl imaging. The presence of transient ischemic dilatation of the left ventricle provides further long-term risk stratification over planar ^{201}Tl imaging in a group of 753 patients. Mean follow-up was 15 months. Event is defined as a nonfatal myocardial infarction or cardiac death. (*Adapted from* Lette *et al.* [23]).

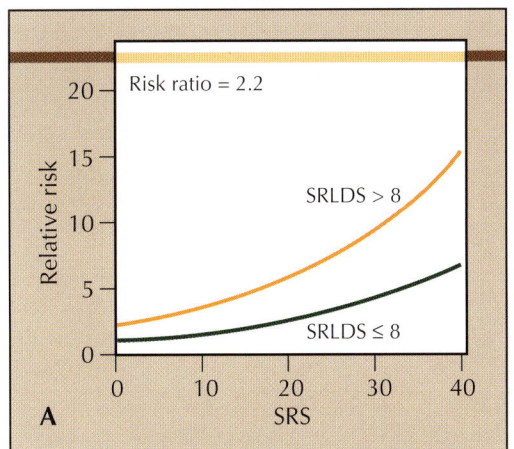
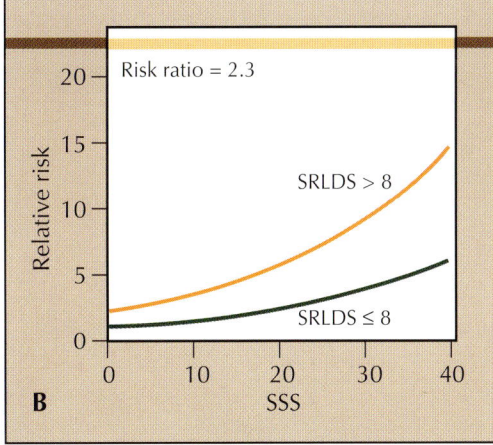

FIGURE 6-23. Resting ^{201}Tl reversibility: added value over summed stress score and summed rest score. In patients with chronic coronary artery disease, the added prognostic value of resting ^{201}Tl reversibility in dual isotope myocardial perfusion SPECT is shown. The two curves represent differing amounts of resting reversibility as measured by the summed rest late difference score (SRLDS). When this score is greater than 8 (extensive resting ischemia), the relative risk with respect to subsequent cardiac events is clearly higher than when less resting reversibility is present. **A**, The incremental prognostic value of resting reversibility persists when either the summed rest score (SRS) or, **B**, the summed stress score (SSS) is considered. These data suggest that a combination of assessing both stress-induced ischemia and resting ischemia might be more effective than assessing stress-induced ischemia alone in evaluating the risk of patients with chronic coronary artery disease. (*Adapted from* Sharir *et al.* [24].)

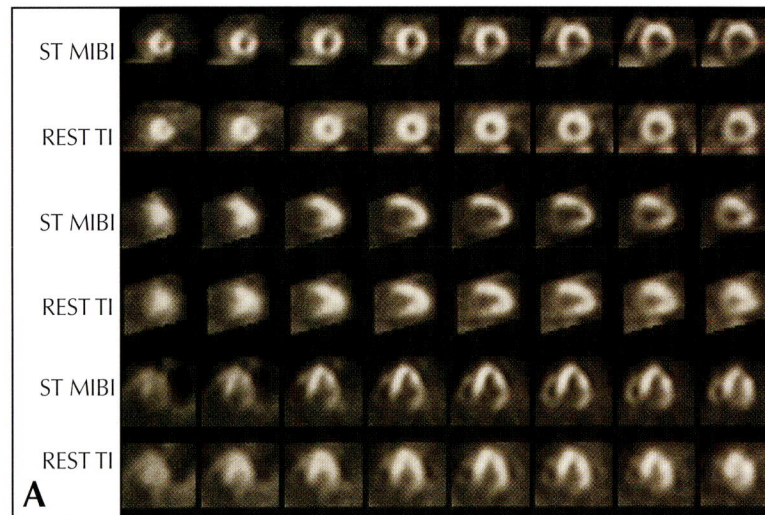
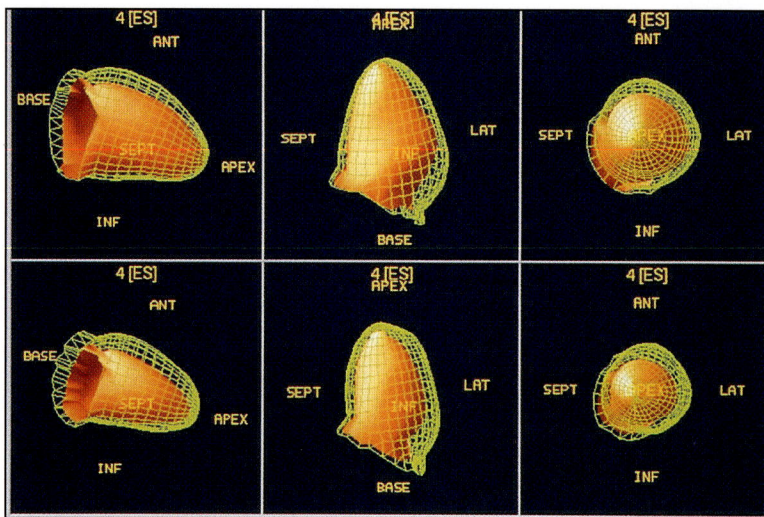

FIGURE 6-24. Assessment of risk using gated myocardial perfusion SPECT. A, Perfusion results from a 73-year-old patient with atypical chest pain who had undergone coronary artery bypass surgery at a remote time and angioplasty 5 years prior to this SPECT study. The patient had hypertension and hypercholesterolemia, and there was no history of prior myocardial infarction. Adenosine stress testing demonstrated ST segment depression (–1.5 mm downsloping in lead V5), and there was no ST segment depression at rest. Exercise stress ^{99m}Tc-sestamibi (ST MIBI) and rest ^{201}Tl (REST Tl) images are interlaced in the alternate rows, which show short-axis images (*top two rows*), vertical long-axis images (*middle two rows*), and horizontal long-axis images (*bottom two rows*). The stress and rest images demonstrate extensive ischemia in the right coronary territory and evidence of ischemia in the diagonal coronary territory. The stress perfusion defects alone indicate a high-risk state. There is also evidence of transient ischemic dilation in the left ventricle, further adding to the concept that ischemia is severe in this patient.

B, Stress (*top row*) and rest (*bottom row*) of the gated SPECT study. Shown are the vertical long-axis (*left column*), horizontal long-axis (*middle column*), and short-axis (*right column*) views. The white grid is the computer-defined endocardial surface from the gated SPECT study at end-diastole, and the shaded gray surface represents the computer-defined endocardial surface at end-systole. This patient demonstrates septal wall motion abnormality at rest (with normal thickening not shown) consistent with prior bypass surgery. Following stress, there is the development of a new wall motion abnormality in the anterior apical and inferior left ventricular walls.

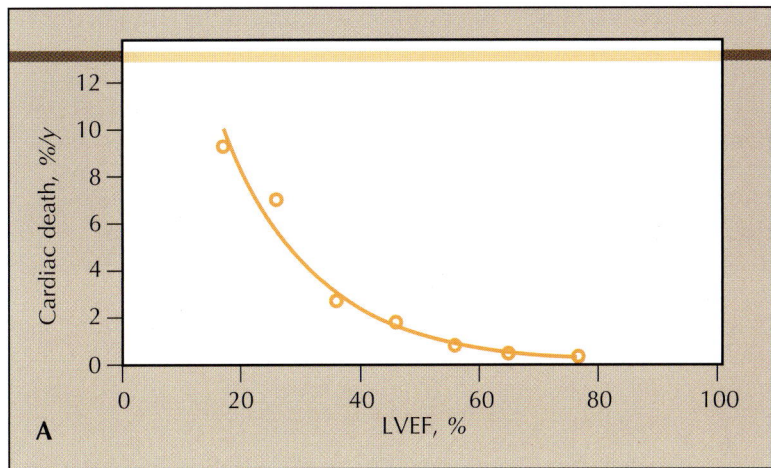
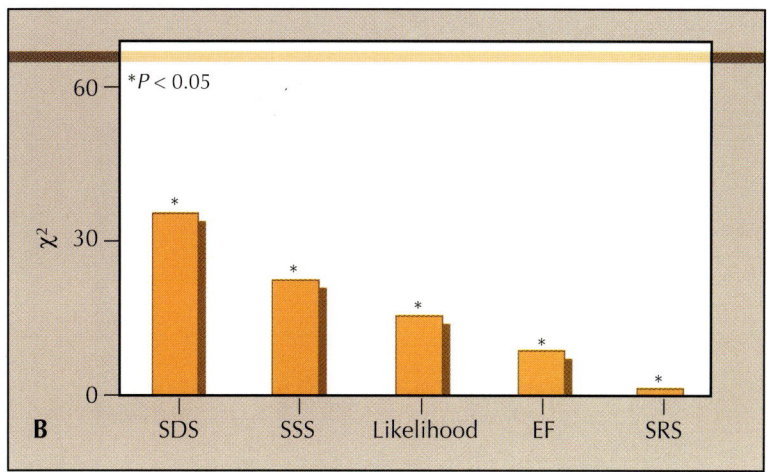
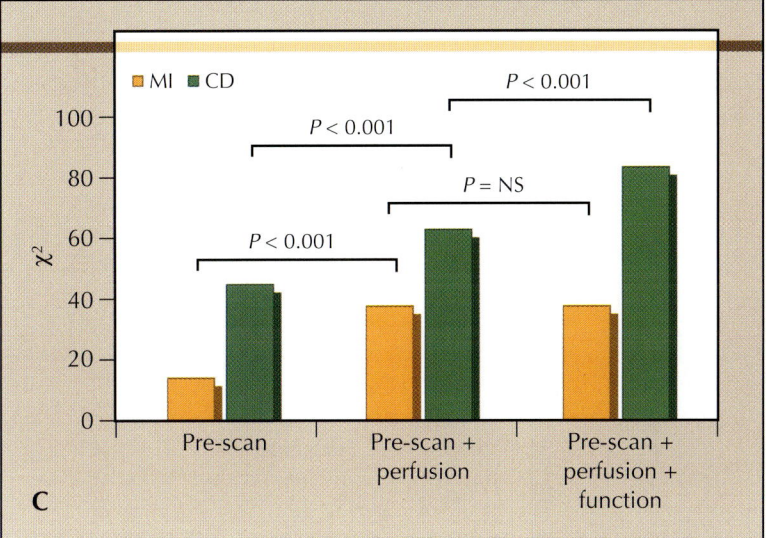

FIGURE 6-25. Relationship between left ventricular ejection fraction (LVEF) easured by gated SPECT and mortality rate and nonfatal myocardial infarction. **A,** In 2686 consecutive patients undergoing stress ^{99m}Tc myocardial perfusion gated SPECT, there is a curvilinear inverse relationship between LVEF at rest and cardiac death [25]. The LVEF was the strongest predictor of mortality in this group. The findings are similar to those reported for LVEF acquired with radionuclide angiography in patients after MI. **B,** When the predictors of nonfatal MI are considered, while LVEF remains a significant predictor, the extent of reversible ischemia as measured by the summed difference score (SDS) is the strongest univariate predictor. Previous studies have also shown that the extent of reversible ischemia is more predictive for cardiac events than the extent of coronary artery disease as assessed by coronary angiography [26]. **C,** When considered from the standpoint of incremental information, stress SPECT perfusion data add significantly to clinical information for predicting nonfatal MI, and there is no further information gained from other variables provided by gated SPECT (*orange bars*). However, when the risk of cardiac death is considered (*green bars*), incremental information is provided over clinical data not only by the stress perfusion findings but also by LVEF assessed by gated SPECT. EF—ejection fraction; SSS—summed stress score; SRS—summed rest score. (*Adapted from* Sharir *et al.* [25].)

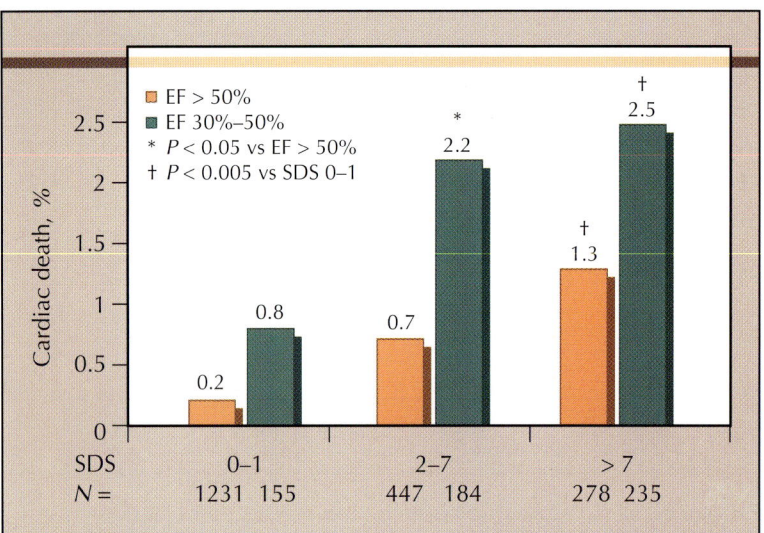

FIGURE 6-26. Cardiac death rate as a function of the amount of ischemia. In 564 patients with post-stress ejection fractions between 30% and 50%, only those with no evidence of reversible defects fell into the category of low risk for cardiac death (0.8% per year), whereas the patients with moderate or severe ischemia as assessed by the summed difference score (SDS) did not have low annual rates of cardiac death. In the patients with post-stress ejection fraction (EF) above 50%, the low 1% annual cardiac death rate was only exceeded when extensive reversible defects were present (SDS > 7). NS—not significant. (*Adapted from* Sharir *et al.* [25].)

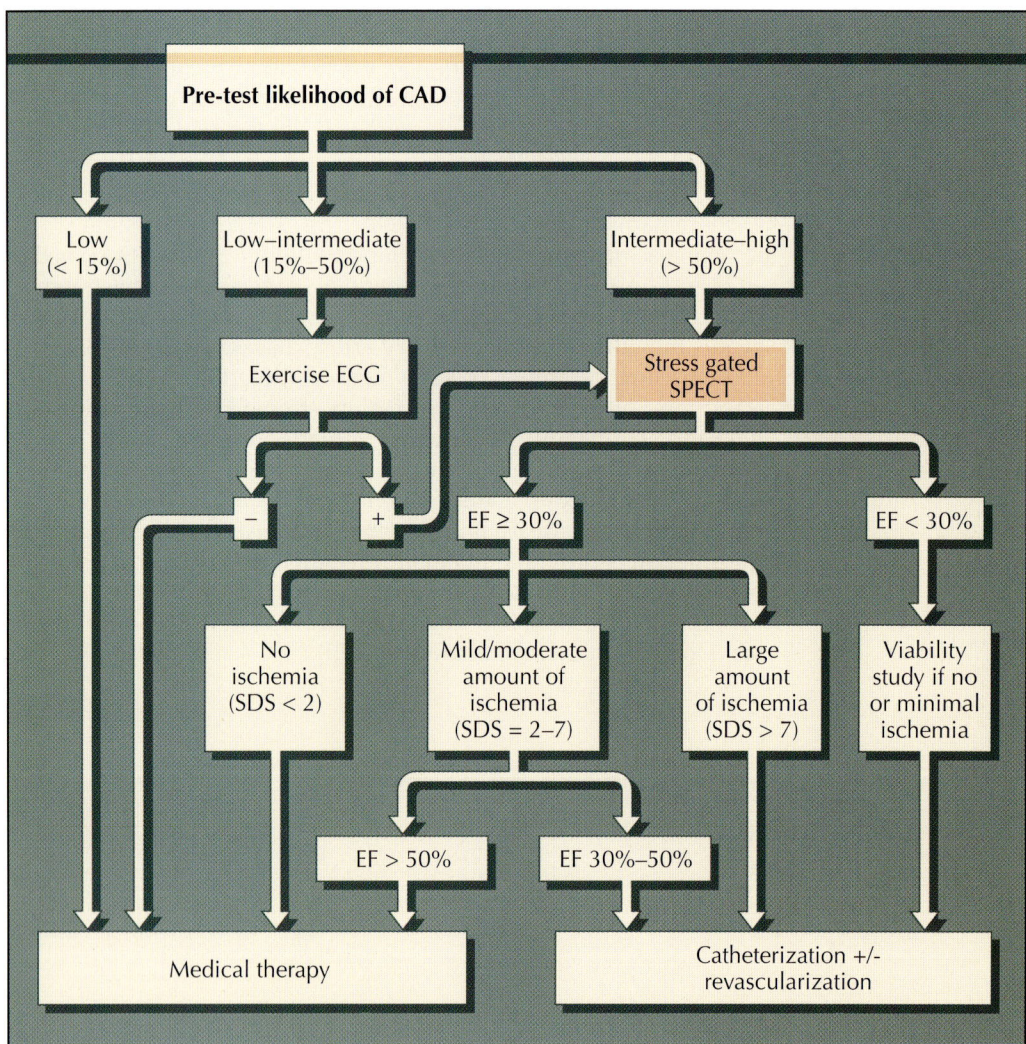

FIGURE 6-27. Role of gated SPECT in the management of coronary artery disease (CAD). Patients with a low likelihood of CAD (< 15%) would not require testing for prognostic purposes. Patients with a low–intermediate likelihood of CAD (15%–50%) and a normal resting electrocardiogram would be considered candidates for exercise testing without imaging. For patients with an intermediate risk (or even high risk) based on the Duke treadmill score, further testing with stress gated SPECT would be useful. Patients with a high–intermediate to high likelihood of CAD (> 50% likelihood of angiographically significant CAD) should proceed directly to gated stress myocardial perfusion SPECT. Following gated SPECT, those known to be at low risk for cardiac death (< 1% per year) would be referred for medical therapy. These include patients with an ejection fraction (EF) of 30% or more with no ischemia, or an EF above 50% with mild to moderate ischemia (summed difference score [SDS] = 2–7). Patients with an intermediate (1%–3% per year) or high (> 3% per year) likelihood of cardiac death would be referred for cardiac catheterization for possible revascularization. These include patients with a large amount of ischemia (SDS > 7) (regardless of EF), those with mild to moderate left ventricular dysfunction (post-stress EF 30%–50%) with any ischemia (SDS ≥ 2), or patients with severely decreased left ventricular function (EF < 30%). Additional viability testing should be considered in patients with EF below 30%. (*Adapted from* Berman *et al.* [26].)

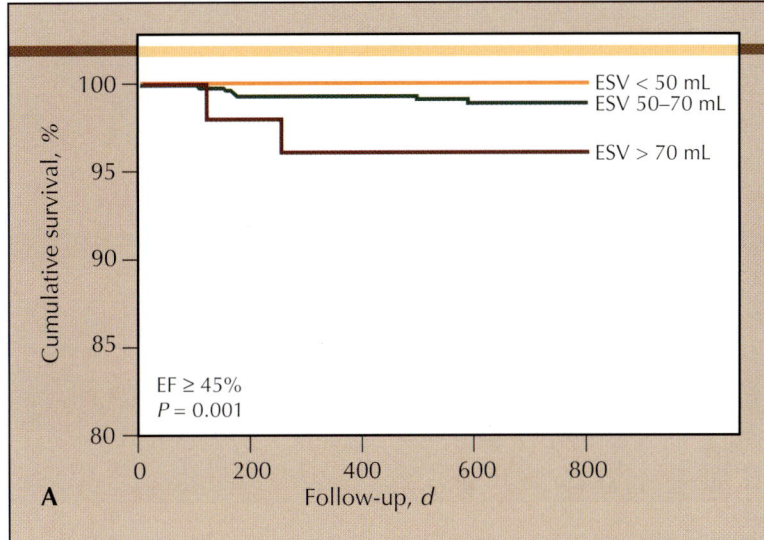
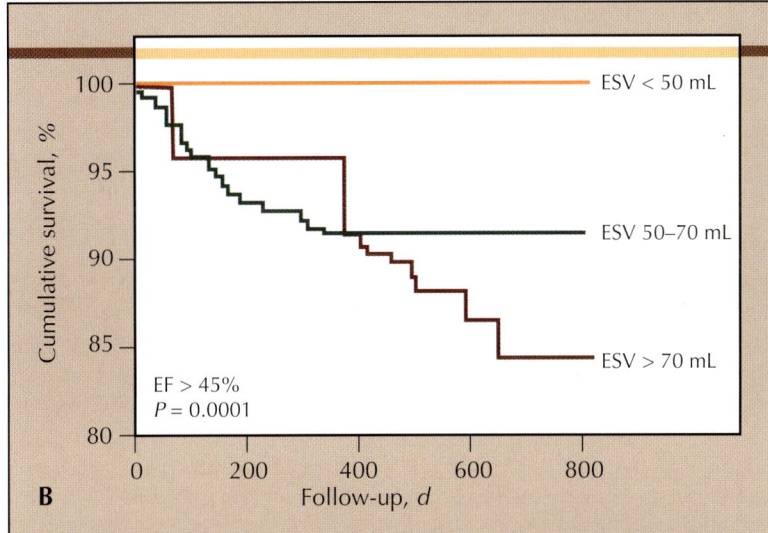
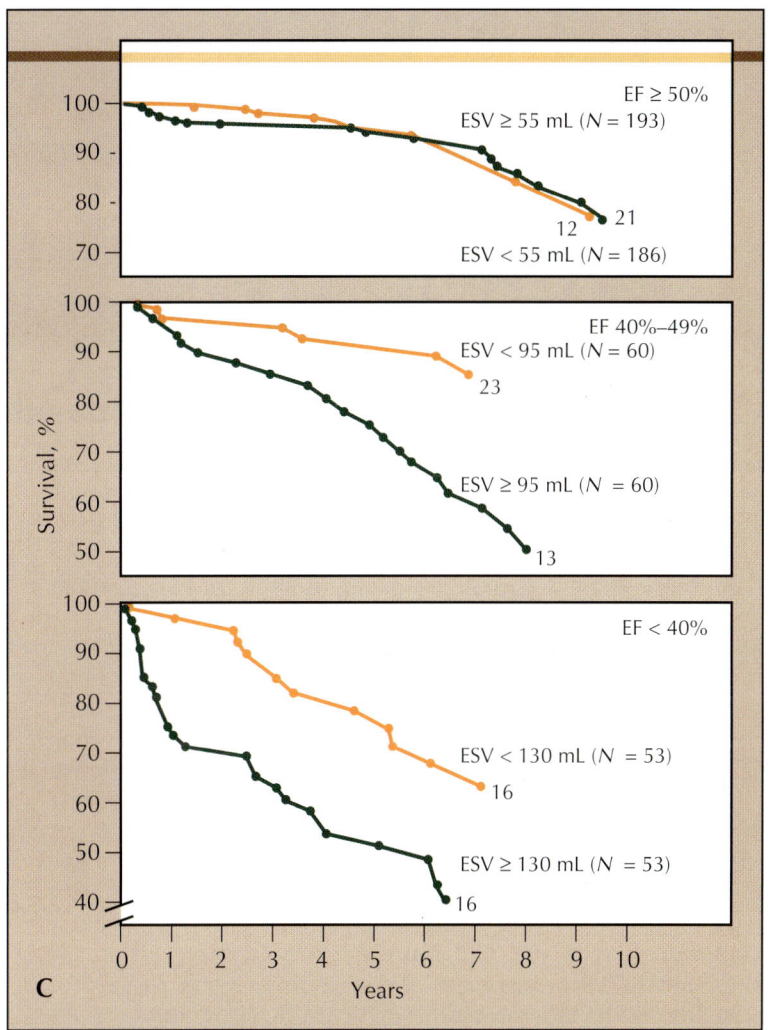

FIGURE 6-28. Left ventricular end-systolic volume (ESV) as the major determinant of survival after myocardial infarction. Beyond assessment of left ventricular ejection fraction (LVEF), gated SPECT also provides information on left ventricular volumes, which may be useful in prognostic stratification. In 1680 patients, ESV assessed by gated SPECT provided significant information over the extent and severity of perfusion defect as measured by the summed stress score in prediction of cardiac death. **A**, Patients with normal LVEF by gated SPECT. **B**, Patients with abnormal LVEF by gated SPECT. Within each LVEF group, patients are then subdivided according to ESV by gated SPECT. In both LVEF groups, ESV further stratified patients with respect to survival. Similar to the findings with contrast ventriculography, this stratification was particularly strong in patients with reduced LVEF. **C**, Using contrast ventriculography, the influence of large versus small ESV on mortality rate is shown in three different LVEF groups of patients following myocardial infarction. In patients with normal LVEF (*top panel*), ventricular volume is not a predictor of death. However, in patients with mild to moderate (*middle panel*) or low (*bottom panel*) LVEF, those with large ESV have distinctly lower survival rates that those with smaller volumes. Similar results were obtained when ESV was measured by gated SPECT. (*Panels A and B adapted from* Sharir et al. [27]; *panel C adapted from* White et al. [28].)

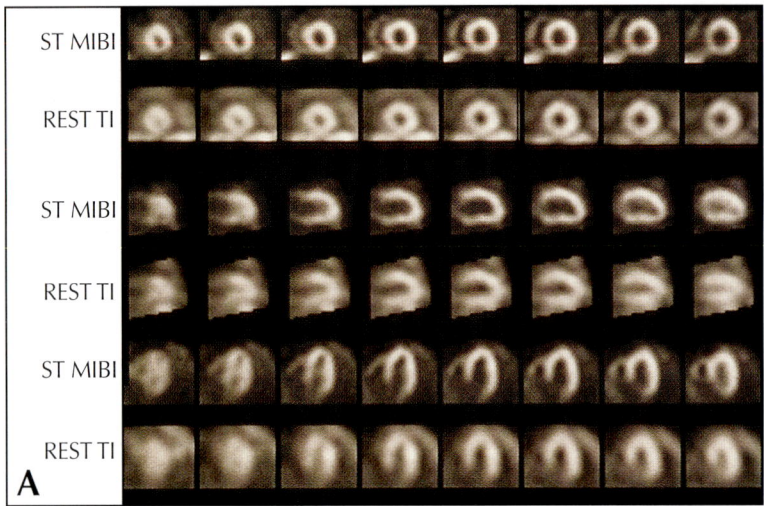
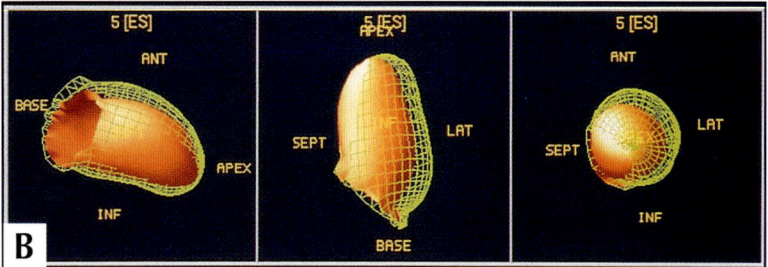

FIGURE 6-29. Incremental prognostic value of gated SPECT. An 84-year-old man was admitted to the hospital with exertional shortness of breath and paroxysmal nocturnal dyspnea. He had nonanginal chest pain, and his cardiac enzymes were negative. After being pain-free for 48 hours, he was referred for adenosine myocardial perfusion scintigraphy. Risk factors included hypertension, diabetes, and hypercholesterolemia, and the resting ECG showed nonspecific ST-T wave abnormalities that did not change over the 2-day period. The patient underwent coronary artery bypass grafting 5 years prior to this admission. The adenosine stress test revealed no clinical or ECG evidence of ischemia. A, Exercise stress ^{99m}Tc-sestamibi (ST MIBI) and rest ^{201}Tl (REST Tl) images are interlaced in the alternate rows, which show short-axis images (*top two rows*), vertical long-axis images (*middle two rows*), and horizontal long-axis images (*bottom two rows*). The stress myocardial perfusion SPECT shows dilated left ventricular cavity and a mild stress perfusion defect (summed stress and rest scores were 4). B, Three-dimensional representation of the left ventricular myocardium from the post-stress gated SPECT studies. The white grid represents the computer-derived endocardial surface at end diastole. The shaded inner surface represents the computer-defined endocardial surface at end systole. The study demonstrates distal anterior apical and inferior hypokinesis. The septal wall motion abnormality was associated with normal septal thickening and thus most likely represented a normal postoperative finding. However, this process would not explain the anterior apical and inferior hypokinesis. Additionally, the patient's left ventricular ejection fraction was moderately reduced at 39%. The end-systolic volume was moderately elevated at 97 mL. Based on the combined perfusion and function studies, the patient was considered high-risk, whereas based on the perfusion study alone the patient would be considered low-risk. Based on these test results, his discharge diagnosis was ischemic cardiomyopathy. The patient was managed medically, and 30 months following admission he suffered a sudden, unexpected death presumed to be cardiac in origin. This case illustrates how gated SPECT classifies risk in a patient with mild perfusion abnormality.

RISK ASSESSMENT IN CHRONIC CORONARY ARTERY DISEASE

NON-NUCLEAR	NUCLEAR
Symptoms/clinical presentation	Extent and severity of perfusion defects
Exercise duration	Lung uptake
Exercise hypotension	TID
Duke treadmill score	LV function
Type of stress	LVEF
Angiographic findings	LV volume
	Wall motion

FIGURE 6-30. Importance of integration of test results in risk assessment in chronic coronary artery disease. Many factors are important in assessing the nuclear test to determine risk of a cardiac event. These include the lung uptake of ^{201}Tl, transient ischemic dilatation (TID), and the rest and post-stress left ventricular (LV) function measurements of the left ventricular ejection fraction (LVEF), end-systolic and end-diastolic left ventricular volumes, and regional wall motion. It should be emphasized, however, that the decision to proceed with invasive management does not rest solely on objective findings provided by nuclear examination, but requires an integration of clinical and test results. Important non-nuclear findings include symptoms and clinical presentation, exercise duration, the presence of exercise hypotension, the Duke treadmill score, the type of stress performed (pharmacologic stress implying higher risk), the presence of co-morbidities such as diabetes, and prior angiographic findings. Despite the strong power of objective measurements provided by gated myocardial perfusion SPECT, the decisions regarding patient management involves the combination of objective measurements (science) and clinical assessment (art).

REFERENCES

1. Yusuf S, Zucker D, Peduzzi P, *et al.*: Effect of coronary artery bypass graft surgery on survival: overview of 10-year results from randomised trials by the Coronary Artery Bypass Graft Surgery Trialists Collaboration. *Lancet* 1994, 344:563–570.

2. Gibbons RJ, Chatterjee K, Daley J, *et al.*: ACC/AHA/ACP-ASIM guidelines for the management of patients with chronic stable angina: a report of the American College of Cardiology/American Heart Association Task Force on Practice Guidelines (Committee on Management of Patients With Chronic Stable Angina) [published correction appears in *J Am Coll Cardiol* 1999, 34(1):314]. *J Am Coll Cardiol* 1999, 33:2092–2197.

3. Comparison of coronary bypass surgery with angioplasty in patients with multivessel disease. The Bypass Angioplasty Revascularization Investigation (BARI) Investigators. *N Engl J Med* 1996, 335:217–225.

4. Little WC, Constantinescu M, Applegate RJ, *et al.*: Can coronary angiography predict the site of a subsequent myocardial infarction in patients with mild-to-moderate coronary artery disease? *Circulation* 1988, 78:1157–1166.

5. Ambrose JA, Tannenbaum MA, Alexopoulos D, *et al.*: Angiographic progression of coronary artery disease and the development of myocardial infarction. *J Am Coll Cardiol* 1988, 12:56–62.

6. Hasdai D, Gibbons RJ, Holmes DR, Jr., *et al.*: Coronary endothelial dysfunction in humans is associated with myocardial perfusion defects. *Circulation* 1997, 96:3390–3395.

7. Ladenheim ML, Pollock BH, Rozanski A, *et al.*: Extent and severity of myocardial hypoperfusion as predictors of prognosis in patients with suspected coronary artery disease. *J Am Coll Cardiol* 1986, 7:464–471.

8. Berman DS, Kiat H, Friedman JD, *et al.*: Separate acquisition rest thallium-201/stress technetium-99m sestamibi dual-isotope myocardial perfusion single-photon emission computed tomography: a clinical validation study. *J Am Coll Cardiol* 1993 22:1455–1464.

9. Mazzanti M, Germano G, Kiat H, *et al.*: Identification of severe and extensive coronary artery disease by automatic measurement of transient ischemic dilation of the left ventricle in dual-isotope myocardial perfusion SPECT. *J Am Coll Cardiol* 1996, 27:1612–1620.

10. Matzer L, Kiat H, Van Train K, *et al.*: Quantitative severity of stress thallium-201 myocardial perfusion single-photon emission computed tomography defects in one-vessel coronary artery disease. *Am J Cardiol* 1993, 72:273–279.

11. Sharir T, Bacher-Stier C, Dhar S, *et al.*: Identification of severe and extensive coronary artery disease by postexercise regional wall motion abnormalities in Tc-99m sestamibi gated single-photon emission computed tomography. *Am J Cardiol* 2000, 86:1171–1175.

12. Ladenheim ML, Kotler TS, Pollock BH, *et al.*: Incremental prognostic power of clinical history, exercise electrocardiography and myocardial perfusion scintigraphy in suspected coronary artery disease. *Am J Cardiol* 1987, 59:270–277.

13. Berman DS, Hachamovitch R, Kiat H, *et al.*: Incremental value of prognostic testing in patients with known or suspected ischemic heart disease: a basis for optimal utilization of exercise technetium-99m sestamibi myocardial perfusion single-photon emission computed tomography. *J Am Coll Cardiol* 1995, 26:639–647.

14. Hachamovitch R, Berman DS, Shaw LJ, *et al.*: Incremental prognostic value of myocardial perfusion single photon emission computed tomography for the prediction of cardiac death: differential stratification for risk of cardiac death and myocardial infarction. *Circulation* 1998, 97:535–543.

15. Vanzetto G, Ormezzano O, Fagret D, *et al.*: Long-term additive prognostic value of thallium-201 myocardial perfusion imaging over clinical and exercise stress test in low to intermediate risk patients: study in 1137 patients with 6-year follow-up. *Circulation* 1999, 100:1521–1527.

16. Galassi AR, Azzarelli S, Tomaselli A, *et al.*: Incremental prognostic value of technetium-99m-tetrofosmin exercise myocardial perfusion imaging for predicting outcomes in patients with suspected or known coronary artery disease. *Am J Cardiol* 2001, 88:101–106.

17. Hachamovitch R, Berman DS, Kiat H, *et al.*: Exercise myocardial perfusion SPECT in patients without known coronary artery disease: incremental prognostic value and use in risk stratification. *Circulation* 1996, 93:905–914.

18. Gibbons RJ, Hodge DO, Berman DS, *et al.*: Long-term outcome of patients with intermediate-risk exercise electrocardiograms who do not have myocardial perfusion defects on radionuclide imaging. *Circulation* 1999, 100:2140–2145.

19. Giri S, Shaw LJ, Murthy DR, *et al.*: Impact of diabetes on the risk stratification using stress single-photon emission computed tomography myocardial perfusion imaging in patients with symptoms suggestive of coronary artery disease. *Circulation* 2002, 105:32–40.

20. Kang X, Berman DS, Lewin HC, *et al.*: Incremental prognostic value of myocardial perfusion single photon emission computed tomography in patients with diabetes mellitus. *Am Heart J* 1999, 138:1025–1032.

21. Wagdy HM, Hodge D, Christian TF, *et al.*: Prognostic value of vasodilator myocardial perfusion imaging in patients with left bundle-branch block. *Circulation* 1998, 97:1563–1570.

22. Cottin Y, Rezaizadeh K, Touzery C, *et al.*: Long-term prognostic value of 201Tl single-photon emission computed tomographic myocardial perfusion imaging after coronary stenting. *Am Heart J* 2001, 141:999–1006.

23. Lette J, Tatum JL, Fraser S, *et al.*: Safety of dipyridamole testing in 73,806 patients: the Multicenter Dipyridamole Safety Study. *J Nucl Cardiol* 1995, 2:3–17.

24. Sharir T, Berman DS, Lewin HC, *et al.*: Incremental prognostic value of rest-redistribution (201)Tl single-photon emission computed tomography. *Circulation* 1999, 100:1964–1970.

25. Sharir T, Germano G, Kang X, *et al.*: Prediction of myocardial infarction versus cardiac death by gated myocardial perfusion SPECT: risk stratification by the amount of stress-induced ischemia and the poststress ejection fraction. *J Nucl Med* 2001, 42:831–837.

26. Berman DS, Hayes SW, Shaw LJ, *et al.*: Recent advances in myocardial perfusion imaging. *Curr Probl Cardiol* 2001, 26:1–140.

27. Sharir T, Germano G, Kavanagh PB, *et al.*: Incremental prognostic value of post-stress left ventricular ejection fraction and volume by gated myocardial perfusion single photon emission computed tomography. *Circulation* 1999, 100:1035–1042.

28. White HD, Norris RM, Brown MA, *et al.*: Left ventricular end-systolic volume as the major determinant of survival after recovery from myocardial infarction. *Circulation* 1987, 76:44–51.

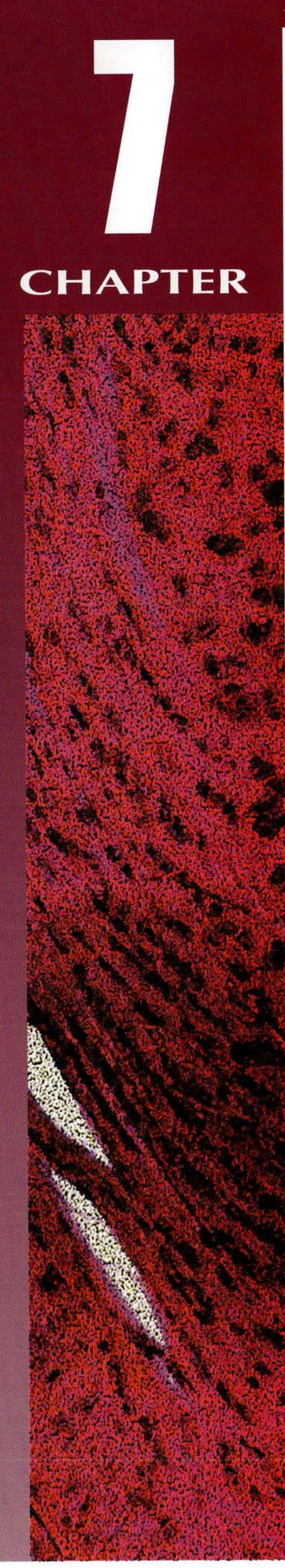

CHAPTER 7

Diagnosis and Risk Stratification in Acute Coronary Syndromes

James E. Udelson

Since the 1970s, radionuclide myocardial perfusion imaging (MPI) has played an important role in diagnosis as well as in risk stratification for patients suffering from acute ischemic coronary syndromes (ACS). Early studies using planar ^{201}Tl imaging documented the superior ability of this technique to assess both the presence and location of myocardial infarction (MI) and to predict the site of coronary disease involvement in unstable syndromes more accurately than ECG findings alone [1]. More recently, the use of ^{99m}Tc-based agents such as sestamibi in the early hours of an infarct has provided important information on areas at risk in the setting of the coronary occlusion, while a follow-up study done several days later provided information on final infarct size and myocardial salvage when both sets of images were compared [2].

Stress MPI in the early aftermath of both unstable angina syndromes as well as acute MI carries powerful prognostic information for risk-stratifying stable post-ACS patients. Imaging for ischemia has been incorporated into numerous randomized clinical trials to better define the roles of different ACS management strategies [3,4]. Over the last few years, MPI has also been used to rule ACS in or out among patients with chest pain syndromes who do not have diagnostic ischemic ECG changes upon presentation to the emergency room. Several published studies now consistently demonstrate very high negative predictive value for ruling out acute ischemia, as well as powerful risk stratification information for those with positive tests in the emergency setting [5–8]. Thus, SPECT MPI techniques are widely used in the setting of ACS, both for initial detection of abnormal blood flow underlying the clinical syndrome and for decision-making regarding conservative versus invasive interventional management.

Recent advances in hardware and software technology have allowed the combined assessment of stress and rest MPI with measures of regional and global left ventricular function using gated SPECT imaging [9]. Based on the wide availability of gated SPECT MPI of both perfusion and left ventricular function, obtaining the incremental value of adding functional information to the perfusion information in ACS is now routine.

In this chapter, the role of radionuclide imaging techniques in the broad setting of ACS will be reviewed, with emphasis on decision points where the imaging data has been shown to enhance the clinician's information base in order to optimally manage patients in this setting.

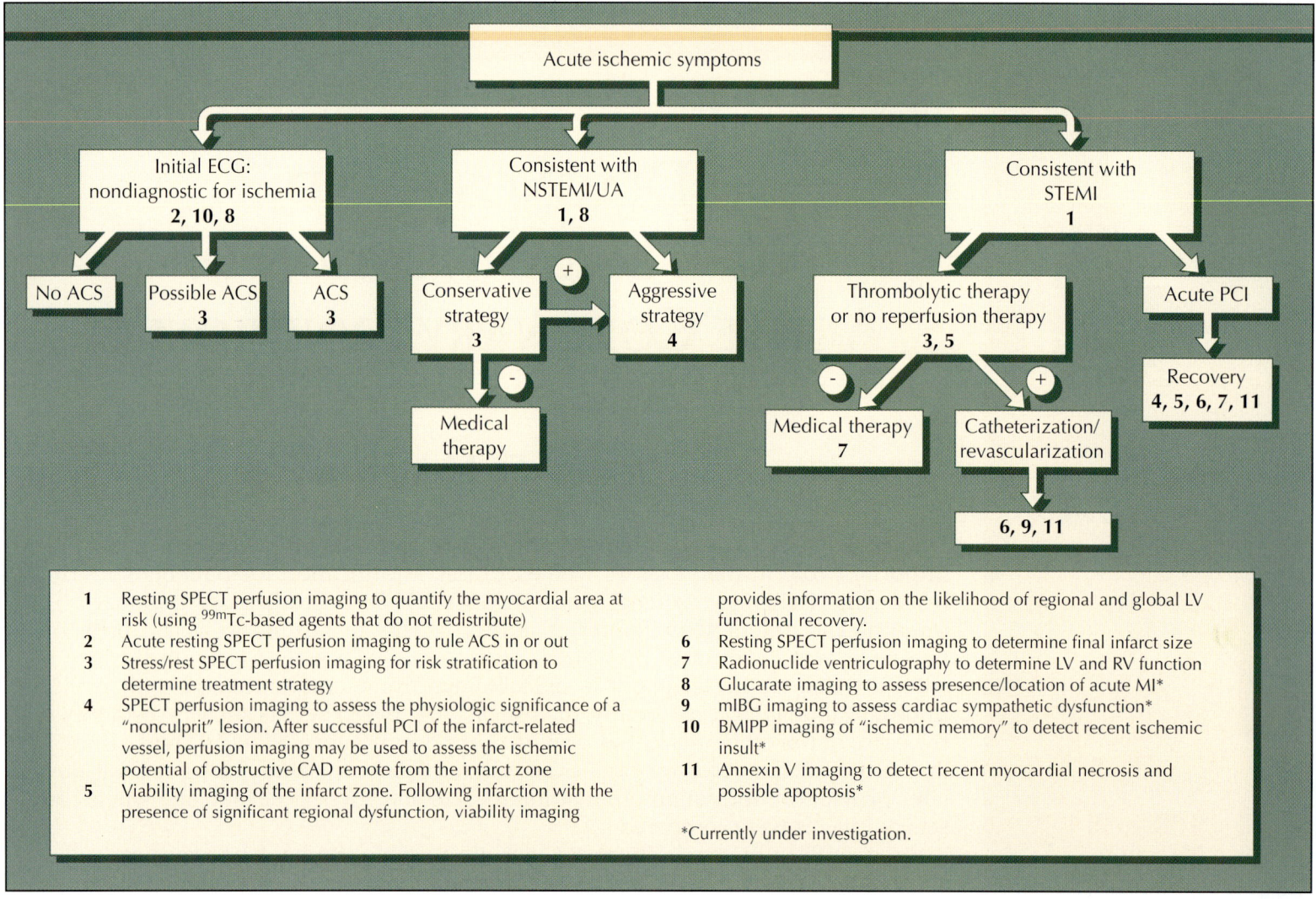

FIGURE 7-1. Diagnostic and therapeutic decision points in three categories of acute ischemic coronary syndromes (ACS). This schematic demonstrates the role of radionuclide techniques in patients seen in the emergency department with suspected ACS who have nondiagnostic ECG changes, patients with non–ST segment elevation myocardial infarction/unstable angina (NSTEMI/UA), and patients with ST segment elevation myocardial infarction (STEMI). Radionuclide imaging techniques that have been applied in either a research or clinical setting are listed, keyed to the appropriate clinical time points where they would be most useful. BMIPP—15-(p-[iodine-123] iodophenyl)-3-(R,S) methyl-pentadecanoic acid; CAD—coronary artery disease; LV—left ventricle; mIBG—metaiodobenzylguanidine; PCI—percutaneous coronary intervention; RV—right ventricle.

ASSESSMENT OF PATIENTS WITH SUSPECTED ACUTE CORONARY SYNDROME

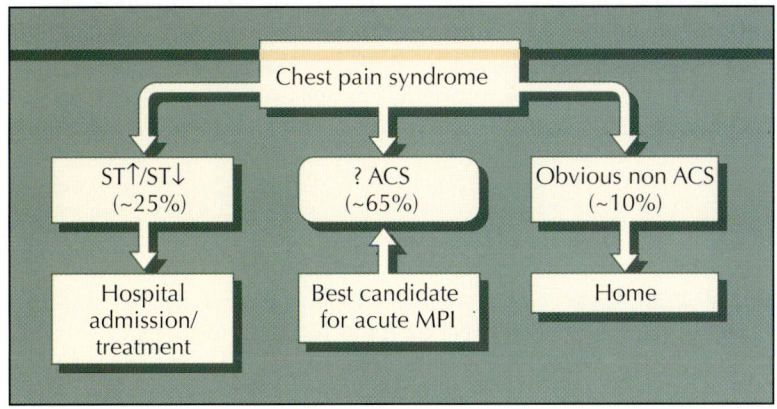

FIGURE 7-2. Initial classification of patients presenting to the emergency room (ER) with symptoms suspicious for acute coronary syndrome (ACS). Patients with initial ECGs demonstrating obvious ST segment elevation or ST segment depression (approximately 25% of all patients presenting with symptoms of possible ischemia) should be admitted promptly and managed according to contemporary practice guidelines [10,11]. In surveys of ER patients with chest pain syndromes, approximately 10% have symptoms that are very unlikely to be due to ischemia after initial history and examination. The remaining population of patients whose initial ECGs are not diagnostic for ACS (60%–70% of all patients presenting to ERs with possible ischemic symptoms) are candidates for acute resting myocardial perfusion imaging (MPI) to better stratify those patients whose symptoms are likely to be ischemic from those whose symptoms are most likely not due to ischemia. The former group (abnormal scan) may be considered candidates for more aggressive therapy, while the latter group (normal resting perfusion scan) may be considered candidates for early discharge from the ER.

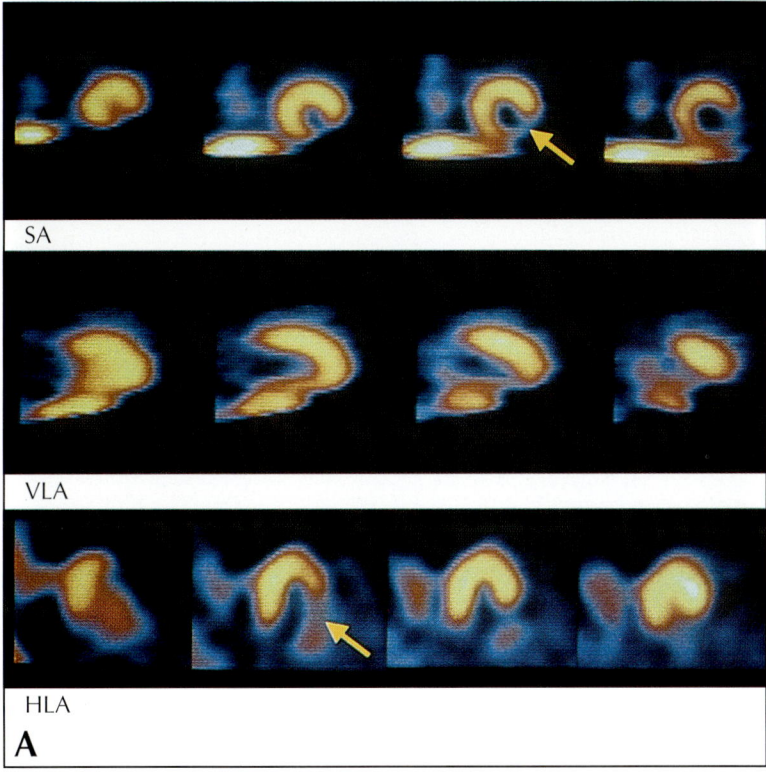

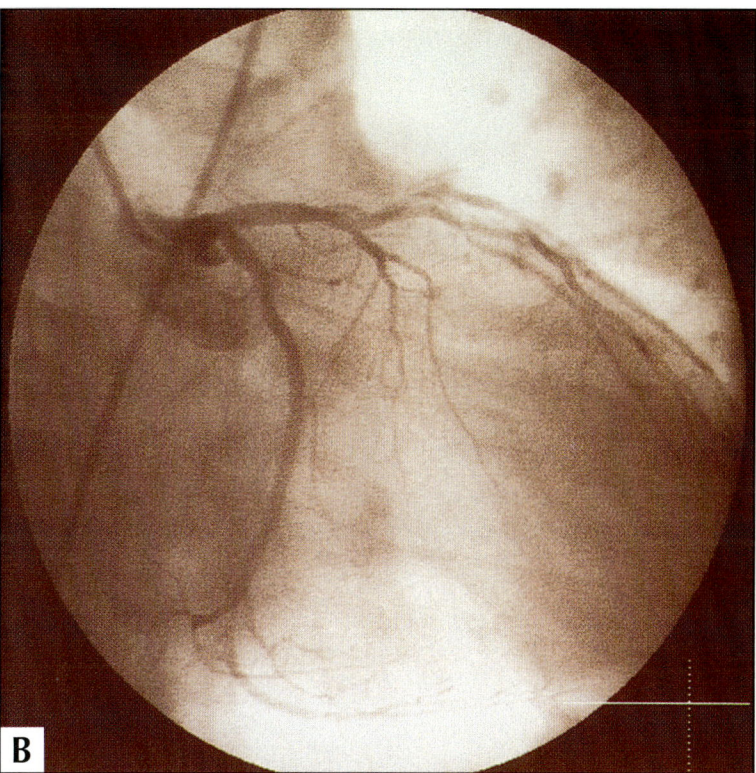

FIGURE 7-3. Significant myocardial perfusion abnormalities in patients with chest pain but nondiagnostic electrocardiographic alterations. **A**, Short-axis (SA), vertical long-axis (VLA), and horizontal long-axis (HLA) resting SPECT myocardial perfusion images (MPIs) of a 39-year-old-man who presented to the emergency room (ER) with chest pain atypical for angina and a normal initial ECG. He was injected with ^{99m}Tc-sestamibi at rest in the ER and underwent SPECT imaging soon thereafter. The images show a dense inferolateral resting perfusion defect (*arrows*), which in the setting of ongoing symptoms was most suggestive of resting ischemia and acute coronary syndrome (ACS). He was immediately triaged to the catheterization laboratory.

B, Right anterior oblique view of the left coronary artery injection showing an acutely occluded left circumflex artery in the patient in *panel A*. Left circumflex occlusions are not always well seen on the standard 12-lead ECG. The patient subsequently underwent successful percutaneous coronary intervention of the left circumflex artery, with an excellent anatomic result. Had MPI not been performed, he may have been admitted for observation, and serial enzyme analysis may have been positive for a myocardial infarction. The use of MPI likely allowed significantly earlier intervention in this case.   *Continued on next page*

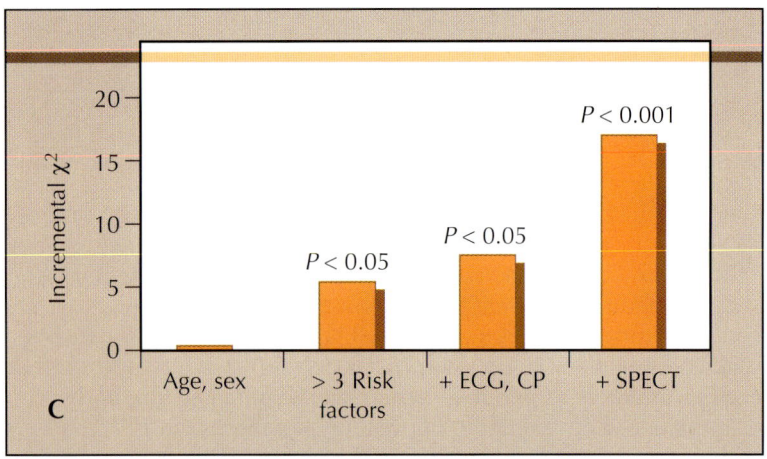

FIGURE 7-3. *(Continued)* **C,** Analysis of the incremental value of resting MPI data to predict cardiac events in patients presenting to the ER with suspected ischemia. The incremental χ^2 value measures the strength of the association between individual factors added to a clinician's knowledge base in incremental fashion and unfavorable cardiac events. Addition of resting SPECT MPI data (+ SPECT) in the ER setting adds highly statistically significant value on detection of ACS and events even given knowledge of age, sex, multiple (> 3) risk factors for coronary artery disease, and ECG changes and the presence or absence of chest pain (CP). (*Panel C adapted from* Heller *et al.* [8].)

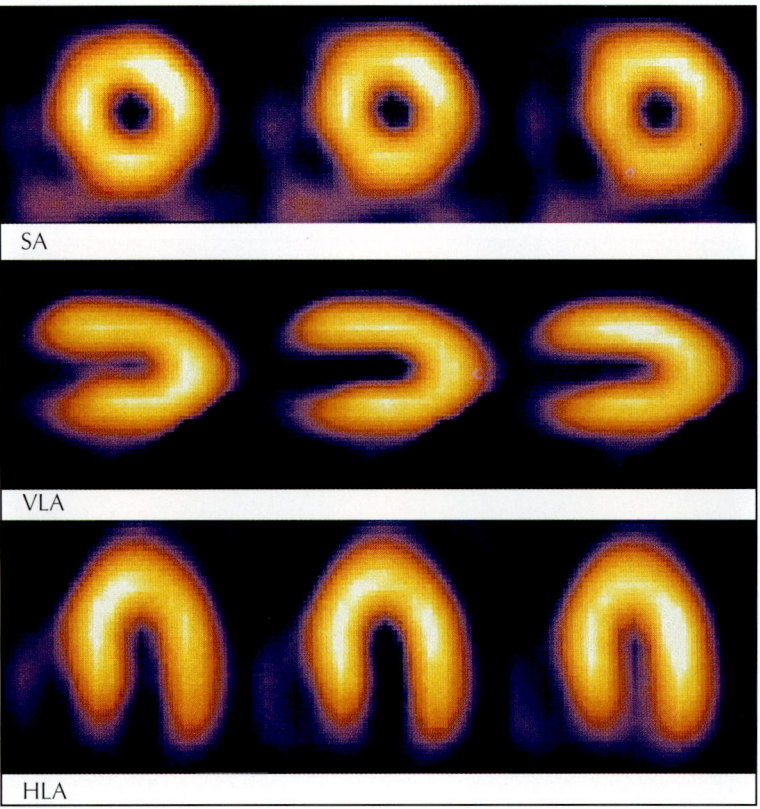

FIGURE 7-4. Absence of myocardial perfusion abnormality in a patient presenting with chest pain but nondiagnostic ECG changes. Short-axis (SA), vertical long-axis (VLA), and horizontal long-axis (HLA) SPECT images of a 52-year-old-man who presented to the emergency room (ER) with chest pain atypical for angina and an initial electrocardiogram with nonspecific ST segment abnormalities not diagnostic for acute ischemia. He was injected with ^{99m}Tc-sestamibi at rest in the ER, and underwent SPECT imaging soon thereafter. The images show a completely normal resting perfusion pattern, and the gated SPECT imaging of resting left ventricular function (not shown) was also normal. This finding is associated with a very low probability of myocardial infarction and acute ischemic syndrome (*see* Fig. 7-5), suggesting that such a patient may be discharged directly from the ER.

MAJOR CLINICAL STUDIES INVOLVING MYOCARDIAL PERFUSION IN ACUTE CHEST PAIN

AUTHOR	N	SENSITIVITY	SPECIFICITY	PPV	NPV	ENDPOINT
Wackers et al. [1]	203	100	63	55	100	MI
Bilodeau et al. [12]	45	96	76	86	94	CAD (by angiography)
Varetto et al. [5]	64	100	67	43	100	MI
		100	92	90	100	CAD
Hilton et al. [6]	102	100	78	38	99	MI
		94	83	44	99	All events
Tatum et al. [7]	438	100	78	7	100	MI
		82	83	32	98	MI, revasc
Kontos et al. [13]	532	93	71	15	99	MI
		81	76	40	95	MI, revasc
Heller et al. [8]	357	90	60	12	99	MI
Duca et al. [14]	75	100	73	33	100	MI
		73	93	89	81	CAD
Kosnik et al. [15]	69	71	92	50	97	MI, revasc, or cardiac death

FIGURE 7-5. Summary of major clinical studies involving myocardial perfusion imaging for endpoint events in patients with chest pain syndromes but nondiagnostic ECGs. All published studies demonstrate a very high negative predictive value (NPV), suggesting that when such a patient has a normal resting perfusion study (as in Fig. 7-4), the risk of myocardial infarction (MI) or ischemic event is relatively small. CAD—coronary artery disease; PPV—positive predictive value; revasc—revascularization by coronary artery bypass grafting or percutaneous transluminal coronary angioplasty.

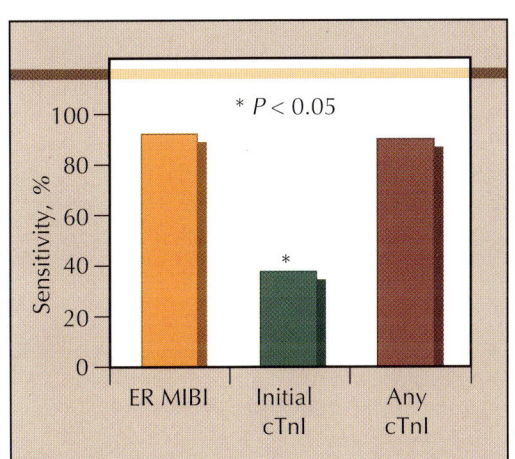

FIGURE 7-6. Comparative role of myocardial perfusion imaging (MPI) and serial analysis of cardiospecific enzymes in patients with chest pain in the emergency room (ER) setting. ^{99m}Tc-sestamibi MPI (ER MIBI) was performed and serial analysis of cardiac troponin I (cTnI) was undertaken in patients presenting with suspected acute coronary syndrome (ACS) but no obvious ischemic ECG changes (low to moderate risk for ACS). The sestamibi perfusion studies, performed very early during the initial evaluation, had 92% sensitivity to detect myocardial infarction, while the initial troponin I value, drawn at a similarly early time in the evaluation, had a sensitivity of only 39%.

The sensitivity of any troponin I value on serial testing over 24 hours ultimately achieved similar sensitivity as the perfusion study. This study illustrates that in the presence of ACS, MPI likely will be positive earlier than serial analysis of enzymes, allowing the opportunity for earlier intervention. (*Adapted from* Kontos et al. [13].)

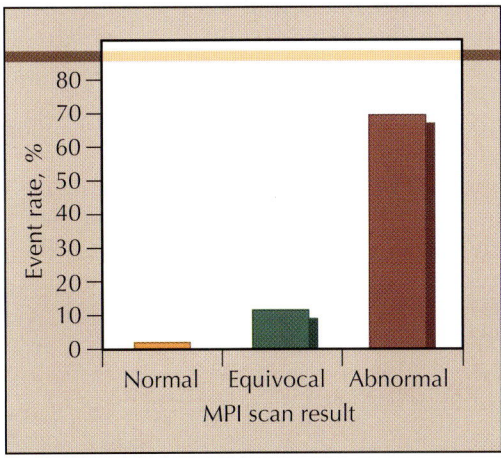

FIGURE 7-7. Cardiac event rate as a function of results of resting ^{99m}Tc-sestamibi SPECT myocardial perfusion imaging (MPI) in patients presenting to emergency room with suspected ischemia. Patients with a normal scan demonstrate a very low event rate, and patients with an abnormal scan had a significantly higher event rate [6], consistent with numerous studies from the literature in this population. Patients with "equivocal" results on resting MPI, *ie*, results that were neither completely normal nor definitely abnormal, likely reflect some patients whose scans were influenced by attenuation artifacts, or those who had small areas of ischemia or infarct, driving an intermediate event rate. Based on such data, equivocal scans should be considered mildly positive for purposes of clinical decision-making, because the event rate is not as low as with patients who have a "normal" scan. (*Adapted from* Hilton et al. [6].)

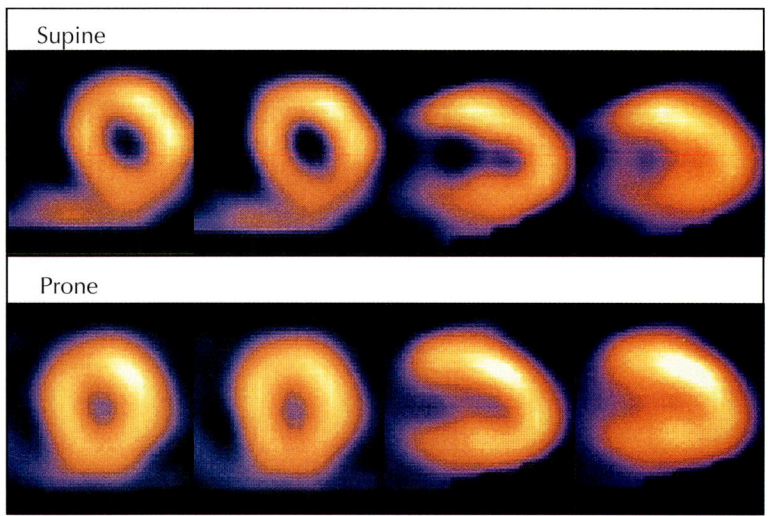

FIGURE 7-8. Characterization of equivocal myocardial perfusion study results. Various strategies can be employed for clarification of equivocal studies. For instance, in a patient who presented to the emergency room with symptoms suspicious for ischemia but a nondiagnostic ECG, initial supine resting ^{99m}Tc-sestamibi imaging demonstrated a possible inferobasal defect consistent with either acute ischemia in that territory or diaphragmatic attenuation artifact (*top row*). Subsequently, imaging was performed in the prone position (*bottom row*). In this set of images, inferobasal myocardial perfusion appears normal, suggesting that the initial study represented diaphragmatic attenuation artifact and not ischemia. Other alternatives to clarify equivocal images include using attenuation correction algorithms in laboratories with the appropriate equipment and experience.

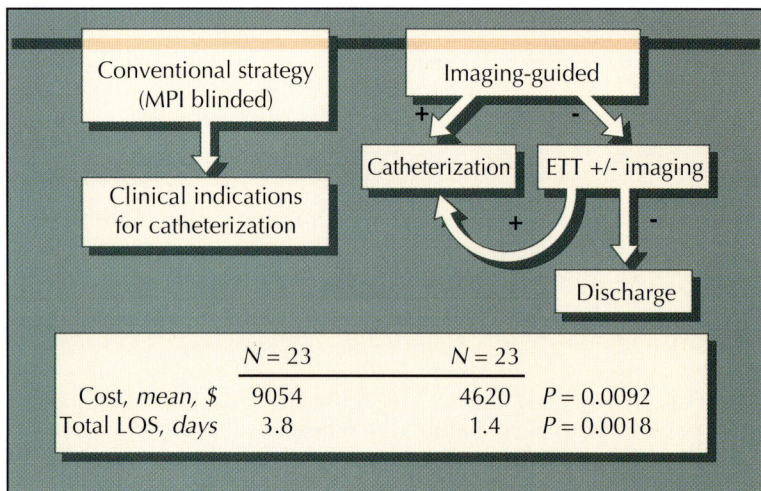

FIGURE 7-9. Myocardial perfusion imaging (MPI) and the management of patients with nondiagnostic ECG changes. Although MPI has been shown in observational studies to have very high negative predictive value for ruling out acute coronary syndrome (ACS) (Fig. 7-5), in none of those studies was the imaging information allowed to affect the management, *ie*, the triage decision on whether to admit the patient to the hospital for observation or to discharge directly home from the emergency room. In order to optimally assess the value of imaging (or any test) in this setting, a randomized trial is needed to compare the decisions made using imaging with those made with a strategy not incorporating imaging. In one such study, a small group of patients presenting to an emergency room with a suspected ischemic syndrome were randomized to an imaging-guided strategy or a conventional strategy (control) not incorporating imaging. In the imaging-guided strategy, perfusion studies were reviewed and management was based on the results; in the control arm, imaging results were kept blinded. The study endpoints included length of hospital stay (LOS) and overall costs of care, with the hypothesis that both would be lower if imaging were used to guide decisions. Among patients randomized to the test arm, LOS as well as costs were reduced by approximately 50% because fewer patients underwent catheterization. The results suggest that MPI could favorably affect management and lower costs in the setting of suspected ACS. ETT—exercise stress testing. (*Adapted from* Stowers *et al.* [16].)

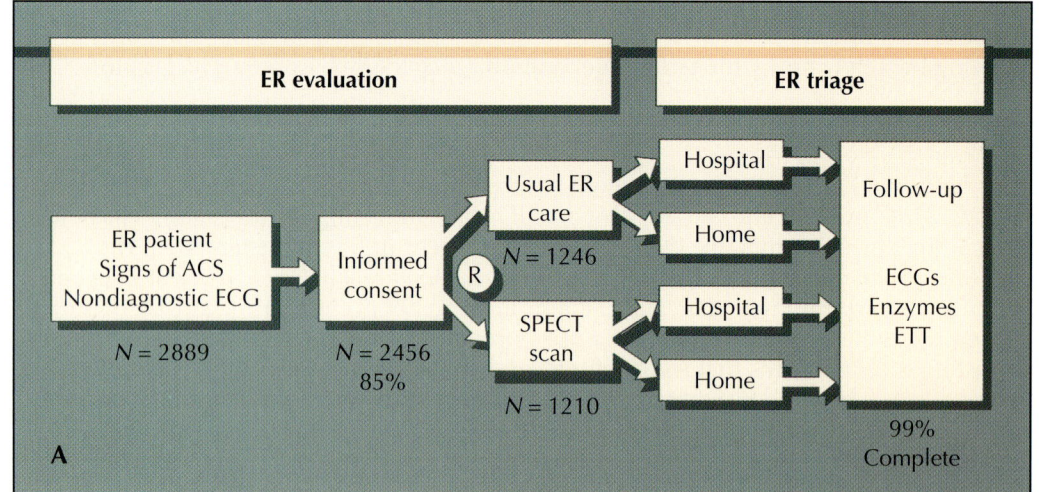

FIGURE 7-10. Assessment of the role of myocardial perfusion imaging in chest pain with nondiagnostic ECG changes. **A,** In a large prospective, randomized study, the ERASE (Emergency Room Assessment of Sestamibi for the Evaluation of Chest Pain) trial [17], investigators at seven sites enrolled 2475 patients with chest pain or other symptoms suggestive of acute cardiac ischemia and a normal or nondiagnostic initial ECG in the emergency room (ER). Patients were randomly assigned to receive either the usual ER evaluation strategy or the usual strategy supplemented by acute resting ^{99m}Tc-sestamibi SPECT imaging. The physician incorporated the imaging information into the decision-making either to admit the patient to the hospital for observation or to discharge directly home from the ER. The "correctness" of that decision was based on all follow-up information (available in 99% of patients at 1 month after presentation), so that the effect of incorporating the imaging information on clinical decision-making could be assessed rigorously [17].

Continued on next page

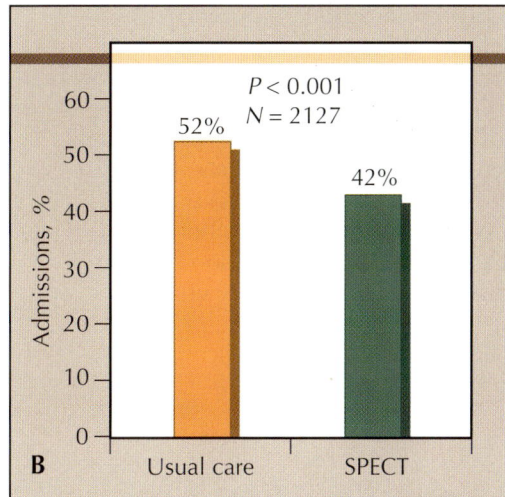
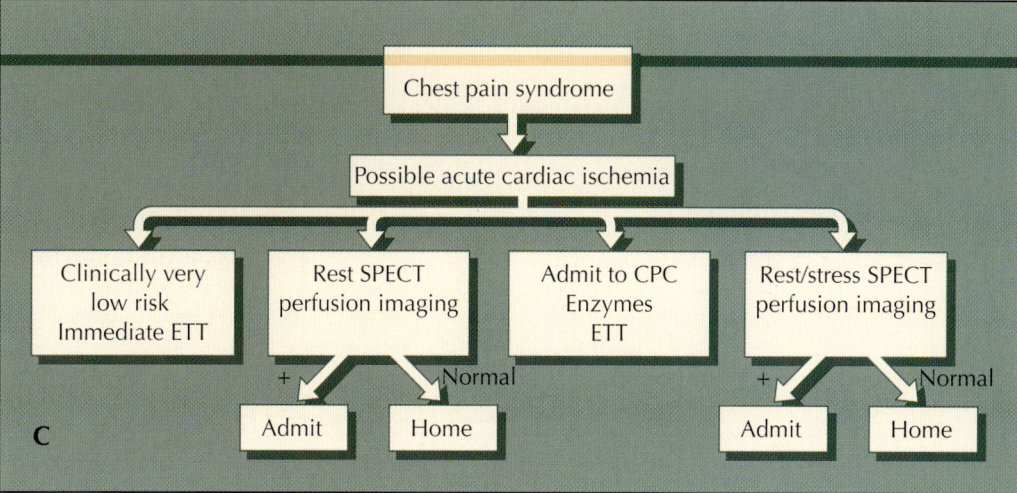

FIGURE 7-10. *(Continued)* **B**, For those patients ultimately determined not to have cardiac ischemia as the presenting syndrome, hospitalization was reduced from 52% with usual care to 42% with ^{99m}Tc-sestamibi imaging (odds ratio 0.68), *ie*, imaging was associated with a 32% reduction in the odds of being admitted unnecessarily to the hospital for admission or observation. On 30-day follow-up, there were no differences in outcomes between the usual care group or imaging group. This study demonstrated that the incorporation of ^{99m}Tc-sestamibi imaging into ER triage decision-making provided a clear benefit in reducing unnecessary hospital admissions without inappropriately reducing admission for patients with acute ischemia [17].

C, Myocardial perfusion imaging (rest SPECT MPI) has been studied rigorously for application in the ER setting, specifically for patients with suspected acute coronary syndrome (ACS) but a nondiagnostic initial ECG. There are several acceptable evaluation strategies for such patients: the "chest pain center" (CPC) protocol (serial evaluation of cardiac specific enzymes over 12 to 24 hours followed by stress testing [ETT] if negative), very early stress testing for clinically very low-risk patients, and a full stress and rest imaging protocol. MPI in this setting potentially can allow earlier triage than serial enzyme evaluation, but it must be performed with meticulous attention to high-quality acquisition, be interpreted by experienced readers, and be associated with prompt reporting of results, as well as good follow-up after discharge. The data suggest that if MPI studies are normal, the risk of ACS or negative events is very low, and early discharge from the ER to home may be considered. If imaging tests suggest acute infarction or ischemia, then rapid admission and entry into an appropriate evidence-based treatment pathway for ACS is in order.

ASSESSMENT OF PATIENTS WITH ST SEGMENT ELEVATION MYOCARDIAL INFARCTION

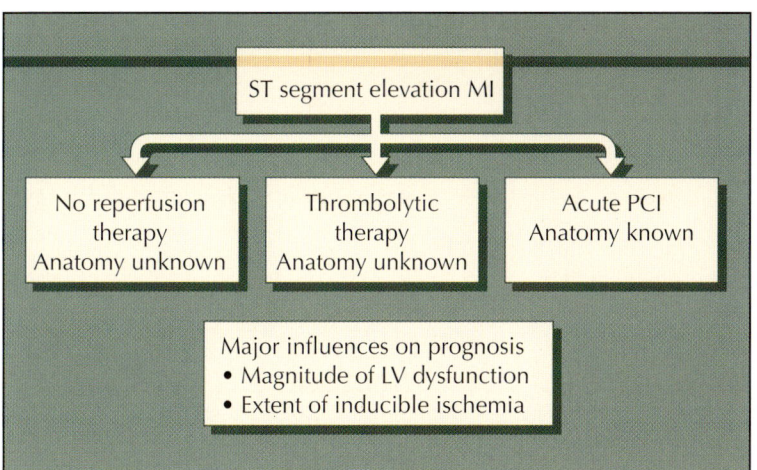

FIGURE 7-11. Therapeutic pathways for patients with ST segment elevation myocardial infarction. In the contemporary therapeutic era, patients with acute ST segment elevation myocardial infarction (MI) may be classified by the initial treatment strategy to assess the potential application of imaging modalities to subsequent management strategy. Based on numerous factors, some patients may receive no initial reperfusion therapy and may not have initial catheterization data; therefore, their anatomy will be unknown. Others may be treated with thrombolytic therapy and not sent to the catheterization laboratory, while a third group may be managed with primary percutaneous coronary intervention (PCI) of the infarct-related vessel, and thus full coronary anatomic information will be at hand. For all groups, however, post-MI prognosis is predicted by the magnitude of residual left ventricular (LV) dysfunction and the presence and magnitude of inducible ischemia. An imaging study in the post-MI setting can assess these variables, which in turn may allow classification and risk-stratification of patients regarding potential long-term post-MI outcomes, information that readily translates into clinical management strategies. Thus, imaging techniques can provide data that can be used specifically to direct patient management.

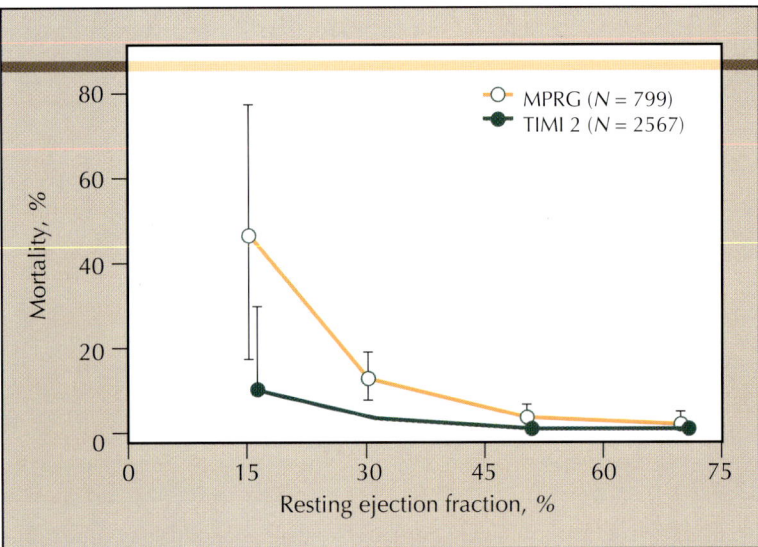

FIGURE 7-12. Relation of post-myocardial infarction (MI) cardiovascular mortality to resting ejection fraction in the pre- and post-thrombolytic era. Data from the MPRG (Multicenter Post Infarction Research Group) and the TIMI 2 (Thrombolysis in Myocardial Infarction Phase 2) trials demonstrate that as the magnitude of left ventricular dysfunction increases, the late mortality post-MI increases. At any given ejection fraction, the mortality is lower in patients receiving thrombolytic reperfusion therapy, but a relation between ejection fraction and survival remains evident in the thrombolytic era. (*Adapted from* Zaret *et al.* [18].)

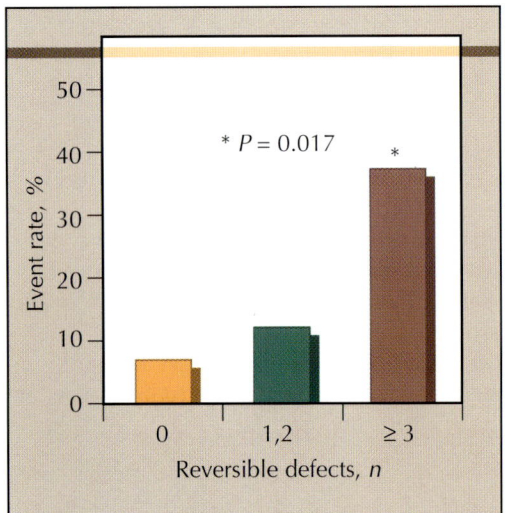

FIGURE 7-13. Relation between the post-myocardial infarction (MI) extent of inducible ischemia and the cardiac event rate. Patients with more extensive ischemia (documented as the number of reversible perfusion defects on ^{99m}Tc-sestamibi imaging) are at progressively higher risk of unfavorable outcome during late post-MI follow-up. These data, confirming the value of knowledge of the extent of ischemia in patients after MI, suggest that patients with a significant degree of inducible ischemia after MI are at risk of death or reinfarction, and thus are candidates for a more aggressive interventional post-MI treatment strategy. (*Adapted from* Travin *et al.* [19].)

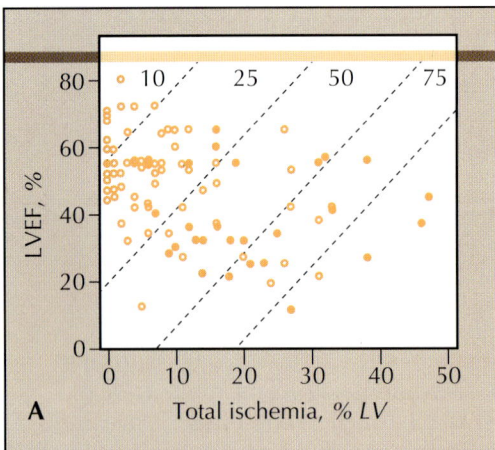
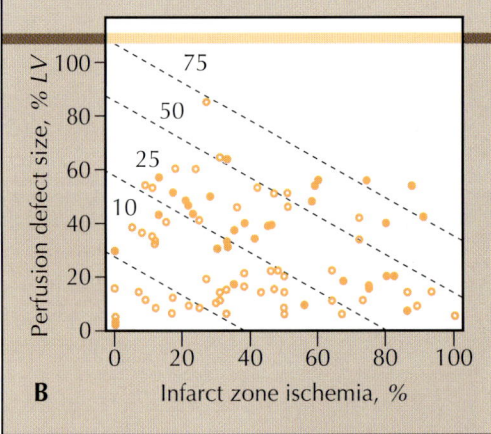
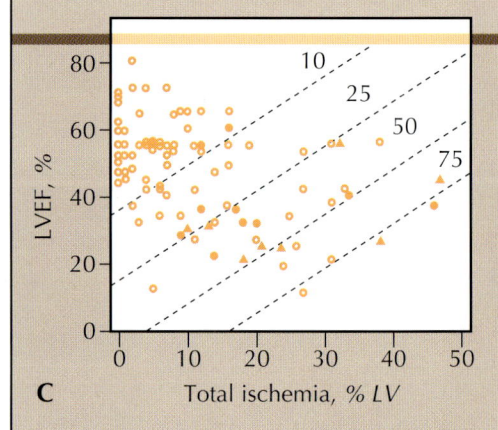

FIGURE 7-14. The independent but complementary nature of the information provided by imaging evaluation of the extent of inducible ischemia and the magnitude of left ventricular (LV) dysfunction. **A**, Cox regression models displaying 1-year risk for cardiac event according to left ventricular ejection fraction (LVEF) and total LV ischemia or, **B**, scintigraphic variables alone. **C**, Cox regression model for predicting infarct-free survival [20]. Diagonal lines denote representative isobars of percent risk of event. Patient risk for any cardiac event (*panel A*), or specifically death and nonfatal reinfarction (*panel C*), increases as total LV ischemia increases and LVEF decreases, or as total perfusion defect size and percent infarct zone ischemia increase (*panel B*). For any given LVEF (*panels A and C*) or perfusion defect size (*panel B*), risk varies widely depending on the extent of ischemia. Left ventricular ejection fraction and scintigraphic results for each of 92 patients who did (*solid circles*) or did not (*open circles*) have subsequent cardiac events over the entire follow-up period are plotted against calculated risk at 1 year (*panels A and B*). Patients are plotted (*panel C*) according to death (*triangles*), nonfatal reinfarction (*solid circles*), or neither of these events (*open circles*). These data suggest that knowledge of LV function and the extent of inducible ischemia by noninvasive imaging techniques in the post-myocardial infarction (MI) setting creates a powerful and comprehensive basis for risk-stratification and delineation of subsequent management strategies. *Continued on next page*

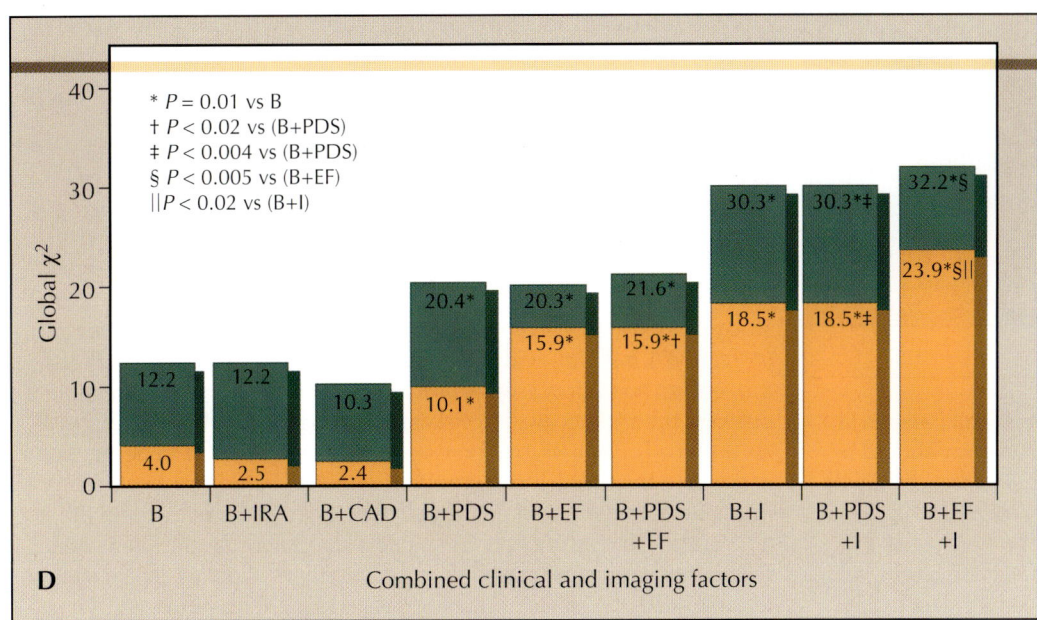

FIGURE 7-14. *(Continued)* **D**, Incremental prognostic power of perfusion variables and ejection fraction information over baseline clinical variables (B) for predicting all events (*entire bar*) or death and reinfarction (*orange portion of bar*). The χ^2 analysis represents the quantified risk of outcome event after MI, based on individual or combined clinical and imaging factors. LVEF and perfusion defect size (PDS), as well as extent of inducible ischemia (I), independently and incrementally predict risk beyond the baseline clinical model. Also, extent of ischemia improved the predictive power of the combined baseline clinical model and PDS (B+PDS) or baseline model and left ventricular ejection fraction (B+EF) for all events and for death and reinfarction. Left ventricular ejection fraction added significant power to the combined baseline model and PDS (B+PDS), as well as to the baseline model and extent of ischemia (B+I) for predicting death and reinfarction. These data confirm that knowledge of the magnitude of LV dysfunction as well as the scintigraphic extent of inducible ischemia carry powerful as well as independent prognostic value in the post-MI setting. CAD—coronary artery disease; IRA—infarct artery patency. (*Adapted from* Mahmarian *et al.* [20].)

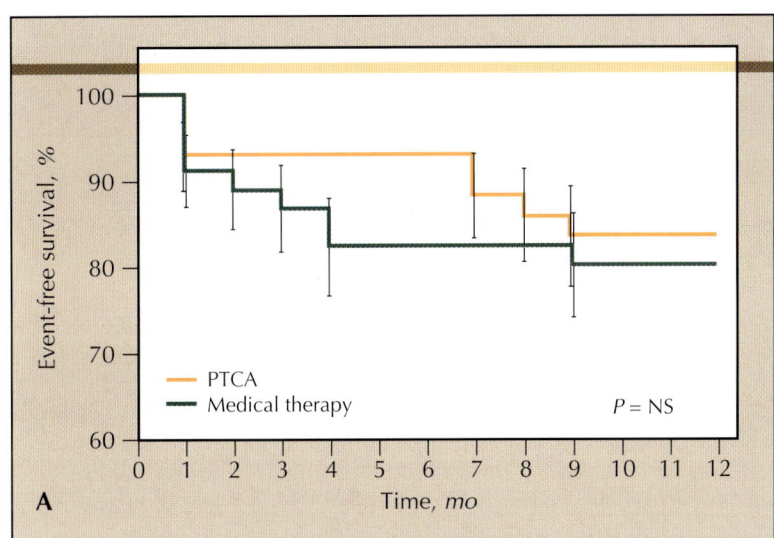

FIGURE 7-15. Importance of demonstrating residual ischemia in the infarct zone after thrombolytic therapy as a guide to the potential benefit of revascularization. **A**, Some cardiologists advocated angioplasty of any residual stenosis present after the administration of thrombolytic therapy. In a study designed to rigorously assess that notion [21], patients who had received thrombolytic therapy for acute myocardial infarction (MI) and also had a residual stenosis of the infarct-related artery but no inducible ischemia in the infarct territory by myocardial perfusion imaging were randomized to either a strategy of percutaneous transluminal coronary angioplasty (PTCA) of the residual stenosis or a strategy of no PTCA. Shown is a plot of actuarial freedom from cardiac death, MI, coronary bypass surgery, or PTCA after randomization to PTCA (*solid line*) or medical therapy (*dashed line*). There is no difference in outcome between the groups. Hence, identification of inducible ischemia (or lack thereof) within the infarct zone by myocardial perfusion imaging after acute MI and reperfusion therapy can guide management decisions regarding revascularization strategy. In the absence of any residual infarct-zone ischemia, there appears to be little benefit from a strategy of revascularization. This concept is being readdressed in a more contemporary era by the OAT (Open Artery Trial), in which patients with an occluded infarct artery in the weeks following MI will be randomized to a strategy of contemporary medical therapy versus PCI to open the occluded infarct-related artery.   *Continued on next page*

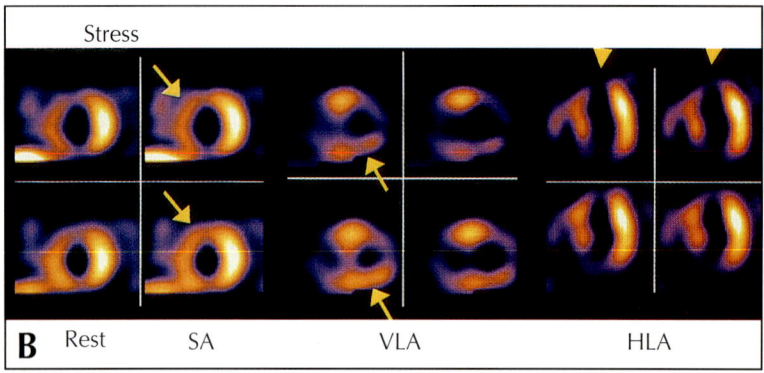

FIGURE 7-15. *(Continued)* **B**, To address the concept that all patients in the aftermath of acute MI treated with thrombolytic therapy should be catheterized, the TIMI 2 (Thrombolysis in Myocardial Infarction [TIMI] 2) [22] study randomized such patients to a strategy of catheterization in the days after presentation, with PTCA or coronary artery bypass grafting based on anatomic considerations, or to an "ischemia-guided" strategy, in which patients underwent noninvasive imaging to detect ischemia within or remote from the infarct zone, with subsequent catheterization based on the presence and extent of ischemia. At 6 months' follow-up, there was no difference between the groups in any outcome measure, and fewer patients in the ischemia-guided group underwent catheterization and revascularization, suggesting lower costs. These data suggest that routine catheterization after initial thrombolytic reperfusion strategy in all patients will not necessarily lead to better outcomes. In this figure, stress and resting SPECT images from a 74-year-old patient who presented with an anterior ST segment elevation MI are depicted. The patient initially had been treated with thrombolytic therapy with subsequent stabilization clinically, with no heart failure, recurrent ischemic symptoms, or arrhythmias. The SPECT study demonstrates an apical fixed defect consistent with infarction (*arrowheads*), but also evidence of extensive inducible ischemia involving the septum and inferior walls (*arrows*), as well as a partially reversible defect of the anterior wall (consistent with ischemia within the infarct zone [*arrow*]). Ejection fraction was 38% by gated SPECT imaging. Thus, in this case the post-MI risk stratification SPECT study suggested very high outcome risk based on the extent of inducible ischemia and the left ventricular dysfunction. Despite the stable clinical state, this patient was referred for catheterization and revascularization (as anatomically feasible) with the expectation of improved long-term outcome. HLA—horizontal long axis; SA—short axis; VLA—vertical long axis. (*Panel A adapted from* Ellis *et al.* [21].)

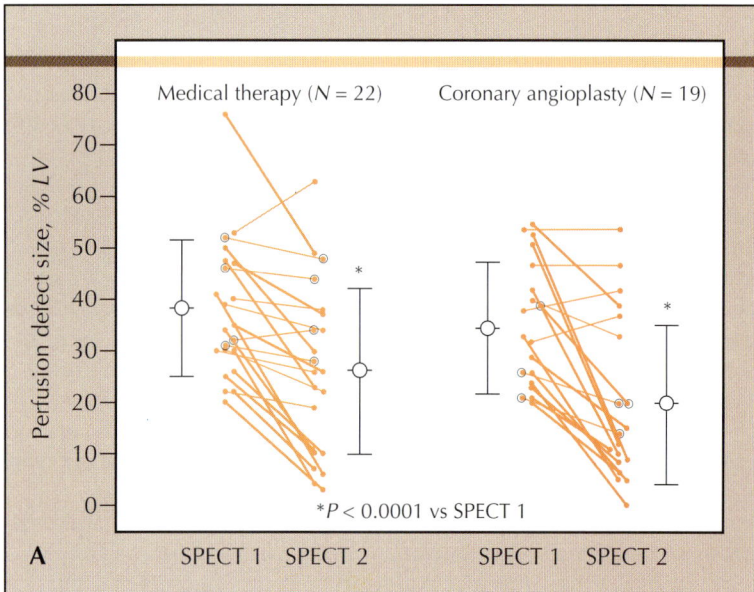

FIGURE 7-16. Suppression of ischemia by medical or interventional therapies after myocardial infarction (MI) and subsequent outcome events. While many studies have demonstrated an important correlation between the presence and extent of ischemia and subsequent outcome after acute MI, the specificity of such determinations is often low. Among patients with "high-risk" scintigraphic or clinical signs, only a minority will suffer an important cardiac event during follow-up, while the majority of patients categorized in this way will remain event-free. Thus, to the extent that common practice dictates most if not all of these "high-risk" patients should undergo catheterization and intervention, many patients are being intervened upon who would otherwise not have an event to prevent such events in the minority. This may be particularly relevant in the contemporary era of aggressive secondary prevention, resulting in a greater degree of plaque stabilization than may have been present in past studies prior to the aggressive use of statins and other therapies in the post-MI setting.

A, In a pilot study designed to address this question, Dakik *et al.* [23] reported on 44 stable survivors of acute MI who underwent adenosine SPECT ^{201}Tl imaging approximately 4 days after MI. Patients who had large total and ischemic perfusion defect size on SPECT quantitative analysis (*ie*, "high-risk" patients who would usually be referred for revascularization) were randomized to either aggressive and intensive medical therapy or percutaneous transluminal coronary angioplasty (PTCA) with a goal of suppressing myocardial ischemia as much as possible. Changes in perfusion defect size (PDS) during repeat adenosine SPECT imaging 6 weeks following randomization to medical or invasive therapy are shown. Similar reduction in PDS was achieved in both groups. Only one of 24 patients with a reduction in PDS of greater than 9% (*dark orange bars*) had a cardiac event on follow-up. Patients who had a recurrent event are indicated by *circled points*.

Continued on next page

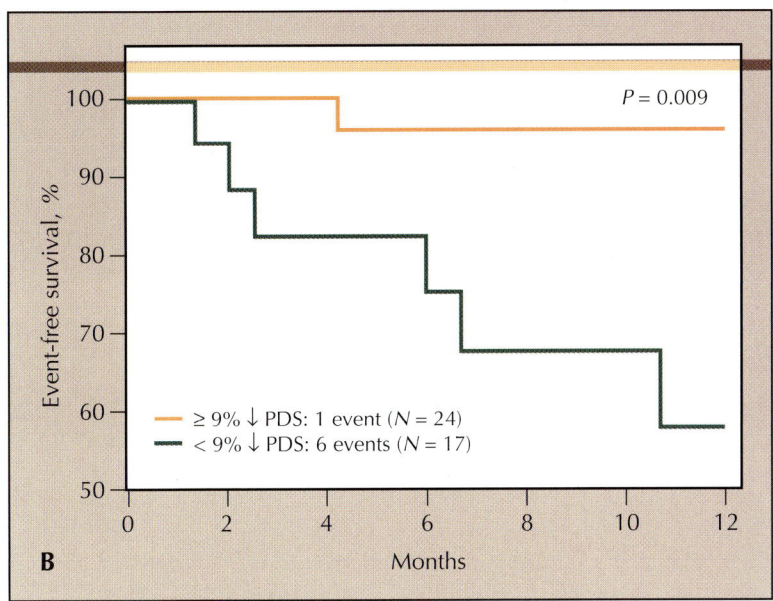

FIGURE 7-16. *(Continued)* **B**, Survival is favorably influenced by reduction in PDS accomplished by either medical or invasive therapy. Patients with a reduction in PDS greater than 9% had a significantly more favorable event-free survival compared with patients who did not experience that magnitude of change in PDS. These data suggest that the response of patients with scintigraphic SPECT ischemia to medical therapy parallels those seen with PTCA. To the extent that the change in ischemic defect size is related to outcome independent of the intervention, these data would suggest that even "high-risk" patients identified by stress scintigraphic imaging after MI may not all benefit from an invasive strategy. The relatively large proportion of patients within the high-risk cohort who are destined to remain stable might be identified on the basis of the response of scintigraphic ischemia to medical therapy. These important and encouraging pilot data are now being extrapolated to a large randomized multicenter trial, the results of which may affect the way patients with uncomplicated MI are treated in coming years. LV—left ventricle. (*Adapted from* Dakik et al. [23].)

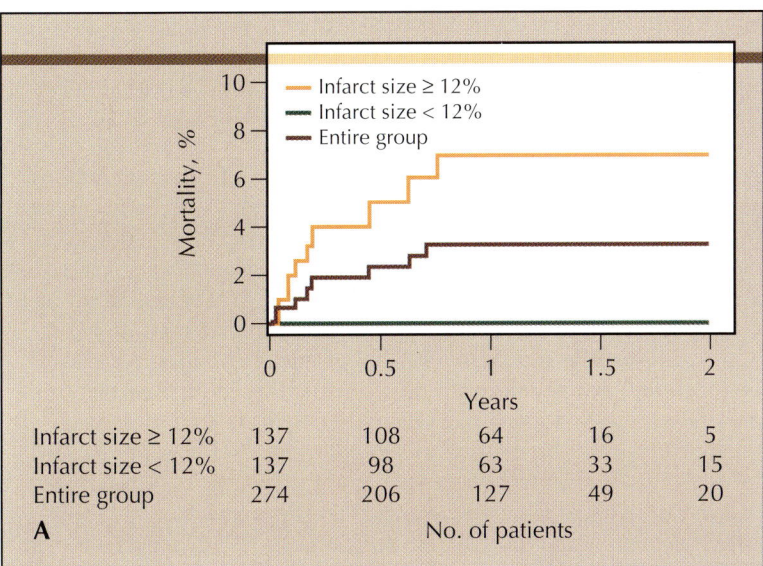

B. VALIDATION OF ^{99m}TC-SESTAMIBI TOMOGRAPHIC INFARCT SIZE

METHOD FOR MEASURING INFARCT SIZE	R VALUE	P VALUE
Discharge ejection fraction	−0.8	< 0.0001
6-week ejection fraction	−0.81	< 0.0001
1-year ejection fraction	−0.78	< 0.0001
Discharge regional wall motion	−0.75	< 0.0001
6-week regional wall motion	−0.81	< 0.0001
1-year end-systolic volume	0.80	< 0.0001
Peak creatinine kinase levels	0.78	0.002
^{201}Tl perfusion defect	0.73	0.002
Human disease	0.91	0.002

FIGURE 7-17. Estimation of post-myocardial infarction (MI) infarct size and clinical outcomes. A substantial body of literature exists supporting the concept that estimation of infarct size by quantitative SPECT ^{99m}Tc-sestamibi myocardial perfusion imaging (MPI) has powerful prognostic value in the aftermath of acute MI. Miller *et al.* [24] studied 274 patients with acute MI who underwent imaging prior to reperfusion therapy (to measure the area of myocardium at risk) and at discharge (to measure final infarct size and myocardial salvage). **A**, Mortality curves are shown for the entire group and those with final infarct size 12% or greater of the left ventricle and less than 12% of the left ventricle by quantitative analysis. The magnitude of infarct size was associated significantly with subsequent mortality. Based on studies such as this, detection of final infarct size by SPECT MPI may be used as an intermediate surrogate marker in trials of new reperfusion strategies in acute MI. Therapies that are shown to result in smaller final infarct size by this technique in phase 2 studies have a higher probability of success in subsequent phase 3 outcome studies. **B**, Validation of ^{99m}Tc-sestamibi tomographic infarct size. Final infarct size using SPECT MPI has been correlated with several other measures reflective of outcome after MI. (*Panel A adapted from* Miller et al. [24]; *panel B adapted from* Christian [25].)

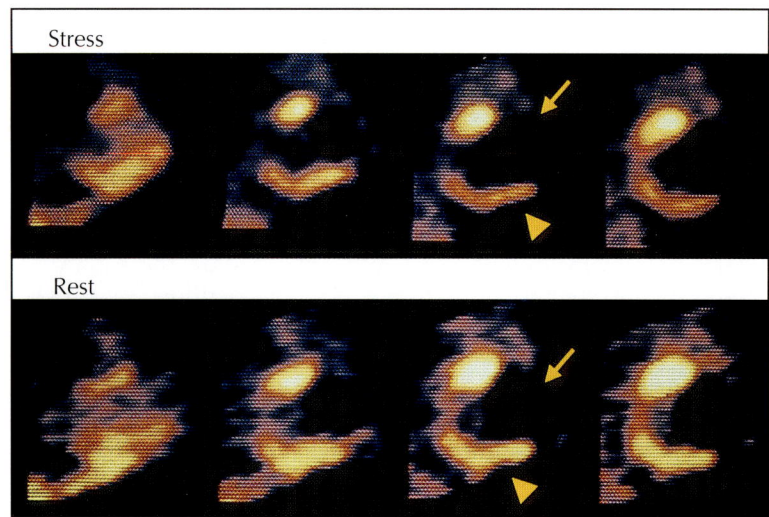

FIGURE 7-18. Vertical long-axis SPECT images in a patient following acute anterior myocardial infarction treated with primary percutaneous coronary intervention. The stress and rest images demonstrate a very large, severe, fixed defect in the anterior wall and apex (*arrows*) with evidence of inducible ischemia of the inferior wall (*arrowhead*). The severity of the anterior wall and apical defect would suggest that very little myocardial viability exists in those territories, and the large infarct size would suggest high risk for mortality, based on data depicted in Figure 7-17A.

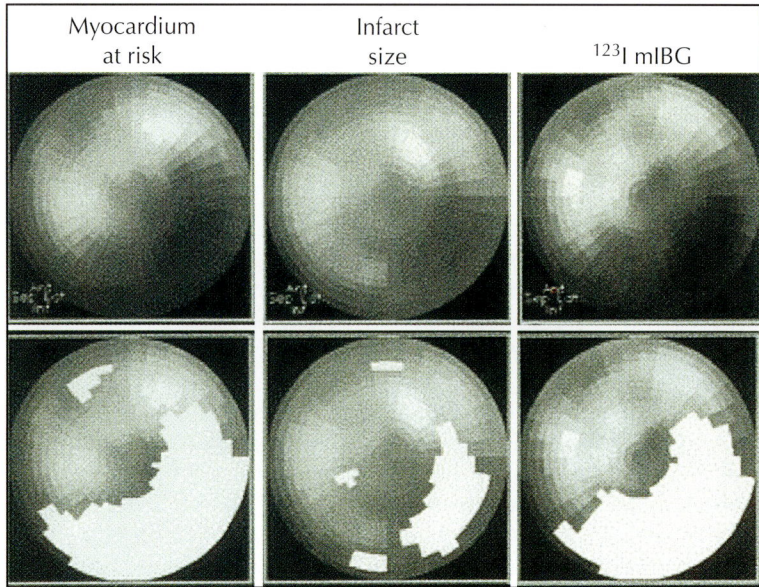

FIGURE 7-19. ^{123}I metaiodobenzylguanidine (mIBG) imaging. An emerging area of scintigraphic risk stratification in the post-myocardial infarction (MI) setting involves the use of ^{123}I mIBG imaging of cardiac sympathetic innervation. In the post-MI setting, several studies have shown that the territory of abnormal ^{123}I mIBG uptake, corresponding to sympathetic denervation, may often exceed the final infarct size, and that such patients may be at higher risk for subsequent ventricular arrhythmias. Matsunari *et al.* [26], using SPECT ^{99m}Tc-sestamibi imaging of infarct risk area and final infarct size as well as ^{123}I mIBG imaging in patients with acute MI, demonstrated that the territory of sympathetic denervation (^{123}I mIBG defect, *right column*) corresponded more closely to the initial MI risk area (*left column*) than the final infarct size (*middle column*). Should such findings in the contemporary therapeutic era prove prognostic for late post-MI outcomes, as suggested by earlier studies, ^{123}I mIBG imaging may prove useful in selecting post-MI patients who may optimally benefit from implantable defibrillators. *Top row*, Polar maps of imaging data depict inferior and lateral defects (darker areas). *Bottom row*, White areas represent defect sizes. The mIBG defect is more similar in magnitude to the initial myocardium at risk than to the final infarct size.

In addition to the role of myocardial perfusion imaging, several methods for early scintigraphic identification of myocardial necrosis are under investigation. ^{99m}Tc-glucarate may be taken up by early necrotic myocardium relatively soon after the onset of ischemia, and far earlier than older techniques using antimyosin antibodies or pyrophosphate [27]. Another exciting new approach to evaluating patients following myocardial necrosis utilizes ^{99m}Tc-labeled annexin V for in vivo visualization of apoptosis [28] (*see* Chapter 12, *Imaging Myocardial Necrosis and Apoptosis*). Should the role of apoptosis in acute MI be confirmed in larger studies, it will allow development of novel therapeutic approaches to attenuate impending myocellular death.

ASSESSMENT OF PATIENTS WITH NON–ST SEGMENT ELEVATION MYOCARDIAL INFARCTION/UNSTABLE ANGINA

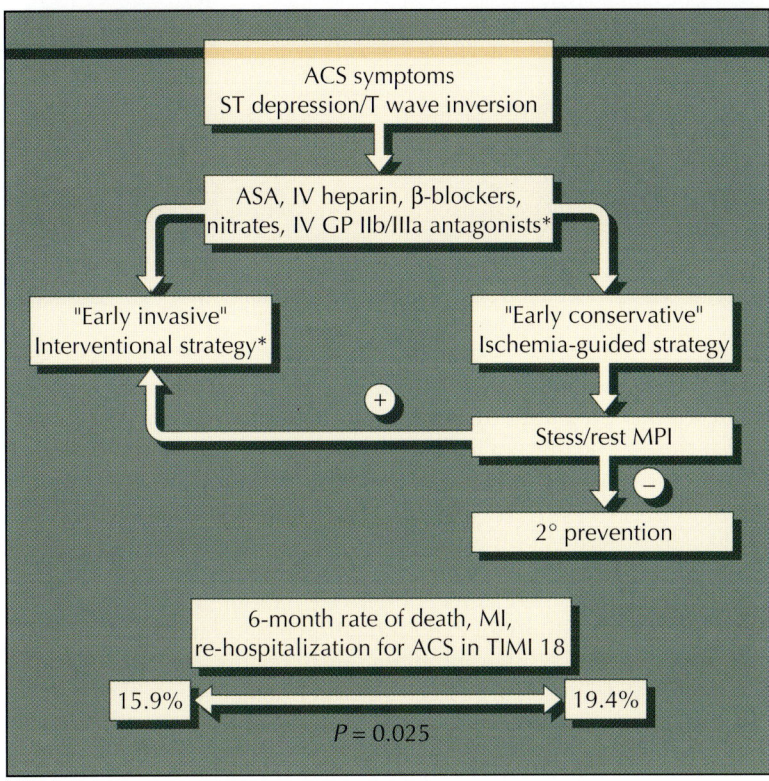

FIGURE 7-20. Use of perfusion imaging for identification of non–ST elevation in patients with acute coronary syndrome (ACS) likely to benefit from intervention. In patients presenting with symptoms consistent with ACS in whom the diagnosis is clear on initial presentation (*ie*, there are clear ischemic initial ECG changes such as ST segment depression or T-wave inversion), initial management consists of aspirin (ASA), intravenous heparin, β-blockers, and nitrates [11]. The current evidence-based paradigm suggests that such patients may derive overall benefit from an "invasive" management strategy, with administration of intravenous platelet inhibitors and referral to catheterization with subsequent revascularization, particularly for the subset of patients with elevated troponin levels or other higher risk clinical markers, such as the TIMI (Thrombolysis in Myocardial Infarction) Risk Score [29]. The role of radionuclide imaging is predominantly within the "conservative" strategy, wherein patients are risk-stratified, followed by more selective referral to catheterization and revascularization based on the extent of inducible ischemia. In the TACTICS (Treat Angina with Aggrastat and Determine Cost of Therapy with an Invasive or Conservative Strategy)–TIMI 18 trial [30], patients with symptoms of ACS and ECG changes supportive of the diagnosis received the platelet inhibitor tirofiban and were randomized to an "early invasive" management strategy (referral to catheterization and revascularization based on anatomic findings at angiography) or an "early conservative" strategy (stress testing with referral to catheterization based on the extent of ischemia or on the basis of spontaneous ischemia). In this contemporary trial, outcomes favored the invasive strategy. Because the absolute benefit of the invasive management strategy was relatively small, subgroup analysis was performed to examine whether any clinical findings could identify a subgroup in which the benefits were larger (or smaller). Subgrouping by troponin status suggested that most of the benefit of the invasive strategy was seen in the subgroup of patients identified by elevated troponins or a higher TIMI risk score, and that TACTICS-type patients without elevation of troponin derived little benefit from the invasive strategy. These latter patients may be best managed by a more conservative approach, with risk stratification using imaging techniques followed by more selective referral to catheterization. GP— glycoprotein; IV—intravenous; MPI—myocardial perfusion imaging; minus—absence of significant inducible ischemia; plus—presence of significant inducible ischemia.

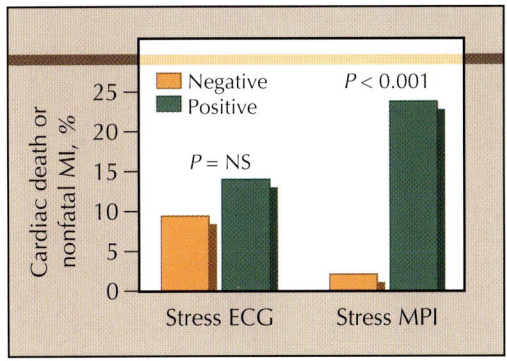

FIGURE 7-21. Use of myocardial perfusion imaging as the decision point in a "conservative" management strategy in non–ST segment elevation acute coronary syndrome. The predictive value of stress myocardial perfusion imaging (MPI) and stress ECG is shown in patients studied after initial stabilization of unstable angina with medical therapy. This figure summarizes the results of three studies in which the incidence of cardiac death or nonfatal myocardial infarction (MI) were assessed as endpoints during follow-up after stabilization of unstable angina. The presence of reversible perfusion defects reflective of ischemia ("positive" stress MPI) was strongly predictive of cardiac events in this setting. The absence of inducible ischemia on MPI ("negative" stress MPI) identifies a low-risk group, suggesting that such patients can be managed conservatively. Data are less consistent on the use of exercise ECG in this setting. NS—not significant. (*Adapted from* Brown [31].)

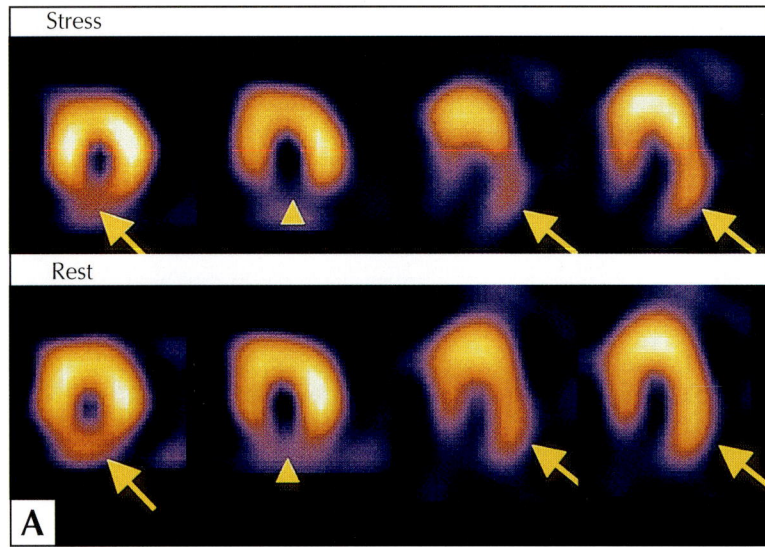
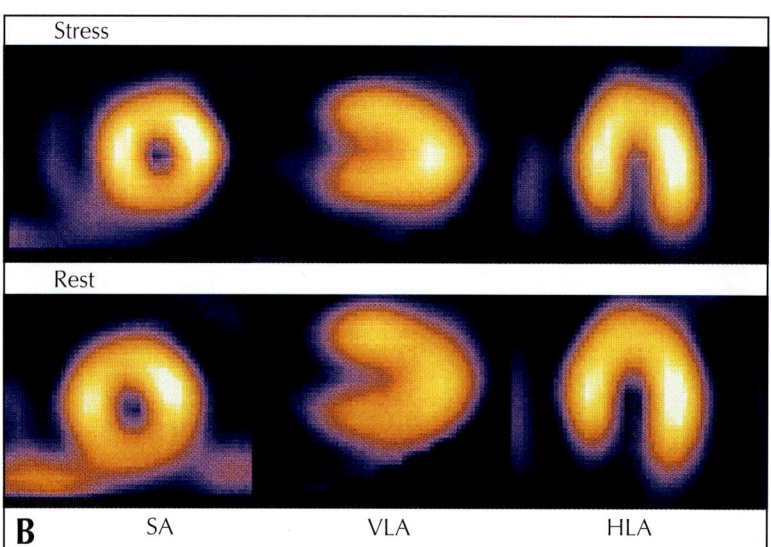

FIGURE 7-22. Examples of myocardial perfusion imaging in non–ST elevation acute coronary syndrome. **A,** Positive myocardial perfusion imaging (MPI) study in a patient with medically stabilized unstable angina. After presentation, the patient's symptoms were controlled with initial medical therapy, and stress MPI was performed. There is evidence of an inferobasal infarct (*arrowhead*), but the extent of inducible ischemia involving the inferoapical and lateral walls (*arrows*) suggests the patient is at high risk for future events, and the patient was subsequently referred to catheterization. **B,** Normal stress and rest SPECT MPI in a 63-year-old woman who presented with a clinical syndrome consistent with unstable angina but nonspecific electrocardiographic changes. Symptoms abated after treatment with aspirin, heparin, β-blockers, and nitrates. The normal MPI study suggests a very low risk for subsequent ischemic events, and catheterization/revascularization is unlikely to improve that risk. In clinical trials of unstable angina, up to 30% of some populations of patients are found to have normal or near-normal coronary arteries after routine catheterization. In a nonclinical high-risk patient, MPI will allow more optimal selection for catheterization based on the risk stratification information inherent in the image results. HLA—horizontal long axis; SA—short axis; VLA—vertical long axis.

Thus, there is potential for imaging the ongoing abnormality in fatty acid metabolism as a signal of "ischemic memory." In 111 patients presenting with symptoms of acute coronary syndrome but no myocardial infarction, BMIPP SPECT imaging performed 1 to 5 days after presentation was more sensitive than rest myocardial perfusion imaging (performed within 24 hours of presentation) in identifying the presence and site of the culprit coronary stenosis or spasm (74% vs 38% respectively; $P < 0.05$) at similar high specificity.

In this example, the *top row* depicts normal resting perfusion by ^{201}Tl SPECT imaging in short-axis tomograms. The *middle row* demonstrates extensive stress-induced ^{201}Tl perfusion abnormalities consistent with inducible ischemia of the anterior, septal, and inferior walls. Thus, in the setting of a recent clinical syndrome of unstable angina, the presence and particularly the extent of inducible ischemia would suggest a very high-risk prognosis, and referral for catheterization and revascularization would be in order. In the *bottom row*, the BMIPP SPECT images of the analogous short-axis tomograms, obtained at rest, demonstrate ongoing abnormality in fatty acid metabolism in the anterior wall, septum, and inferior wall, temporally distinct from the presenting ischemic insult. Although the extent of abnormality in the BMIPP resting image is somewhat less than in the stress ^{201}Tl study, the BMIPP images still suggest the presence of a previous extensive ischemic insult, also suggesting a potential high-risk prognosis. Thus, this technique may provide risk stratification information based on the magnitude of abnormal fatty acid metabolism, to the extent that it may reflect the recent extent of ischemia during the symptomatic episode, using rest imaging alone without the need for a stress test. This concept is currently under study. (*From* Kawai *et al.* [32]; with permission.).

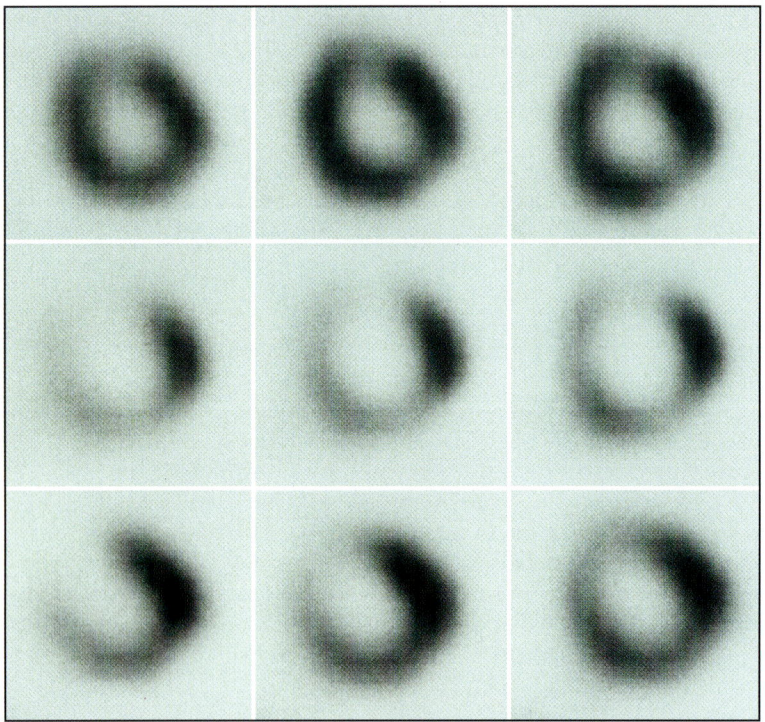

FIGURE 7-23. Potential use of fatty acid imaging for risk stratification in unstable angina. In the aftermath of the acute ischemic symptoms, a radioiodinated fatty acid analogue, 15-(p-[iodine-123] iodophenyl)-3-(R,S) methylpentadecanoic acid (BMIPP), has been used to assess fatty acid utilization in the myocardium. Following an ischemic insult, fatty acid metabolism may be abnormal for a prolonged time, far beyond the time when flow returns to normal and signs and symptoms of regional ischemia have resolved.

References

1. Wackers FJ, Lie KI, Liem KL, et al.: Potential value of thallium-201 scintigraphy as a means of selecting patients for the coronary care unit. *Br Heart J* 1979, 41:111–117.

2. Gibbons RJ, Verani MS, Behrenbeck T, et al.: Feasibility of tomographic 99mTc-hexakis-2-methoxy-2-methylpropyl-isonitrile imaging for the assessment of myocardial area at risk and the effect of treatment in acute myocardial infarction. *Circulation* 1989, 80:1277–1286.

3. Boden WE, O'Rourke RA, Crawford MH, et al.: Outcomes in patients with acute non–Q-wave myocardial infarction randomly assigned to an invasive as compared with a conservative management strategy [published correction appears in *N Engl J Med* 1998, 339:1091]. *N Engl J Med* 1998, 338:1785–1792.

4. Effects of tissue plasminogen activator and a comparison of early invasive and conservative strategies in unstable angina and non–Q-wave myocardial infarction: results of the TIMI IIIB trial: Thrombolysis in Myocardial Ischemia. *Circulation* 1994, 89:1545–1556.

5. Varetto T, Cantalupi D, Altieri A, et al.: Emergency room technetium-99m sestamibi imaging to rule out acute myocardial ischemic events in patients with nondiagnostic electrocardiography. *J Am Coll Cardiol* 1993, 22:1804–1808.

6. Hilton TC, Thompson RC, Williams H, et al.: Technetium-99m sestamibi myocardial perfusion imaging in the emergency room evaluation of chest pain. *J Am Coll Cardiol* 1994, 23:1016–1022.

7. Tatum JL, Jesse Rl, Kontos MC, et al.: Comprehensive strategy for the evaluation and triage of the chest pain patient. *Ann Emerg Med* 1997, 29:116–125.

8. Heller GV, Stowers SA, Hendel RC, et al.: Clinical value of acute rest technetium-99m tetrofosmin tomographic myocardial perfusion imaging in patients with acute chest pain and nondiagnostic electrocardiograms. *J Am Coll Cardiol* 1998, 31:1011–1017.

9. Jafary F, Udelson JE: Assessment of myocardial perfusion and left ventricular function in acute coronary syndromes: implications for gated SPECT imaging. In *Clinical Gated Cardiac SPECT*. Edited by Germano G, Berman DS. Armonk, NY: Futura; 1999.

10. Ryan TJ, Antman EM, Brooks NH, et al.: 1999 Update: ACC/AHA Guidelines for the Management of Patients With Acute Myocardial Infarction: Executive Summary and Recommendations: A report of the American College of Cardiology/American Heart Association Task Force on Practice Guidelines (Committee on Management of Acute Myocardial Infarction). *Circulation* 1999, 100:1016–1030.

11. Braunwald E, Antman EM, Beasley JW, et al.: ACC/AHA guidelines for the management of patients with unstable angina and non-ST-segment elevation myocardial infarction: a report of the American College of Cardiology/American Heart Association Task Force on Practice Guidelines (Committee on the Management of Patients with Unstable Angina). *J Am Coll Cardiol* 2000, 36:970–972

12. Bilodeau L, Theroux P, Gregoire J, et al.: Technetium-99m sestamibi tomography in patients with spontaneous chest pain: correlations with clinical, electrocardiographic and angiographic findings. *J Am Coll Cardiol* 1991, 18:1684–1691.

13. Kontos MC, Jesse RL, Anderson P, et al.: Comparison of myocardial perfusion imaging and cardiac troponin I in patients admitted to the emergency department with chest pain. *Circulation* 1999, 99:2073–2078.

14. Duca MD, Giri S, Wu AHB, et al.: Comparison of acute rest myocardial perfusion imaging and serum markers of myocardial injury in patients with chest pain syndromes. *J Nucl Cardiol* 1999, 6:570–576.

15. Kosnik JW, Zalenski RJ, Shamsa F, et al.: Resting sestamibi imaging for the prognosis of low-risk chest pain. *Acad Emerg Med* 1999, 6:998–1004.

16. Stowers SA, Eisenstein EL, Wackers FJ, et al.: An economic analysis of an aggressive diagnostic strategy with single photon emission computed tomography myocardial perfusion imaging and early exercise stress testing in emergency department patients who present with chest pain but nondiagnostic electrocardiograms: results from a randomized trial. *Ann Emerg Med* 2000, 35:17–25.

17. Udelson JE, Beshansky JR, Ballin DS, et al.: Myocardial perfusion imaging for evaluation and triage of patients with suspected acute cardiac ischemia: a randomized controlled trial. *JAMA* 2002, 288:2693–2700.

18. Zaret BL, Wackers FJ, Terrin ML, et al.: Value of radionuclide rest and exercise left ventricular ejection fraction in assessing survival of patients after thrombolytic therapy for acute myocardial infarction: results of Thrombolysis in Myocardial Infarction (TIMI) phase II study. *J Am Coll Cardiol* 1995, 26:73–79.

19. Travin MI, Dessouki A, Cameron T, Heller GV: Use of exercise technetium-99m sestamibi SPECT imaging to detect residual ischemia and for risk stratification after acute myocardial infarction. *Am J Cardiol* 1995, 75:665–669.

20. Mahmarian JJ, Mahmarian AC, Marks GF, et al.: Role of adenosine thallium-201 tomography for defining long-term risk in patients after acute myocardial infarction. *J Am Coll Cardiol* 1995, 25:1333–1340.

21. Ellis SG, Mooney MR, George BS, et al.: Randomized trial of late elective angioplasty versus conservative management for patients with residual stenoses after thrombolytic treatment of myocardial infarction (TOPS trial). *Circulation* 1992, 86:1400–1406.

22. Comparison of invasive and conservative strategies after treatment with intravenous tissue plasminogen activator in acute myocardial infarction. Results of the thrombolysis in myocardial infarction (TIMI) phase II trial. The TIMI Study Group. *N Engl J Med* 1989, 320:618–627.

23. Dakik HA, Kleiman NS, Farmer JA, et al.: Intensive medical therapy versus coronary angioplasty for suppression of myocardial ischemia in survivors of acute myocardial infarction. A prospective, randomized pilot study. *Circulation* 1998, 98:2017–2023.

24. Miller TD, Christian TF, Hopfenspirger MR, et al.: Infarct size after acute myocardial infarction measured by quantitative tomographic 99mTc sestamibi imaging predicts subsequent mortality. *Circulation* 1995, 92:334–341.

25. Christian TF: The use of perfusion imaging in acute myocardial infarction: applications for clinical trials and clinical care. *J Nucl Cardiol* 1995, 2:423–436.

26. Matsunari I, Schricke U, Bengel FM et al.: Extent of cardiac sympathetic neuronal damage is determined by the area of ischemia in patients with acute coronary syndromes. *Circulation* 2000, 101:2579–2585.

27. Narula J, Petrov A, Pak KY, et al.: Very early noninvasive detection of acute experimental nonreperfused myocardial infarction with 99mTc-labeled glucarate. *Circulation* 1997, 95:1577–1584.

28. Hofstra L, Liem IH, Dumont EA, et al.: Visualisation of cell death in vivo in patients with acute myocardial infarction. *Lancet* 2000, 356(9225):209–212.

29. Antman EM, Cohen M, Bernink PJ, et al.: The TIMI risk score for unstable angina/non-ST elevation MI: a method for prognostication and therapeutic decision making. *JAMA* 2000, 284:835–842.

30. Cannon CP, Weintraub WS, Demopoulos LA, et al.: Comparison of early invasive and conservative strategies in patients with unstable coronary syndromes treated with the glycoprotein IIb/IIIa inhibitor trofiban. *N Engl J Med* 2001, 344:1879–1887.

31. Brown KA: Management of unstable angina: The role of noninvasive risk stratification. *J Nucl Cardiol* 1997, 4:S164–S168.

32. Kawai Y, Tsukamoto E, Nozaki Y, et al.: Significance of reduced uptake of iodinated fatty acid analogue for the evaluation of patients with acute chest pain. *J Am Coll Cardiol* 2001, 38:1888–1894.

CHAPTER 8

MYOCARDIAL VIABILITY: REVERSIBLE LEFT VENTRICULAR DYSFUNCTION

Vasken Dilsizian

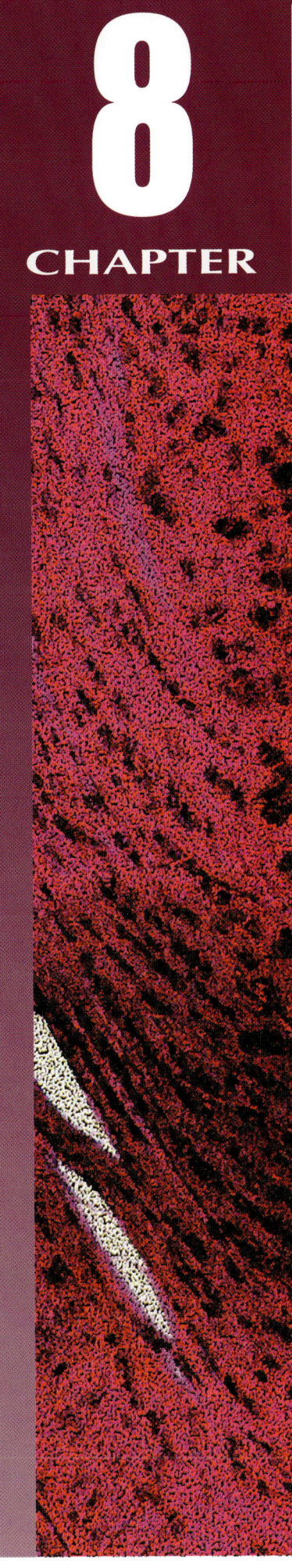

The objective of myocardial viability assessment is to identify prospectively patients with potentially reversible left ventricular dysfunction in whom prognosis may be favorably altered with coronary artery revascularization. The concept that impaired left ventricular function at rest may be reversible after revascularization is now well established. Pathophysiologic paradigms have emerged that describe the relationships between myocardial perfusion and ventricular function, leading to the concepts of stunning and hibernation. In these paradigms, myocardial function is depressed but myocytes remain viable, and therefore left ventricular dysfunction may be completely reversible. Considerable advances in basic research and clinical science since the 1980s have helped clarify the underlying mechanisms of the functional alterations in stunned and hibernating myocardium. These advances have altered clinical practice and have led to improved patient management and survival. However, despite significant advances in our understanding and medical management of patients with left ventricular dysfunction, the prevalence of heart failure and the resultant death rates have almost tripled since the 1970s.

Coronary artery disease is responsible for approximately two thirds of cases of heart failure, and is now the leading etiology of left ventricular dysfunction and heart failure in the United States. After the initial ischemic injury, left ventricular dysfunction may continue to decompensate even in the absence of clinical signs and symptoms of heart failure. This has been attributed to a combination of factors that include left ventricular remodeling, impaired energetics, myocyte dysfunction, and cell death due to necrosis and apoptosis. Pathophysiologic processes involved in left ventricular remodeling and progressive systolic dysfunction may be related to the presence and extent of myocardial viability. Because impaired energetics may play an important role in the pathophysiology of heart failure, treatment with pharmacologic agents that improve heart failure symptoms at the expense of an increase in cardiac energy expenditure may worsen prognosis. On the other hand, therapeutic strategies that cause negative inotropy and preserve or reduce cardiac energy expenditure (such as β-adrenergic blocking agents and ACE inhibitors) or restore myocardial blood flow improve patient survival. Myocardial reperfusion in ischemic cardiomyopathy via revascularization reduces ischemic injury, recruits hibernating regions, and prevents future infarction and left ventricular remodeling.

Parallel advances in the development of new radiotracers and techniques in nuclear cardiology have resulted in remarkable breakthroughs that contribute importantly to our understanding of mechanisms involved in dysfunctional but viable myocardium. Biologically derived radiopharmaceuticals have been synthesized that provide insight into the regulation of metabolic processes and upregulation of receptors in the failing human heart. A number of strategies have emerged in the literature for differentiating viable from nonviable myocardium in dysfunctional regions. Techniques that assess intact cellular metabolic processes, *eg*, [^{18}F]-fluorodeoxyglucose, or cell membrane integrity, *eg*, ^{201}Tl, have inherent advantages over indexes of resting function and regional blood flow, *eg*, ^{99m}Tc-labeled perfusion tracers. It has been demonstrated that patients with extensive myocardial viability assessed by PET or ^{201}Tl have significantly lower nonfatal infarction and cardiac death with revascularization than with medical therapy alone. These new advances have lent themselves to more rational and efficient management of patients with ischemic left ventricular dysfunction and heart failure.

In this chapter, clinical experience of recent years, histomorphologic and structural changes in ischemic cardiomyopathy, left ventricular remodeling, and nuclear techniques that are most useful in clinical practice are presented. Such precise knowledge of myocardial viability is used to guide cardiologists in treating patients with ischemic left ventricular dysfunction and heart failure. To reduce the risk of heart failure and associated high mortality in such patients, attenuation of myocardial ischemia via revascularization and prevention of left ventricular remodeling with medical therapy may be the optimum goals for managing such patients clinically.

MYOCARDIAL ISCHEMIA AND VIABILITY

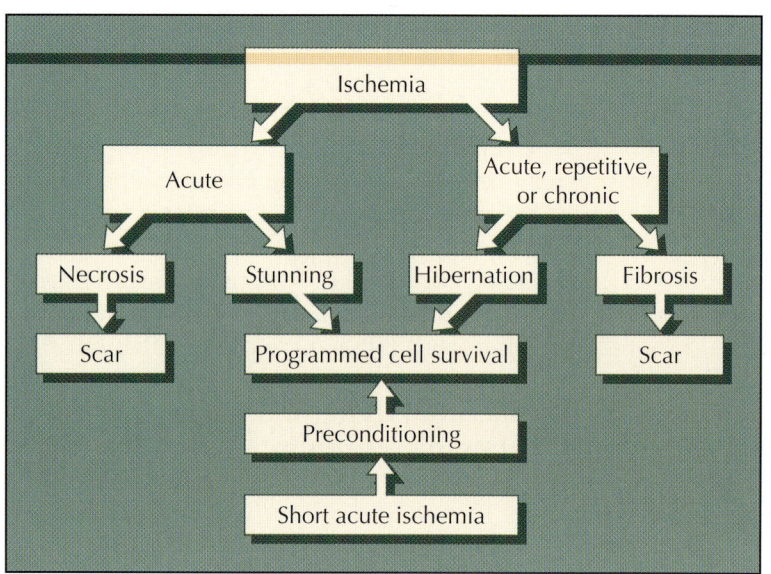

FIGURE 8-1. Imbalance between oxygen supply, usually due to reduced myocardial perfusion, and oxygen demand, determined primarily by the rate and force of myocardial contraction, is termed *ischemic myocardium*. If the oxygen supply-demand imbalance is transient (*ie*, triggered by exertion), it represents reversible ischemia. On the other hand, if regional oxygen supply-demand imbalance is prolonged, high-energy phosphates will be depleted, regional contractile function will progressively deteriorate, and cell membrane rupture with cell death will follow (myocardial necrosis and fibrosis). The phenomena of stunning, hibernation, and ischemic preconditioning represent different mechanisms of acute and chronic adaptation to a temporary or sustained reduction in coronary blood flow. Such modulated responses to ischemia are regulated to preserve sufficient energy to protect the structural and functional integrity of the cardiac myocyte. In contrast to programmed cell death, or apoptosis, Taegtmeyer [1] has coined the term *programmed cell survival* to describe the commonality between myocardial stunning, hibernation, and ischemic preconditioning independent from their disparate myocardial responses to acute and chronic ischemia. (*Adapted from* Taegtmeyer [1].)

REQUIREMENTS FOR CELLULAR VIABILITY

Adequate myocardial blood flow
Sarcolemmal membrane integrity
Preserved metabolic activity

FIGURE 8-2. Requirements for cellular viability. To date, the most common definition of myocardial viability has been the temporal improvement in contractile function of a dysfunctional region after restoration of blood flow. Requirements for cellular viability include sufficient myocardial blood flow, intact sarcolemmal membrane function, and preserved metabolic activity. Myocardial blood flow has to be adequate to deliver substrate to the myocyte to be used in the metabolic process, as well as to remove the end products of the metabolic process. If regional blood flow is severely reduced or absent, then the metabolites and end products will accumulate, causing inhibition of the enzymes of the metabolic pathway, depletion of high-energy phosphates, cell membrane disruption, and cell death. Thus, at either extreme of the range of blood flow, myocardial perfusion tracers provide information regarding myocardial viability. However, in regions in which the reduction in blood flow is of intermediate severity, perfusion information alone may be insufficient to determine viability, and additional pieces of data such as metabolic indexes would be necessary. Intact sarcolemmal membrane function to maintain electrochemical gradients across the cell membrane is a requirement for myocyte viability. Because cell membrane integrity is highly dependent on preserved intracellular metabolic activity to generate high-energy phosphates, tracers that reflect sarcolemmal cation flux as well as perfusion, such as ^{201}Tl and ^{82}Rb, should parallel the viability information provided by markers of metabolic activity, *eg*, [^{18}F]-fluorodeoxyglucose. Thus, in the setting of reduced regional blood flow and function, techniques that assess intact cellular sarcolemmal function or metabolic processes provide unique insight into the presence or absence of myocardial viability.

LEFT VENTRICULAR DYSFUNCTION AND HEART FAILURE

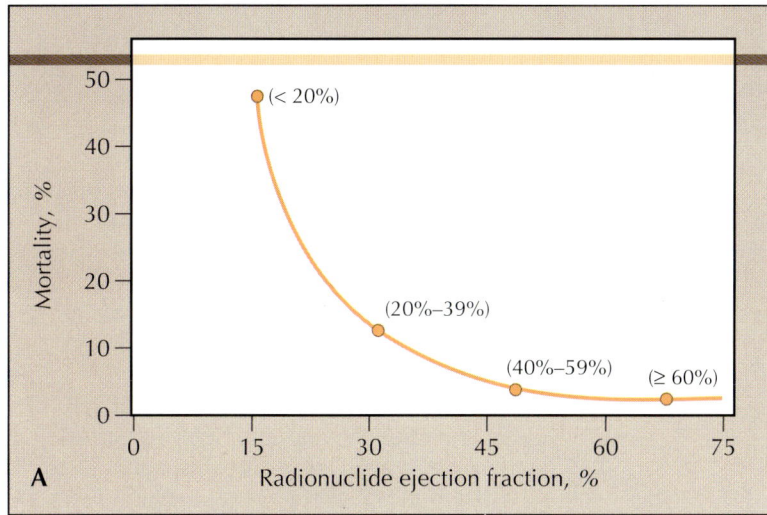
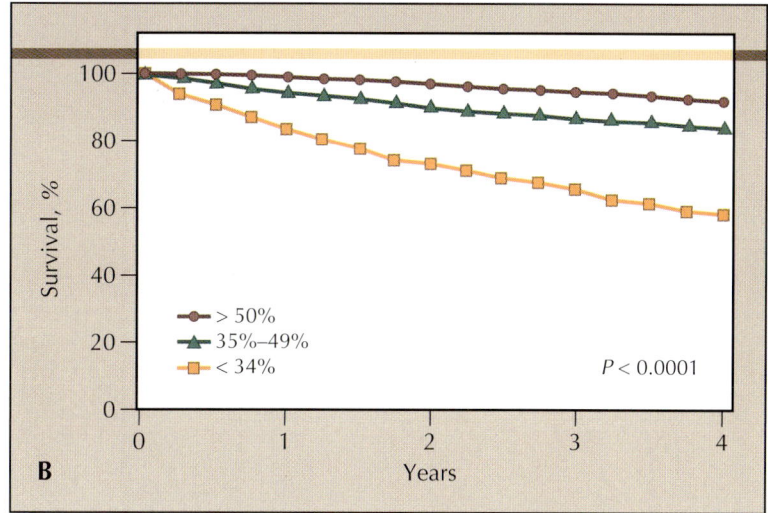

FIGURE 8-3. Left ventricular ejection fraction. Left ventricular ejection fraction (LVEF) is a major determinant of survival in patients with acute and chronic coronary artery disease. **A,** In patients with acute myocardial infarction, the Multicenter Postinfarction Trial showed a curvilinear relationship between mortality rates in the first year after myocardial infarction and predischarge LVEF. This relationship has been demonstrated conclusively in virtually every study assessing patient outcome after myocardial infarction. It is apparent from the curve that attempts to risk-stratify patients with preserved left ventricular function ($\geq 50\%$) further will be problematic, because this cohort will have few cardiac-related deaths during the subsequent year after infarction. On the other hand, among patients with moderate-to-severe left ventricular dysfunction, further risk stratification is both feasible and clinically relevant. **B,** In chronic stable coronary artery disease, the cumulative 4-year survival of the medically treated Coronary Artery Surgery Study registry patients based on LVEF at rest is shown. Patients with normal ($\geq 50\%$) or mildly reduced (35%–49%) left ventricular function have an excellent 4-year survival on medical therapy (92% and 83%, respectively). On the other hand, patients with moderate to severely reduced (< 35%) left ventricular function have a significantly lower 4-year survival (58%) when treated with medical therapy alone. (*Adapted from* [2] and Mock *et al.* [3].)

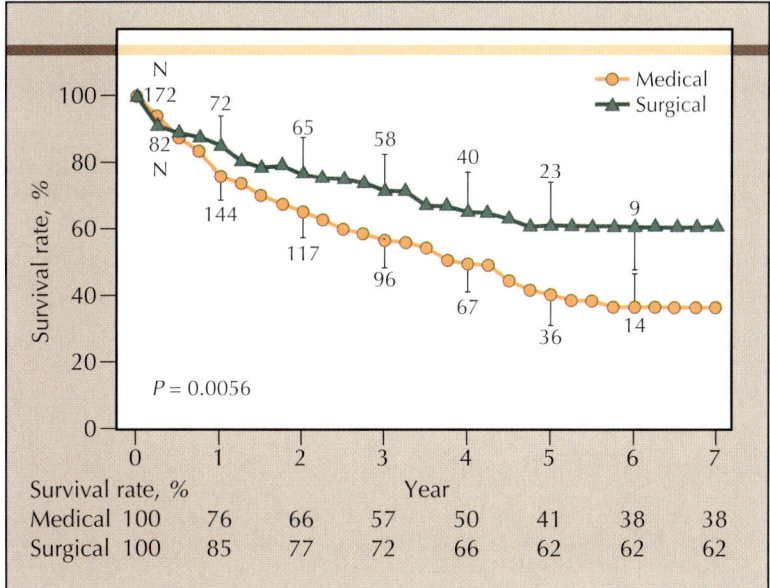

FIGURE 8-4. Life-table cumulative survival for surgically and medically treated Coronary Artery Surgery Study registry patients with severely reduced left ventricular ejection fraction (LVEF). Short- and long-term surgical survival benefits are greatest in patients with the most severe left ventricular dysfunction. Among the patients with LVEF of 25% or lower, the 5-year survival rate is 62% with surgical treatment and 41% with medical treatment. The 1- and 2-year survival rates of surgically treated patients is 85% and 77%, in contrast to 76% and 66% in the medically treated patients, respectively. Myocardial reperfusion via revascularization ameliorates ischemic injury, recruits hibernating regions, and prevents future infarction. However, the operative risk of coronary artery bypass surgery is increased in this patient population, which explains the reluctance of cardiac surgeons to operate on these patients without evidence of myocardial viability. With increased surgical expertise and improved intraoperative myocardial preservation techniques, combined with accurate prospective assessment of myocardial viability, surgical mortality rates have decreased substantially since the 1980s. (*Adapted from* Alderman *et al.* [4].)

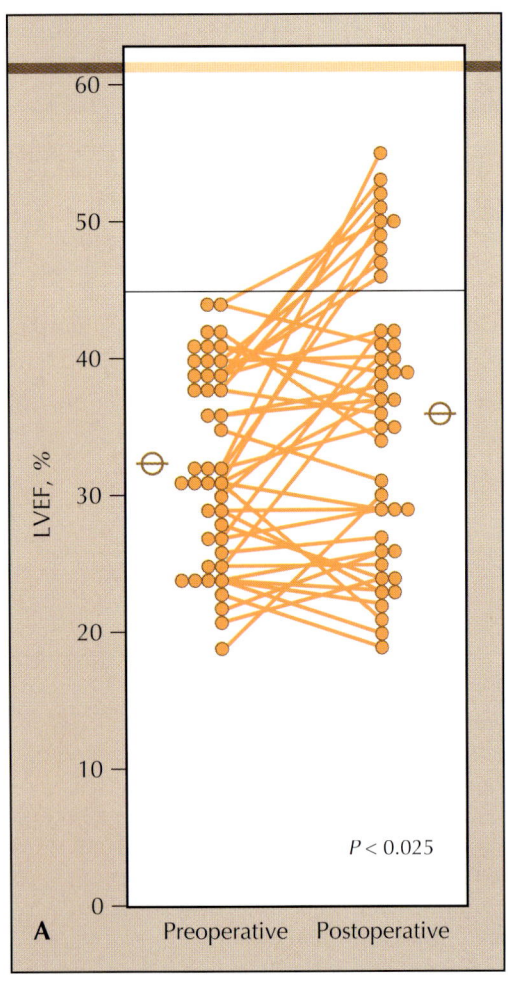
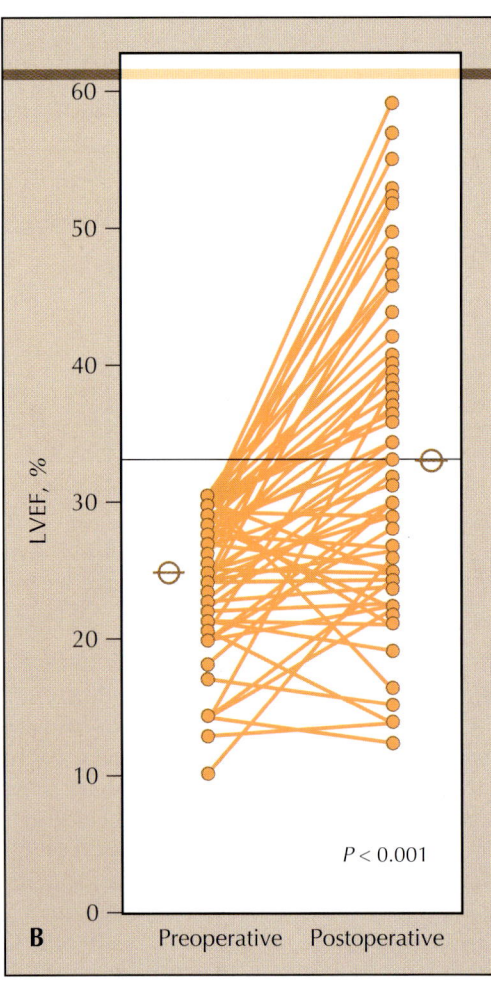

FIGURE 8-5. Change in left ventricular ejection fraction at rest before (preoperative) and after (postoperative) coronary artery bypass surgery. In patients with moderate (A) and severe (B) left ventricular dysfunction, successful coronary artery revascularization resulted in improved left ventricular function at rest in approximately one third of patients. Thus, the conventional wisdom that impaired left ventricular function at rest is an irreversible process has been challenged by such observations. Substantial data now exist to indicate that under certain conditions, when viable myocytes are subjected to hypoperfusion or transient periods of ischemia, prolonged alterations in regional and global left ventricular function may occur and this dysfunction may be completely reversible. (*Adapted from* Bonow and Dilsizian [5] and Elefteriades *et al*. [6].)

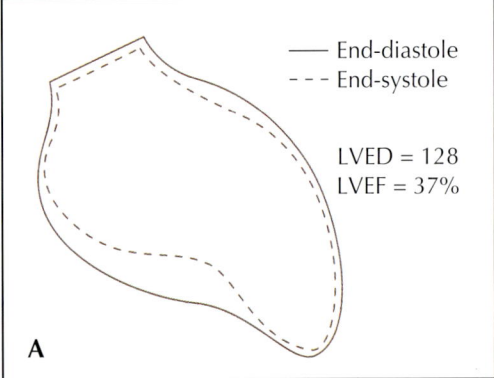
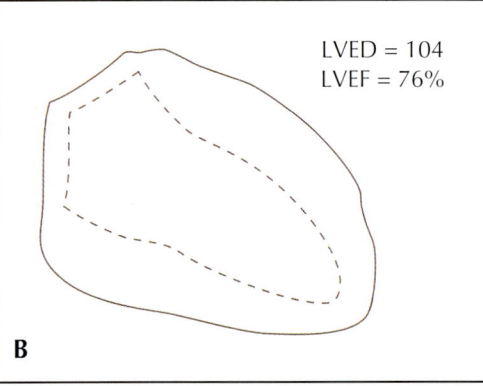

FIGURE 8-6. Hibernating myocardium. Recovery of regional and global left ventricular function at rest following revascularization is shown in a patient with totally occluded left anterior descending coronary artery and left ventricular dysfunction. End-diastolic and end-systolic silhouettes of the left ventricle from the right anterior oblique contrast ventriculography before (A) and 8 months after (B) coronary artery bypass surgery are shown. Preoperatively, the anteroapical region is akinetic, associated with a left ventricular ejection fraction (LVEF) of 37% at rest. Postoperatively, the anteroapical regional contraction is normal and the LVEF at rest has nearly doubled to 76%. LVED—left ventricular end-diastolic volume. (*Adapted from* Rahimtoola [7].)

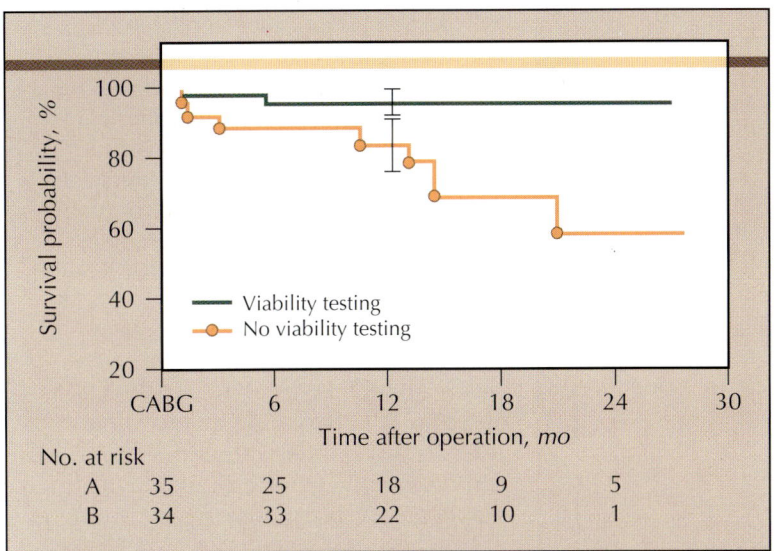

FIGURE 8-7. Myocardial viability testing prior to surgical revascularization. Determination of myocardial viability evaluation in patients with coronary artery disease and severe left ventricular dysfunction before referral to coronary artery revascularization affects clinical outcome with respect to both in-hospital mortality and 1-year survival rate. In this retrospective study, the perioperative and postoperative event-free survival rate was significantly lower in patients who were referred to revascularization on the basis of clinical presentation and angiographic data but without viability testing (group A) compared with those who were selected according to the extent of viable tissue determined by PET (group B) in addition to clinical presentation and angiographic data. There were four in-hospital deaths (11.4%) in group A and none in group B ($P = 0.04$). Moreover, after 12 months, the survival rate was 79% in group A and 97% in group B ($P = 0.01$). (*Adapted from* Haas *et al.* [8].)

CONTRACTION–PERFUSION MISMATCH AND MATCH: STUNNING AND HIBERNATION

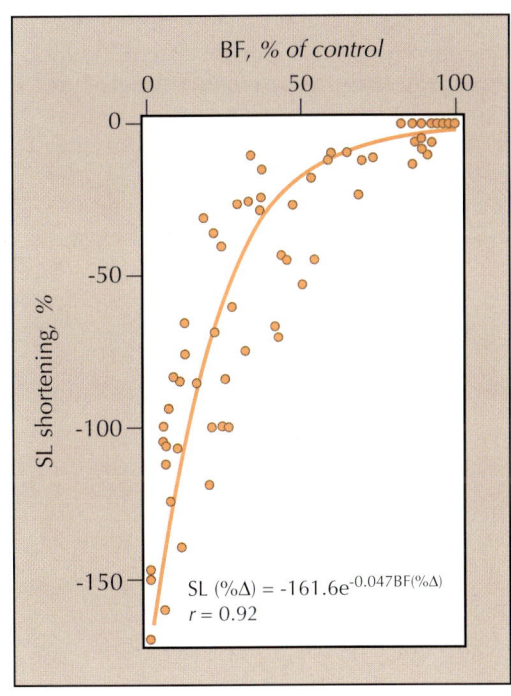

FIGURE 8-8. Coupling between acute reductions in myocardial blood flow and function in conscious dogs with acute graded levels of coronary artery stenosis. There is an exponential relationship between the decreases in myocardial blood flow (BF) (radioactive microsphere technique) and segmental length (SL) shortening (ultrasonic dimension technique). Whereas only slight (10%–20%) decreases in blood flow are required to reduce segmental function initially, some segmental shortening is maintained until blood flow is severely reduced (> 90% of control), at which point there is complete loss of segmental function. (*Adapted from* Vatner [9].)

MYOCARDIAL VIABILITY: REVERSIBLE LEFT VENTRICULAR DYSFUNCTION

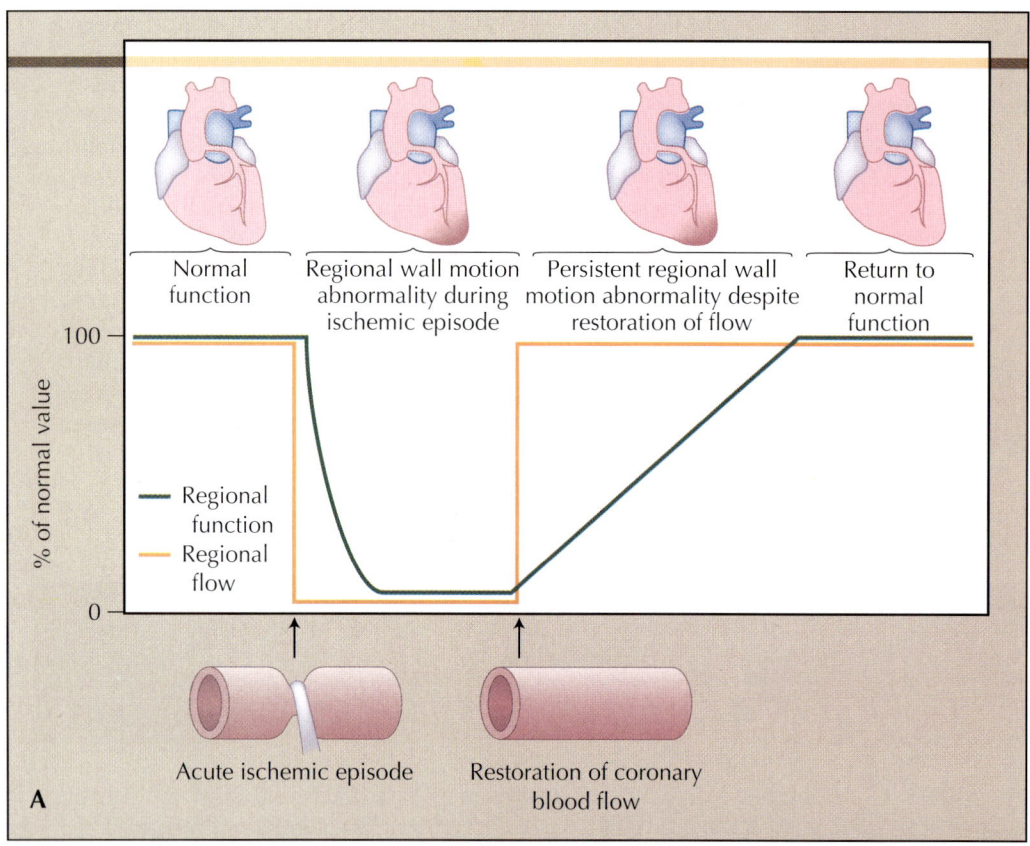
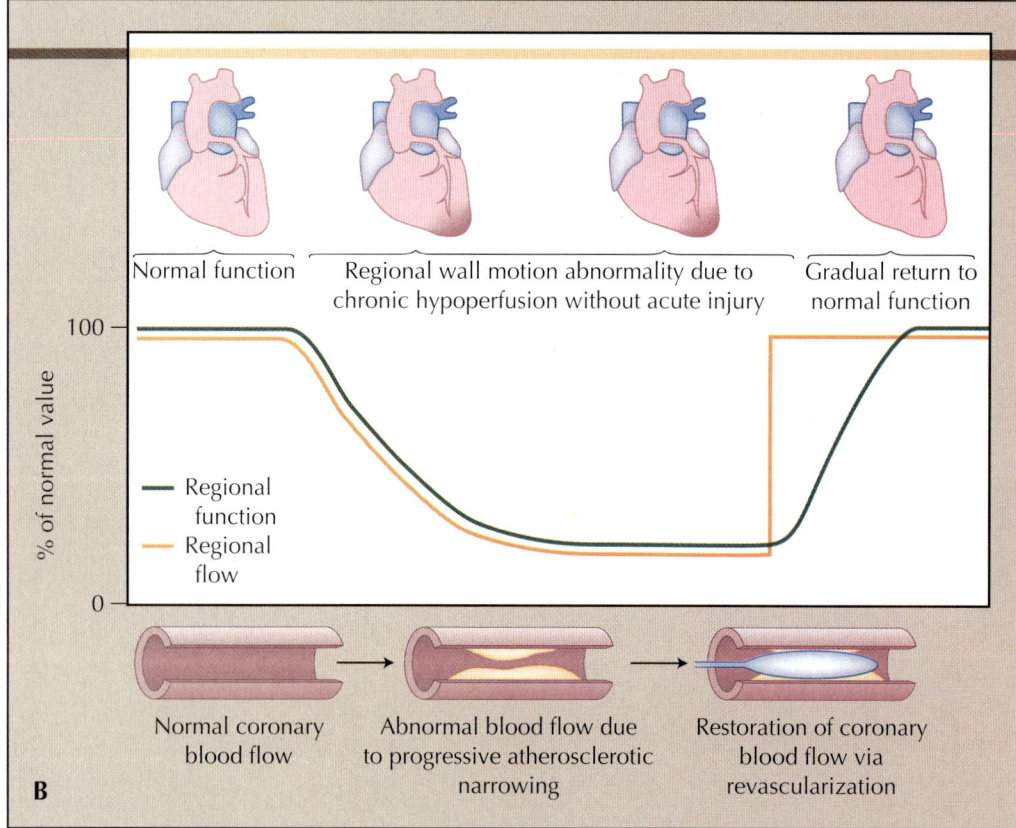

FIGURE 8-9. Pathophysiologic paradigms concerning the relationship between myocardial perfusion and left ventricular function in stunned and hibernating myocardium. **A,** Stunned myocardium refers to the state of delayed recovery of regional left ventricular dysfunction after a transient period of ischemia that has been followed by reperfusion [10]. The ischemic episodes that ultimately lead to myocardial stunning can be single or multiple, brief or prolonged, but never severe enough to result in myocardial necrosis. **B,** Hibernating myocardium refers to an adaptive rather than injurious response of the myocardium, in which viable but dysfunctional myocardium arises from prolonged myocardial hypoperfusion at rest in the absence of clinically evident ischemia [7]. In stunning, interventions aimed at decreasing the frequency, severity, or duration of ischemic episodes would result in improved contractile function. In hibernation, interventions that favorably alter the supply/demand relationship of the myocardium, either improvement in blood flow or reduction in demand, would be expected to improve contractile function. It is very likely, however, that in patients with chronic coronary artery disease, the adaptive responses of hibernation and injurious responses of stunning coexist.

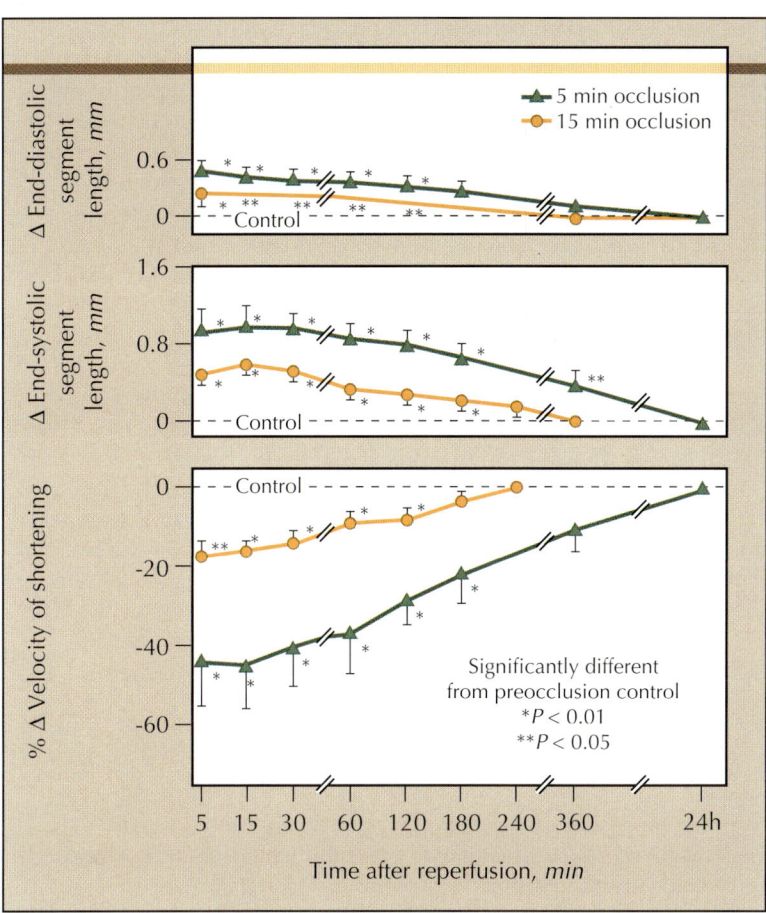

FIGURE 8-10. Experimental evidence for stunned myocardium. Conscious dogs were subjected to 5 or 15 minutes of coronary artery occlusion followed by reperfusion. Recovery times for end-diastolic and end-systolic segment length and velocity of shortening are shown after 5-minute (*circles*) and 15-minute (*triangles*) occlusions. Recovery times from 5 minutes to 24 hours after reperfusion are also shown. During the occlusion phase, regional systolic thickening was absent in the ischemic zone, and the ECG showed ST segment elevation. During the reperfusion phase, ST segments returned to baseline within 1 minute, and reactive hyperemia was observed within the ischemic zone. Systolic thickening, however, remained depressed for more than 3 hours after the 5-minute coronary occlusion and for more than 6 hours after the 15-minute occlusion. (*Adapted from* Heyndrickx *et al.* [11].)

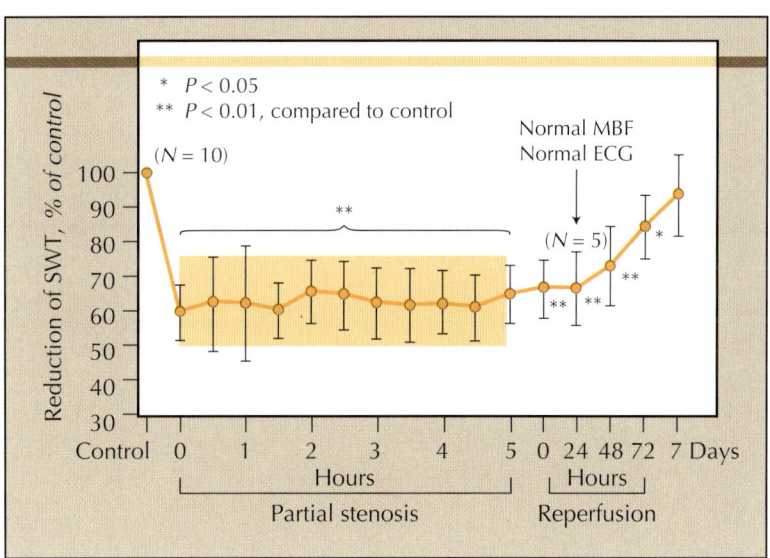

FIGURE 8-11. Experimental model for short-term hibernation demonstrating balanced reduction of myocardial function and blood flow (MBF) (contraction-perfusion match). Changes in systolic wall thickening (SWT) in the ischemic area during 5-hour partial coronary artery occlusion and after reperfusion are plotted as a percent of control at frequent intervals to indicate the sustained nature of the regional dysfunction. Data points are ± 1 SD, which is within the limits of a 25% to 50% decrease in function (*shaded area*). After reperfusion, regional dysfunction initially remained depressed but showed late recovery. At 24 hours after reperfusion, five of the 10 dogs had dysrhythmia. Thus, only the data obtained from the remaining five dogs were analyzed. The findings in this canine model indicate that prolonged moderate regional dysfunction caused by nontransmural ischemia during partial stenosis can be sustained for 5 hours. Furthermore, after reperfusion, there is complete recovery of regional and global contractile function within a period of 7 days. (*Adapted from* Matsuzaki *et al.* [12].)

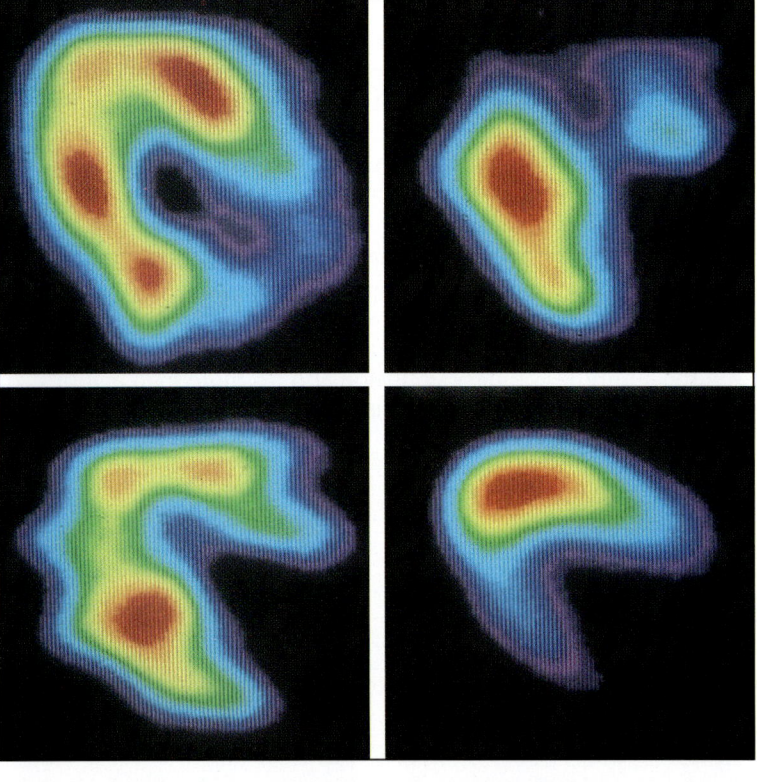

FIGURE 8-12. Positron emission tomograms demonstrating metabolic alterations in post-ischemic myocardium of a patient with exercise-induced angina. Physical exercise is probably the most common precipitating factor responsible for myocardial ischemia in patients with coronary artery disease, manifested as angina and, most importantly, left ventricular dysfunction. Although recovery of such stress-induced left ventricular dysfunction is thought to occur within minutes after the termination of exercise, persistent contractile dysfunction has been observed in some patients up to 90 minutes after the termination of exercise, which has been attributed to stunned myocardium. Transaxial rubidium-82 (^{82}Rb) images reflecting myocardial blood flow at rest, during exercise, and after exercise are shown along with [^{18}F]-fluorodeoxyglucose (FDG) images after exercise. At rest (*top, left*), the distribution of myocardial blood flow is homogeneous in all myocardial regions. During exercise (*top, right*), there are extensive blood flow abnormalities in the apical and anteroseptal regions that improve on the postexercise images (*bottom, left*) and are comparable to the ^{82}Rb rest image (*top left*). FDG was injected 8 minutes after the termination of exercise. The FDG image recorded 60 minutes after tracer injection (*bottom, right*) shows metabolic alterations in the previously ischemic regions. (*From* Camici *et al.* [13]; with permission.)

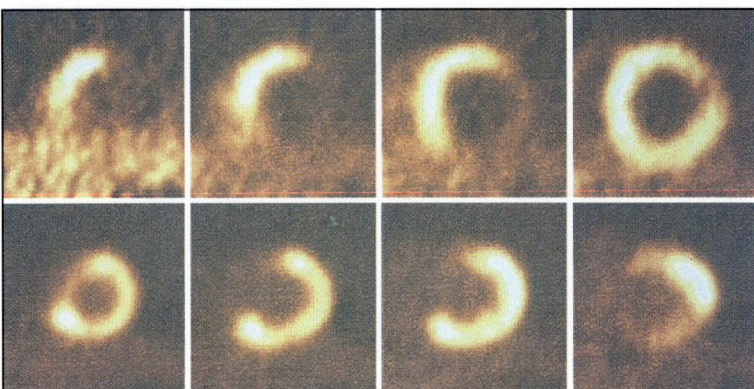

FIGURE 8-13. Positron emission tomograms demonstrating perfusion-metabolism mismatch (reduced blood flow with preserved or enhanced [^{18}F]-fluorodeoxyglucose [FDG] uptake) in a patient with chronic ischemic left ventricular dysfunction and heart failure symptoms. The principle of using a metabolic tracer, such as FDG, is based on the concept that viable myocytes in hypoperfused and dysfunctional regions are metabolically active, while scarred or fibrotic tissue is metabolically inactive. Although fatty acids are the primary source of myocardial energy production in the fasting state, in the setting of reduced oxygen supply (a consequence of hypoperfusion at rest), the myocytes compensate for the loss of oxidative potential by shifting toward greater glucose utilization to generate high-energy phosphates. Thus, in chronic ischemia, aerobic metabolism is slowed while the anaerobic metabolism is accelerated, a reversal of the well-known Pasteur effect [14]. Such increased FDG uptake (anaerobic metabolism) in asynergic myocardial regions with reduced blood flow at rest has become a scintigraphic marker of hibernation. *Top row*, Short-axis [^{13}N]-ammonia scans demonstrate large lateral and inferior perfusion defects at rest. *Bottom row*, The corresponding FDG images acquired under fasting conditions demonstrate that FDG metabolic activity is preserved in the lateral and inferior regions (mismatch pattern). On the other hand, the lack of FDG metabolic activity in the anterior and septal regions reflects the utilization of fatty acid rather than glucose as the primary fuel in such normally perfused myocardial regions.

HISTOMORPHOLOGIC AND STRUCTURAL CHANGES UNDERLYING LEFT VENTRICULAR DYSFUNCTION

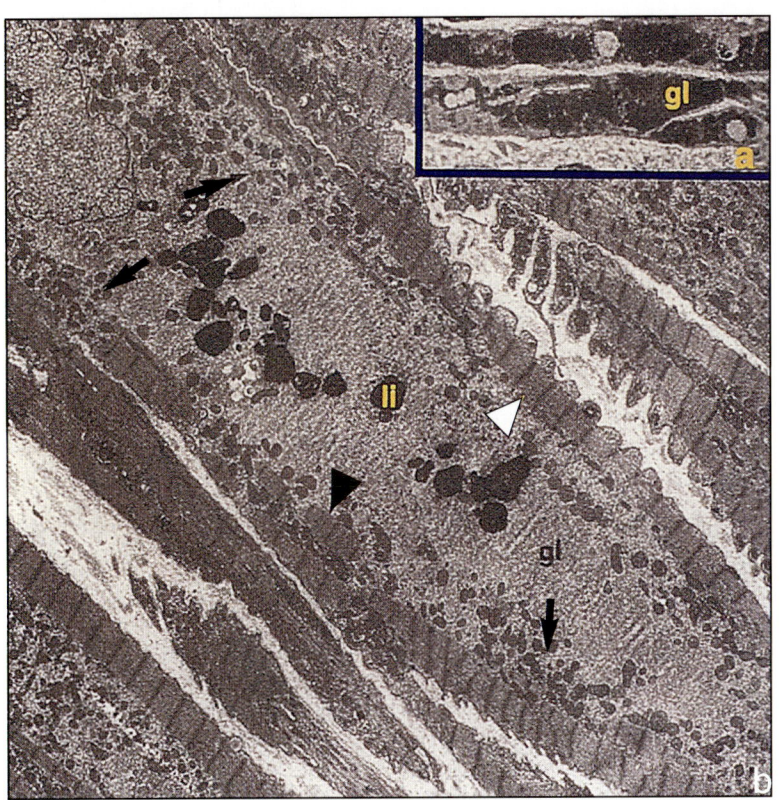

FIGURE 8-14. Subcellular changes in cardiomyocytes of hibernating myocardium. **A**, **B**, Light and electron micrographs show depletion of sarcomeres (present only at the cell periphery [*arrowhead*]) and contractile filament material, accumulation and storage of glycogen (gl), and the appearance of numerous small mitochondria (*arrows*). Because some of these structural changes of altered myocytes resemble those of embryonic cells, such changes have been attributed to a dedifferentiation process. Moreover, altered myocytes have been shown to re-express contractile proteins that are specific to the fetal heart, such as the α-smooth muscle cell, actin. Whether these phenotypic changes are the result of prolonged hypoperfusion or ischemia or secondary to prolonged contractile loading and are reversible after revascularization is unknown ($\times$ 350; *inset*, $\times$ 3250). li—lipfuscin. (*From* Borgers and Ausma [15]; with permission.)

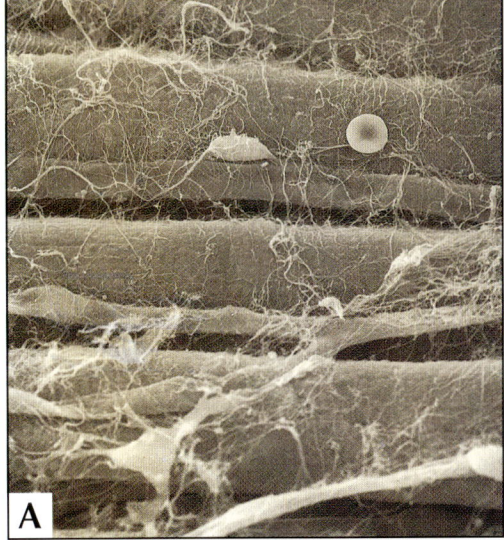
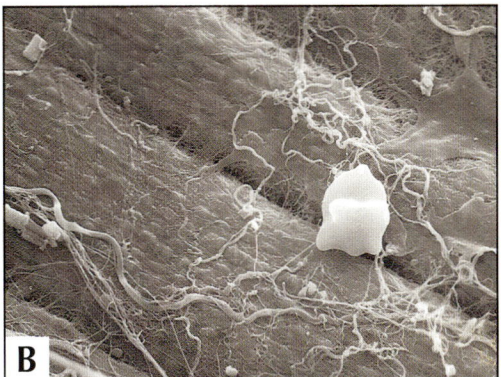
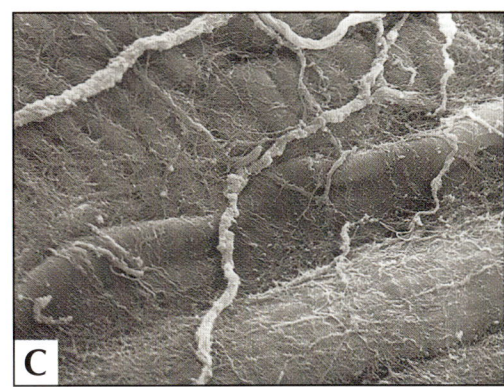
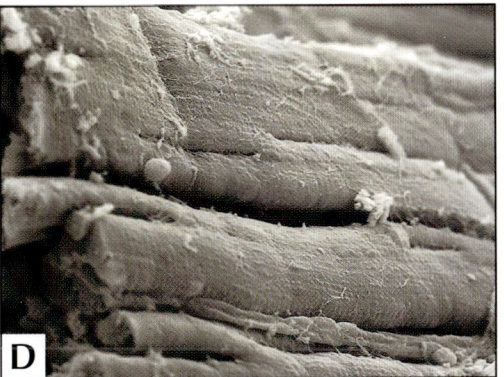

FIGURE 8-15. Scanning electron micrographs from normal tissue, a nonischemic region, and stunned myocardial regions. **A**, Normal tissue shows the usual dense and florid collagen weave enveloping the individual myocytes. There are abundant collagen struts that interconnect myocyte to myocyte and myocyte to capillary. The collagen struts are also connected to collagen weave ($\times$ 3000). **B**, In the nonischemic myocardial region, collagen cables are smooth and continuous, branch off into smaller cables, and connect with the underlying collagen weave on the surface of the myocyte ($\times$ 5700). **C**, In the stunned myocardial region, the collagen cables are characterized by a rough, irregular, notched appearance. The collagen weave is generally matted with a beaded and granular appearance, suggestive of degeneration ($\times$ 9000). **D**, In another example of stunned myocardium, the normally ubiquitous myocyte to myocyte struts are minimal to absent, with nodular or nublike structures likely indicative of broken collagen struts. In addition, there is almost complete absence of the perimysial weave ($\times$ 2100). (*Courtesy of* Calvin Eng; *from* Zhao *et al.* [16]; with permission.)

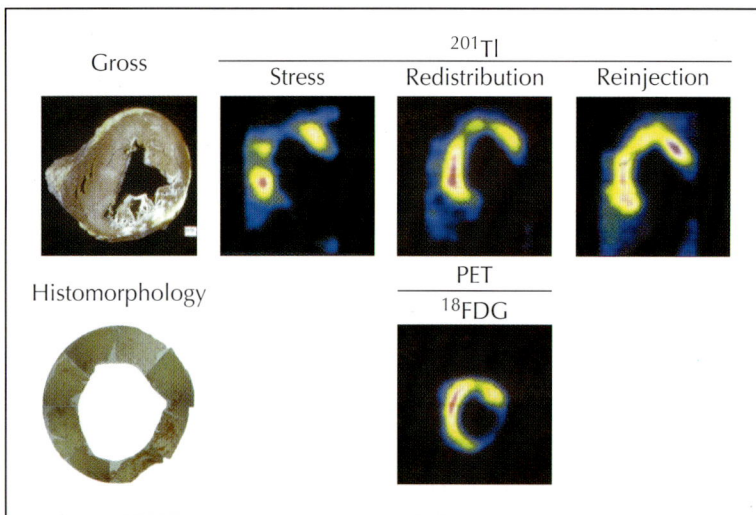

FIGURE 8-16. Disparity between left ventricular contractile dysfunction and the extent of myocardial injury assessed by thallium scintigraphy. Correlation between gross pathology, histomorphology, ^{201}Tl and [^{18}F]-fluorodeoxyglucose (FDG) PET studies from a patient with stable chronic ischemic heart disease, and severe left ventricular dysfunction who underwent orthotopic cardiac transplantation is demonstrated. Gross pathology and histomorphology of a midventricular slice is shown, *left*, with corresponding thallium and FDG PET images, *right*. On the thallium study, there are extensive abnormalities in the anterior, septal, and inferolateral regions during stress. On the redistribution image, there is partial reversibility of the anterior region, complete reversibility of the septum, and irreversible defect in the inferolateral region. After ^{201}Tl reinjection, there is complete reversibility of the septal and anterior regions with persistent irreversible defect in the inferolateral region. The corresponding FDG PET image shows preserved metabolic activity and hence viability in all regions except for the inferolateral region. On gross pathology, there is white fibrotic myocardium in the inferolateral region, and histomorphologic analysis shows a significant amount of red-stained collagen intermixed within normal tissue. Because structural changes in hibernating myocardium are chronic in nature and have developed over a prolonged period, some regions viable by scintigraphic or echocardiographic techniques may be irreversible despite successful revascularization [17]. (*Courtesy of* Jamshid Shirani, Albert Einstien College of Medicine, Bronx, NY.)

LEFT VENTRICULAR REMODELING

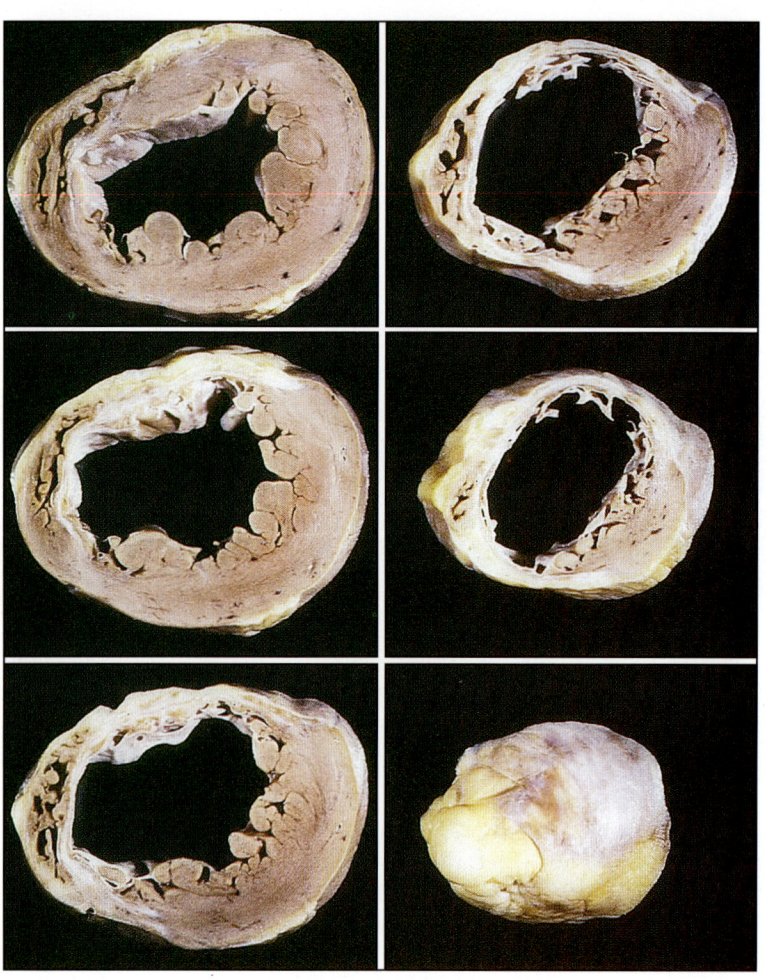

FIGURE 8-17. Gross pathology of a heart removed from a cardiac transplant recipient with ischemic cardiomyopathy. There is evidence of left ventricular cavity dilatation, large anterior, septal, and apical infarction, characterized as thinning and elongation of the infarcted region, and hypertrophy of the remaining regions secondary to remodeling. After an acute myocardial infarction, the myocardium is replaced by scarred tissue, which is susceptible to further thinning and elongation due to infarct expansion. It has been demonstrated that this process of infarct expansion involves slippage of muscle bundles within ischemic as well as nonischemic myocardial regions. In addition to the infarct expansion, left ventricular dilatation and remodeling ensues within days and months after the acute myocardial injury. The morphologic and geometric changes of the left ventricle as a result of remodeling affect regions of scarred as well as nonischemic, viable myocardium. The cardiac interstitium may also play a role in modulating muscle configuration after ischemic insults. (*Courtesy of* Jamshid Shirani, Albert Einstein College of Medicine, Bronx, NY.)

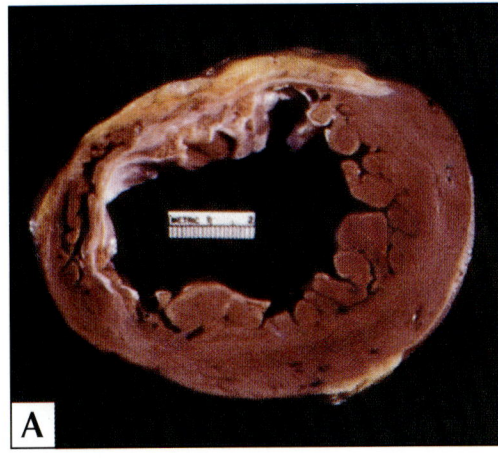
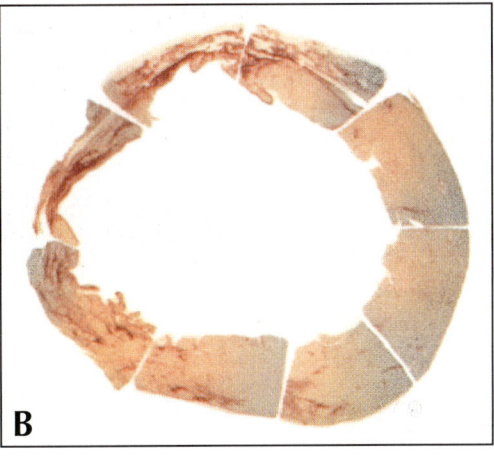
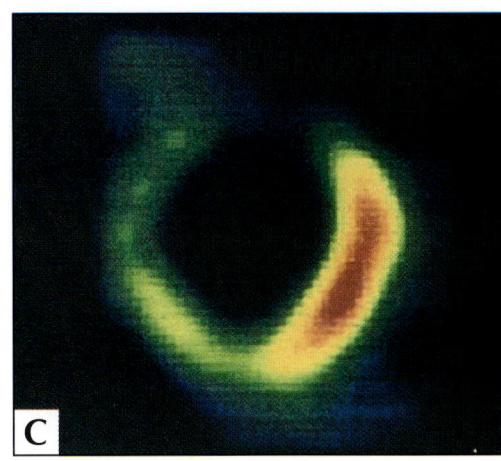

FIGURE 8-18. Correlation between short-axis tomograms from a patient with stable chronic ischemic heart disease and severe left ventricular dysfunction who underwent orthotopic cardiac transplantation. **A**, On gross pathology, there is white fibrotic myocardium in the anterior extending to the anteroseptal region, with corresponding red-stained collagen on histomorphologic analysis (**B**), and severe thallium defects in the anterior and anteroseptal regions on the redistribution-reinjection tomogram (**C**) [17]. (*Courtesy of* Jamshid Shirani, Albert Einstein College of Medicine, Bronx, NY.)

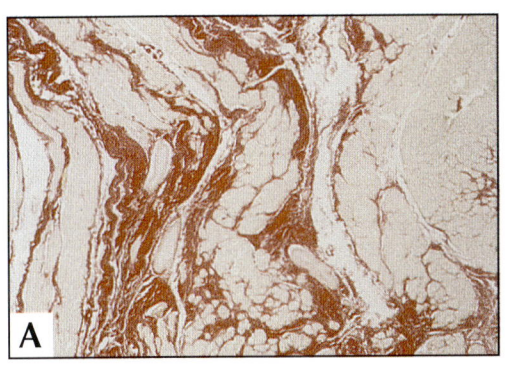
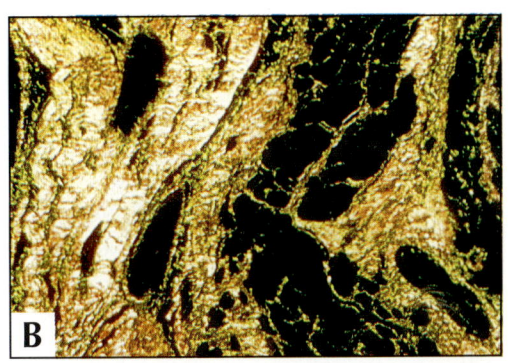
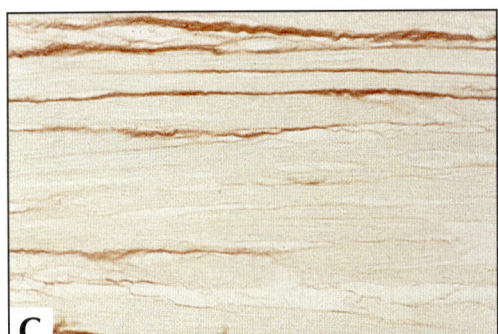
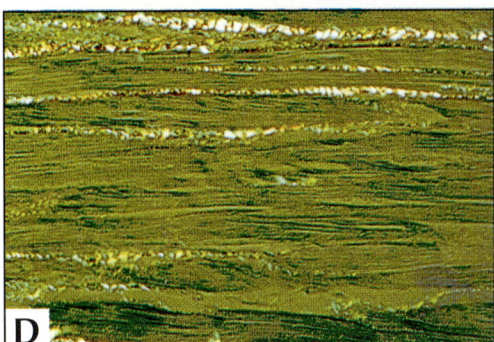

FIGURE 8-19. Histomorphologic analysis of infarcted and noninfarcted myocardial segments: insight into myocyte viability and remodeling of the nonmyocyte compartment. Microscopic sections from (**A, B**) infarcted and (**C, D**) noninfarcted segments stained with picrosirius red are shown. The dark red areas of *panels A* and *C* represent collagen replacement, and the green and yellow areas of *panels B* and *D* represent birefringence of collagen under polarized light. The infarcted segments (transmural scar by gross pathology) demonstrate morphologically normal-appearing myocytes that could be detected by ^{201}Tl scintigraphy, [^{18}F]-fluorodeoxyglucose (FDG) PET, and gross pathology. Conversely, a microscopic section from the noninfarcted segment (normal by gross pathology) shows layers of collagen within normal-appearing myocytes that could not be detected by ^{201}Tl scintigraphy, FDG PET, or gross pathology [17]. (*Courtesy of* Jamshid Shirani, Albert Einstein College of Medicine, Bronx, NY.)

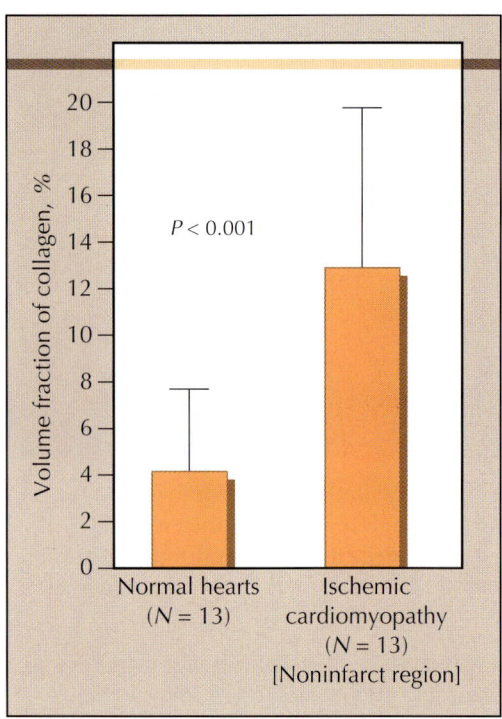

FIGURE 8-20. Mean volume fraction of collagen in noninfarcted myocardial segments from 13 patients with chronic ischemic cardiomyopathy and age-matched control hearts obtained at autopsy from individuals who fulfilled the criteria for normalcy by preautopsy, autopsy, and histologic criteria. Mean volume fraction of collagen in the noninfarcted segments significantly exceeds that in the age-matched control hearts. It is likely that the patchy areas of replacement fibrosis in the remodeled segments represent myocyte necrosis due to prolonged persistent myocardial hypoperfusion or microvascular atherothrombotic or embolic occlusion. This is supported by the observation that the severity of coronary artery narrowing is significantly worse in remodeled noninfarcted myocardium compared with the nonremodeled segments. (*Adapted from* Shirani *et al*. [17].)

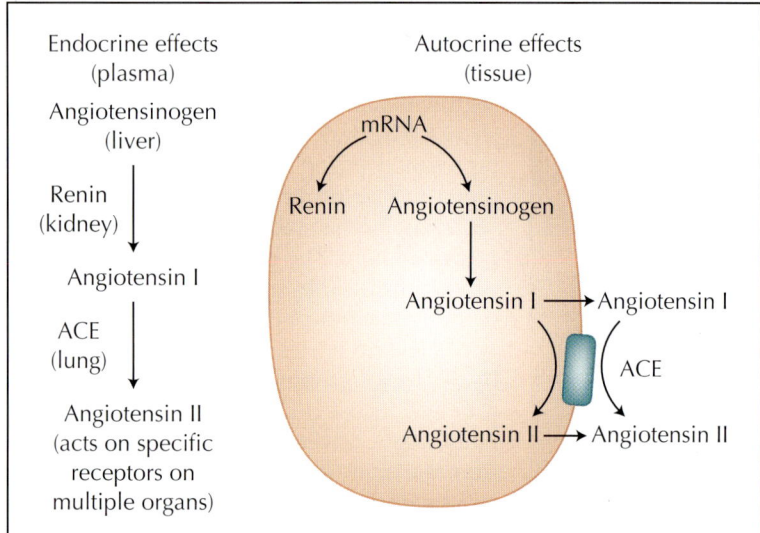

FIGURE 8-21. Renin-angiotensin system. The renin-angiotensin system is frequently activated in patients with ischemic left ventricular dysfunction and heart failure. Angiotensin II, a potent vasoconstrictor, has been implicated in left ventricular remodeling, interstitial fibrosis, and cell death in heart failure. ACE inhibitors have been proven to reduce the risk of morbidity and mortality in large clinical trials of patients with coronary artery disease and left ventricular dysfunction who have symptoms of congestive heart failure. ACE inhibitors impact left ventricular remodeling and thereby improve prognosis in patients with heart failure. The traditional concept of the renin-angiotensin system is a circulation-borne endocrine system whose components are secreted by different organs: angiotensinogen from the liver, renin from the kidney, and ACE from the lung. The product of this biochemical cascade, angiotensin II, acts on specific receptors on multiple organs. However, recent data demonstrate that renin and angiotensin are synthesized locally in the myocyte. The discovery of the tissue-ACE system and its ability to convert angiotensin I to angiotensin II (autocrine effects) as opposed to the plasma/endocrine effects of angiotensin II has led investigators to study the potential of ACE inhibition in preventing or reversing left ventricular remodeling. This emerging concept implies a role of local tissue effects of angiotensin on myocytes, left ventricular remodeling, and vascular tone that may exceed those of circulating plasma effects.

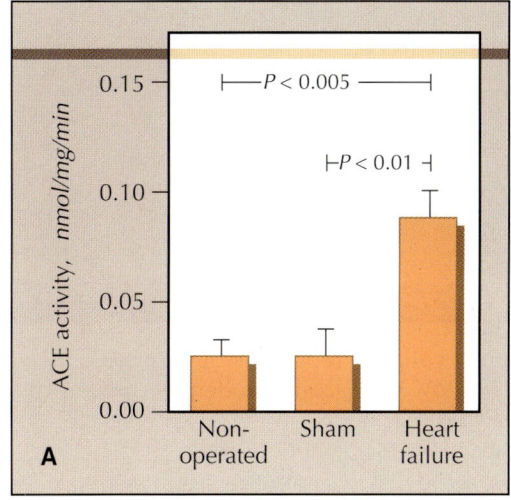 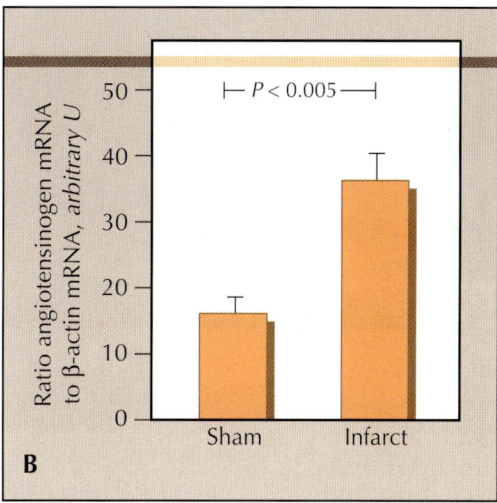 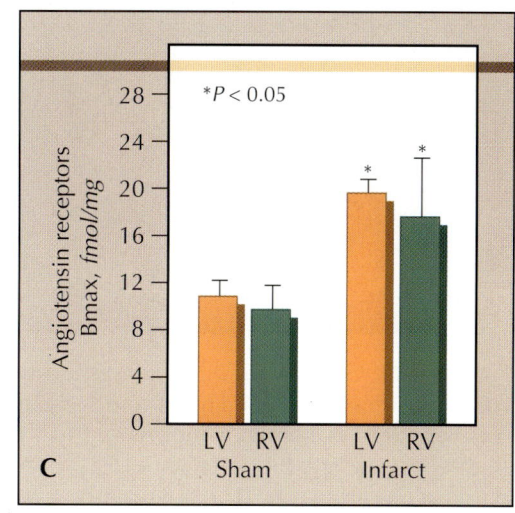

FIGURE 8-22. Upregulation of several components of the tissue renin-angiotensin system in the noninfarcted myocardium of rats after myocardial infarction. There is increasing evidence that in heart failure there is activation of the tissue renin-angiotensin system associated with increased expression of several components of the pathway, including ACE, angiotensinogen, and angiotensin II type I receptors. These data show (**A**) a significant increase in ACE activity, (**B**) the level of angiotensinogen mRNA, and (**C**) the density of angiotensin II receptors. Although serum renin-angiotensin activity often returns to relatively normal levels in well-compensated heart failure, tissue renin-angiotensin activity may remain elevated in the myocardium and vasculature, and thereby contribute significantly to the progression of myocardial remodeling. LV—left ventricle; RV—right ventricle. (*Adapted from* Hirsch *et al.* [18]; Lindpaintner *et al.* [19]; and Meggs *et al.* [20].)

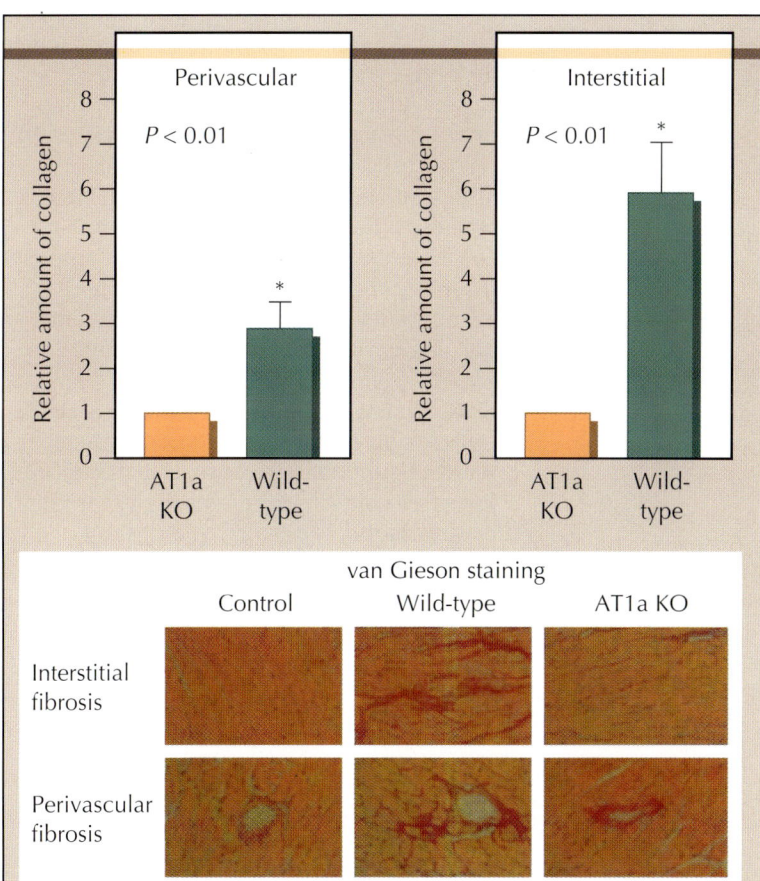

FIGURE 8-23. The role of angiotensin II type 1A (AT1a) receptor in reactive fibrosis and remodeling in noninfarcted myocardium. The extent of interstitial fibrosis and perivascular fibrosis is shown in AT1a receptor knockout (KO) mice and wild-type mice at 1 and 4 weeks after large acute myocardial infarction. At 4 weeks after infarction, control mice showed more marked left ventricular remodeling and fibrosis than did the AT1a KO mice. In addition, the cumulative 4-week mortality rate for the AT1a KO mice was reduced from 22.7% to 5.9% compared with controls, despite similar initial infarct size. These findings indicate that AT1a receptors play a pivotal role in the progression of left ventricular remodeling after myocardial infarction. (*From* Harada *et al.* [21]; with permission.)

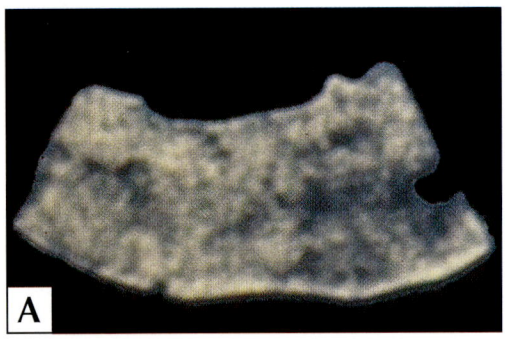 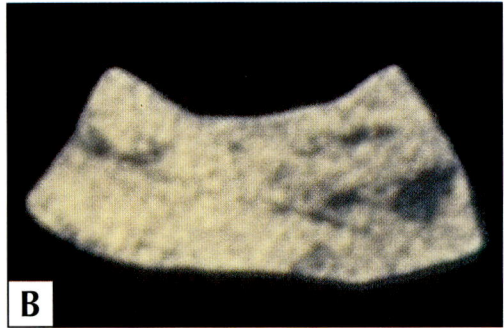 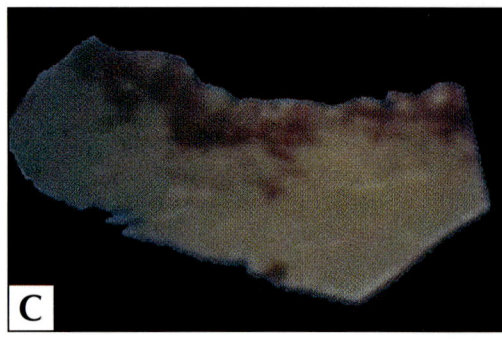

FIGURE 8-24. Specific binding of [^{18}F]fluorobenzyl-linsinopril to ACE in human tissue of a heart removed from a cardiac transplant recipient with ischemic cardiomyopathy. Contiguous myocardial segments incubated in vitro with [^{18}F]fluorobenzyl-linsinopril, without (**A**) and with (**B**) 10^{-6} M lisinopril, are shown. The former solution should give binding at ACE and nonspecific sites, whereas the latter should block binding at ACE. **C**, The corresponding segment stained with picrosirius red reveals the presence and distribution of collagen replacement in relation to ACE binding. The images show that [^{18}F]fluorobenzyl-linsinopril binds specifically to ACE and that there is apparent increased ACE in the juxtaposed areas of replacement fibrosis. If ACE upregulation is reversible, *eg*, by ACE inhibitors, noninvasive imaging with PET may allow monitoring of both the progression of disease and the effect of medical and interventional therapies in such patients [22].

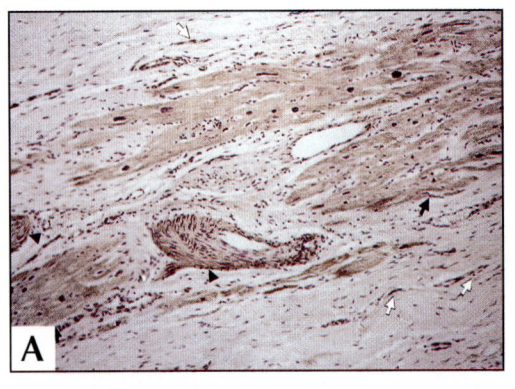 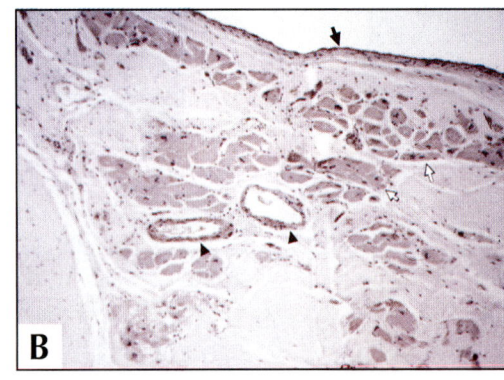

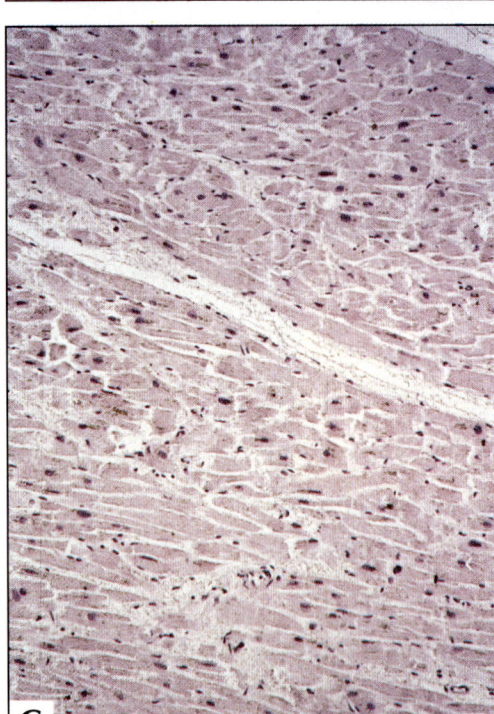 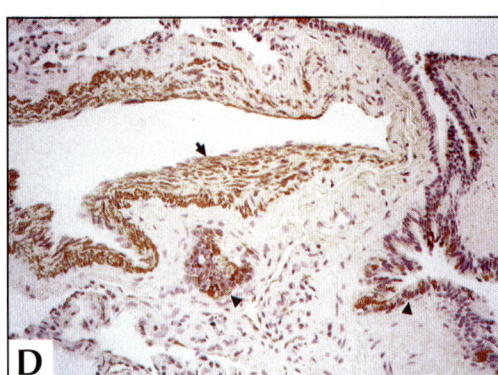

FIGURE 8-25. Micrographs showing immunolabeling of angiotensin II type I receptor (AT1, shown in *brown*) in human tissue of a heart removed from a cardiac transplant recipient with ischemic cardiomyopathy compared to normal control heart and lung. **A**, An island of surviving myocytes within an infarct area and, **B**, peri-infarct area exhibit increased immunoreactivity to AT1. Note that smooth muscle cells of vessels and fibroblasts are also positive for the reaction (original magnification, ×100 and ×200, respectively). **C**, Healthy control heart obtained at autopsy from an patient who fulfilled the criteria for normalcy by preautopsy, autopsy, and histologic criteria showing nonreactivity for AT1 (original magnification, ×100). **D**, Bronchial epithelial and vascular smooth muscle cells from lung tissue in a patient without pulmonary disease used as control for AT1 receptor immunoreactivity (original magnification, ×200) [23]. (*Courtesy of Maria L. Loredo, National Heart, Lung, and Blood Institute, Bethesda, MD.*)

REFERENCES

1. Taegtmeyer H: Modulation of responses to myocardial ischemia: metabolic features of myocardial stunning, hibernation, and ischemic preconditioning. In *Myocardial Viability: A Clinical and Scientific Treatise*. Edited by Dilsizian V. Armonk, New York: Futura; 2000:25–36.
2. Risk stratification and survival after myocardial infarction. *N Engl J Med* 1983, 309:331–336.
3. Mock MB, Ringqvist I, Fisher LD, *et al.*: Survival of medically treated patients in the coronary artery surgery study (CASS) registry. *Circulation* 1982, 66:562–568.
4. Alderman EL, Fisher LD, Litwin P, *et al.*: Results of coronary artery surgery in patients with poor left ventricular function (CASS). *Circulation* 1983; 68:785–795.
5. Bonow RO, Dilsizian V: Thallium-201 for assessment of myocardial viability. *Sem Nucl Med* 1991, 21:230–241.
6. Elefteriades JA, Tolis G Jr, Levi E, *et al.*: Coronary artery bypass grafting in severe left ventricular dysfunction: excellent survival with improved ejection fraction and functional state. *J Am Coll Cardiol* 1993, 22:1411–1417.
7. Rahimtoola SH: A perspective on the three large multicenter randomized clinical trials of coronary bypass surgery for chronic stable angina. *Circulation* 1985, 72(suppl V):V123–V135.
8. Haas F, Haehnel CH, Picker W, *et al.*: Preoperative positron emission tomography viability assessment and perioperative and postoperative risk in patients with advanced ischemic heart disease. *J Am Coll Cardiol* 1997, 30:1693–1700.
9. Vatner S: Correlation between acute reduction in myocardial blood flow and function in conscious dogs. *Circ Res* 1980, 47:201–207.
10. Braunwald E, Kloner RA: The stunned myocardium: prolonged, postischemic ventricular dysfunction. *Circulation* 1982, 66:1146–1149.
11. Heyndrickx GR, Millard RW, McRitchie RJ, *et al.*: Regional myocardial functional and electrophysiological alterations after brief coronary artery occlusion in conscious dogs. *J Clin Invest* 1975, 56:978–985.
12. Matsuzaki M, Gallagher KP, Kemper S, *et al.*: Sustained regional dysfunction produced by prolonged coronary stenosis: gradual recovery after reperfusion. *Circulation* 1983, 68:170–182.
13. Camici P, Araujo LI, Spinks T, *et al.*: Increased uptake of ^{18}F-fluorodeoxyglucose in postischemic myocardium of patients with exercise-induced angina. *Circulation* 1986, 74:81–88.
14. Krebs H: The Pasteur effect and the relation between respiration and fermentation. *Essays Biochem* 1972, 8:1–34.
15. Borgers M, Ausma J: Structural aspects of the chronic hibernating myocardium in man. *Basic Res Cardiol* 1995, 90:44–46.
16. Zhao M, Zhang H, Robinson TF, *et al.*: Profound structural alterations of the extracellular collagen matrix in postischemic dysfunction ("stunned") but viable myocardium. *J Am Coll Cardiol* 1987, 10:1322–1334.
17. Shirani J, Lee J, Quigg RJ, *et al.*: Relation of thallium uptake to morphologic features of chronic ischemic heart disease: evidence for myocardial remodeling in non-infarct myocardium. *J Am Coll Cardiol* 2001, 38:84–90.
18. Hirsch AT, Talsness CE, Schunkert H, *et al.*: Tissue-specific activation of cardiac angiotensin converting enzyme in experimental heart failure. *Circ Res* 1991, 69:475–482.
19. Lindpaintner K, Lu W, Niedermajer N, *et al.*: Selective activation of cardiac angiotensinogen gene expression in post-infarction ventricular remodeling in the rat. *J Mol Cell Cardiol* 1993, 25:133–143.
20. Meggs LG, Coupet J, Huang H, *et al.*: Regulation of angiotensin II receptors on ventricular myocytes after myocardial infarction in rats. *Circ Res* 1993, 72:1149–1162.
21. Harada K, Sugaya T, Murakami K, *et al.*: Angiotensin II type 1A receptor knockout mice display less left ventricular remodeling and improved survival after myocardial infarction. *Circulation* 1999, 100:2093–2099.
22. Dilsizian V, Shirani J, Lee YHC, *et al.*: Specific binding of [^{18}F] fluorobenzoyl-lisinopril to angiotensin converting enzyme in human heart tissue of ischemic cardiomyopathy. *Circulation* 2001, 104:II-694.
23. Dilsizian V, Loredo ML, Ferrans VJ, *et al.*: Evidence for increased angiotensin II type I receptor immunoreactivity in peri-infarct myocardium of human explanted hearts. *J Am Coll Cardiol* 2002, 39:365A.

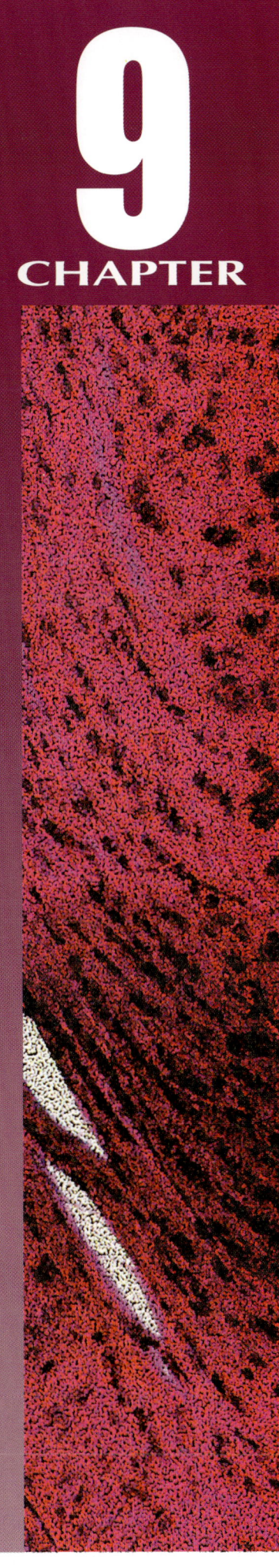

FIRST-PASS AND EQUILIBRIUM RADIONUCLIDE ANGIOGRAPHY

Jeffrey S. Borer

The field of nuclear cardiology originated with the assessment of cardiac performance. From nonimaging experiments in the 1920s, methodology gradually evolved to allow ventricular angiography first by invasive methods in the 1960s, with administration of radionuclide via catheter placed in the left ventricle (LV) [1], followed soon thereafter by noninvasive methodology using intravenous radionuclide administration. The earliest noninvasive approaches also were nonimaging: time-activity curves, relating isotope activity within the LV to specific instants during the cardiac cycle, were achieved by placement of a radiation detector on the chest wall directly over the region occupied predominantly by the LV [2]. These early efforts also featured a first-pass approach, *ie*, radionuclide injected as a relatively tight bolus into the LV or a peripheral vein was followed during its passage through the heart, where it resided in each chamber in concentrations sufficient to generate visually interpretable images and, at least for the right and left ventricles, statistically reliable time-activity curves for 10 to 15 seconds. This same first-pass approach, using the most up to date and efficient radiation detectors, continues to be used in clinical studies [3].

Subsequently, development of "gating" devices (mechanisms employing physiologic signals, most commonly generated by the ECG, to allow precise registration and superimposition of sequential cardiac images and resulting time-activity curves) enhanced temporal resolution and quantitative precision of studies comprising multiple gated images compared with first-pass studies. The multi-image, gated approach enabled creation of composite images and time-activity curves acquired after radionuclide had reached equilibrium within the intravascular compartment [4–6]. Application of computer technology to these "cardiac blood pool" studies permitted collection and display of images in real time; when coupled with list-mode collection techniques, it became possible to isolate and interrogate any portion of the collected image sequence, or images collected at any specific heart rate [5–7]. With modest technical variations, this method, too, regularly is in use today. Unlike the first-pass method, the equilibrium approach requires administration of radionuclide in a form that resides continually within the intravascular space during the time that images are collected, with relatively little extravascular leakage. Although several binders can increase the intravascular residence of the isotope, direct binding of the currently employed radionuclide (^{99m}Tc) to red blood cells is the preferred approach [8]. Because of the relatively long biologic half-lives (several hours) of the red cell–bound radionuclide preparations, nonimaging radionuclide probes can be used for continual monitoring of LV function using equilibrium methodology during ambulatory activity once a baseline image has confirmed positioning of the probe [9,10].

Different technical characteristics of first-pass and equilibrium methods account for their respective advantages and disadvantages. However, both provide LV volumes and temporal variations of volume necessary for LV functional assessments. Since chamber blood volumes are proportional to the density of radioactive emissions emanating from the chamber, their determination is independent of geometric formulas [4–6], enabling accurate application to patients with irregular or misshapen LV, to the right ventricle (RV) [11–13], and for studies performed during peak exercise, when diagnostically and prognostically important cardiac functional abnormalities typically are evoked. Consequently, radionuclide angiography has been applied extensively in all areas of cardiac disease, including diagnosis of coronary artery disease [5,6] and cardiomyopathy [3], and for prognosticating, making management decisions, and evaluating therapy in patients with coronary artery disease [6,14–18], valvular heart disease [6,19–27], and heart failure of diverse etiologies. With a nonimaging modification of the equilibrium approach, it also has become possible to monitor LV function over several hours under various physiologic states and activities.

Important technical limitations remain, including the relatively restricted spatial resolution of standard Anger cameras, precluding precise evaluation of regional LV abnormalities, and overlap of atria and ventricles during equilibrium studies, even in the standard left anterior oblique view, limiting precision in measuring LV and RV volumes. SPECT technology has been applied to blood pool imaging to overcome these problems, providing some obvious advantages over planar imaging [28,29]. However, these advantages have not yet been sufficient to justify replacing the less expensive, less time-consuming, and less complex planar approach. Technical research in this area continues.

RADIONUCLIDE ANGIOGRAPHY IN CLINICAL CARDIOLOGY

Useful for patients with
  Chronic stable CAD
    Diagnosis
    Prognostication
    Assessment of efficacy of treatment
  Regurgitant valvular diseases
    Prognostication and timing of valvular surgery
    Assessment of effects of treatment
  Cardiomyopathy
    Determination of functional severity, categorization for treatment selection
    Assessment of effects of treatment
Useful only for highly selected applications in patients with
  Acute CAD
    Diagnosis of acute right ventricular infarction
    Prognostication
  Stenotic valvular diseases
    Mitral stenosis—may be useful in prognostication

FIGURE 9-1. Radionuclide angiography in clinical cardiology. Radionuclide angiography can be employed for diagnosis, prognostication, and evaluation of therapy in a variety of situations as listed here. However, other modalities may be more appropriately applied in specific clinical settings. The most appropriate situations for application of radionuclide angiography are listed, with notation as to whether radionuclide angiography may be considered a primary evaluation method or whether better alternatives clearly exist. *Italicized entities* are those for which radionuclide angiography has the greatest potential applicability in clinical practice. CAD—coronary artery disease.

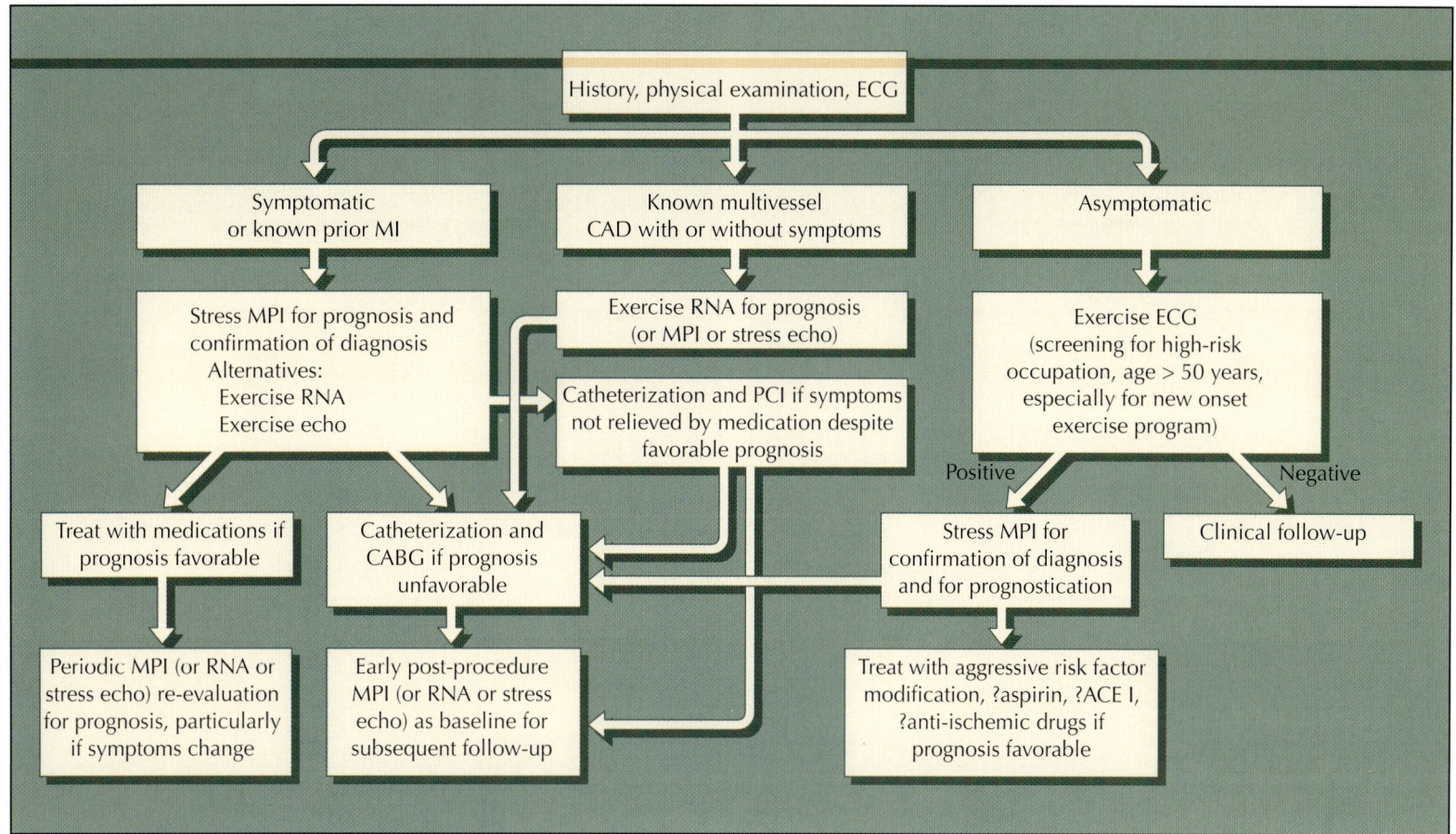

FIGURE 9-2. Role of radionuclide angiography in patients with coronary artery disease. For patients with chronic stable coronary artery disease (CAD), the primary utility of radionuclide angiography (RNA) is in prognostication for definition of management strategy. Prognosis can be defined from myocardial perfusion scintigraphy, the primary noninvasive diagnostic modality, but when the diagnosis otherwise is known (*eg*, when coronary arteriography already has been performed), right and left ventricular ejection fraction determination, at rest and during exercise, provides the most accurate prognostic information. However, the need for application of this method must be determined on a case-by-case basis if myocardial perfusion scintigraphy already has been performed or is likely to be performed. Stress echocardiography (echo) also can be used for prognostication but, because of the inferior precision of this method compared with RNA during exercise, its application for prognostication in chronic stable CAD may be less appropriate than use of RNA. CABG—coronary artery bypass grafting; MI—myocardial infarction; MPI—myocardial perfusion imaging; PCI—percutaneous coronary intervention.

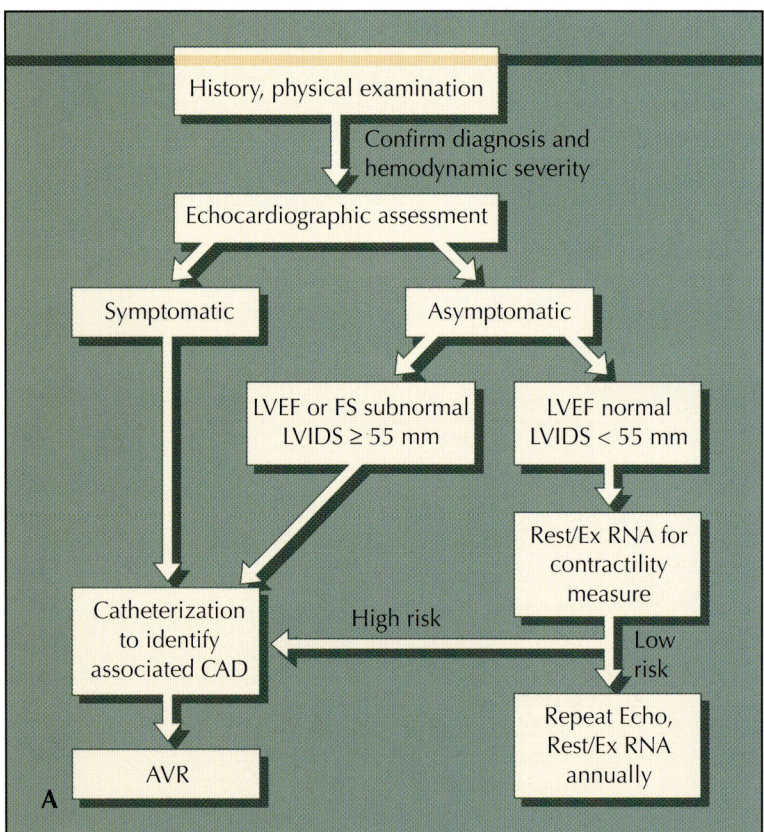 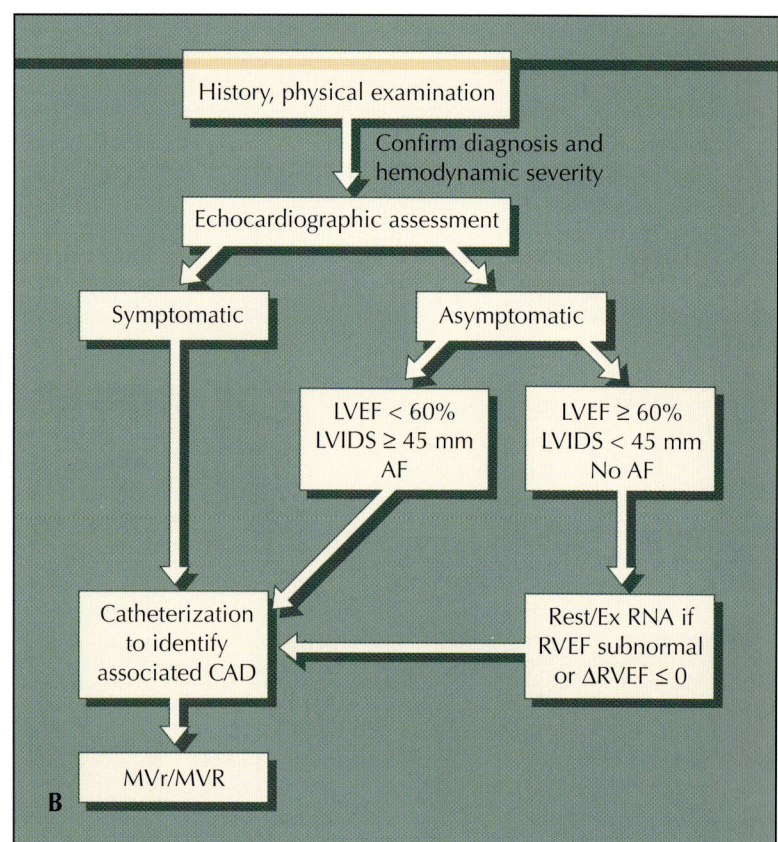

FIGURE 9-3. Role of radionuclide angiography in patients with aortic regurgitation and mitral regurgitation. For asymptomatic patients with regurgitant valvular diseases, echocardiography (echo) is a primary method for diagnosis and for determination of hemodynamic severity of disease. If echocardiography unequivocally demonstrates subnormal left ventricular ejection fraction (LVEF) at rest, or "high-risk" left ventricular systolic or diastolic dimension descriptors, management decisions can be made with confidence. However, for patients with severe aortic regurgitation (**A**), the geometric irregularity and regional functional variability of the large left ventricle can result in ambiguity of ejection fraction determination, obviated by non–geometry-dependent evaluation with radionuclide angiography (RNA); if echocardiographic results do not indicate high risk, contractility determination by additional RNA with exercise can detect prognostically important disease. **B**, For patients with mitral regurgitation, the unique capacity of RNA to interrogate right ventricular performance adds an important prognostic dimension not available with echocardiography. In patients with mitral stenosis, right ventricular ejection fraction (RVEF) determination by RNA carries prognostically important information, but these data have not yet reached routine use in defining management strategies in this setting. Echocardiography remains the primary evaluative modality for mitral stenosis. AF—atrial fibrillation; AVR—aortic valve replacement; CAD—coronary artery disease; Ex—exercise; FS—echocardiographic fractional shortening; LVIDS—left ventricular internal dimension at end systole; MVr—mitral valve repair; MVR—mitral valve replacement.

First-pass Radionuclide Angiography

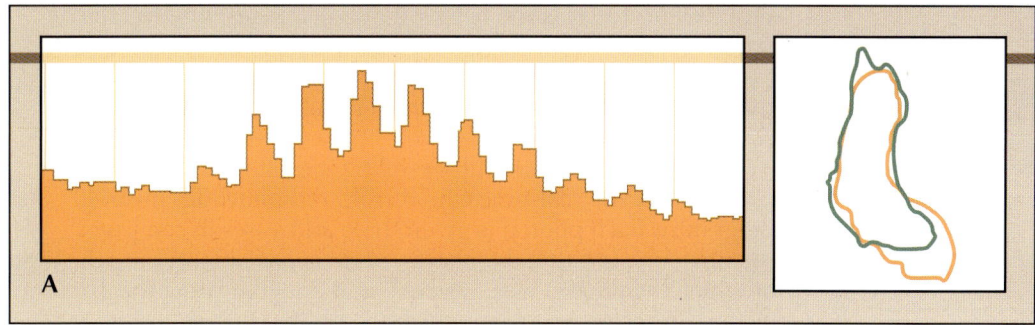

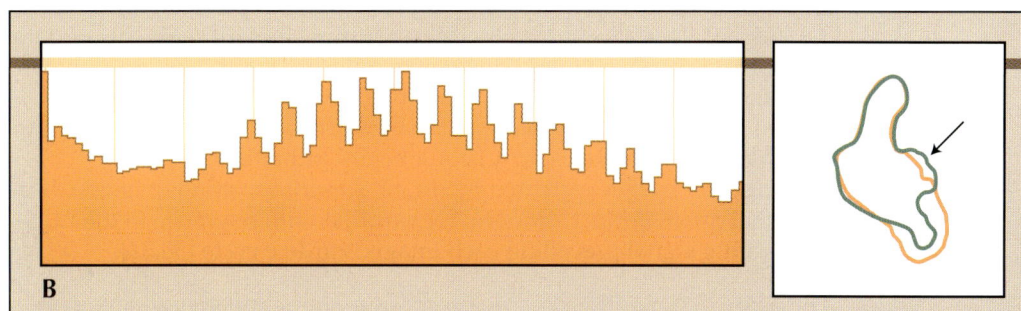

FIGURE 9-4. Left ventricle time-activity curves obtained during first-pass radionuclide angiography performed at rest. **A,** Results from a study done on a healthy patient. **B,** Results from a study done on a patient with mitral regurgitation (MR). Note that the amplitude of the time-activity curve excursion is lower in the patient with MR than in the healthy patient, though the relative volume at end diastole is similar in both studies. Thus, the left ventricular ejection fraction and stroke volume are lower in this patient with MR than in the normal subject.

The associated images reveal enlargement of the left atrium (*arrow*) in the patient with MR, a common finding in this setting. (*Adapted from* Port [3].)

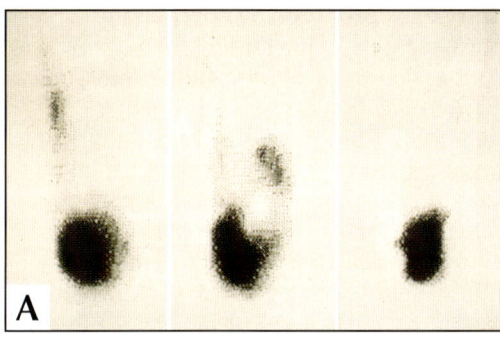

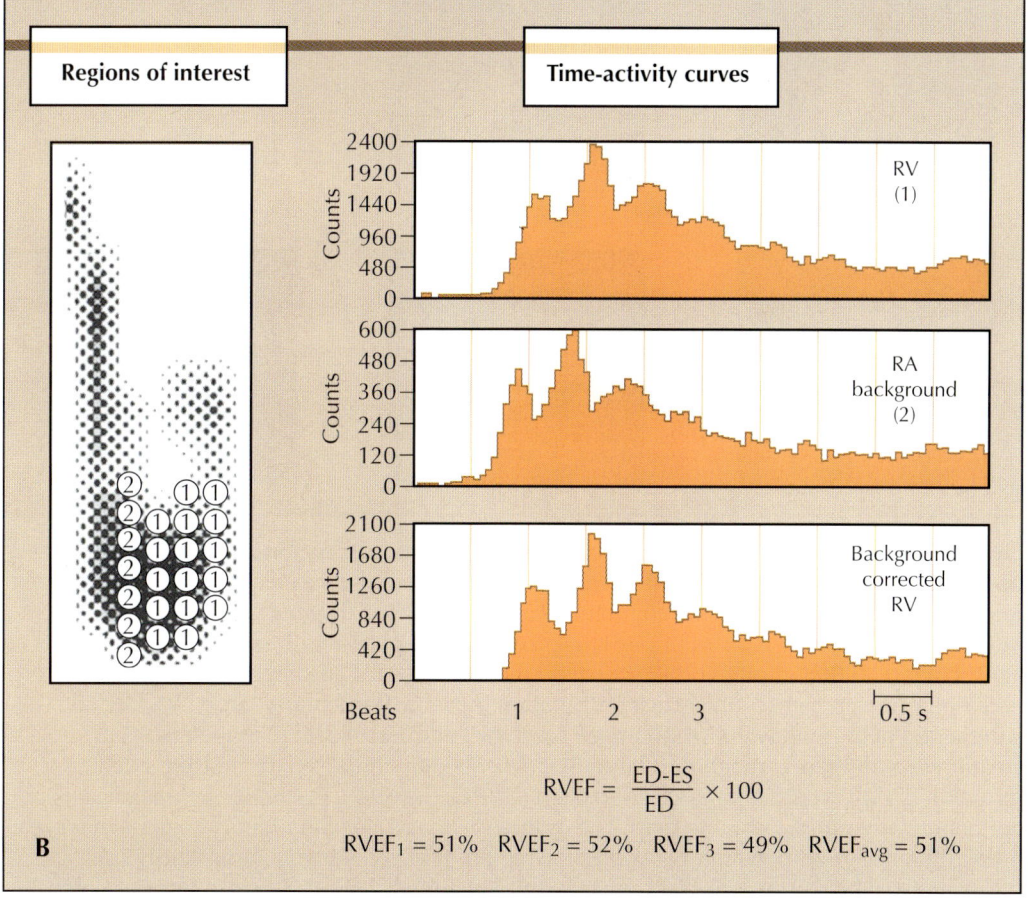

FIGURE 9-5. First-pass radionuclide angiography. **A,** Analog computer-smoothed display of right ventricular (RV) end-diastolic (ED) and end-systolic (ES) frames chosen from the right ventricular portion of the time-activity curve of a first-pass radionuclide angiogram. Single frames were computer-smoothed using a linear extrapolation algorithm. The end-systolic image (*center*) was digitally subtracted from the end-diastolic image (*left*) to create a "difference image" (*right*), used to facilitate definition of the right ventricular region of interest to be used for reanalysis of the time-activity curve for final determination of right ventricular ejection fraction.

B, Right ventricular and right atrial (RA) background regions of interest (*left*) superimposed upon a right heart image. The numeral "1" represents the right ventricular region of interest determined as in *panel A*; the numeral "2" represents the standardized background zone. Note that peak activity in the RV curve occurs when activity in the RA is lowest. The background-corrected RV time-activity curve was obtained by subtracting the RA curve from the RV curve. Peak activity in the background curve is approximately one fourth of maximal RV activity. Beat to beat calculation of right ventricular ejection fraction (RVEF) is taken from background-corrected time-activity curves in three successive cardiac cycles. RVEF is defined as counts at ED minus counts at ES divided by counts at ED, multiplied by 100. (*Panel A from* Berger *et al.* [11]; with permission; *panel B adapted from* Berger *et al.* [11].)

$$RVEF = \frac{ED-ES}{ED} \times 100$$

$RVEF_1 = 51\%$ $RVEF_2 = 52\%$ $RVEF_3 = 49\%$ $RVEF_{avg} = 51\%$

Equilibrium Radionuclide Angiography

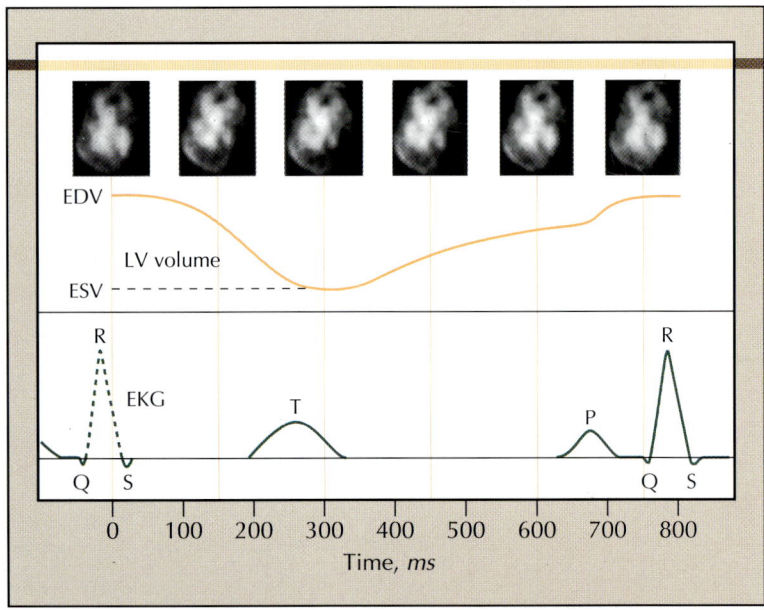

Figure 9-6. The relation between movie images, time versus volume curve, and ECG (gating signal is a portion of the QRS complex). The time versus volume curve is proportional to the time-activity curve, from which it can be derived with a simple correction.

Multiple functions are subserved by the list-mode data set collected during real-time equilibrium radionuclide cineangiography. Each photon is given three addresses in computer memory, one locating the photon in space, one identifying the time at which the photon was detected, and one indicating the duration of the cardiac cycle during which the photon was collected. In addition, the computer also stores the time of the last gating signal. This allows for precise superimposition of segments of data collected during intervals timed similarly after the gating signal in successive cardiac cycles, resulting in production of an endless loop movie display of the composite cardiac cycle [7]. The "picture file" (movie images) in an equilibrium radionuclide cineangiogram is created by digital superimposition of image data that are in perfect temporal registration with reference to the ECG gating signal preceding each imaged cardiac cycle [30,31].

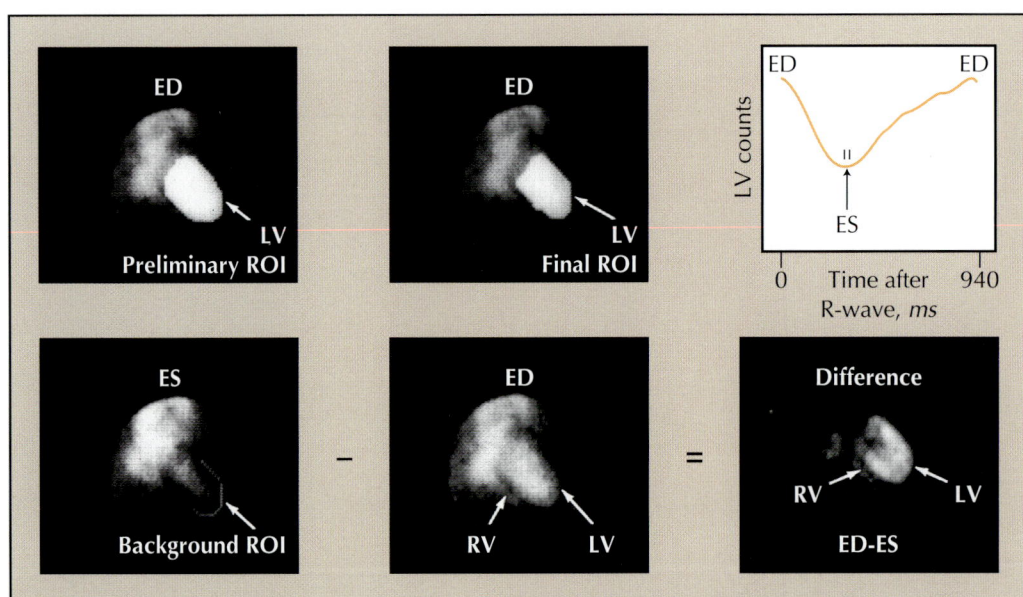

Figure 9-7. Selection of a preliminary and final left ventricular region of interest and background region of interest for definition of a "background-corrected" time-activity curve from which left ventricular ejection fraction can be calculated. The background region of interest (ROI) typically is a rim of pixels approximately 1 pixel-width outside the left ventricular (LV) ROI, though other schemes have been used. The images displayed here were obtained from a patient with aortic regurgitation (note the particularly large LV). Digital subtraction of the end-systolic (ES) image from the end-diastolic (ED) image results in creation of a difference image, similar to that described in Figure 9-5 for first-pass determination of right ventricular ejection fraction (RVEF); the difference image actually is a regional relative stroke volume map. The difference image also can identify regions in which little difference exists between ED and ES, *ie*, regions that are akinetic or markedly hypokinetic, which appear as black areas within the initial LV ROI. This can be very helpful in identifying regional dysfunction from equilibrium radionuclide angiograms, particularly when the regional dysfunction does not affect the edges of the image in the typical 2-D display. Variations on difference images, *eg*, regional EF maps, regional filling rate maps, also can be produced by appropriate normalization of the difference image. Automated edge detection algorithms, based on identification of predetermined reductions from maximum image count density, have been developed, based on "functional images" analogous to the difference image. The automated methods allow rapid creation of LV ROIs for each frame within the movie of the composite cardiac cycle. EF is calculated from equilibrium data as (ED counts minus ES counts)/(ED counts minus background counts). However, for accurate count-based calculation of left ventricular ejection fraction or RVEF, it is necessary to minimize or avoid overlap between LV and RV and between atria and ventricles. This requirement can be achieved only when the camera is oriented in the left anterior oblique (LAO) position. Isolation of the RV cannot be obtained throughout the cardiac cycle when equilibrium methodology is employed. However, isolation can be reasonably approximated in the LAO view at ED and at ES (*see* Fig. 9-9). The LAO view also is useful for assessment of regional LV function (*see* Fig. 9-10). Statistically valid data can be collected within 30 to 45 seconds. (*From* Green *et al.* [31]; with permission.)

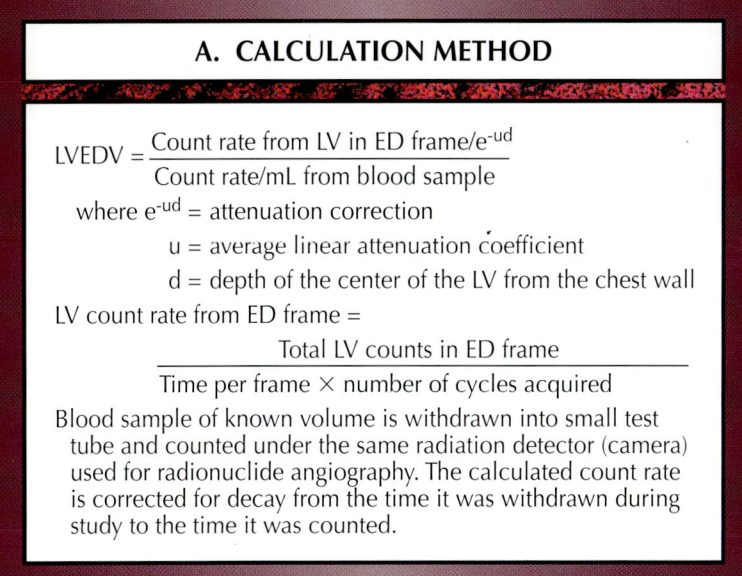
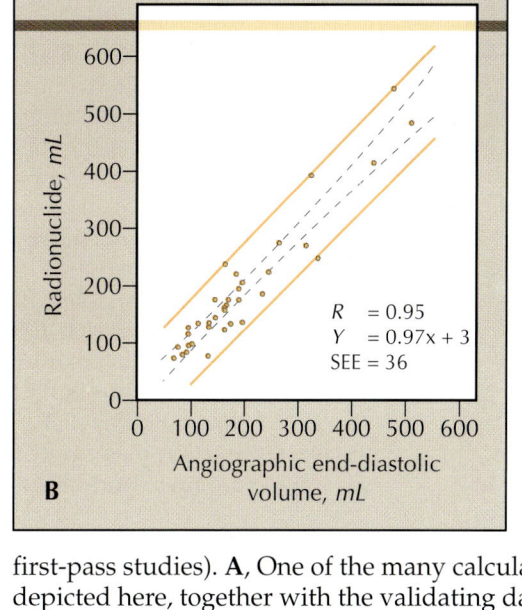

FIGURE 9-8. Calculation of left ventricular end-diastolic volume from equilibrium radionuclide angiograms. When corrected for duration of data collection (*ie*, number of beats collected and frame duration), administered dose and plasma volume, absolute left ventricular (LV) volume can be calculated with relatively high precision from equilibrium radionuclide angiograms (and from first-pass studies). **A**, One of the many calculation methods is depicted here, together with the validating data comparing volumes obtained by equilibrium radionuclide angiography and by contrast angiography at catheterization (**B**). ED—end diastolic; LVEDV—left ventricular end-diastolic volume. (*Adapted from* Links *et al.* [32].)

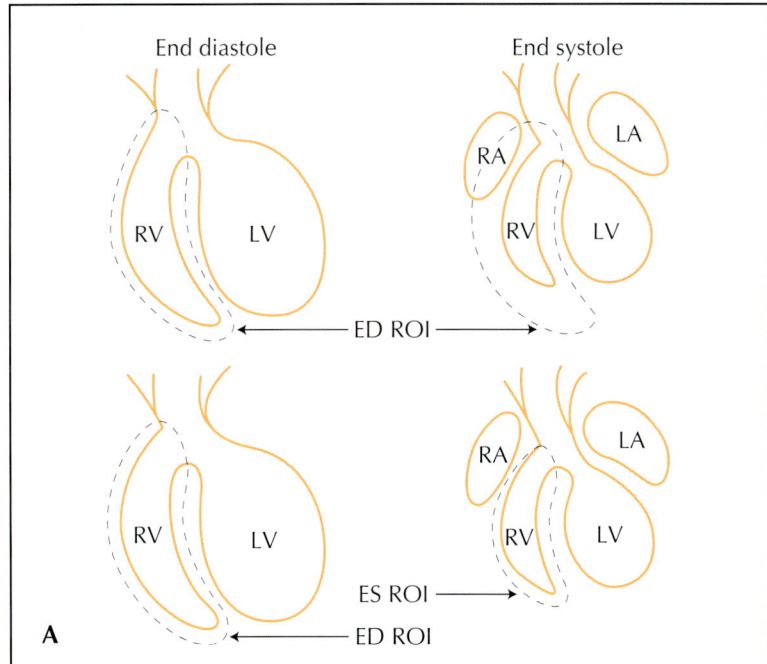
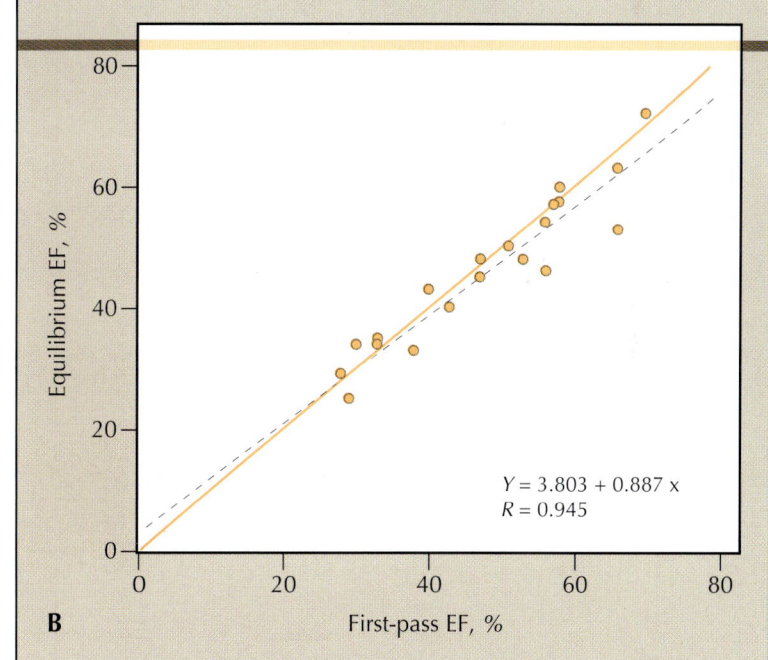

FIGURE 9-9. Right ventricular ejection fraction from equilibrium radionuclide angiograms. The current standard for right ventricular ejection fraction (RVEF) measurement is first-pass radionuclide angiography (*see* Fig. 9-5), although MRI also enables accurate RVEF measurement. However, equilibrium radionuclide angiography also permits accurate RVEF determination. The method is illustrated here, and involves separate identification of end-diastolic (ED) and end-systolic (ES) right ventricular (RV) regions of interest (ROIs). Although RV overlap with the right atrium cannot be avoided completely, the right atrium is posterior to the RV and is almost empty at end diastole; therefore, its contribution to counts from the RV ROI is minimal at end diastole. At end systole, isolation of the RV from the right atrium can be achieved with reasonable accuracy, minimizing the right atrial contribution to counts in the RV ROI at end systole. When carefully performed, RVEF by the equilibrium method correlates well with that obtained by the first-pass approach and with determinations by contrast angiography [13]. **A**, The construction of ROIs for RVEF determination from equilibrium radionuclide angiograms; **B**, the close correlation between RVEF calculated from equilibrium and first-pass studies in the same patients. LA—left atrium; RA—right atrium. (*Adapted from* Maddahi [12].)

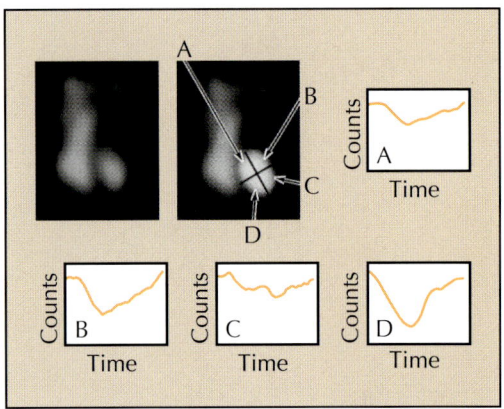

FIGURE 9-10. Determination of regional left ventricular ejection fraction from an equilibrium radionuclide angiogram. Because background is relatively small around the left ventricle (LV) during first-pass studies, this approach is particularly effective in isolating specific regions of the LV for evaluation. It even is possible to isolate regions of distribution of specific coronary arteries, facilitating management decisions. However, only a limited amount of isotope can be administered during a single imaging session; therefore, optimally, the region to be isolated must be known before imaging begins, a requirement that often cannot be achieved. Regional LV assessment by equilibrium methodology is inherently limited because the LV can be isolated only in the left anterior oblique (LAO) position; in this orientation, the specific territories of distribution of the left anterior descending coronary artery overlaps with or is superimposed on the region of distribution of the right coronary artery. Although the left circumflex distribution is reasonably isolated in the LAO view, even this territory may be superimposed on that of the right coronary distribution. Nonetheless, division of the LV into regions can be useful for quantitative evaluation of therapeutic interventions. This figure depicts a system used by the author in which the LV is divided into four regions; time-activity curves are presented for each region. It is clear that the inferolateral region manifests a lower ejection fraction than the other regions (and, in fact, far lower than ejection fractions found for this region in normal subjects).

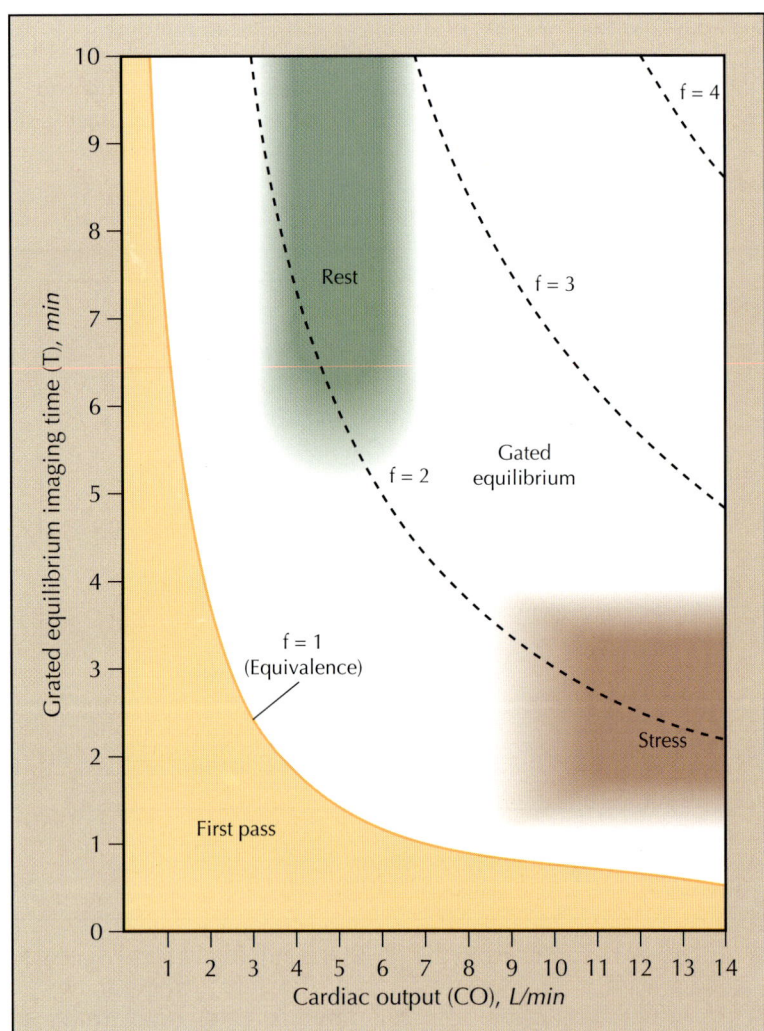

FIGURE 9-11. Relative advantages of first-pass and equilibrium radionuclide angiography. First-pass and equilibrium radionuclide angiography (RNA) share many of the same advantages, including lack of dependence on geometric formulas for determination of chamber volumes (enabling accurate assessment of geometrically irregular cardiac chambers such as the right ventricle, or the left ventricle [LV] in a variety of disease states), and applicability during exercise. Each method also has advantages and disadvantages relative to the other. One of the relative advantages of first-pass RNA is the rapidity of collection (seconds), allowing determinations truly at peak exercise, as compared with the equilibrium approach, which requires at least 30 seconds for a statistically reliable collection and 2 minutes or longer for a high-quality image series. However, if the same radiation detector and isotope are employed for each method, it can be shown that the precision of volume determination (measured as the standard deviation of the net end-diastolic LV counts, where smaller standard deviation indicates greater precision) is greater with the equilibrium method after only 30 seconds of data collection, and that this advantage increases with increasing duration of data collection. The curve $f = 1$ indicates the series of T,CO points for which the standard deviations of the net end-diastolic counts are equal for first-pass and equilibrium studies. This curve divides the T,CO plane into two regions: for points above and to the right of the curve, $f >1$, *ie*, the standard deviation is lower for equilibrium studies than for first-pass and, thus, equilibrium results are more precise; for points below and to the left of the curve, $f <1$, *ie*, the standard deviation is lower for first-pass determinations. The shaded areas indicate portions of the plane typically represented in rest and stress studies. (*Adapted from* Green *et al.* [33].)

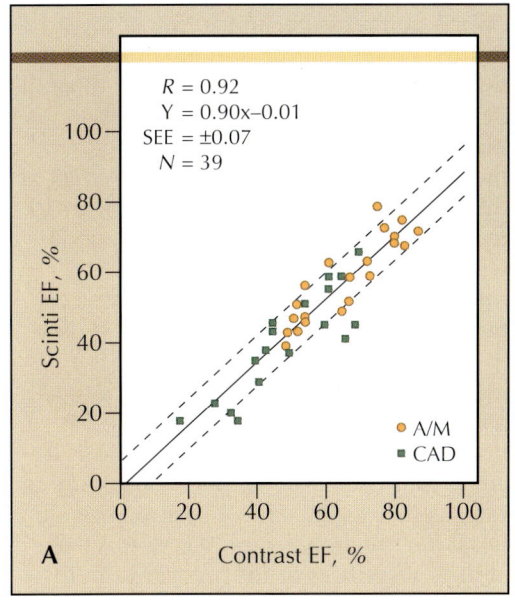
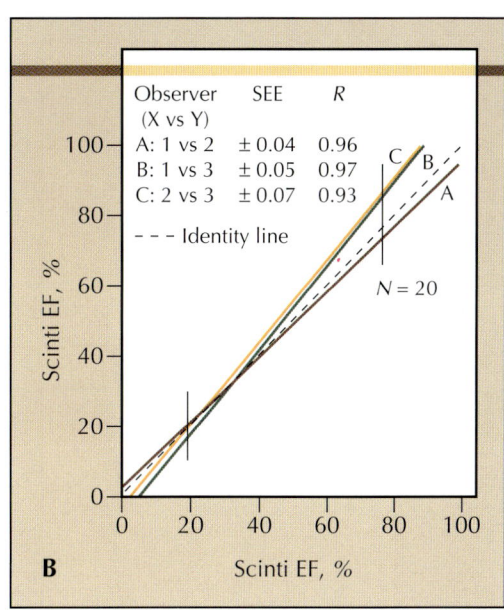
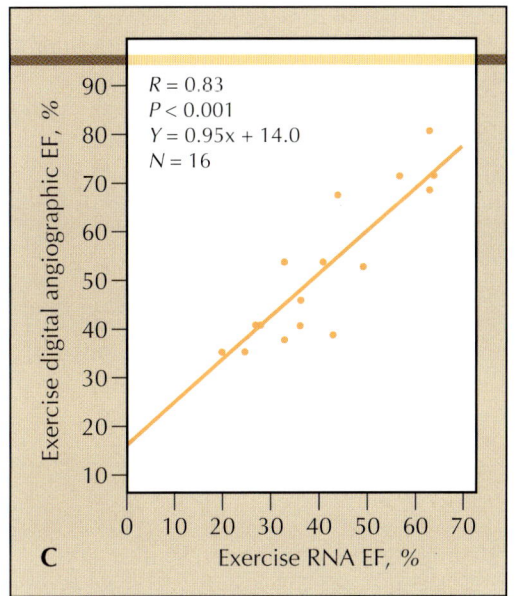
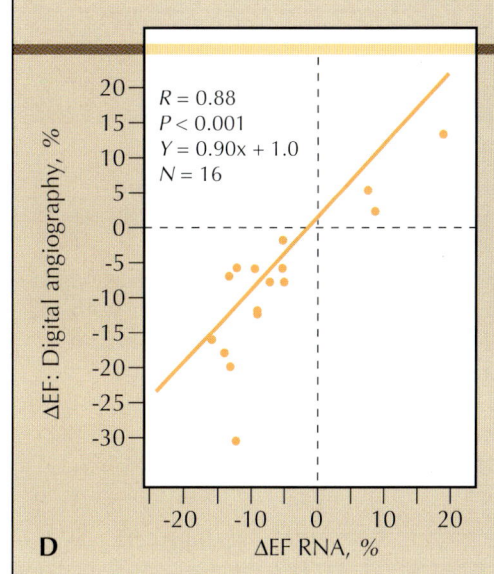

FIGURE 9-12. Accuracy of left ventricular ejection fraction determination from equilibrium radionuclide angiography. Radionuclide angiography (RNA) enables calculation of left ventricular ejection fraction (LVEF), which accurately reproduces the values available by the traditional standard method, contrast angiography at catheterization. From an early study using equilibrium angiography at rest, both the accuracy in reproducing the results of contrast angiography, **A**, and the interobserver reproducibility, **B**, are apparent [34].

C, RNA also is accurate in reproducing the results of LVEF determined from contrast angiography performed during maximal supine bicycle exercise. In this study, contrast was administered intravenously and digital subtraction angiography was performed, utilizing a protocol analogous to that employed during first-pass RNA [35].

D, One of the most powerful parameters available from RNA is a measure of the functional severity of a variety of cardiac diseases, expressed as the change in LVEF from rest to exercise. This measure accurately reproduces the same parameter assessed by digital subtraction angiography performed after intravenous administration of contrast medium [35]. (*Panels A and B adapted from* Green *et al.* [34]; *panels C and D adapted from* Goldberg *et al.* [35].)

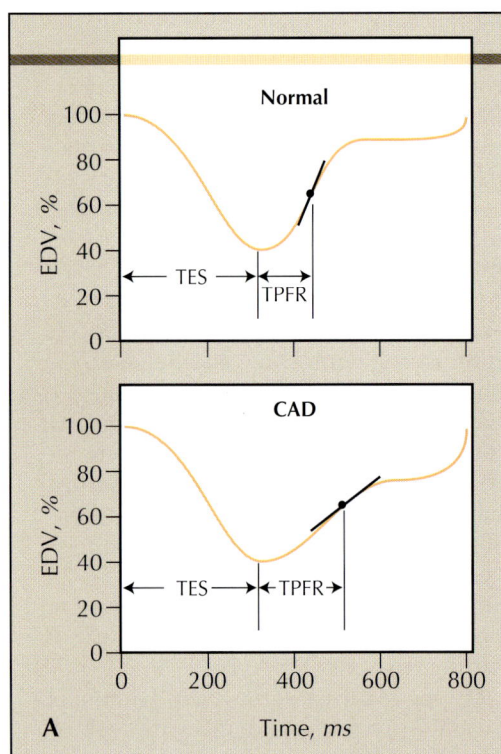
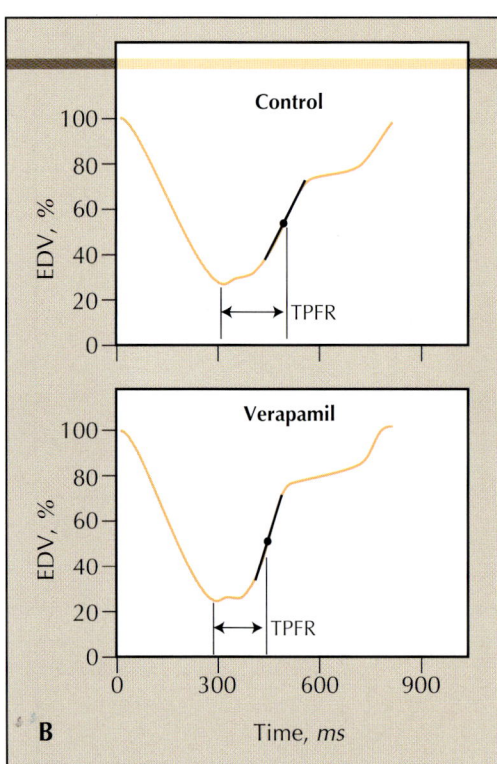

FIGURE 9-13. Measurement of left ventricular diastolic function with equilibrium radionuclide angiography. When equilibrium radionuclide angiographic data are collected in list mode (*see* Fig. 9-8), it is possible to superimpose corresponding frames from successive cardiac cycles beginning from end diastole moving not only forward through systole but also backward through diastole. The utility of this approach is based on the capacity for very fine temporal resolution afforded by list mode, together with the statistical reliability of the high-count density information available from equilibrium collections. These advantages generally are not available from first-pass studies. "Backward framing" potentially is useful in defining diastolic function because variation of diastolic landmarks with heart rate changes is substantially greater than the variation of systolic landmarks; thus, relatively small heart rate variations, such as those encountered during a typical 3-minute data collection, might affect the timing of diastolic events, so that superimposition of forward-framed cycles could result in temporal misregistration sufficient to distort diastolic events and indices while having little impact on systolic phase descriptors. Backward framing can obviate the effect of these variations by bringing diastole into more accurate registration than is possible with forward framing. To optimize information content from both phases of the cardiac cycle, forward framing is used to define the time-activity curve of the initial two thirds of the cardiac cycle, and backward framing is used to define the final third, the portion of the time-activity curve that usually includes the peak filling rate, as well as diastasis and atrial systole. Diastolic function typically is one of the earliest responses of the myocardium to ischemia. Peak filling rate typically is subnormal and time to peak filling rate (TPFR) is prolonged in patients with hemodynamically important coronary artery disease (CAD). **A,** The difference in diastolic phase indices at rest between a healthy patient and a patient with CAD is illustrated. **B,** Normalization of these indices is effected by the anti-ischemic anti-anginal drug, verapamil. Assessment of diastolic function by equilibrium radionuclide angiography is useful both in diagnosis of CAD and in evaluation of effects of therapy. EDV—end-diastolic volume. (*Adapted from* Bonow *et al.* [16,36].)

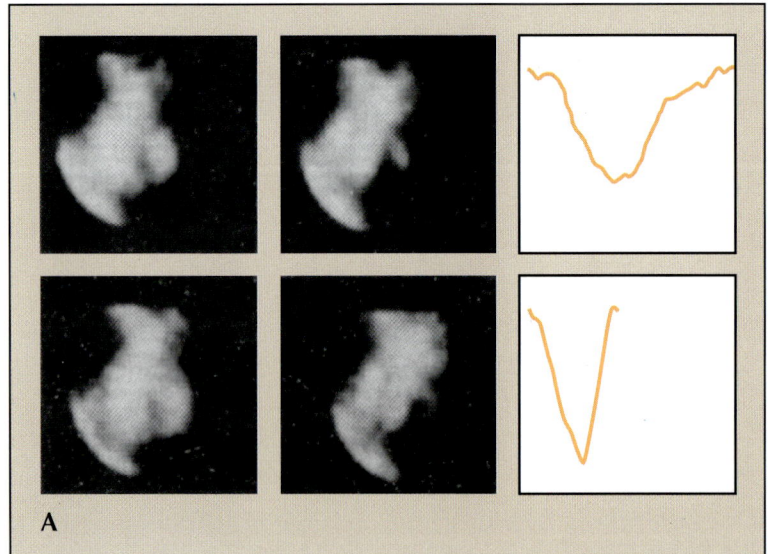

FIGURE 9-14. Radionuclide angiography in the recognition and assessment of severity of ischemic heart disease due to coronary artery obstruction. **A,** Unretouched selected frames in sequence from a radionuclide cineangiogram taken in a healthy patient at rest (*top row*) and during maximal exercise (*bottom row*). End-diastolic images are in the column at *left*, and end-systolic images are to the *right*. Left ventricular emptying is more complete during exercise than at rest.   *Continued on next page*

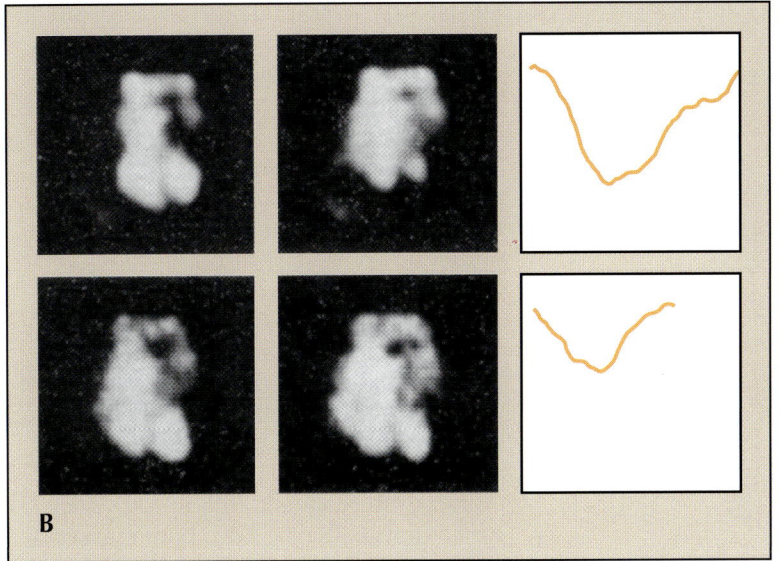

FIGURE 9-14. *(Continued)* **B,** Unretouched selected frames in sequence from a radionuclide angiogram taken in a patient with three-vessel coronary artery disease (CAD) at rest (*top row*) and during maximal exercise (*bottom row*). End-diastolic images are in the column at *left*, and end-systolic images are to the *right*. Emptying is obviously less complete during exercise than at rest (*ie*, left ventricular ejection fraction [LVEF] falls from rest to exercise). From the angiographic display and the difference image not shown here (*see* Fig. 9-8), regional dysfunction could be identified, strongly suggesting that CAD is the basis of exercise-induced dysfunction. These images exemplify the potential utility of radionuclide angiography for evaluation of CAD.

Time-activity curves from the four radionuclide cineangiograms quantify the increase in LVEF from rest to exercise in the healthy patient (61% at rest to 82% during exercise) and the fall from rest to exercise in the patient with CAD (62% at rest to 35% during exercise). (*From* Borer *et al*. [5]; with permission.)

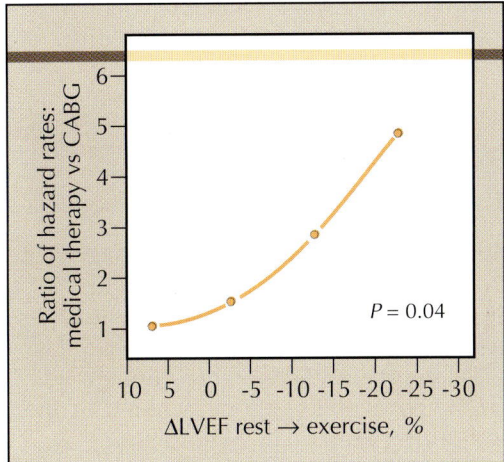

FIGURE 9-15. Equilibrium radionuclide angiography as a prognostic tool in patients with coronary artery disease. Although radionuclide angiography is useful in the diagnosis of coronary artery disease (CAD), its use for this purpose has been limited by the relative lack of disease specificity of changes in left ventricular ejection fraction (LVEF). However, in patients with known CAD, left ventricular function measurement is the most accurate basis for prognostication. Among patients with well-preserved LVEF at rest (*ie*, patients without prior massive myocardial infarction, with LVEF above 30% at rest), the most accurate index of prognosis is the change in LVEF from rest to exercise. This figure depicts the relationship between change in LVEF from rest to exercise and the relative benefit of medical therapy alone versus medical therapy plus coronary artery bypass grafting (CABG) among patients with angiographically defined three-vessel CAD who were followed for 5 years after the index radionuclide study and initiation of therapy. The study from which these data were derived was designed to provide information for clinical decision-making. Thus, prognostic data are most useful for supporting therapeutic decisions when outcome is defined as a function of test results obtained immediately before competing management strategies; the relative benefits of one or the other strategy then also can be defined as a function of the pretreatment test result. This figure indicates that when patients with three-vessel CAD have little or no ischemia (ΔLVEF 0 or more), CABG offers little or no benefit as compared with medical therapy alone (hazard ratio ≈ 1); when severe ischemia is present at index study (ΔLVEF 10% or higher), CABG is associated with significant event-reduction over 5 years (hazard ratio 2 to 5, increasing as ischemia at index study increases). (*Adapted from* Supino *et al*. [14].)

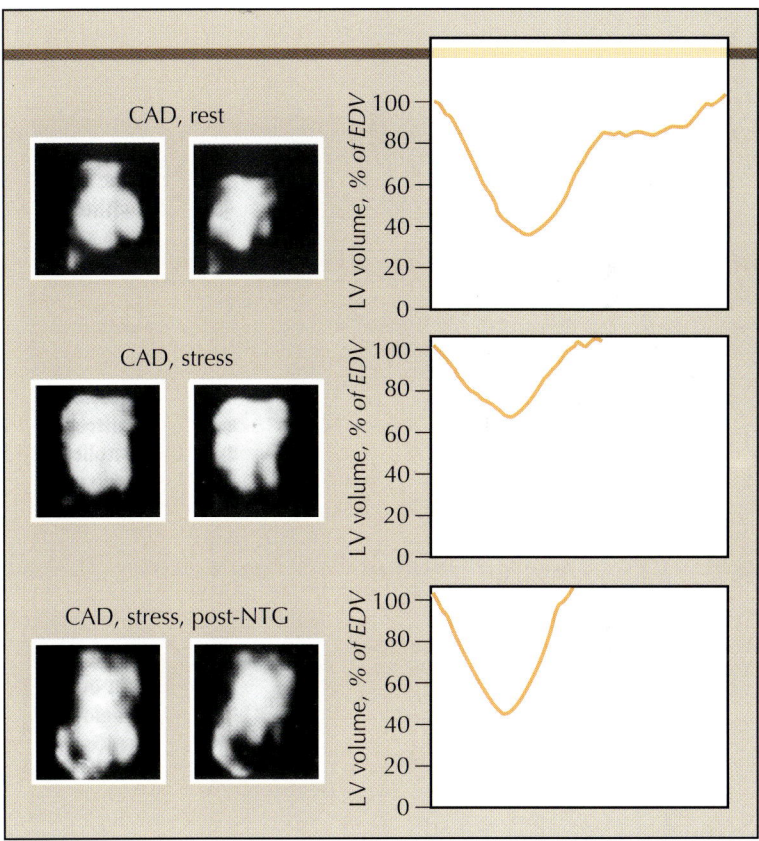

FIGURE 9-16. Radionuclide angiography in the assessment of drug therapy. Radionuclide angiography can be useful in evaluating the effects of therapy on the functional severity of ischemia. Figure 9-14 demonstrated this capacity with reference to global diastolic function. It is far more common to assess drug effects on systolic function. As illustrated here in a patient with coronary artery disease (CAD) and normal left ventricular (LV) function at rest (*top row*), ischemic dysfunction induced by exercise (*center row*) is mitigated by treatment with nitroglycerin (NTG) prior to subsequent exercise (*bottom row*). End-diastolic images are in the column at *left*, and end-systolic images are in the *center*. The study from which these figures were taken demonstrated that this phenomenon is seen in most if not all patients with CAD. The time-activity curves associated with the image series provide quantitative corroboration of the magnitude of the effect of the drug in preventing exercise-induced ischemia. EDV—end-diastolic volume. (*From* Borer *et al*. [15]; with permission.)

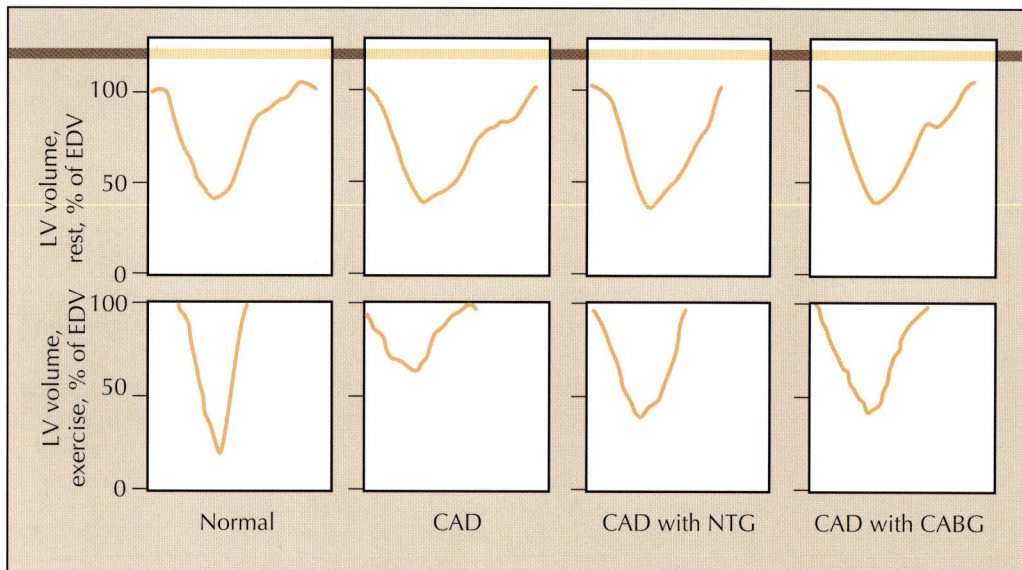

Figure 9-17. Radionuclide angiography in assessment of anti-ischemic therapy. A more extensive depiction of the utility of radionuclide angiography in evaluating the effect of therapy for coronary artery disease (CAD) is seen here, in the data from a single patient with CAD who underwent treatment with nitroglycerin (NTG) before undergoing coronary artery bypass grafting (CABG). As compared with the healthy patient (*left*), the patient's left ventricular ejection fraction (LVEF) was indistinguishable at rest; this normal value was little affected by nitroglycerin or CABG. However, during exercise, the patient was markedly subnormal prior to therapy. Pretreatment with nitroglycerin, as well as subsequent CABG, both markedly improved LVEF during exercise, bringing this value into the normal range [5,15,17]. EDV—end-diastolic volume. (*Adapted from* Borer *et al*. [5].)

VALVULAR HEART DISEASE

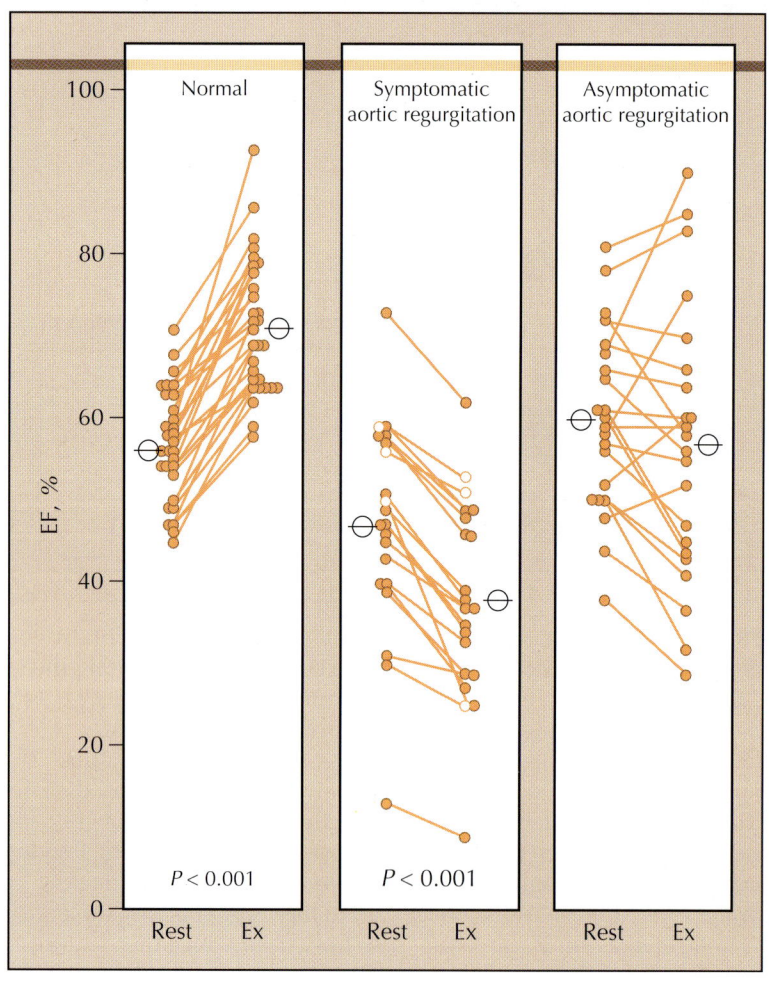

Figure 9-18. Radionuclide angiography in patients with aortic regurgitation. In 1978, the observations depicted in this figure in patients with aortic regurgitation demonstrated that radionuclide angiography could be used during exercise (Ex) to unmask myocardial dysfunction due to processes other than coronary artery disease. Although left ventricular ejection fraction (EF) often was subnormal at rest and during exercise in symptomatic patients, the appearance of exercise-induced left ventricular dysfunction in patients who were asymptomatic and had normal LVEF at rest suggested a potential role for exercise radionuclide angiography in prognostication among patients with aortic regurgitation. (*Adapted from* Borer *et al*. [37].)

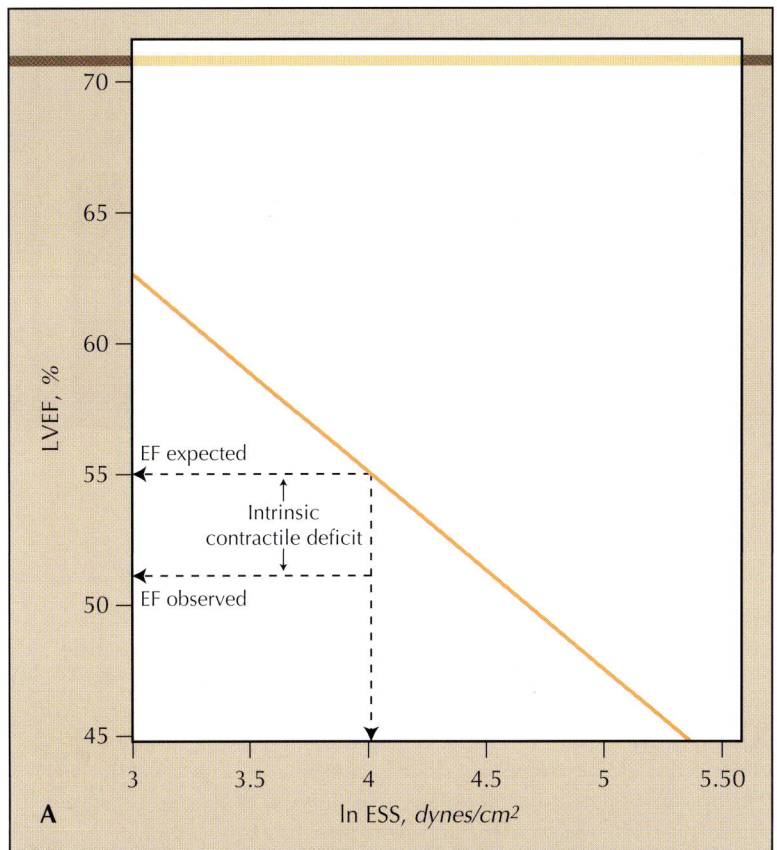
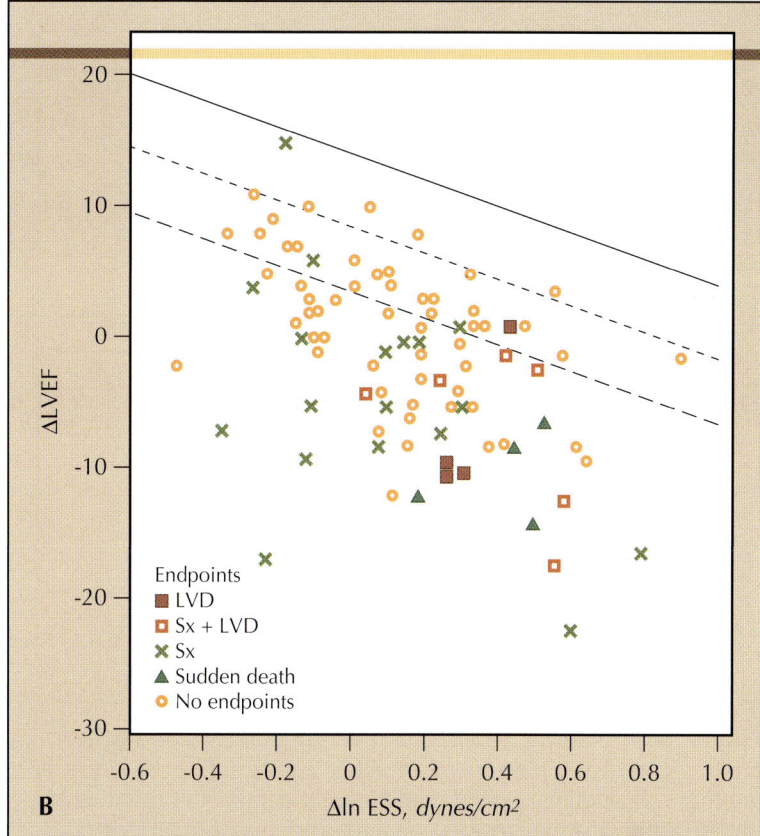
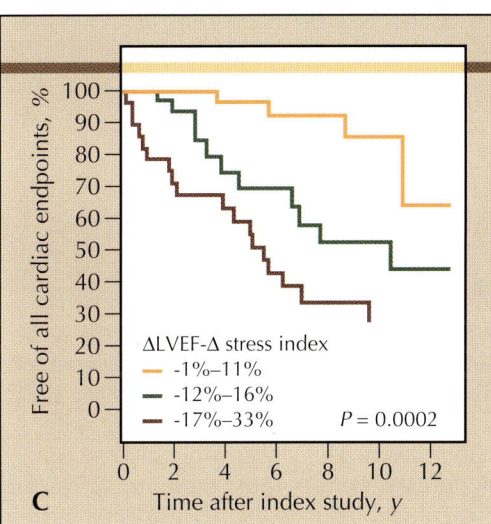

FIGURE 9-19. Prognostication in aortic regurgitation using radionuclide angiography. The prognostic value of radionuclide angiographic ΔLVEF (left ventricular ejection fraction) from rest to exercise ultimately was borne out in several studies. However, a more powerful approach to prognostication in this disease can be achieved by adjusting ΔLVEF for the change in LV wall stress from rest to exercise by combining echocardiographic and radionuclide angiographic data. The resulting index of intrinsic myocardial contractility is particularly valuable in prognostication, as seen in *panel C* and Figure 9-20.

A, The solid line indicates the relationship between end-systolic wall stress (ESS, a measure of LV afterload) and LVEF in normal subjects. From this relationship, for any given ESS, the LVEF expected in a normal subject can be determined (*eg*, for ln ESS = 4, LVEF normally is 55%). If the LVEF actually observed in a patient differs from that expected, the difference is an index of the "contractility excess" if the value is higher than expected, and of the "contractility deficit" if the value is lower than expected. **B**, A similar relationship was constructed for ΔLVEF and ΔESS for normal subjects, and is represented by the solid line; the dashed lines represent 1 and 2 standard deviations below the average relation. Superimposed on these normal standards are the actual values obtained at entry into a study of natural history of severe aortic regurgitation and its predictors in patients with normal LVEF at rest and either no symptoms (the great majority) or minimal symptoms that were not clearly attributable to cardiac causes. Data points are coded for outcome events during multiyear follow-up while patients remained free of aortic valve replacement surgery.

C, When the patients in Figure 9-3 were followed for up to 15 years after study entry (and were censored if aortic valve replacement was performed), outcome events occurred at an average rate of 6.2% per year. However, when the study population was divided arbitrarily into terciles based on the contractility descriptor, progression rate in the third with the poorest contractility was approximately 15% per year, almost tenfold greater than the rate in the third with the best preserved contractility at study entry. Moreover, sudden death occurred only among those with markedly compromised contractility. LVD—left ventricular dysfunction; Sx—symptoms. (*Adapted from* Borer *et al.* [19].)

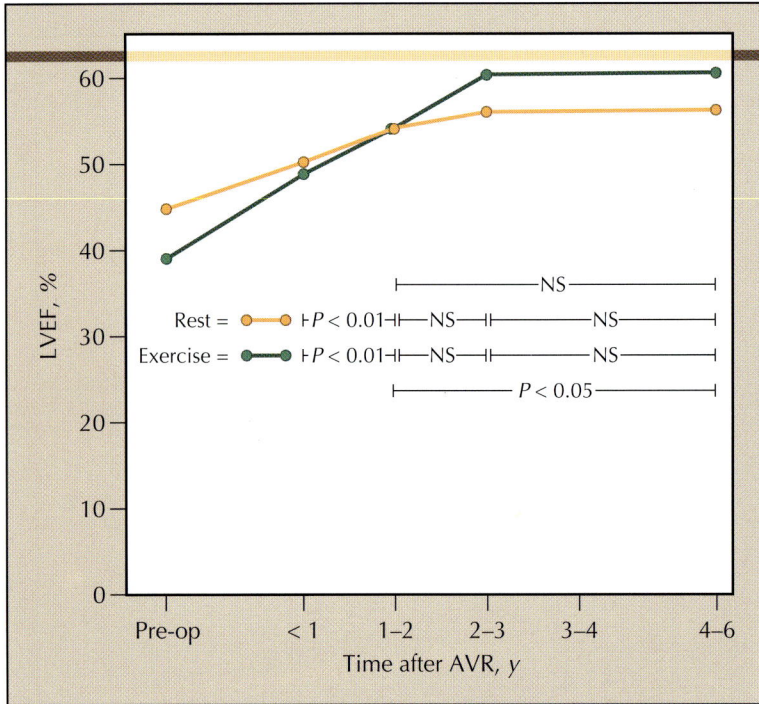

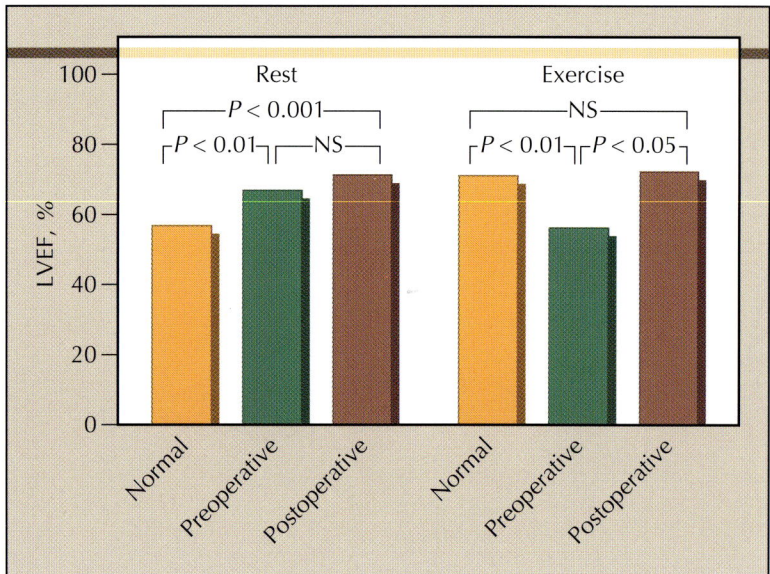

FIGURE 9-20. Natural history of left ventricular ejection fraction after aortic valve replacement for aortic regurgitation. Radionuclide angiography can be applied to evaluate the impact of treatment in patients with aortic regurgitation and other noncoronary diseases. The natural history of recovery of left ventricular function after aortic valve replacement (AVR) is illustrated in this figure. Importantly, maximal recovery required 3 years, by which time average left ventricular ejection fraction (LVEF) values at rest and during exercise had returned to within the normal range. The duration of the LV remodeling process suggests the involvement of multiple cellular and molecular changes, at least some with particularly prolonged kinetic constants. NS—not significant; Pre-op—preoperative. (*Adapted from* Borer *et al.* [38].)

FIGURE 9-21. Natural history of left ventricular ejection fraction after aortic valve replacement for aortic stenosis. Radionuclide angiography also has defined the effect of aortic valve replacement among patients with aortic stenosis. For this group of 26 symptomatic patients with severe aortic stenosis, average left ventricular ejection fraction (LVEF) at rest was supernormal (preoperative) and remained so after valve replacement (postoperative). However, LVEF fell from rest to exercise before operation; this deficit disappeared after surgical removal of the abnormal impedence to LV outflow. NS—not significant. (*Adapted from* Borer *et al.* [26].)

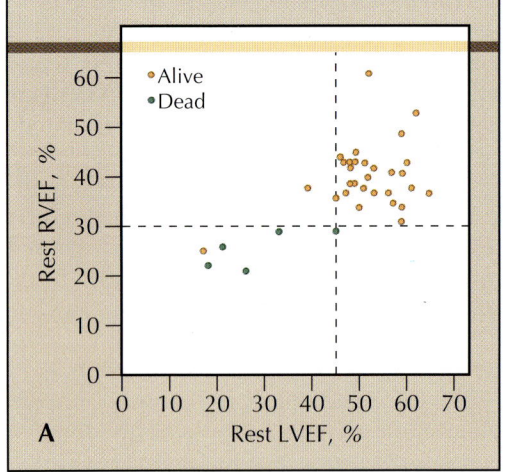

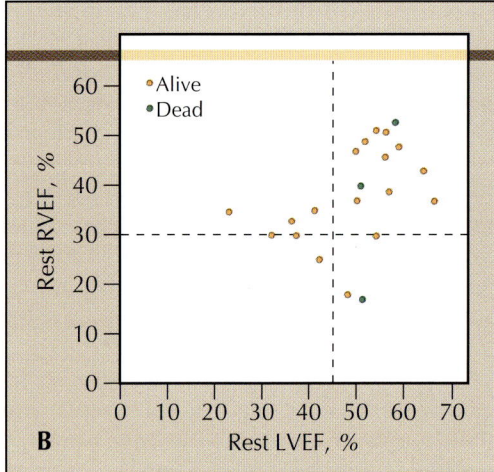

FIGURE 9-22. Prognostication in patients with mitral regurgitation. In patients with severe mitral regurgitation, shock organs include both the left ventricle and the right ventricle. Functional assessment of both ventricles carries prognostic information not only for unoperated patients, **A**, but for patients who subsequently undergo mitral valve surgery, **B**. *Continued on next page*

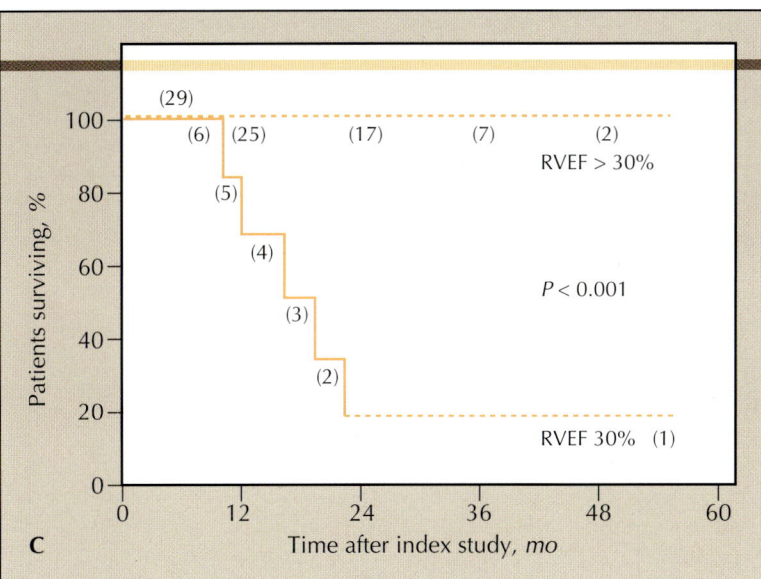

FIGURE 9-22. *(Continued)* **C,** When right ventricular ejection fraction (RVEF) is less than 30% at rest by equilibrium radionuclide angiography (lower limit of normal = 35%), survival is particularly compromised. This is true even if left ventricular ejection fraction (LVEF) is well preserved. (*Adapted from* Hochreiter *et al.* [24].)

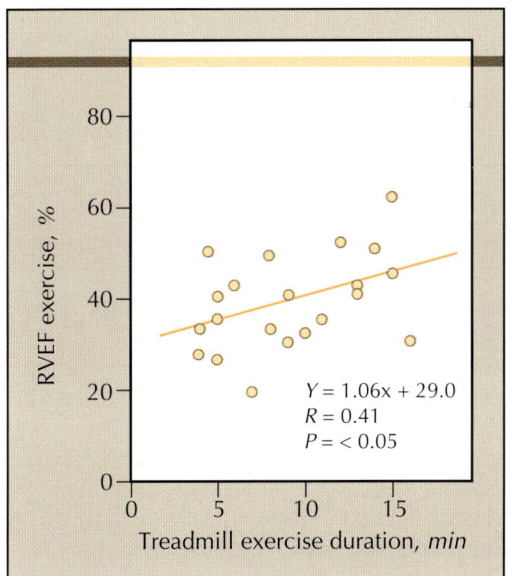

FIGURE 9-23. Exercise tolerance in patients with severe mitral regurgitation as a function of right ventricular ejection fraction (RVEF) during exercise by equilibrium radionuclide angiography [24]. Although there was very modest but significant relation of exercise tolerance and left ventricular ejection fraction exercise, a far stronger and significant relation was apparent when RVEF exercise was evaluated. This relationship derives from the impact of pulmonary artery pressure both on RVEF and on pulmonary vascular congestion/dyspnea on exertion. NS—not significant. (*Adapted from* Borer *et al.* [22].)

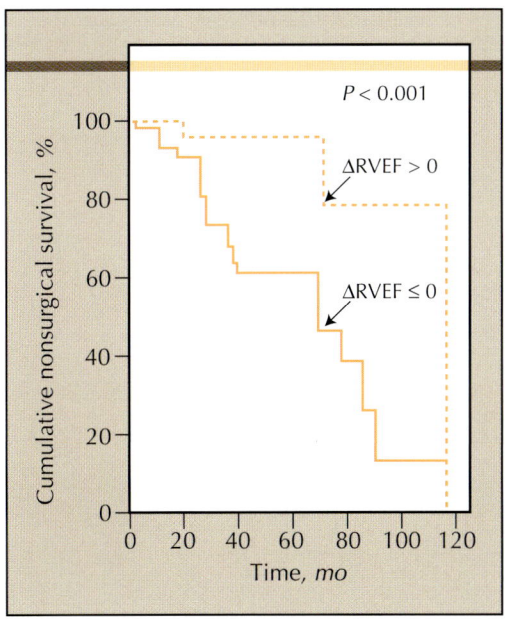

FIGURE 9-24. Prognostication in asymptomatic/minimally symptomatic patients with mitral regurgitation and normal left and right ventricular ejection fractions at rest. The importance of right ventricular functional reserve in patients with severe mitral regurgitation is illustrated in this figure, constructed with data from patients with no symptoms (the majority) or minimal symptoms not clearly of cardiac origin who were entered into a study of the natural history of mitral regurgitation and its predictors. Although all patients had normal left ventricular ejection fraction and right ventricular ejection fraction (RVEF) at rest, those who manifested an increase in RVEF from rest to exercise had a fourfold slower rate of progression to overt heart failure than those who did not. (*Adapted from* Rosen *et al.* [23].)

CARDIOMYOPATHIC DISORDERS

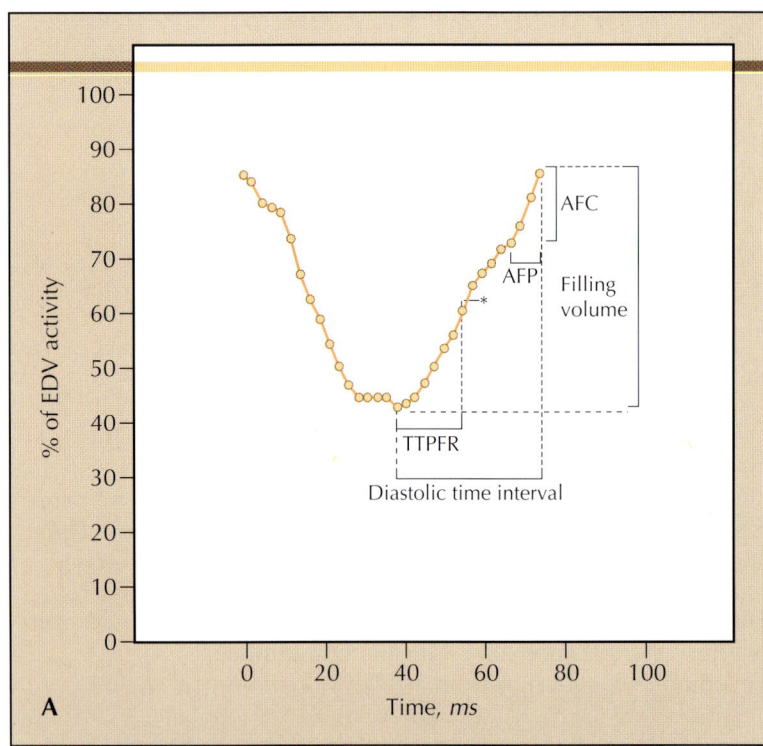 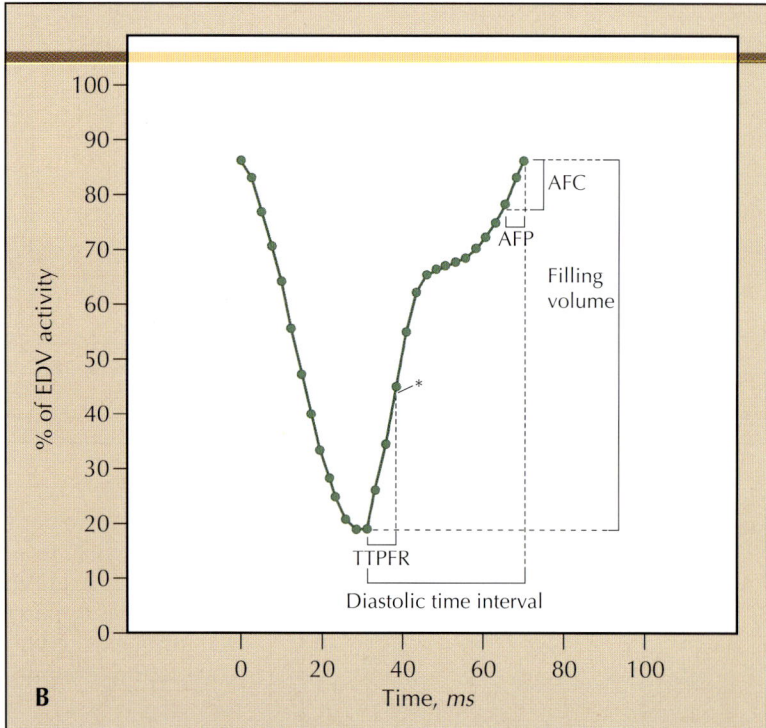

FIGURE 9-25. Distinction between restrictive and constrictive processes using radionuclide angiography. The diastolic portion of the time-activity curve can be employed to assess the pathophysiology and functional impact of various forms of cardiomyopathy. Here, diastolic phase analysis of first-pass radionuclide angiograms has been used to differentiate between **A**, restrictive cardiomyopathy and **B**, pericardial constriction. As compared with restrictive cardiomyopathy, pericardial constriction features very short time to peak left ventricular (LV) filling rate (TTPFR), more rapid peak filling rate (*asterisk*), smaller atrial contribution to LV filling (AFC), shorter atrial filling period (AFP), and greater LV filling fraction between 10% and 70% of the diastolic time interval. Filling fraction in pericardial constriction also was greater than normal, while restrictive cardiomyopathy filling fraction was less than normal; TTPFR in pericardial constriction was shorter than normal, while AFC was greater than normal in restrictive myopathy and near normal in pericardial constriction. EDV—end-diastolic volume. (*Adapted from* Aroney *et al.* [39].)

LEFT VENTRICULAR EJECTION FRACTION DURING DOXORUBICIN THERAPY

BASELINE EF	PERFORM EQUILIBRIUM RADIONUCLIDE ANGIOGRAPHY	AT RISK FOR CHF
Normal (≈ 50%)	At baseline At ≈ 450 mg/m^2 At 250–300 mg/m^2*	≥ 10% EF fall from baseline to < 50%
≥ 30% to < 50%	At baseline Prior to each subsequent dose	≥ 10% EF fall from baseline or EF < 30%
< 30%	Avoid doxorubicin	

FIGURE 9-26. Directing doxorubicin therapy. Radionuclide angiography (RNA) is the most widely accepted method for serial evaluation of cardiac function in patients undergoing doxorubicin therapy. Left ventricular ejection fraction (LVEF) is an important and universally accepted index of cardiac function. Overt congestive heart failure due to doxorubicin cardiotoxicity is preceded by a progressive fall in LVEF. Serial studies can detect a change in cardiac function over time, and doxorubicin administration can be stopped when a predetermined fall in LVEF is observed. Both the absolute LVEF and the magnitude of fall are important strategic determinants. The guidelines for using serial RNA at rest, during the course of doxorubicin therapy, are standardized and are based upon experience with nearly 1500 patients over a 7-year period. A greater than fourfold reduction in the incidence of overt cardiac failure was observed when these guidelines were followed. Moreover, if congestive heart failure (CHF) develops, it was mild and rapidly responsive to medical therapy. A recent study has reestablished the clinical relevance and cost-effectiveness of serial LVEF monitoring with equilibrium RNA for the prevention of congestive heart failure during the course of doxorubicin therapy [40]. Exercise RNA also has been used in patients undergoing treatment with doxorubicin. However, patients with malignancies often are unable to undergo exercise testing because of generalized debility, fever, anemia, or musculoskeletal problems. Moreover, exercise testing does not appear to provide additional information compared with resting RNA. Some caution may be required in interpreting changes in LVEF during the course of chemotherapy, since these values also are affected by several noncardiac conditions such as anemia, fever, and sepsis. Resting RNA continues to be the most practical and effective way of monitoring doxorubicin cardiotoxicity. (*Adapted from* Schwartz *et al.* [41].)

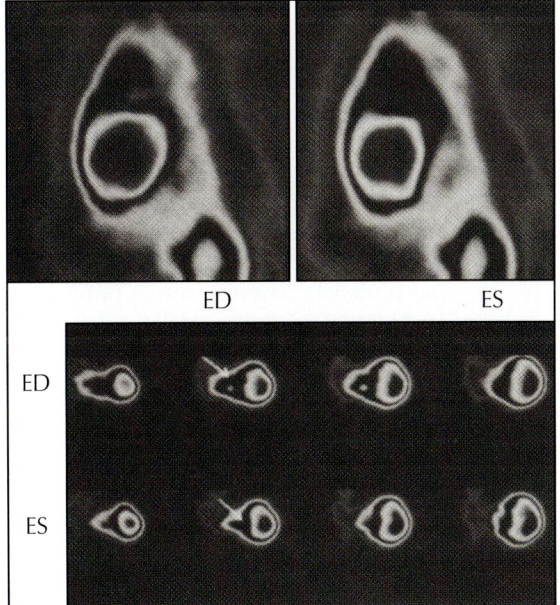

FIGURE 9-27. SPECT radionuclide angiography. SPECT has been applied to blood pool imaging. Although this approach has not yet achieved widespread clinical application, the potential value of the method, as compared with standard planar imaging, is illustrated here. The precision of tomography in defining regional left ventricular function can be helpful in several clinical settings and, most dramatically, in evaluating patients with left ventricular aneurysms, in whom the likely success of surgery depends on an accurate definition of the extent and function of nonaneurysmal myocardium. ED—end diastole; ES—end systole. (*From* Lu *et al.* [29]; with permission.)

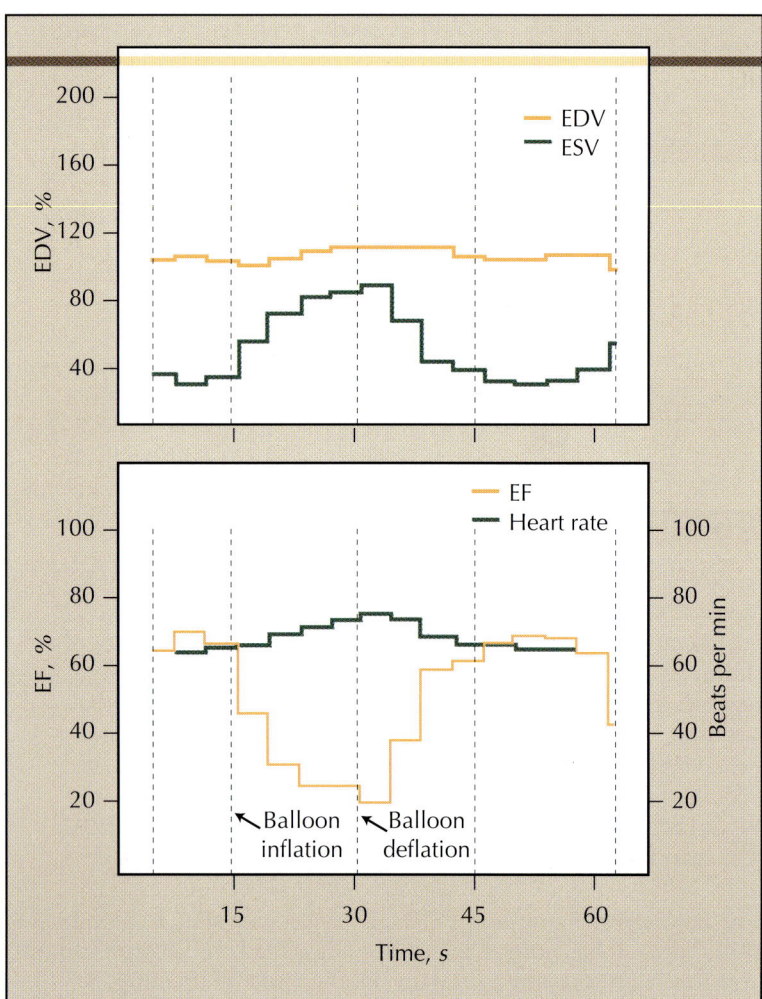

FIGURE 9-28. Validation of ambulatory left ventricular function monitoring device. Continuous left ventricular function monitoring was carried out in the cardiac catheterization laboratory during balloon angioplasty of the left anterior descending coronary artery. With inflation of the balloon, left ventricular ejection fraction (LVEF) fell, preceding symptoms and ST segment depression. The LVEF returned to baseline after deflation of the balloon. EDV—end-diastolic volume; EF—ejection fraction; ESV—end-systolic volume. (*Adapted from Kayden et al.* [42].)

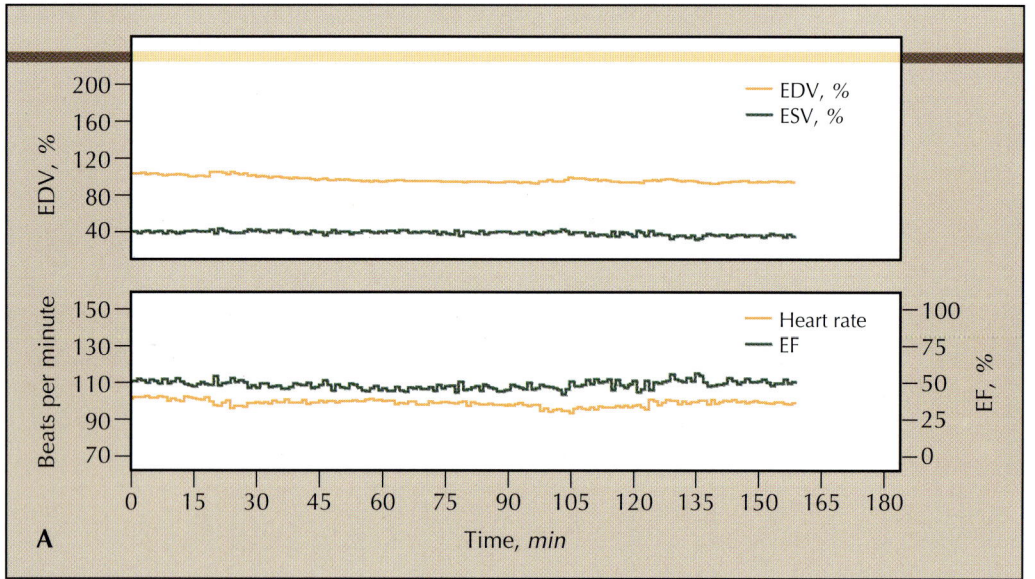

FIGURE 9-29. Continuous left ventricular function monitoring data. **A,** Left ventricular ejection fraction (LVEF), heart rate, and relative end-diastolic volume (EDV) and end-systolic volume (ESV) over a period of nearly 3 hours from a patient admitted with non–Q-wave myocardial infarction. LVEF is normal, and there is no clinically meaningful change in the ejection fraction (EF) during the period of monitoring. *Continued on next page*

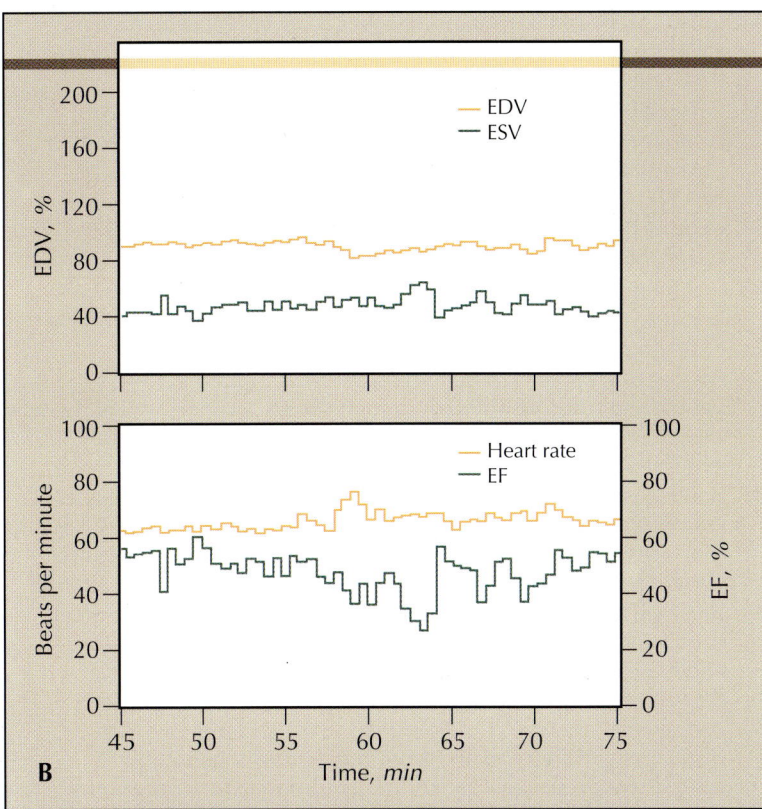

FIGURE 9-29. *(Continued)* **B**, LVEF, heart rate, and relative EDV and ESV over a period of over 30 minutes are shown from a patient admitted with unstable angina. There are several episodes of fall in LVEF which were asymptomatic and were associated with a small increase in heart rate. (*Courtesy of* Diwakar Jain, MD, Hahnemann Hospital, Philadelphia.)

REFERENCES

1. Folse R, Braunwald E: Determination of fraction of left ventricular volume ejected per beat and of ventricular end-diastolic and residual volumes. *Circulation* 1962, 25:674–684.
2. Hoffmann G, Kleine N: Die methode der radiokardiographischen funktions analyse. *Nuklearmedizin* 1968, 7:350–370.
3. Port SC: Recent advances in first-pass radionuclide angiography. *Cardiol Clin North Am* 1994, 12:359–372.
4. Green MV, Ostrow HG, Doulas MA, *et al.*: *Scintigraphic cineangiography of the heart.* Proceedings of MEDINFO 74. Amsterdam: North Holland Publishing Co.; 1974:827–830.
5. Borer JS, Bacharach SL, Green MV, *et al.*: Real-time radionuclide cineangiography in the noninvasive evaluation of global and regional left ventricular function at rest and during exercise in patients with coronary artery disease. *N Engl J Med* 1977, 296:839–844.
6. Borer JS, Supino PG: Radionuclide angiography: equilibrium imaging. In *Nuclear Cardiac Imaging: Principles and Applications*, edn 3. Edited by Iskandrian A, Verani M. New York: Oxford; 2002:323–367.
7. Bacharach SL, Green MV, Borer JS, *et al.*: A real-time system for multi-image gated cardiac studies. *J Nucl Med* 1977, 18:79–84.
8. Hegge FN, Hamilton GW, Larson SM, *et al.*: Cardiac chamber imaging: a comparison of red blood cells labeled with technetium-99m in-vitro and in-vivo. *J Nucl Med* 1978, 19:129–134
9. Bacharach SL, Green MV, Borer JS, *et al.*: ECG-gated scintillation probe measurement of left ventricular function. *J Nucl Med* 1977, 18:1176–1183.
10. Tamaki N, Yasuda T, Moore RH, *et al.*: Continuous monitoring of left ventricular function by an ambulatory radionuclide detector in patients with coronary artery disease. *J Am Coll Cardiol* 1988, 12:669–679.
11. Berger HJ, Matthay RA, Loke J, *et al.*: Assessment of cardiac performance with quantitative radionuclide angiography: right ventricular ejection fraction with reference to findings in chronic obstructive pulmonary disease. *Am J Cardiol* 1978, 41:897.
12. Maddahi J, Berman D, Matsuoka DT, *et al.*: A new technique for assessing right ventricular ejection fraction using rapid multiple gated equilibrium cardiac blood pool scintigraphy. *Circulation* 1979, 60:581–589.
13. Goldberg HL, Herrold EM, Hochreiter C, *et al.*: Videodensitometric determination of right ventricular and left ventricular ejection fraction. *Am J Noninvasive Cardiol* 1987, 1:18–23.
14. Supino PG, Borer JS, Herrold EM, Hochreiter C: Prognostication in 3-vessel coronary artery disease based on left ventricular ejection fraction during exercise: influence of coronary artery bypass grafting. *Circulation* 1999, 100:924–932.
15. Borer JS, Bacharach SL, Green MV, *et al.*: Effect of nitroglycerin on exercise-induced abnormalities of left ventricular regional function and ejection fraction in coronary artery disease: assessment by radionuclide cineangiography in symptomatic and asymptomatic patients. *Circulation* 1978, 57:314–320.
16. Bonow RO, Leon MB, Rosing DR, *et al.*: Effect of verapamil and propranolol on left ventricular systolic function and diastolic filling in patients with coronary artery disease: radionuclide angiographic studies at rest and exercise. *Circulation* 1982, 65:1337–1350.
17. Kent KM, Borer JS, Green MV, *et al.*: Effects of coronary artery bypass on global and regional left ventricular function during exercise. *N Engl J Med* 1978, 1434–1439.
18. Wallis JB, Supino PG, Borer JS: Prognostic value of left ventricular ejection fraction response to exercise during long-term follow-up after coronary bypass graft surgery. *Circulation* 1993, 88:99–109.
19. Borer JS, Hochreiter C, Herrold EM, *et al.*: Prediction of indications for valve replacement among asymptomatic or minimally symptomatic patients with chronic aortic regurgitation and normal left ventricular performance. *Circulation* 1998, 97:525–534.
20. Borer JS, Wencker D, Hochreiter C: Management decisions in valvular heart disease: the role of radionuclide-based assessment of ventricular function and performance. *J Nucl Cardiol* 1996, 3:72–81.

21. Wencker D, Borer JS, Hochreiter C, *et al*.: Preoperative predictors of late postoperative outcome among patients with non-ischemic mitral regurgitation with "high risk" descriptors, and comparison with unoperated patients. *Cardiology* 2000, 93:37–42.

22. Borer JS, Hochreiter CA, Supino PG, *et al*.: The importance of right ventricular performance measurement in selecting asymptomatic patients with mitral regurgitation for valve surgery. *Adv Cardiol* 2002, 39:144–152.

23. Rosen S, Borer JS, Hochreiter C, *et al*.: Natural history of the asymptomatic/minimally symptomatic patient with normal right and left ventricular performance and severe mitral regurgitation due to mitral valve prolapse. *Am J Cardiol* 1994, 74:374–380.

24. Hochreiter C, Niles N, Devereux RB, *et al*.: Mitral regurgitation: relationship of non-invasive descriptors of right and left ventricular performance to clinical and hemodynamic findings and to prognosis in medically and surgically treated patients. *Circulation* 1986, 73:900–912.

25. Niles N, Borer JS, Kamen M, *et al*.: Pre-operative left and right ventricular performance in combined aortic and mitral regurgitation and comparison with isolated aortic or mitral regurgitation. *Am J Cardiol* 1990, 65:1372–1378.

26. Borer JS, Jason M, Devereux RB, *et al*.: Function of the hypertrophied left ventricle at rest and exercise: hypertension and aortic stenosis. *Am J Med* 1983, 75(suppl III):III-34–III-39.

27. Morise AP, Goodwin C: Exercise radionuclide angiography in patients with mitral stenosis: value of right ventricular response. *Am Heart J* 1986, 112:509–517.

28. Corbett JR, Jansen DE, Lewis SE, *et al*.: Tomographic gated blood pool radionuclide ventriculography: analysis of wall motion and left ventricular volumes in patients with coronary artery disease. *J Am Coll Cardiol* 1985, 6:349–358.

29. Lu P, Liu X-J, Shi R, *et al*.: Comparison of tomographic and planar radionuclide ventriculography in assessment of regional left ventricular function in patients with LV aneurysm before and after surgery. *J Nucl Cardiol* 1994, 1:537–545.

30. Green MV, Ostrow HG, Douglas MA, *et al*.: High temporal resolution ECG-gated scintigraphic angiocardiography. *J Nucl Med* 1975, 16:95–98.

31. Green MV, Bacharach SL, Douglas MA, *et al*.: The measurement of left ventricular function and the detection of wall motion abnormalities with high temporal resolution ECG-gated scintigraphic angiocardiography. *IEEE Trans Nucl Sci* 1976, NS–23.

32. Links JM, Becker LC, Shindledecker JG, *et al*.: Measurement of absolute left ventricular volume from gated blood pool studies. *Circulation* 1982, 65:82–91.

33. Green MV, Bacharach SL, Borer JS, Bonow RO: A theoretical comparison of first pass and gated equilibrium methods in the measurement of systolic left ventricular function. *J Nucl Med* 1991, 32:1801–1807.

34. Green MV, Brody WR, Douglas MA, *et al*.: Ejection fraction by count rate from gated images. *J Nucl Med* 1978, 19:880–883.

35. Goldberg HL, Moses JW, Borer JS, *et al*.: Exercise left ventriculography utilizing intraveneous digital angiography. *J Am Coll Cardiol* 1983, 3:1092–1098.

36. Bonow RO, Bacharach SL, Green MV, *et al*.: Impaired left ventricular diastolic filling in patients with coronary artery disease: assessment with radionuclide cineangiography. *Circulation* 1981, 64:315–323.

37. Borer JS, Bacharach SL, Green MV, *et al*.: Exercise-induced left ventricular dysfunction in symptomatic and asymptomatic patients with aortic regurgitation: Assessment by radionuclide cineangiography. *Am J Cardiol* 1978, 42:351–357.

38. Borer JS, Herrold EM, Hochreiter C, *et al*.: Natural history of left ventricular performance at rest and during exercise after aortic valve replacement for aortic regurgitation. *Circulation* 1991, 84(Suppl III):III-133–III-139.

39. Aroney CN, Ruddy TD, Dighero H, *et al*.: Differentiation of restrictive cardiomyopathy from pericardial constriction: assessment of diastolic function by radionuclide angiography. *J Am Coll Cardiol* 1989, 13:1007–1014.

40. Mitani I, Jain D, Joska TM, *et al*.: Doxorubicin cardiotoxicity: Prevention of congestive heart failure with serial cardiac function monitoring with equilibrium radionuclide angiocardiography in the current era. *J Nucl Cardiol*. In press.

41. Schwartz RG, McKenzie WB, Alexander J, *et al*.: Congestive heart failure and left ventricular dysfunction complicating doxorubicin therapy. Seven-year experience using serial radionuclide angiocardiography. *Am J Med* 1987, 82:1109–1118.

42. Kayden DS, Remetz MS, Cabin HS, *et al*.: Validation of continuous radionuclide left ventricular functioning monitoring in detecting silent myocardial ischemia during balloon angioplasty of the left anterior descending coronary artery. *Am J Cardiol* 1991, 67:1339–1343.

CHAPTER 10

GATED MYOCARDIAL PERFUSION SPECT

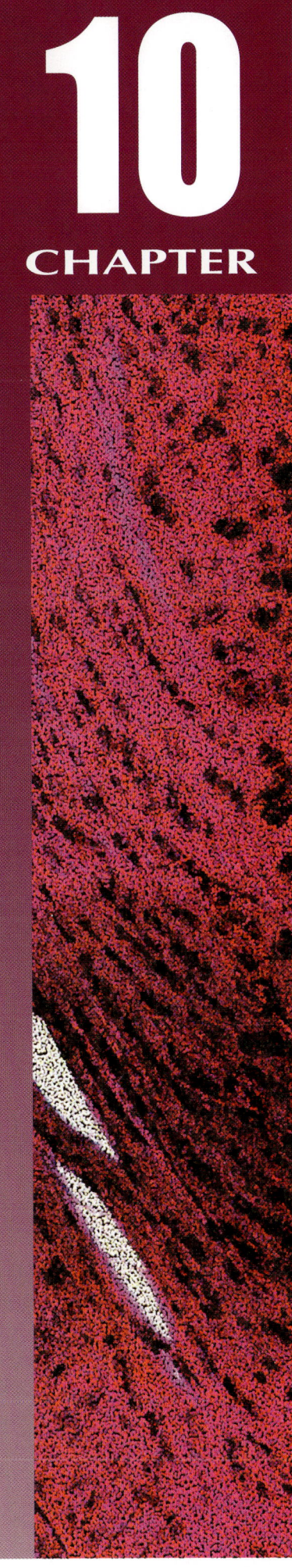

Guido Germano and Daniel S. Berman

Computer advances in the field of nuclear cardiology in the 1990s allowed the technology of gated myocardial perfusion SPECT to become a routine part of myocardial perfusion SPECT assessment. With this approach, accurate measurements are made of left ventricular end-diastolic and end-systolic volumes as well as of left ventricular ejection fraction. Additionally, this method provides a validated technique for assessing regional ventricular function both at rest and following stress. From a variety of vendors, software approaches have been developed which allow quantitation of volumes and ejection fraction, adding to the objectivity of analyses provided by gated SPECT assessments. Due to the complementary nature of assessments of perfusion and function, acceptance of gated SPECT has been rapid in clinical nuclear cardiology.

Clinical research has documented that gated SPECT improves the information provided by nongated myocardial perfusion SPECT in many areas. Several articles have documented increased specificity of the overall interpretation of myocardial perfusion SPECT when the functioning of segments with questionable perfusion abnormalities (versus attenuation artifacts) is considered [1,2]. In addition to assessment of rest and stress myocardial perfusion, gated SPECT provides incremental prognostic information through assessment of the post-stress ejection fraction. Additionally, numerous manuscripts have now demonstrated the potent incremental prognostic information provided by gated SPECT through assessment of the post-stress ejection fraction in addition to assessment of rest and stress myocardial perfusion [3,4]. These prognostic applications are more fully addressed in Chapter 6, *Risk Stratification and Patient Management*. Beyond this routine application, a more elaborate form of gated SPECT assessment could be provided by the use of gated SPECT at rest and during low-dose dobutamine stress, yielding information regarding the recruitment of regional function similar to that provided by low-dose dobutamine echocardiography. The potential of gated SPECT to assess diastolic function is now beginning to be explored. Gated SPECT can provide insight into the severity of coronary artery obstructions through its ability to provide information regarding the development of early post-stress wall motion abnormalities, a sign of critical coronary stenosis. In the area of overall disease detection, it is likely that the added information provided by assessment of regional function following stress will add to the ability of the technique of myocardial perfusion SPECT to identify individual coronary artery stenoses, and thus to assess the overall extent of coronary artery disease. In the area of myocardial viability, if a region of the myocardium moves and thickens, it can be considered viable. This analysis, which is provided by gated SPECT, can provide information in areas where viability is in question.

In this chapter, the technique of gated SPECT is described, important areas of quality control are emphasized, the validation of the various measurements provided are reviewed, and potential assessments such as diastolic function are addressed. Additionally, the chapter evaluates the contributions of gated SPECT to diagnostic assessment (including the use of gated SPECT to increase specificity through recognition of attenuation artifacts) and the added information provided by gated SPECT regarding the severity of coronary stenoses through the observation of post-stress stunning. Modification of protocols are discussed that might be of clinical interest, such as stress-only protocols, or fast gated acquisitions, that might be most useful for the assessment of viability. Finally, the technique of gated blood pool SPECT, considered to be the technique of choice for the radionuclide assessment of ventricular function using blood pool scintigraphy, is explored.

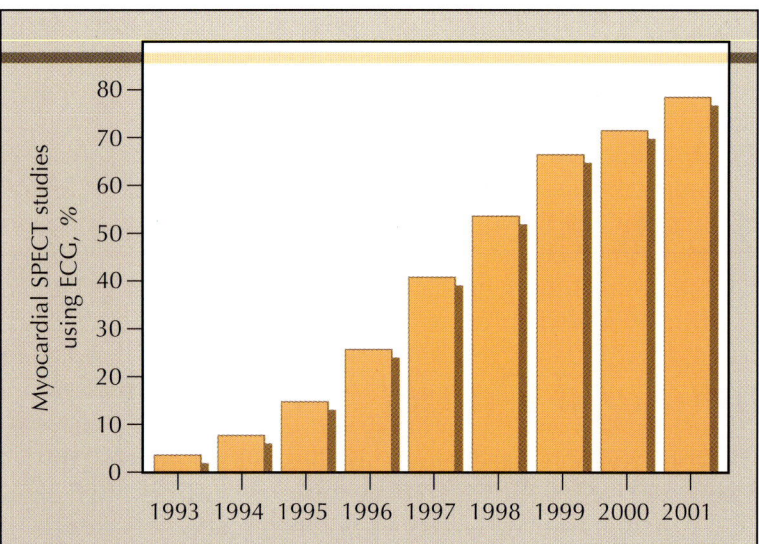

FIGURE 10-1. Gated myocardial perfusion SPECT as percentage of all myocardial SPECT performed in the United States. Over 5 million myocardial SPECT studies were performed in the United States in 2001. Of these, almost 80% utilized ECG gating, compared to almost none in 1993. The enormous growth in the use of gated myocardial perfusion SPECT is linked to several technical breakthroughs. Among these are the recent availability of ^{99m}Tc-based radiopharmaceuticals that can be injected in higher doses and produce higher count statistics compared to ^{201}Tl, as well as the widespread diffusion of multidetector cameras that allow the acquisition of a high–count rate SPECT study in shorter times compared to traditional single-detector cameras. The clinical reason for the exceptional growth of gated SPECT is its ability to provide both perfusion and function information with a single radiopharmaceutical injection and a single acquisition sequence. Powerful computers make it possible to process this wealth of information speedily and collect it into 3-D and 4-D images, a task that only a few years ago required a minimum of 30 minutes on dedicated workstations. The incremental cost for gating a myocardial SPECT study is minimal, consisting mainly of additional computer storage requirements and the need for placing ECG leads on the patient prior to acquisition.

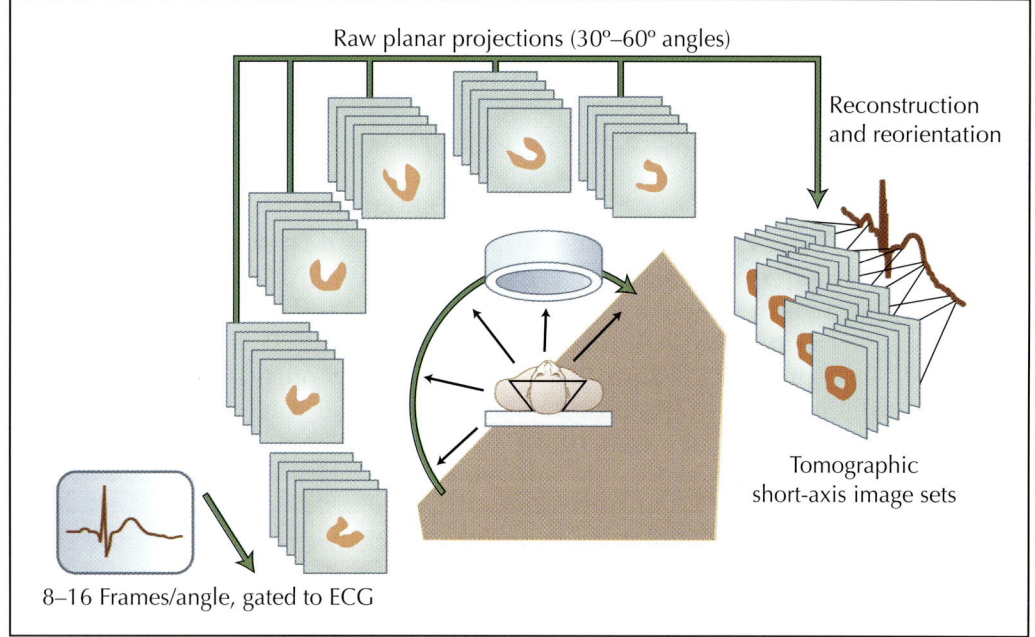

FIGURE 10-2. Gated myocardial perfusion SPECT: acquisition. A gated cardiac SPECT acquisition proceeds almost exactly like an ungated one: the camera detector(s) rotate around the patient, collecting projection images at equally spaced angles along a 180° or 360° arc, and these projections are then filtered and reconstructed into tomographic short- and long-axis images [5,6]. The distinguishing feature of gated SPECT imaging is that at each angle, several (8, 16, or even 32) projection images are acquired, each corresponding to a specific phase of the cardiac cycle. Reconstruction of all same-phase projections produces a 3-D "snapshot" of the patient's heart, frozen in time at that particular phase. Doing so for all phases results in 4-D image volumes (x, y, z, and time, tomographic short-axis image sets) from which cardiac function can be readily assessed.

Typical parameters used are low-energy, high-resolution collimator(s), patient weight-based injection of 25 to 40 mCi of ^{99m}Tc-sestamibi/tetrofosmin or 3 to 4.5 mCi of ^{201}Tl, 3 degrees spacing between adjacent projections, and 25 seconds (^{99m}Tc) or 35 seconds (^{201}Tl) acquisition time per projection [3]. The resulting total acquisition time can be as short as 12.5 minutes (^{99m}Tc) or 17.5 minutes (^{201}Tl), if a dual detector camera with the detectors at a 90-degree angle is used. (*Adapted from* Germano et al. [7].)

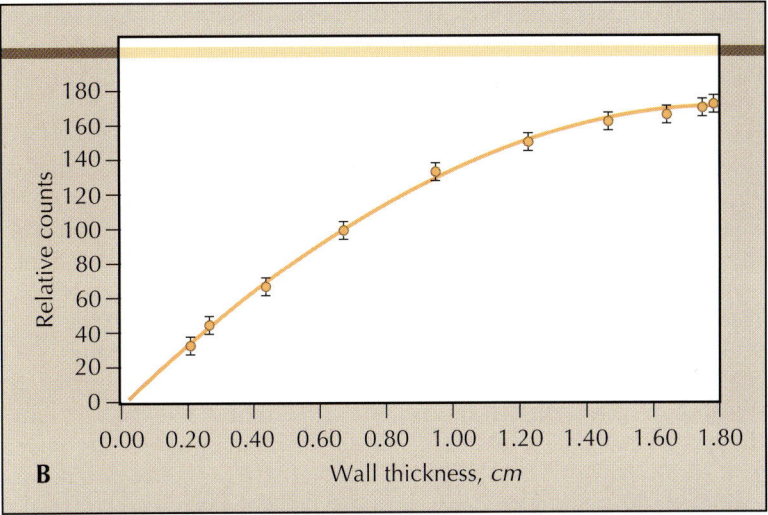

Figure 10-11. *(Continued)* **B,** The relationship between myocardial wall thickness and corresponding maximum count value, the recovery coefficient curve, is shown [14,61]. To the extent that the recovery coefficient curve is linear in the range of myocardial thicknesses spanned during the cardiac cycle, myocardial brightening may be considered an accurate proxy for, and linearly proportional to, actual thickening. (Panel B *adapted from* Smith *et al.* [56].)

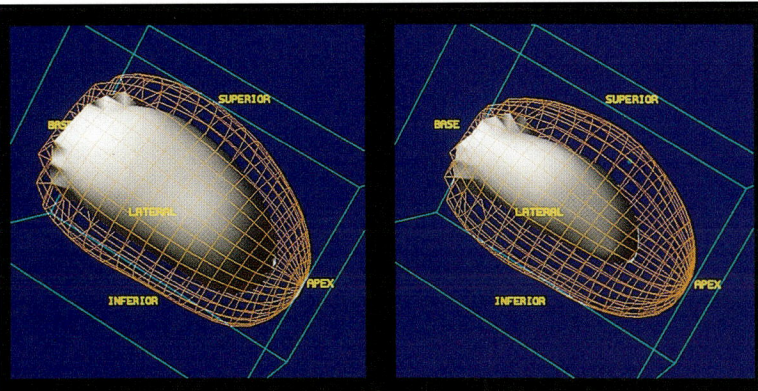

Figure 10-12. Three-dimensional display of gated SPECT images. Three-dimensional displays in gated SPECT are particularly appealing as an aid in the assessment of myocardial motion, and can be implemented through surface rendering techniques [62]. As shown in the figure, surfaces can be approximated by a wire mesh tiled with a mosaic of polygons (epicardium), or by the outward faces of the voxels belonging to the surface itself (endocardium); the main depth cue can be derived from simulated illumination of the surface by a light source in the upper left corner of the image. "Endless loop cineing" of the surfaces through all gating intervals gives the illusion of a 3-D pulsating heart. A fixed grid representing the location of the endocardium at end diastole is often substituted for the epicardial grid to make it easier to assess endocardial motion. Three-dimensional images are frequently presented in standard orientations, like the right anterior oblique view shown in the figure.

Surface rendering is the least computationally demanding form of rendering because it discards all nonsurface information about the rendered object. That notwithstanding, interactive manipulation of surface-rendered images requires real-time redrawing of all the polygons in the wire mesh, and until a few years ago, this computational burden required specialized display hardware. (*From* Germano *et al.* [21].)

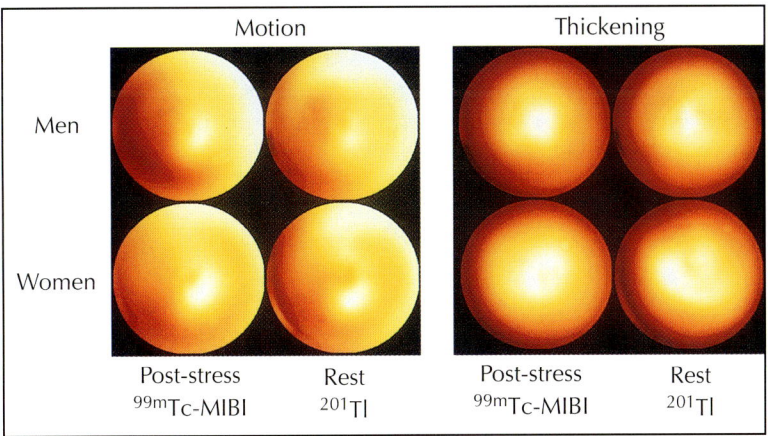

Figure 10-13. Normal patterns of regional myocardial function. SPECT perfusion assessments have traditionally included the use of polar maps, a 2-D parametric representation of perfusion in the entire 3-D myocardium based on a finite number of samples [15,63]. Gated SPECT imaging extends that approach by representing regional myocardial motion and thickening in polar maps; specifically, motion is expressed by the endocardial excursion from end diastole to end systole, and thickening is expressed by the percent myocardial count increase from end diastole to end systole.

While it is reasonable to assume that normal myocardial perfusion will result in a uniform perfusion polar map, the same cannot be said for myocardial motion and thickening. Indeed, in absolute terms, "normal" endocardial excursion is smaller at the septum than at the lateral wall level (due to the anterior translational motion of the heart during systole), and a normal motion polar map will contain lower values in its septal region [64]. Similarly, the normal myocardial apex has been reported to thicken more than the basal myocardium [1], and its relative thinness makes it particularly susceptible to the partial volume effect, which enhances its apparent thickening [64]. Consequently, a normal thickening polar map will contain higher values in its central area. It is recommended that assessment of regional myocardial function should not be based on the function polar maps alone, and normal limits are required for quantitation. Unlike perfusion, however, limits are not heavily dependent on patient gender, radioisotope, or imaging protocol used. MIBI—sestamibi.

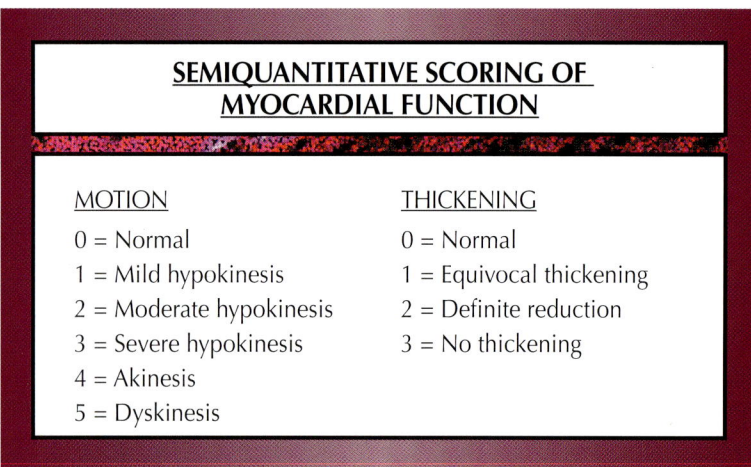

FIGURE 10-14. Semiquantitative scoring of myocardial function. Endocardial motion is categorized according to a six-point scoring system (0 = normal to 5 = dyskinesis), based on what is "normal" for a given region. This approach assumes that the observer is familiar with the range of motion normal for a given segment, just as he would be expected to be familiar with the range of "normal" perfusion in a given segment. Wall motion analysis is performed by visualizing the endocardial edge of the left ventricle, a process that is aided by the alternation between "contours on" and "contours off," if quantitation is available. As a general rule, most experts recommend the use of a gray scale for the interpretation of regional wall motion.

For purposes of wall thickening evaluation, many investigators recommend the use of a 10-step color scale as opposed to a gray scale. The degree of regional thickening is scored similarly to that of regional motion, but using a four-point system (0 = normal, 3 = absent thickening). In general, for a given short axis slice, there is greater uniformity of myocardial thickening than there is of endocardial motion, due to the greater effect of translational motion of the heart's long axis during systole on perceived regional wall motion rather than on thickening.

FIGURE 10-15. Clinical value of gated SPECT: better diagnostic accuracy and agreement. The incremental value of gated SPECT for the differentiation of true perfusion defects from attenuation artifacts was further demonstrated in patients with equivocal fixed perfusion defects on stress-rest ^{99m}Tc-tetrofosmin SPECT [2]. Two independent observers classified the defects as true or artifactual in three separate steps by visually assessing the stress-rest perfusion images (tomography), the stress-rest perfusion images plus the stress-rest rotating projection images (projection view), and all of the above plus myocardial wall motion from the rest gated SPECT images (gated image). The diagnostic accuracy for each observer (measured by the area under the receiver operating characteristic curve) increased at each step; moreover, the kappa coefficient of agreement between the two observers improved with each step, signifying an increase in interobserver reproducibility.

Thus, gated SPECT is frequently useful in determining whether nonreversible defects in regions of possible attenuation artifact (*eg*, breast, diaphragm) are artifactual or real. This improvement in specificity, however, is largely limited to the situation where questionable nonreversible defects are found. When a questionable reversible defect is found, a normal motion pattern on post-stress gated SPECT could be consistent with either ischemia or artifact. In this circumstance, a possible manner for improving specificity is to combine supine and prone imaging with the ^{99m}Tc-perfusion agents, rather than to simply rely on gating. (*Adapted from* Choi *et al*. [2].)

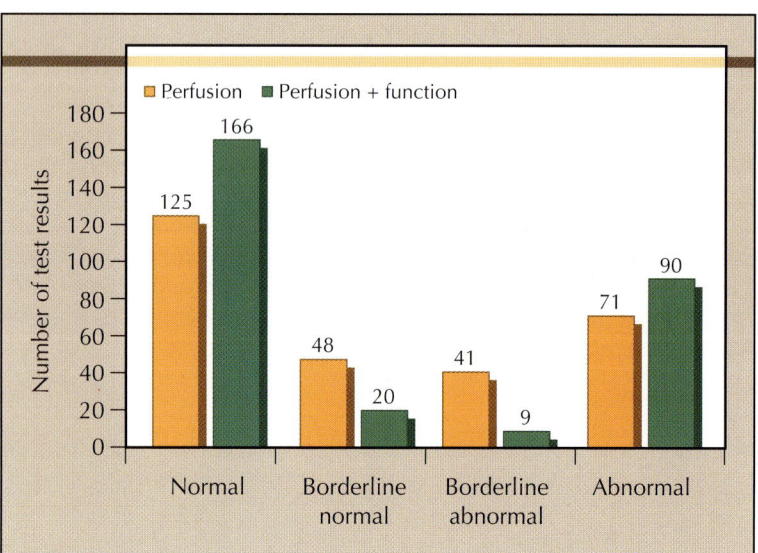

FIGURE 10-16. Clinical value of gated SPECT: reduction of equivocal diagnoses. In 285 consecutive patients (142 men, 143 women) studied with same-day rest and gated post-stress ^{99m}Tc-sestamibi SPECT, 89 patients (31%) had a "borderline" interpretation using the perfusion images alone. However, when wall motion from the gated SPECT images was also considered, the number of borderline interpretations fell to 29 (10%). Of note, the increase in normal interpretations occurred mostly in the subset of patients with a low (< 10%) pretest likelihood of disease, whereas the increase in abnormal interpretations was associated with the subsample of patients with documented coronary artery disease [65].

A limitation of gated SPECT in the context of this analysis is that regions with subendocardial infarction and recanalized infarct-related arteries may contract normally or near normally and demonstrate only nonreversible defects. Clinical correlations are particularly useful in arriving at the correct diagnosis in this setting. (*Adapted from* Smanio *et al*. [65].)

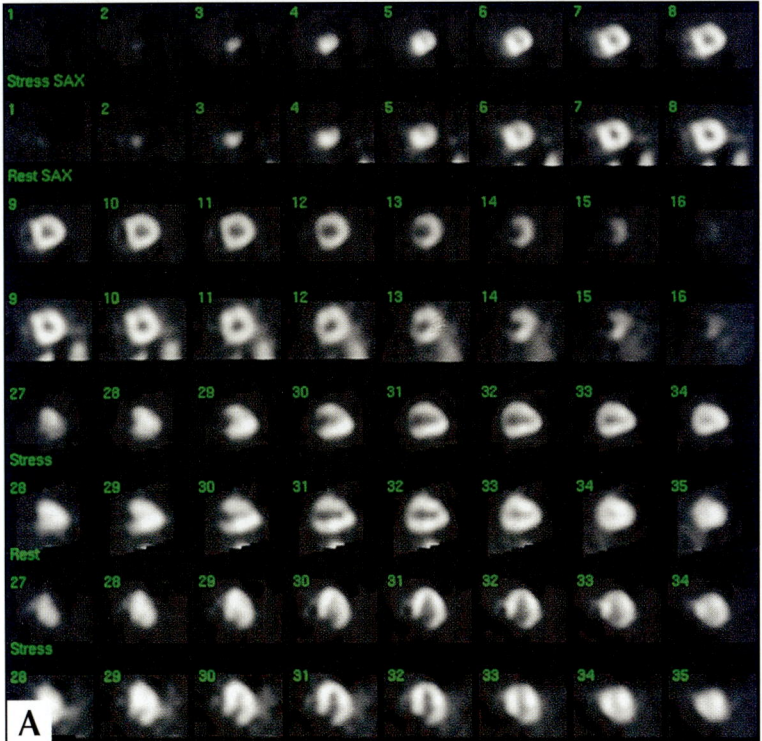

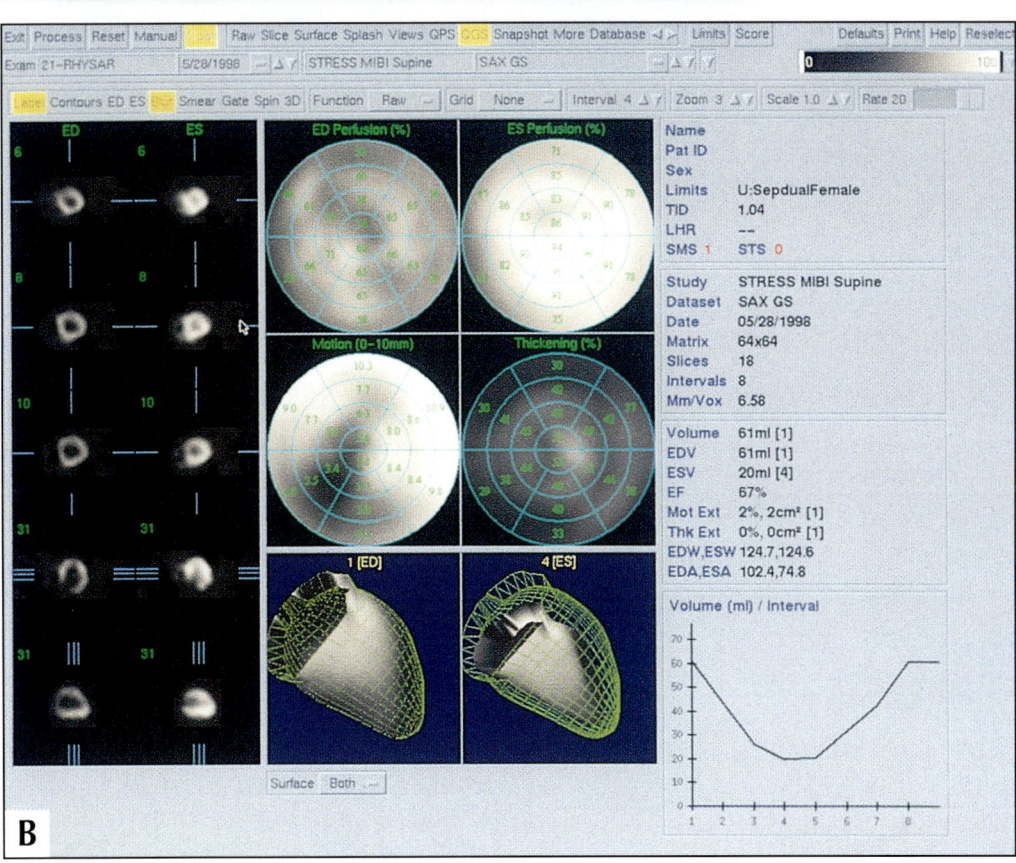

FIGURE 10-17. Example of breast attenuation in a 72-year-old woman with a history of shortness of breath who underwent a rest ^{201}Tl/gated post-stress ^{99m}Tc-sestamibi SPECT study. Risk factors included hypertension, hypercholesterolemia, smoking, and family history of coronary artery disease. The stress electrocardiogram revealed no ST segment depression. **A**, Visual assessment of the interleaved perfusion images (*top 4 rows*, short axis images; *bottom 4 rows*, long axis images) reveals a small, mild, fixed defect in the distal anterior myocardial wall in both the rest and the post-stress images. This perfusion defect could be artifactual, consistent with breast tissue attenuation.

B, The function component of the study as derived from quantitative and visual analysis of the gated post-stress ^{99m}Tc-sestamibi SPECT images shows normal post-stress left ventricular ejection fraction of 67%. The time-volume curve from which it is derived has a canonical shape, suggesting that gating errors have not occurred. Regional myocardial wall motion and thickening in the segments corresponding to the small, mild perfusion defect are both normal. The combined perfusion and function assessment suggests that the small perfusion defect in the distal anterior myocardium represents soft tissue (breast) attenuation. In cases such as this, an attenuating breast shadow may be also visualized on the rotating projection images display, confirming the normal diagnosis. The final report considers the SPECT study normal and identifies this patient as having a low (< 10%) likelihood for the presence of angiographically significant coronary artery disease.

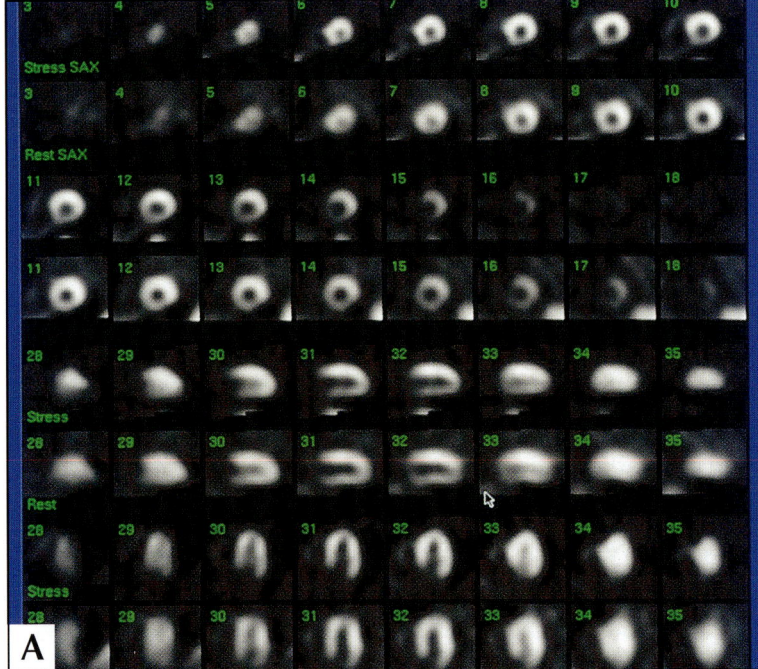
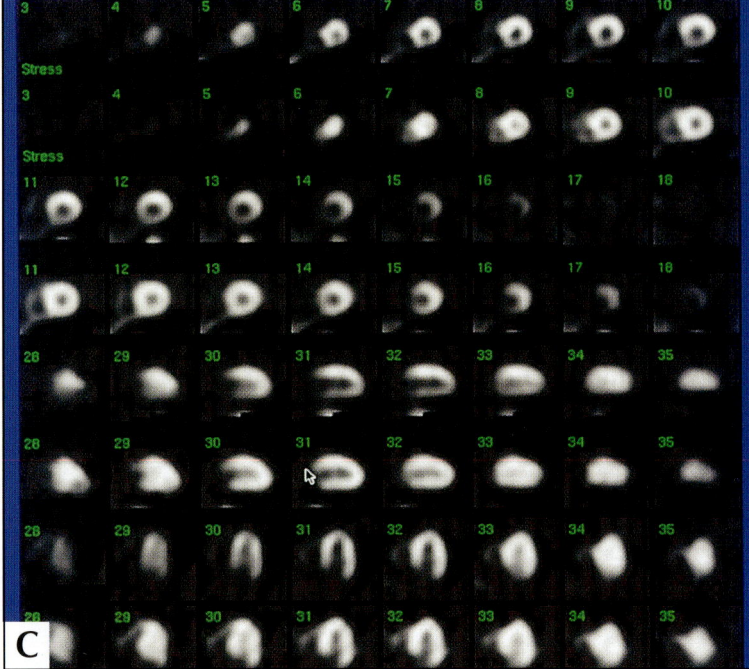
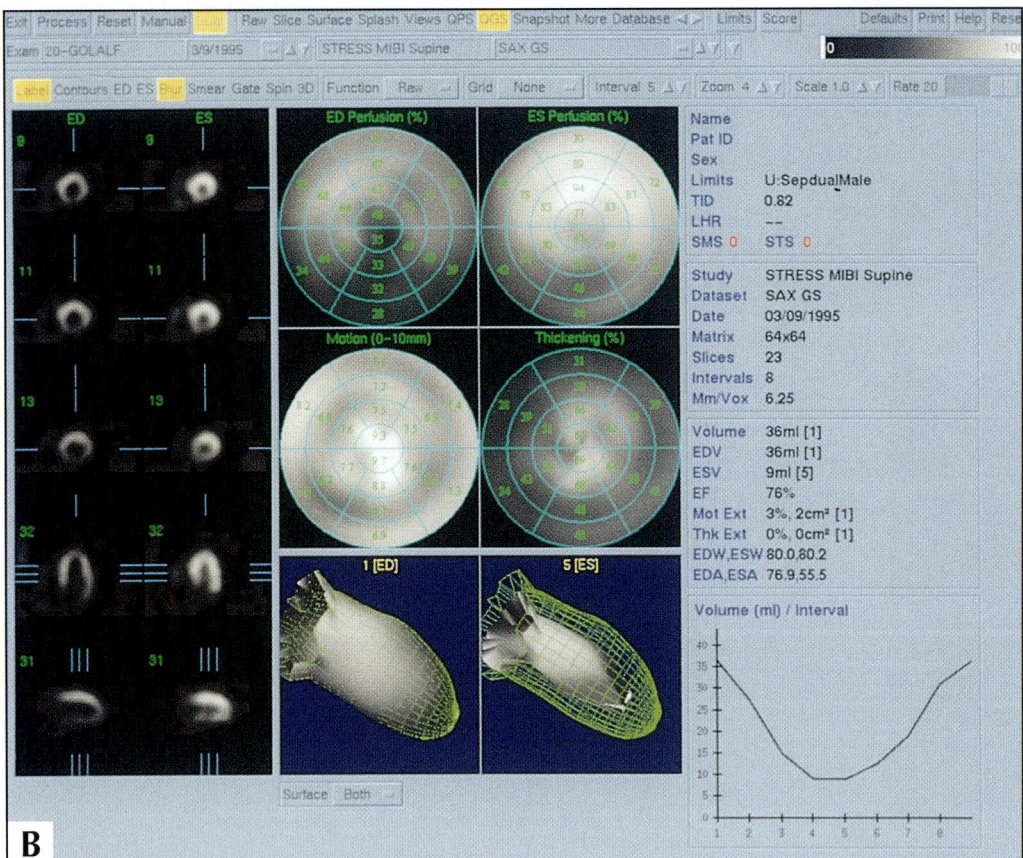

FIGURE 10-18. Example of diaphragmatic attenuation in a 78-year-old man with hypertension, hypercholesterolemia, and a history of nonanginal chest discomfort who underwent a rest ^{201}Tl/gated post-adenosine stress ^{99m}Tc-sestamibi SPECT study. The resting ECG showed low voltage and inferior Q waves, while the clinical response to adenosine stress and the ECG response were nonischemic. A, Visual assessment of the interleaved perfusion images (*top 4 rows*, short-axis images; *bottom 4 rows*, long-axis images) reveals an equivocal nonreversible perfusion defect in the inferior portion of the myocardial wall. This perfusion defect could be artifactual, consistent with diaphragmatic attenuation, since this patient has no history of inferior myocardial infarction.

B, The function component of the study as derived from quantitative and visual analysis of the gated post-adenosine stress ^{99m}Tc-sestamibi SPECT images shows normal post-stress left ventricular ejection fraction of 75%. The time-volume curve from which it is derived has a canonical shape, suggesting that gating errors have not occurred. Regional myocardial wall motion and thickening in the segments corresponding to the perfusion defect are both normal. The combined perfusion and function assessment suggests that the small perfusion defect in the inferior myocardium represents diaphragmatic attenuation. The final report considers the SPECT study normal and identifies this patient as having a low (< 10%) likelihood for the presence of angiographically significant coronary artery disease.

C, When the patient was imaged in the prone position immediately after the post-stress gated SPECT supine acquisition, visual assessment of the interleaved perfusion images (*odd rows*, supine images; *even rows*, corresponding prone images) reveals that the perfusion defect in the inferior portion of the myocardial wall is not present. Thus, prone SPECT imaging decreases the number of false-positive studies by reducing patient motion and providing a proxy for attenuation correction.

With ^{99m}Tc-sestamibi or ^{99m}Tc-tetrofosmin, prone SPECT imaging can help clarify questionable supine perfusion abnormalities. Since these radiotracers do not redistribute appreciably during the time necessary to perform back-to-back supine and prone SPECT acquisitions, the actual uptake pattern in the myocardium would not be expected to change. Prone imaging is frequently associated with artifactual anteroseptal perfusion defects, and therefore should not be used alone in place of supine imaging. Instead, its role is that of allowing a second view of equivocal inferior myocardial wall defects apparent in the supine images by providing a different myocardium-diaphragm spatial relationship and attenuating characteristics. Prone imaging is less useful for ^{201}Tl imaging, since this tracer may redistribute during the performance of the prone SPECT acquisition, and false-negative results may be produced in patients with true ischemia on the supine images.

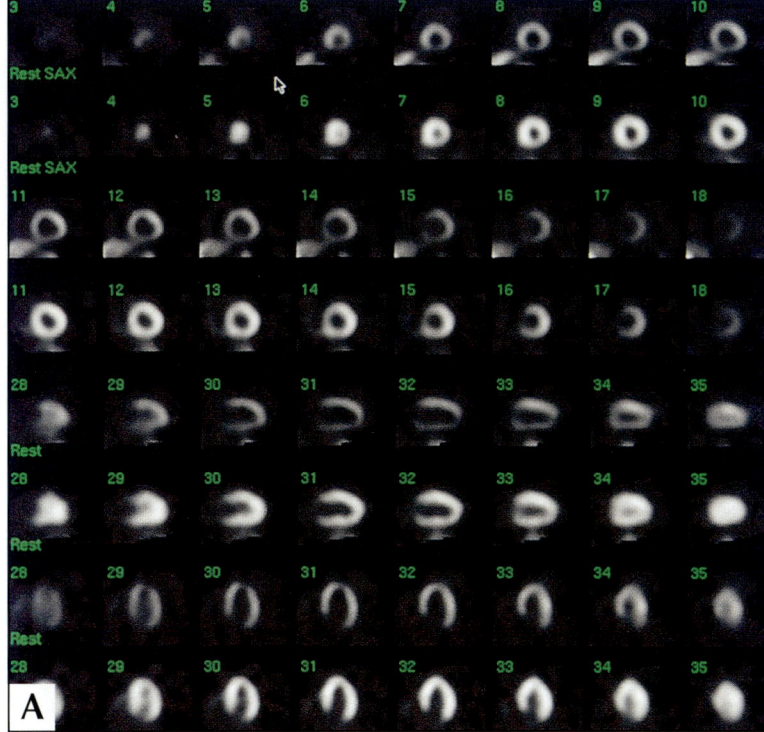

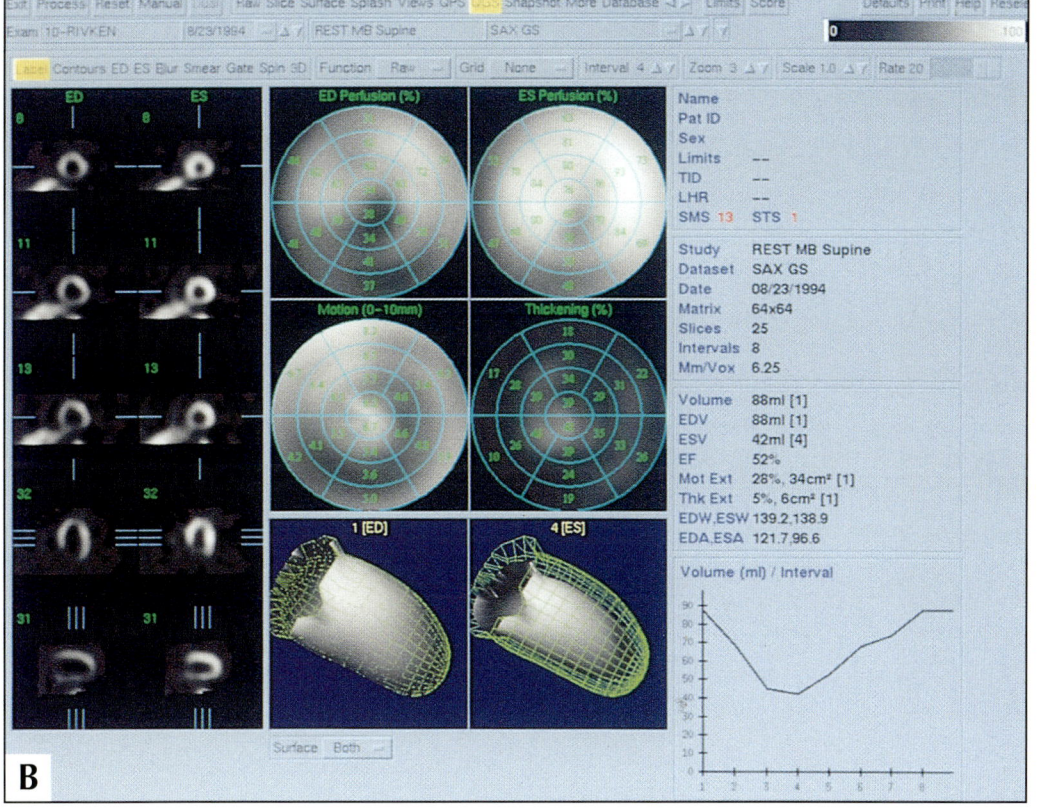

FIGURE 10-19. Example of extracardiac activity in a 55-year-old man with a history of hypertension, presenting to the emergency room with persistent resting chest pain, and consequently referred for a rest ^{99m}Tc-sestamibi SPECT study to rule out an acute coronary syndrome. The patient had no history of coronary artery disease and his electrocardiogram was normal. **A**, Visual assessment of the perfusion images (*odd rows*, supine images; *even rows*, corresponding prone images) reveals a small perfusion defect in the inferior myocardial wall. However, this perfusion defect could be artifactual, since it is known that high extracardiac activity in conjunction with filtered backprojection reconstruction may lead to the cancellation of counts in the myocardial areas adjacent to the extracardiac activity [66]. Possible options to reduce this effect of extracardiac activity include the use of a tomographic reconstruction technique other than filtered backprojection, specifically, iterative reconstruction [66,67]. Also, prone SPECT imaging can be performed in addition to supine SPECT imaging. In this patient, perfusion assessment from prone images was normal.

B, The function component of the study as derived from quantitative and visual analysis of the gated rest ^{99m}Tc-sestamibi SPECT images shows a normal left ventricular ejection fraction (52%). The time-volume curve from which it is derived has a canonical shape, suggesting that gating errors have not occurred. Regional myocardial wall motion and thickening in the segments corresponding to the small perfusion defect are both normal. The combined perfusion and function assessment suggests that the small perfusion defect in the inferior myocardial wall is artifactual and is caused by the combination of high extracardiac activity and filtered backprojection reconstruction. The final report considers the SPECT study normal and identifies this patient as having a low (< 10%) likelihood for the presence of angiographically significant coronary artery disease.

Rest myocardial perfusion SPECT imaging has been shown to have a high sensitivity (97%) and a high negative predictive value (99%) for patients with resting chest pain and possible acute coronary syndromes (unstable angina or acute myocardial infarction) [68]. The high sensitivity reduces the number of inappropriate discharges of patients who truly have an acute coronary syndrome, thus improving patient care and limiting physician liability. In addition, the high negative predictive value reduces unnecessary hospital admissions for patients with noncardiac chest pain. Gated SPECT and prone imaging may increase accuracy and observer confidence in interpreting subtle cases in an acute syndrome setting.

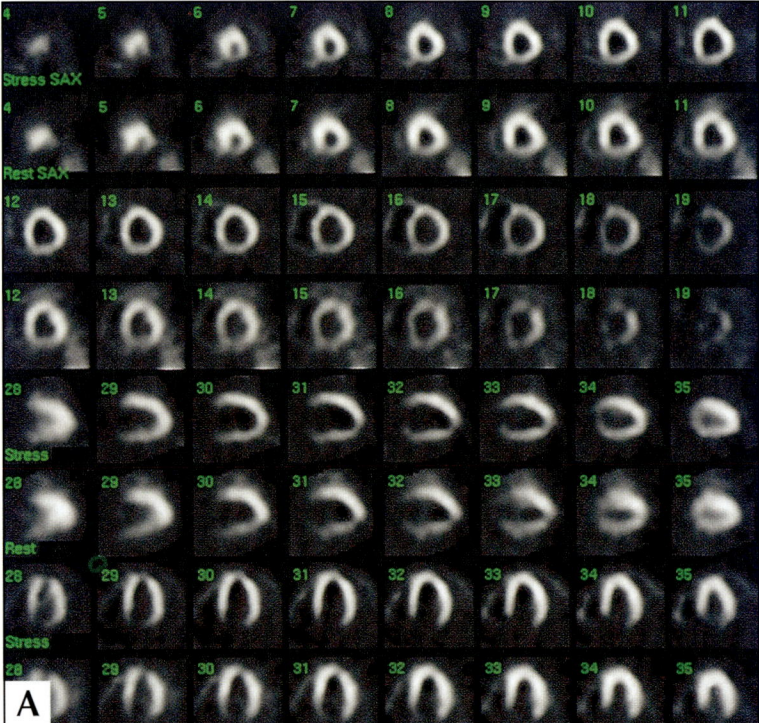

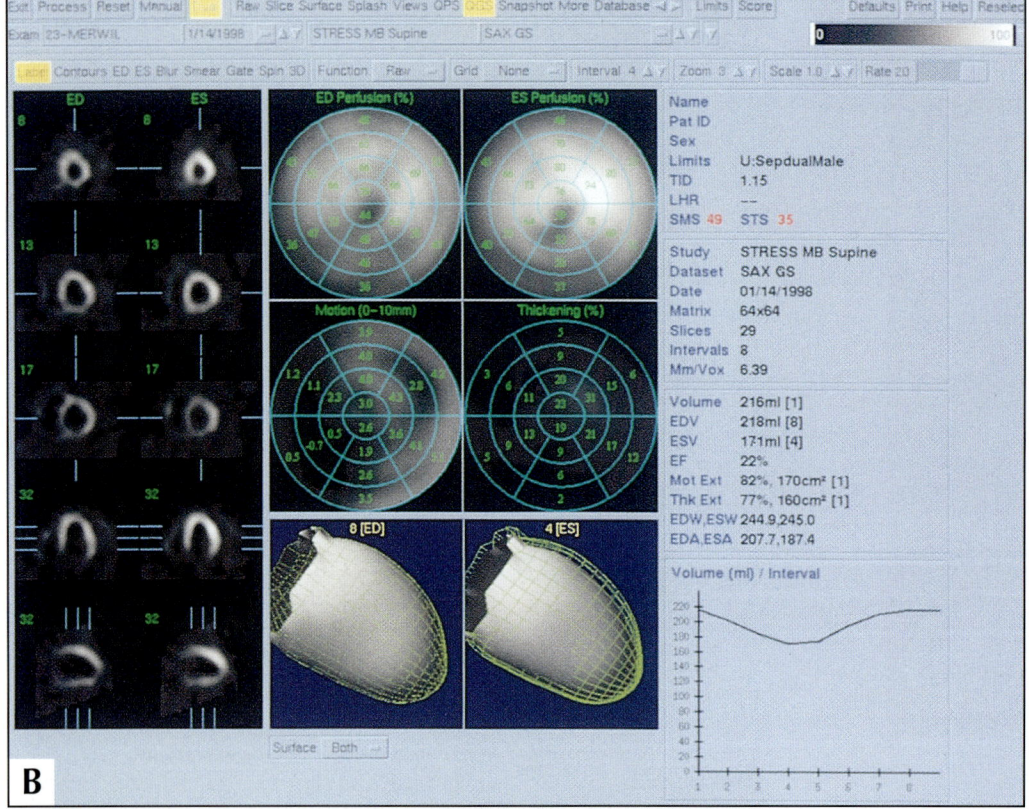

FIGURE 10-20. Example of a 51-year-old man with nonischemic cardiomyopathy who was admitted to the hospital with atypical chest pain. Risk factors included a family history of coronary artery disease. When the cardiac enzymes were negative, the patient underwent rest ^{201}Tl/gated post-stress ^{99m}Tc-sestamibi SPECT imaging the following day. The resting ECG revealed left anterior fascicular block, possible anterior myocardial infarction, and left atrial enlargement, while the stress ECG showed no ST segment depression.

A, Visual assessment of the interleaved perfusion images (*top 4 rows*, short axis images; *bottom 4 rows*, long axis images) demonstrates a mildly decreased uptake in the inferior myocardial wall in both the rest and the post-stress images.

B, The function component of the study as derived from quantitative and visual analysis of the gated post-exercise ^{99m}Tc-sestamibi SPECT images shows severely reduced post-stress left ventricular ejection fraction at 21%. Left ventricular wall motion assessed on gated SPECT shows severe hypokinesis in the apical, lateral, inferior, septal, and anterior myocardial walls, accompanied by severely reduced thickening. Moreover, the end-diastolic left ventricular cavity volume is 218 mL, confirming the visual assessment of resting enlargement (without further dilation during stress) drawn from the perfusion images. The combined perfusion and function assessment is consistent with a nonischemic cardiomyopathic process, suggesting that catheterization is unnecessary and should be avoided for this type of patient.

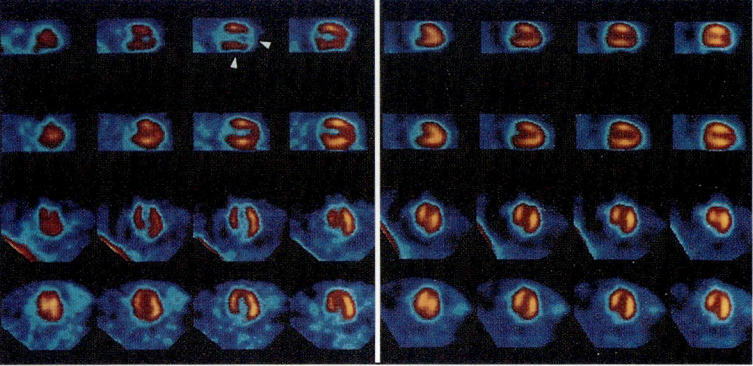

FIGURE 10-21. Gated SPECT for diastolic imaging. The conventional nongated myocardial SPECT study from which perfusion is assessed averages together the various phases of the cardiac cycle, therefore somewhat smoothing the radioactivity distribution and potentially hiding small perfusion defects. In women patients with suspected coronary artery disease who underwent 2-day gated post-stress/gated rest ^{99m}Tc-sestamibi SPECT and 16 gating frames, end-diastolic images (*left*) were constructed by summing, before tomographic reconstruction, data from the three gating frames corresponding to end diastole, while conventional images (*right*) utilized summed data from all 16 frames.

Continued on next page

FIGURE 10-21. *(Continued)* When two expert observers evaluated both image series in blinded fashion, it was found that end-diastolic imaging identified 39% more ischemic myocardial segments compared with conventional imaging. Although the differences in sensitivity and specificity were not statistically significant based on an angiographic standard, there was a trend towards better sensitivity for the end-diastolic images, as shown for the apical perfusion defect in the figure. (*From* Taillefer *et al.* [69]; with permission.)

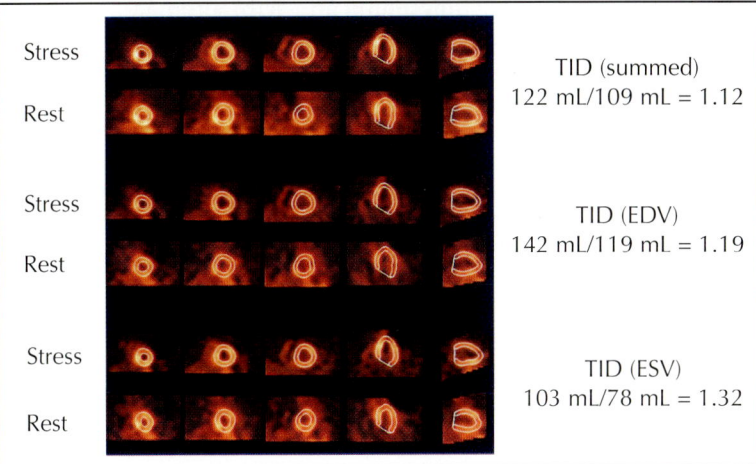

FIGURE 10-22. The SPECT transient ischemic dilation (TID) ratio: gated and nongated. As much as diastolic perfusion imaging may allow identification of subtle perfusion defects, use of the end-diastolic or end-systolic information may allow for better characterization of TID of the left ventricular cavity. The TID ratio traditionally has been calculated from nongated images as the ratio of stress (post-stress) to rest left ventricle cavity volumes, and has been demonstrated to represent an extremely specific and moderately sensitive marker of severe and extensive coronary artery disease [70]. The optimal threshold for TID abnormality is known to depend on the type of protocol used, with rest/post-exercise dual isotope SPECT requiring a higher value compared to same-day post-exercise/rest ^{99m}Tc-sestamibi SPECT [71], and pharmacologic stress currently being investigated [72]. As illustrated, calculations of TID based on the end-diastolic volume (EDV) or end-systolic volume (ESV) generally result in different values from the nongated volumes. Because measurement of nongated volumes may be problematic in certain subpopulations of patients (for example, patients with small left ventricles), it is likely that gated SPECT TID measurements will be of incremental diagnostic and prognostic utility in those patients.

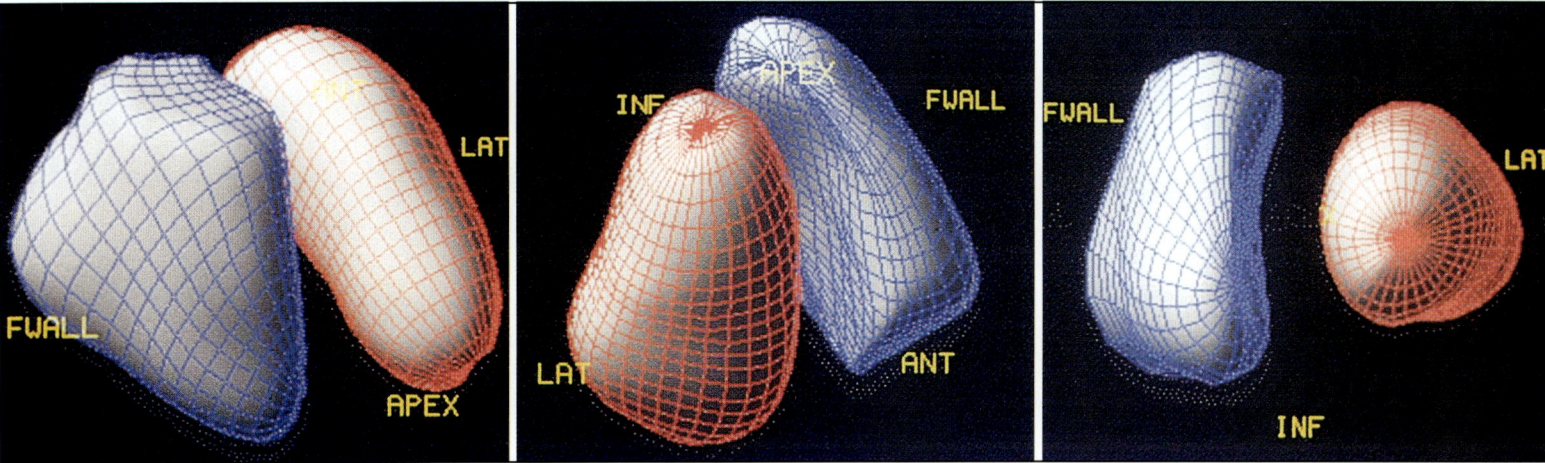

FIGURE 10-23. Gated blood pool SPECT: left ventricle (LV) and right ventricle (RV). With the increase in the use of echocardiographic procedures and the widespread acceptance of gated myocardial perfusion SPECT, gated planar blood pool imaging has decreased to less than 10% of all nuclear cardiac studies performed in the United States, although the percentage may be substantially higher in other countries. Conversely, the case for gated blood pool SPECT has considerably strengthened, due to the increase in computer speed, the greater diffusion of multidetector cameras, and the general acceptance of state of the art 3-D analysis and display techniques. We believe that gated blood pool SPECT will become the most commonly utilized nuclear cardiology method for blood pool scintigraphy, the main rationale for its use being its ability to assess both left ventricular and right ventricular function parameters, without need for background subtraction. Gated blood pool SPECT images can be displayed in parametric 3-D format, much like gated perfusion SPECT; because the epicardium is not visualized in blood pool imaging, a standard display will represent the LV and RV endocardium as shaded surfaces, and their location at end-diastole as wire grids.

The clinical circumstances in which this procedure is likely to become effective are the same as those in which resting blood pool scintigraphy is currently applied, chief among them the assessment of adriamycin cardiotoxicity. Blood pool scintigraphy is also commonly employed in serial assessment of patients with aortic insufficiency, congestive heart failure, and patients who have undergone cardiac transplantation. Promising recent data have suggested that phase analysis from blood pool scintigraphy may clinical value in selecting patients who might benefit from bi-ventricular pacing for resynchronization. ANT—anterior; FWALL—free wall; INF—inferior; LAT—lateral.

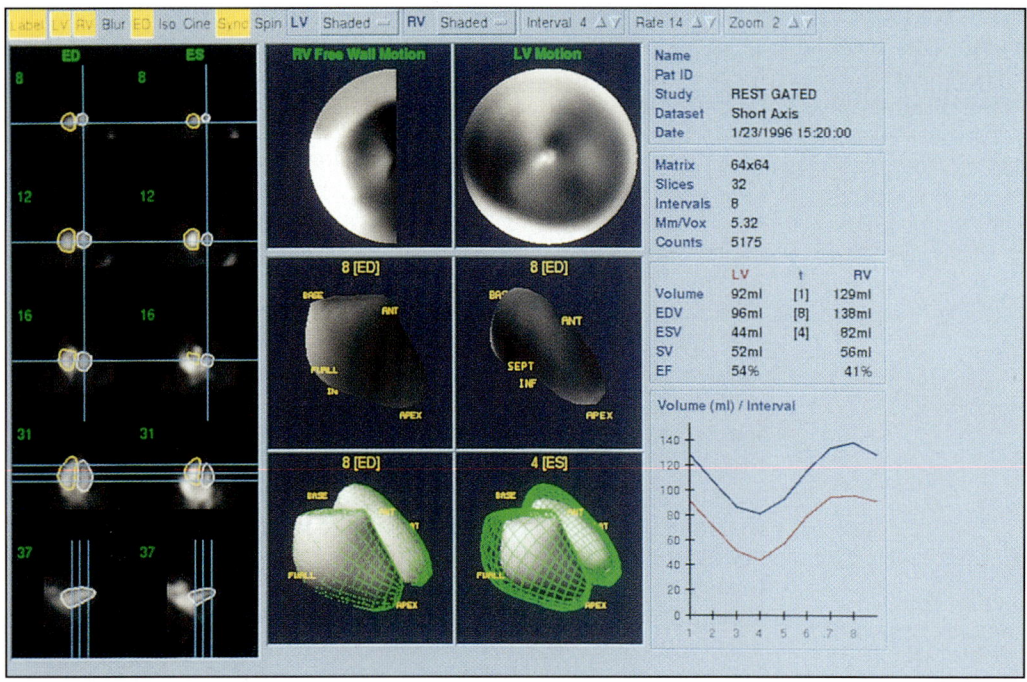

FIGURE 10-24. Gated blood pool SPECT: quantitation. Quantitation of left and right ventricular ejection fractions, left and right ventricular volumes, and left and right regional endocardial motion is possible with gated blood pool SPECT imaging.

Despite the fact that the right ventricle geometry is more difficult to model than that of the left ventricle, and that fewer gold standards exist for the study of right ventricular function, a number of automated and semiautomated algorithms for gated blood pool SPECT quantitation have been developed and are being validated and compared [73]. Unlike planar blood pool, many of these approaches rely on space-based rather than count-based analysis, although hybrid approaches have also been proposed [74]. Most of the technical issues discussed for gated perfusion SPECT also apply to gated blood pool SPECT imaging, and usually the same acquisition and processing parameters are used for the two modalities. A notable exception is the setting of the cardiac beat length acceptance window to 20% to 30% in the latter, to minimize the effects of arrhythmia, because no perfusion information is acquired.

REFERENCES

1. Berman D, Germano G, eds: An approach to the interpretation and reporting of gated myocardial perfusion SPECT. In *Clinical Gated Cardiac SPECT*. Armonk, NY: Futura; 1999:147–182.

2. Choi JY, Lee KH, Kim SJ, *et al.*: Gating provides improved accuracy for differentiating artifacts from true lesions in equivocal fixed defects on technetium 99m tetrofosmin perfusion SPECT. *J Nucl Cardiol* 1998, 5(4):395–401.

3. Sharir T, Germano G, Kavanagh PB, *et al.*: Incremental prognostic value of post-stress left ventricular ejection fraction and volume by gated myocardial perfusion single photon emission computed tomography. *Circulation* 1999, 100(10):1035–1042.

4. Sharir T, Germano G, Kang X, *et al.*: Prediction of myocardial infarction versus cardiac death by gated myocardial perfusion SPECT: risk stratification by the amount of stress-induced ischemia and the poststress ejection fraction. *J Nucl Med* 2001, 42(6):831–837.

5. Germano G: Technical aspects of myocardial SPECT imaging. *J Nucl Med* 2001, 42(10):1499–1507.

6. The Cardiovascular Imaging Committee, American College of Cardiology, The Committee on Advanced Cardiac Imaging and Technology, *et al.*: Standardization of cardiac tomographic imaging. *J Am Coll Cardiol* 1992, 20(1):255–256.

7. Germano G, Berman D, eds: Acquisition and processing for gated perfusion SPECT: technical aspects. In *Clinical Gated Cardiac SPECT*. Armonk, NY: Futura; 1999:93–113.

8. Bar Harbor Invitation Meeting 2000. *J Nucl Cardiol* 2001, 8(2):224–316.

9. Germano G, Berman D: Gated SPECT. In *Nuclear Cardiac Imaging: Principles and Applications*, edn 3. Edited by Iskandrian AS, Verani MS. New York: Oxford University Press; 2002..

10. Nichols K, DePuey EG, Rozanski A: Automation of gated tomographic left ventricular ejection fraction. *J Nucl Cardiol* 1996, 3(6 Pt 1):475–482.

11. Everaert H, Bossuyt A, Franken PR: Left ventricular ejection fraction and volumes from gated single photon emission tomographic myocardial perfusion images: comparison between two algorithms working in three-dimensional space. *J Nucl Cardiol* 1997, 4(6):472–476.

12. Yoshioka J, Hasegawa S, Yamaguchi H, *et al.*: Left ventricular volumes and ejection fraction calculated from quantitative electrocardiographic-gated 99mTc-tetrofosmin myocardial SPECT. *J Nucl Med* 1999, 40(10):1693–1698.

13. Manrique A, Koning R, Cribier A, Vera P: Effect of temporal sampling on evaluation of left ventricular ejection fraction by means of thallium-201 gated SPECT: comparison of 16- and 8-interval gating, with reference to equilibrium radionuclide angiography. *Eur J Nucl Med* 2000, 27(6):694–699.

14. Chua T, Yin LC, Thiang TH, *et al.*: Accuracy of the automated assessment of left ventricular function with gated perfusion SPECT in the presence of perfusion defects and left ventricular dysfunction: correlation with equilibrium radionuclide ventriculography and echocardiography. *J Nucl Cardiol* 2000, 7(4):301–311.

15. Kikkawa M, Nakamura T, Sakamoto K, *et al.*: Assessment of left ventricular diastolic function from quantitative electrocardiographic-gated (99)mTc-tetrofosmin myocardial SPET [published correction appears in *Eur J Nucl Med* 2001, 28:1579]. *Eur J Nucl Med* 2001, 28(5):593–601.

16. Everaert H, Franken PR, Flamen P, *et al.*: Left ventricular ejection fraction from gated SPET myocardial perfusion studies: a method based on the radial distribution of count rate density across the myocardial wall. *Eur J Nucl Med* 1996, 23(12):1628–1633.

17. Vera P, Manrique A, Pontvianne V, *et al.*: Thallium-gated SPECT in patients with major myocardial infarction: effect of filtering and zooming in comparison with equilibrium radionuclide imaging and left ventriculography. *J Nucl Med* 1999, 40(4):513–521.

18. Calnon DA, Kastner RJ, Smith WH, *et al.*: Validation of a new counts-based gated single photon emission computed tomography method for quantifying left ventricular systolic function: comparison with equilibrium radionuclide angiography. *J Nucl Cardiol* 1997, 4(6):464–471.

19. Faber TL, Cooke CD, Folks RD, *et al.*: Left ventricular function and perfusion from gated SPECT perfusion images: an integrated method. *J Nucl Med* 1999, 40(4):650–659.

20. Williams KA, Taillon LA: Left ventricular function in patients with coronary artery disease assessed by gated tomographic myocardial perfusion images. Comparison with assessment by contrast ventriculography and first-pass radionuclide angiography. *J Am Coll Cardiol* 1996, 27(1):173–181.

21. Germano G, Kiat H, Kavanagh PB, *et al.*: Automatic quantification of ejection fraction from gated myocardial perfusion SPECT. *J Nucl Med* 1995, 36(11):2138–2147.

22. He ZX, Cwajg E, Preslar JS, *et al.*: Accuracy of left ventricular ejection fraction determined by gated myocardial perfusion SPECT with Tl-201 and Tc-99m sestamibi: comparison with first-pass radionuclide angiography. *J Nucl Cardiol* 1999, 6(4):412–417.

23. Inubushi M, Tadamura E, Kudoh T, *et al.*: Simultaneous assessment of myocardial free fatty acid utilization and left ventricular function using 123I-BMIPP-gated SPECT. *J Nucl Med* 1999, 40(11):1840–1847.

24. Vallejo E, Dione DP, Sinusas AJ, Wackers FJ: Assessment of left ventricular ejection fraction with quantitative gated SPECT: accuracy and correlation with first-pass radionuclide angiography. *J Nucl Cardiol* 2000, 7(5):461–470.

25. Nichols K, DePuey EG, Rozanski A, *et al.*: Image enhancement of severely hypoperfused myocardia for computation of tomographic ejection fraction. *J Nucl Med* 1997, 38(9):1411–1417.

26. Vaduganathan P, He ZX, Vick GW 3rd, *et al.*: Evaluation of left ventricular wall motion, volumes, and ejection fraction by gated myocardial tomography with technetium 99m-labeled tetrofosmin: a comparison with cine magnetic resonance imaging. *J Nucl Cardiol* 1999, 6(1 Pt 1):3–10.

27. Tadamura E, Kudoh T, Motooka M, *et al.*: Assessment of regional and global left ventricular function by reinjection T1-201 and rest Tc-99m sestamibi ECG-gated SPECT: comparison with three-dimensional magnetic resonance imaging. *J Am Coll Cardiol* 1999, 33(4):991–997.

28. Bax JJ, Lamb H, Dibbets P, *et al.*: Comparison of gated single-photon emission computed tomography with magnetic resonance imaging for evaluation of left ventricular function in ischemic cardiomyopathy. *Am J Cardiol* 2000, 86(12):1299–1305.

29. Bavelaar-Croon CD, Kayser HW, van der Wall EE, *et al.*: Left ventricular function: correlation of quantitative gated SPECT and MR imaging over a wide range of values. *Radiology* 2000, 217(2):572–575.

30. Stollfuss JC, Haas F, Matsuhari I, *et al.*: Regional myocardial wall thickening and global ejection fraction in patients with low angiographic left ventricular ejection fraction assessed by visual and quantitative resting ECG-gated 99mTc-tetrofosmin single-photon emission tomography and magnetic resonance imaging. *Eur J Nucl Med* 1998, 25(5):522–530.

31. Stollfuss JC, Haas F, Matsunari H, *et al.*: 99mTc-tetrofosmin SPECT for prediction of functional recovery defined by MRI in patients with severe left ventricular dysfunction: additional value of gated SPECT. *J Nucl Med* 1999, 40(11):1824–1831.

32. Abe M, Kazatani Y, Fukuda H, *et al.*: Left ventricular volumes, ejection fraction, and regional wall motion calculated with gated technecium-99m tetrofosmin SPECT in reperfused acute myocardial infarction at super-acute phase: comparison with left ventriculography. *J Nucl Cardiol* 2000, 7(6):569–574.

33. Atsma DE, Bavelaar-Croon CD, Germano G, *et al.*: Good correlation between gated single photon emission computed myocardial tomography and contrast ventriculography in the assessment of global and regional left ventricular function. *Int J Card Imaging* 2000, 16(6):447–453.

34. Nichols K, Tamas J, DePuey EG, *et al.*: Relationship of gated SPECT ventricular function parameters to angiographic measurements. *J Nucl Cardiol* 1998, 5(3):295–303.

35. Cwajg E, Cwajg J, Keng F, *et al.*: Gated myocardial perfusion tomography for the assessment of left ventricular function and volumes: comparison with echocardiography. *J Nucl Med* 1999, 40(11):1857–1865.

36. Bacher-Stier C, Muller S, Pachinger O, *et al.*: Thallium-201 gated single-photon emission tomography for the assessment of left ventricular ejection fraction and regional wall motion abnormalities in comparison with two-dimensional echocardiography. *Eur J Nucl Med* 1999, 26(12):1533–1540.

37. Nichols K, Lefkowitz D, Faber T, *et al.*: Echocardiographic validation of gated SPECT ventricular function measurements. *J Nucl Med* 2000, 41(8):1308–1314.

38. Nakajima K, Taki J, Kawano M, *et al.*: Gated SPECT quantification of small hearts: mathematical simulation and clinical application. *Eur J Nucl Med* 2000, 27(9):1372–1379.

39. Johnson LL, Verdesca SA, Aude WY, *et al.*: Postischemic stunning can affect left ventricular ejection fraction and regional wall motion on post-stress gated sestamibi tomograms. *J Am Coll Cardiol* 1997, 30(7):1641–1648.

40. Berman D, Germano G, Lewin H, *et al.*: Comparison of post-stress ejection fraction and relative left ventricular volumes by automatic analysis of gated myocardial perfusion single-photon emission computed tomography acquired in the supine and prone positions. *J Nucl Cardiol* 1998, 5(1):40–47.

41. Nakajima T, Nagaoka Y, Handa S, *et al.*: Assessment of the reverse remodeling effect of beta-blocker in chronic heart failure by LV volumes obtained from the quantitative gated SPECT using 99mTc-tetrofosmin [abstract]. *J Nucl Cardiol* 2001, 8(1):S24.

42. Tanaka R, Nakamura T: Serial evaluation of myocardial blood flow and cardiac function using Tc-99m tetrofosmin gated SPECT before and after reperfusion therapy in patients with acute myocardial infarction [abstract]. *J Nucl Med* 2001, 42(5):166P–167P.

43. Tadamura E, Kudoh T, Motooka M, *et al.*: Use of technetium-99m sestamibi ECG-gated single-photon emission tomography for the evaluation of left ventricular function following coronary artery bypass graft: comparison with three-dimensional magnetic resonance imaging. *Eur J Nucl Med* 1999, 26(7):705–712.

44. Zuber E, Rosfors S: Effect of reversible hypoperfusion on left ventricular volumes measured with gated SPECT at rest and after adenosine infusion. *J Nucl Cardiol* 2000, 7(6):655–660.

45. Iskandrian AE, Germano G, VanDecker W, *et al.*: Validation of left ventricular volume measurements by gated SPECT 99mTc-labeled sestamibi imaging. *J Nucl Cardiol* 1998, 5(6):574–578.

46. Germano G, Kavanagh PB, Kavanagh JT, *et al.*: Repeatability of automatic left ventricular cavity volume measurements from myocardial perfusion SPECT. *J Nucl Cardiol* 1998, 5(5):477–483.

47. Everaert H, Vanhove C, Franken PR: Low-dose dobutamine gated single-photon emission tomography: comparison with stress echocardiography. *Eur J Nucl Med* 2000, 27(4):413–418.

48. Itti E, Rosso J, Damien P, *et al.*: Assessment of ejection fraction with Tl-201 gated SPECT in myocardial infarction: Precision in a rest-redistribution study and accuracy versus planar angiography. *J Nucl Cardiol* 2001, 8(1):31–39.

49. Germano G, Berman D, eds: Quantitative gated perfusion SPECT. In *Clinical Gated Cardiac SPECT*. Armonk, NY: Futura; 1999:115–146.

50. Damrongpipatkij Y, Mohammed F, Brown E, *et al.*: Quantitative cardiac SPECT: measuring diastolic function [abstract]. *J Nucl Med* 2000, 41(5):154P.

51. Higuchi T, Taki J, Yoneyama T, *et al.*: Diastolic and systolic parameters obtained by myocardial ECG-gated perfusion study [abstract]. *J Nucl Med* 2000, 41(5):160P.

52. Nakajima K, Taki J, Kawano M, *et al.*: Diastolic dysfunction in patients with systemic sclerosis detected by gated myocardial perfusion SPECT: an early sign of cardiac involvement. *J Nucl Med* 2001, 42(2):183–188.

53. Kumita S, Cho K, Nakajo H, *et al.*: Assessment of left ventricular diastolic function with electrocardiography-gated myocardial perfusion SPECT: comparison with multigated equilibrium radionuclide angiography. *J Nucl Cardiol* 2001, 8(5):568–574.

54. Higuchi T, Nakajima K, Taki J, *et al.*: The accuracy of left-ventricular time volume curve derived from ECG-gated myocardial perfusion SPECT [abstract]. *J Nucl Cardiol* 2001, 8(1):S18.

55. Higuchi T, Nakajima K, Taki J, *et al.*: Assessment of left ventricular systolic and diastolic function based on the edge detection method with myocardial ECG-gated SPET. *Eur J Nucl Med* 2001, 28(10):1512–1516.

56. Smith WH, Kastner RJ, Calnon DA, *et al.*: Quantitative gated single photon emission computed tomography imaging: a counts-based method for display and measurement of regional and global ventricular systolic function. *J Nucl Cardiol* 1997, 4(6):451–463.

57. Hoffman EJ, Huang SC, Phelps ME: Quantitation in positron emission computed tomography: 1. Effect of object size. *J Comput Assist Tomogr* 1979, 3(3):299–308.

58. Wallis JW, Miller TR: Three-dimensional display in nuclear medicine and radiology. *J Nucl Med* 1991, 32(3):534–546.

59. Germano G, Kavanagh PB, Waechter P, *et al.*: A new algorithm for the quantitation of myocardial perfusion SPECT. I: technical principles and reproducibility. *J Nucl Med* 2000, 41(4):712–719.

60. Garcia EV, Van Train K, Maddahi J, *et al.*: Quantification of rotational thallium-201 myocardial tomography. *J Nucl Med* 1985, 26(1):17–26.

61. Sharir T, Berman DS, Waechter PB, *et al.*: Quantitative analysis of regional motion and thickening by gated myocardial perfusion SPECT: normal heterogeneity and criteria for abnormality. *J Nucl Med* 2001, 42(11):1630–1638.

62. Kramer U, Miller S, Helber U, *et al.*: Variability in the MR tomographic determination of myocardial function and perfusion parameters in healthy subjects. *Rofo Fortschr Geb Rontgenstr Neuen Bildgeb Verfahr* 2000, 172(7):609–614.

63. Garcia EV, Van Train K, Maddahi J, *et al.*: Quantification of rotational thallium-201 myocardial tomography. *J Nucl Med* 1985, 26(1):17–26.

64. Ficaro EP, Kritzman JN, Corbett JR: Automatic segmental scoring of myocardial wall thickening and motion: validation of a new semi-quantitative algorithm [abstract]. *J Nucl Med* 2001, 42(5):171P.

65. Smanio PE, Watson DD, Segalla DL, *et al.*: Value of gating of technetium-99m sestamibi single-photon emission computed tomographic imaging. *J Am Coll Cardiol* 1997, 30(7):1687–1692.

66. Germano G, Chua T, Kiat H, *et al.*: A quantitative phantom analysis of artifacts due to hepatic activity in technetium-99m myocardial perfusion SPECT studies. *J Nucl Med* 1994, 35(2):356–359.

67. Buvat I, El Fakhri G, Walter R, *et al.*: Impact of reconstruction algorithms upon activity quantitation in Tc-99m cardiac SPECT [abstract]. *J Nucl Med* 1999, 40(5):148P.

68. Duncan B, Heller G: Acute rest myocardial perfusion imaging in the evaluation of patients with chest pain syndromes. *ACC Curr J Review* 1999, 8(6):52–56.

69. Taillefer R, DePuey EG, Udelson JE, *et al.*: Comparison between the end-diastolic images and the summed images of gated 99mTc-sestamibi SPECT perfusion study in detection of coronary artery disease in women. *J Nucl Cardiol* 1999, 6(2):169–176.

70. Mazzanti M, Germano G, Kiat H, *et al.*: Identification of severe and extensive coronary artery disease by automatic measurement of transient ischemic dilation of the left ventricle in dual-isotope myocardial perfusion SPECT. *J Am Coll Cardiol* 1996, 27(7):1612–1620.

71. Kritzman JN, Ficaro EP, Corbett JR: Post-stress LV dilation: the effect of imaging protocol, gender and attenuation correction [abstract]. *J Nucl Med* 2001, 42(5):50P.

72. Williams K, Schnieder C, Jain A: Transient ischemic dilatation (TID) with pharmacological stress dual isotope SPECT [abstract]. *Circulation* 2000, 102(18): II–546.

73. Germano G, Van Kriekinge S, Berman D: Quantitative gated blood pool SPECT. In *Clinical Gated Cardiac SPECT*. Edited by Germano G, Berman D. Armonk, NY: Futura; 1999:339–347.

74. Nichols K, Saouaf R, Bergmann S: Assessment of different gated blood pool SPECT right ventricle models [abstract]. *J Nucl Cardiol* 2001, 8(4):S130.

CHAPTER 11

MYOCARDIAL INNERVATION

Markus Schwaiger

The heart is innervated by sympathetic and parasympathetic nerve fibers, which modify cardiac performance to respond quickly and effectively to changing demands on cardiovascular performance. The sympathetic nervous system is considered stimulatory, yielding positive inotropic and chronotropic effects, while the parasympathetic nervous system exerts primarily negative chronotropic responses [1]. The autonomic innervation is divided into presynaptic and postsynaptic arms, which interact by release of neurotransmitters. The most common sympathetic neurotransmitter is norepinephrine, which is synthesized, stored, and metabolized within the sympathetic nerve terminal. Upon neurostimulation, the neurotransmitter is released by exocytosis within the synaptic cleft. A small portion of the released neurotransmitter interacts with α- and β-adrenergic receptors; β_1 receptors are the predominant receptors in the heart. Most of the released neurotransmitter undergoes reuptake in the nerve terminals (uptake 1); this norepinephrine transporter (NET, a sodium/chloride-dependent transport protein) has a high affinity to catecholamines and catecholamine analogues. Uptake 2 refers to nonneuronal uptake of catecholamines in cardiac tissue. Inside the nerve terminal, norepinephrine is either metabolized by monoamine oxidase or sequestered in vesicles by the vesicular monoamine transporter, a proton-dependent transport protein localized in the vesicle membrane. Uptake 1 regulates the extraneuronal concentration of adrenergic neurotransmitters and plays an important physiologic and pathophysiologic role in modifying signal transduction and extraneuronal catecholamine concentration. This regulatory role includes the reuptake of locally released norepinephrine as well as the uptake and metabolism of circulating catecholamines, which enter the extracellular space. This high affinity uptake system is of significance in protecting the heart from the deleterious effects of elevated levels of circulating catecholamines [2,3].

The density of sympathetic nerve terminals is highest in the right and left ventricles. Sympathetic nerve fibers travel along the vascular structures, penetrating the myocardial wall from the epicardial surface toward the endocardium. A heterogeneous distribution of nerve terminals has been reported in animals and humans, with a gradient from the base to the apex of the left ventricle [4,5]. In contrast, parasympathetic nerve fibers are found most predominantly in the atria. The nerve fibers travel along endocardial layers within the right and left ventricles. There is a high density of muscarinic receptors (predominantly M_2) that interact with the parasympathetic neurotransmitter acetylcholine released by the parasympathetic nerve terminals.

Several radiolabeled compounds have been synthesized to probe the sympathetic and parasympathetic nervous system at the pre- and postsynaptic levels [6]. SPECT and PET tracers can be divided into radiolabeled catecholamines and catecholamine analogues. The most commonly employed SPECT tracer is metaiodobenzylguanidine (mIBG), which represents an analogue of the antihypertensive drug guanethidine [7]. Radiolabeled catecholamine analogues for PET include metaraminol, metahydroxyephedrine, and phenylephrine [8–10]. These "false adrenergic neurotransmitters" share the same reuptake mechanism and endogenous storage with the true neurotransmitters, but are neither metabolized nor do they interact with postsynaptic receptors [11].

Although there is little tissue uptake of mIBG involving the nonneuronal transport process as well as passive diffusion, retention of mIBG in the myocardium has been found to be specific for the sympathetic nerve terminals [12]. Imaging studies involve a two-step protocol, with early image acquisition after tracer injection followed by delayed imaging (4 or more hours after injection). By comparing initial uptake and delayed retention, regional distribution of nerve terminals as well as washout kinetics can be determined. There is indirect evidence that the rate of mIBG washout from the myocardium represents a parameter of neuronal function [13,14]. Planar and SPECT images are usually acquired, and an activity ratio can be determined by using regions of interest placed over the myocardium and the mediastinum [15]. Most commonly, radiolabeling of mIBG is performed using isotopic exchange reactions. More recently, a non–carrier-added synthesis of ^{123}I-mIBG has been described. This labeling procedure yields a higher specific activity of ^{123}I-mIBG, which may affect the tissue kinetics. However, studies have shown that even in the carrier-added synthesis method, specific activity is high enough to avoid mass effects on the neuronal uptake mechanism [16,17].

The most successful PET radiopharmaceutical agent for the imaging of presynaptic function is C-11 hydroxyephedrine (^{11}C-HED) [18,19]. ^{11}C-HED is produced by N-methylation of metaraminol using C-11 methyliodide. In contrast to mIBG, this tracer uptake primarily reflects the transport by NET. Vesicular storage seems to occur, but binding inside the vesicle is weaker compared with norepinephrine due to its higher lipid solubility. Based on experimental observations, myocardial retention reflects a continuing release and reuptake of ^{11}C-HED in the nerve terminal. Tracer retention is commonly quantitated by calculating the retention index or retention fraction (which reflects myocardial activity at 40 minutes) normalized to the integral of the arterial input function [20]. More recently, a tracer kinetic model for ^{11}C-HED kinetics has been developed that allows calculation of the distribution volume within the myocardium [21].

Modifications of cardiac neuronal function have been reported in the pathophysiology of various cardiovascular diseases such as heart failure, arrhythmias, ischemic heart disease, and diabetes. In patients with heart failure, the presynaptic sympathetic nervous system is altered with decreased reuptake of norepinephrine [22]. In addition, there is down-regulation of β receptors observed in the presence of high levels of circulating catecholamines [2]. The alteration of the sympathetic nervous system within the left ventricle appears to be heterogeneous in patients with congestive heart failure, producing a marked gradient from the base to the apex of the left ventricle in presynaptic dysfunction [23]. An association has been reported between the extent of presynaptic sympathetic denervation in patients with congestive heart failure and clinical outcome [24,25]. Mortality is significantly higher in patients with denervated hearts, documented by reduced mIBG or ^{11}C-HED uptake, compared with patients with preserved presynaptic nerve function. It is unclear if this observation in selected patients represents an independent prognostic indicator, which can be used for risk stratification of heart failure patients. Recent clinical studies suggest that noninvasive characterization of the sympathetic system may be useful for selecting patients with heart failure for β-receptor blocker therapy [26,27].

Several experimental and clinical studies have linked pre- and postsynaptic function of the sympathetic nervous system and the presence of arrhythmias [28–30]. An association between the presence of arrhythmia and regional defects in presynaptic mIBG uptake has been described [31,32]. However, the prognostic value of altered regional or global tracer uptake and clinical outcome of patients with documented arrhythmias has not yet been established [33]. On the other hand, in patients with diabetic neuropathy, regional sympathetic denervation of the left ventricle has been described using mIBG and ^{11}C-HED imaging [34–37]. Starting at the apex and inferior wall of the left ventricle, this abnormality extends toward the inferior wall and base of the left ventricle as the neuropathic process advances. A correlation has been established between the degree of cardiac denervation and clinical parameters of autonomic dysfunction [38]. The scintigraphic determination of presynaptic tracer uptake appears to be more sensitive than clinical parameters in detecting early involvement of the heart in diabetic neuropathy. In addition, myocardial ischemia results in regional denervation of the heart even in the absence of myocardial damage [39,40]. Based on these data, neuronal tissue appears to be more sensitive to ischemia than myocytes. In support of this hypothesis, experimental and clinical data indicate that the area of neuronal damage following myocardial infarction is larger than the area of myocyte necrosis [14,41,42]. This mismatch of innervation and tissue viability has been demonstrated using mIBG as well as ^{11}C-HED imaging. Follow-up studies in patients with prior myocardial infarction reveal reinnervation of the acutely denervated area in about 40% of patients [43].

Finally, imaging approaches to evaluate presynaptic neuronal function have been used in patients following cardiac transplantation [19,44,45]. Low tracer uptake in patients shortly after transplantation documents the low nonspecific uptake of these tracers in the denervated myocardium [46]. However, as time after cardiac transplantation passes, there is evidence for regional reinnervation [19]. Uptake of radiolabeled catecholamines in the anterior wall, septum, and base of the left ventricle indicates the reappearance of functioning sympathetic nerve terminals. The pharmacologic integrity of these nerve terminals has been demonstrated by studies of neurotransmitter released following the intracoronary injection of tyramine [47]. The reinnervation process is beneficial for the exercise performance of patients following heart transplantation [48].

The scintigraphic visualization of cardiac innervation using radiopharmaceutical agents developed for PET or SPECT allows a unique pathophysiologic evaluation of disease processes that affect the autonomic nervous system. However, most of these imaging approaches have been used predominantly for clinical research. The clinical application of these innovative methods will depend on future documentation of their diagnostic and prognostic value in patients with cardiovascular disease. Particularly, the initial results in patients with congestive heart failure are promising but require confirmation in prospective multicenter trials [49].

Autonomic Nervous System

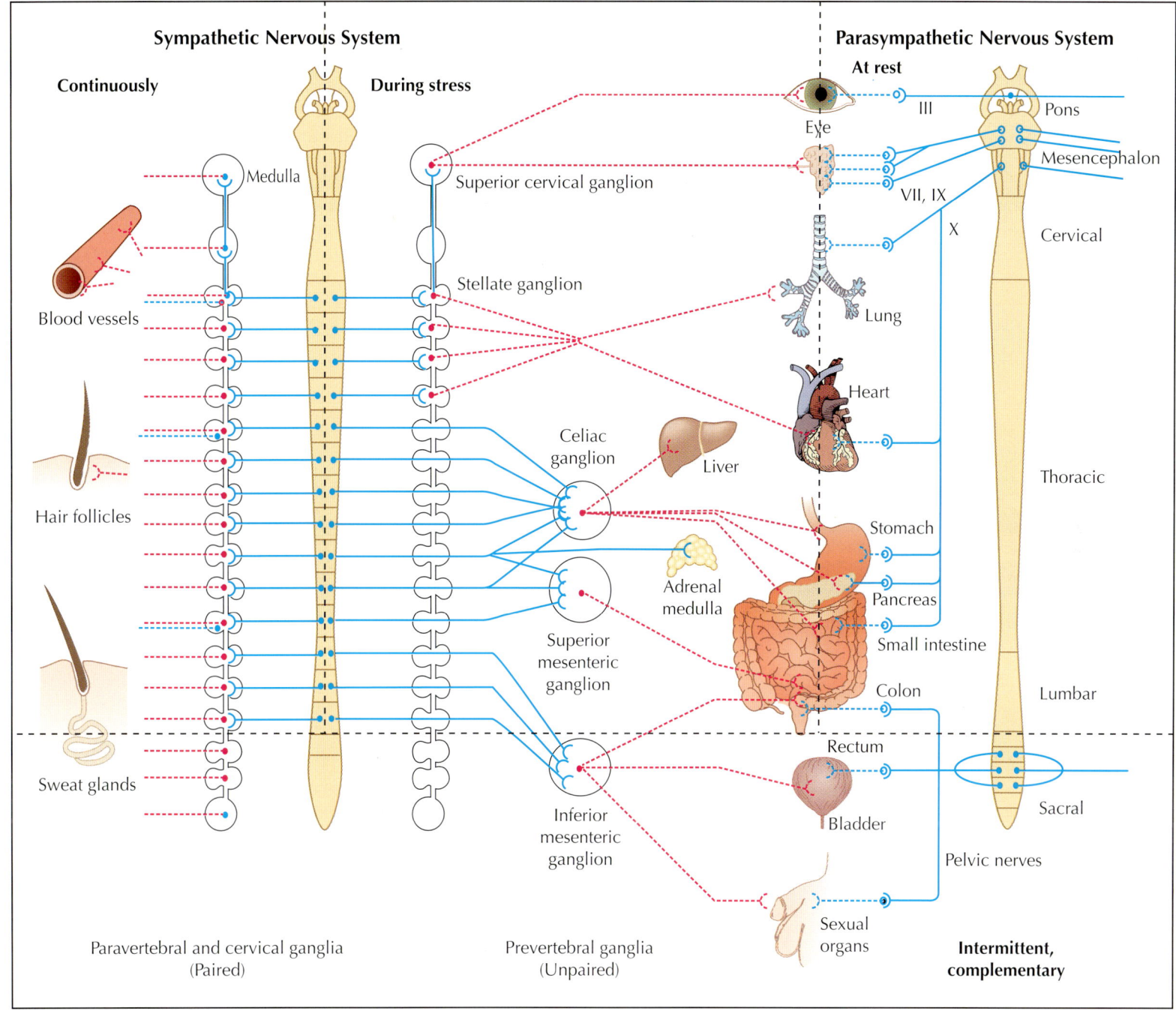

Figure 11-1. Structure of the autonomic nervous system (ANS). The ANS is historically divided in two major efferent components, the sympathetic (cervicothoracic, SNS) and parasympathetic (craniosacral, PNS) nervous systems. In either case, end-organ innervation is provided by nerve fibers originating from autonomic ganglia located outside the central nervous system (CNS), driven by preganglionic cholinergic input from the CNS (*solid blue lines*). Main differences consist of the types of principal transmitter used by postganglionic fibers (PNS: acetylcholine [*dotted blue*]; SNS: norepinephrine [*dotted red*]), the location of the ganglia (PNS: near or within the end organs; SNS: near the spinal cord, either paravertebral [22 pairs] or prevertebral [unpaired]), the degree of divergence and convergence of preganglionic input to post-ganglionic neurons (PNS: very little; SNS: considerable), and their respective functional roles. Most internal organs receive input from both PNS and SNS (*center*). Important exceptions include skin and blood vessels (pilomotor and sudomotor) functions, which are exclusively controlled by noradrenergic and cholinergic post-ganglionic fibers of SNS origin only (*left*), and the adrenal gland, which functions as the equivalent of a sympathetic ganglion, causing systemic catecholamine release (80% epinephrine, 20% norepinephrine) in response to preganglionic cholinergic stimulation. In the case of most internal organs, SNS and PNS exert opposite effects. PNS effects normally prevail at rest, whereas SNS effects predominate during stress or exercise (flight or fight response). In genitourinary organs, SNS and PNS functions are complementary; for example, PNS mediates erection, SNS mediates ejaculation. (*Adapted from* Bannister and Mathias [50].)

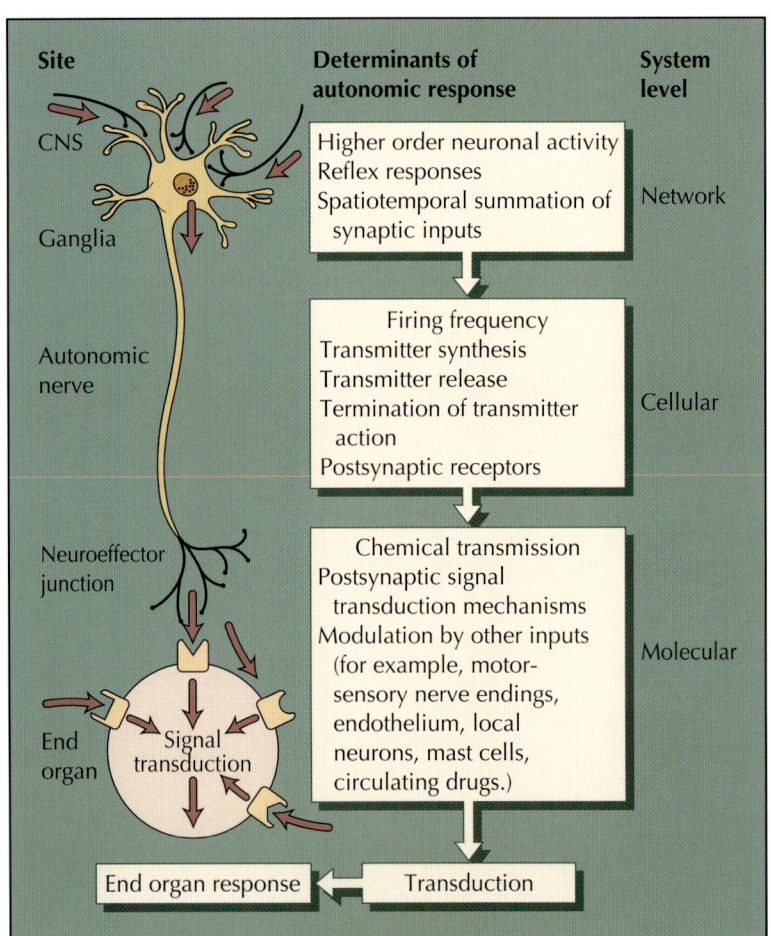

FIGURE 11-2. Determinants of end-organ control by the autonomic nervous system (ANS). Control mechanisms operate concurrently at different system levels. At a neural network level, processing and integration of patterns of neuronal activity (including reflex responses) determine the firing frequency of autonomic efferent nerve fibers. Cellular mechanisms operative at the level of nerve terminals determine the types, amounts, and fates of chemical transmitters released at autonomic synapses and neuroeffector junctions. At a molecular level, membrane receptor and post-synaptic signal transduction mechanisms determine the types and magnitude of cellular effector responses. At each of these system levels, various interactions occur between distinct functional divisions of the ANS (sympathetic, parasympathetic, afferent, enteric, and local neuronal systems) involving classic (cholinergic and adrenergic) transmitters as well as a variety of nonclassic neurotransmitter systems. CNS—central nervous system. (*Adapted from* Milner and Burnstock [51].)

Adrenergic Nerve Terminals

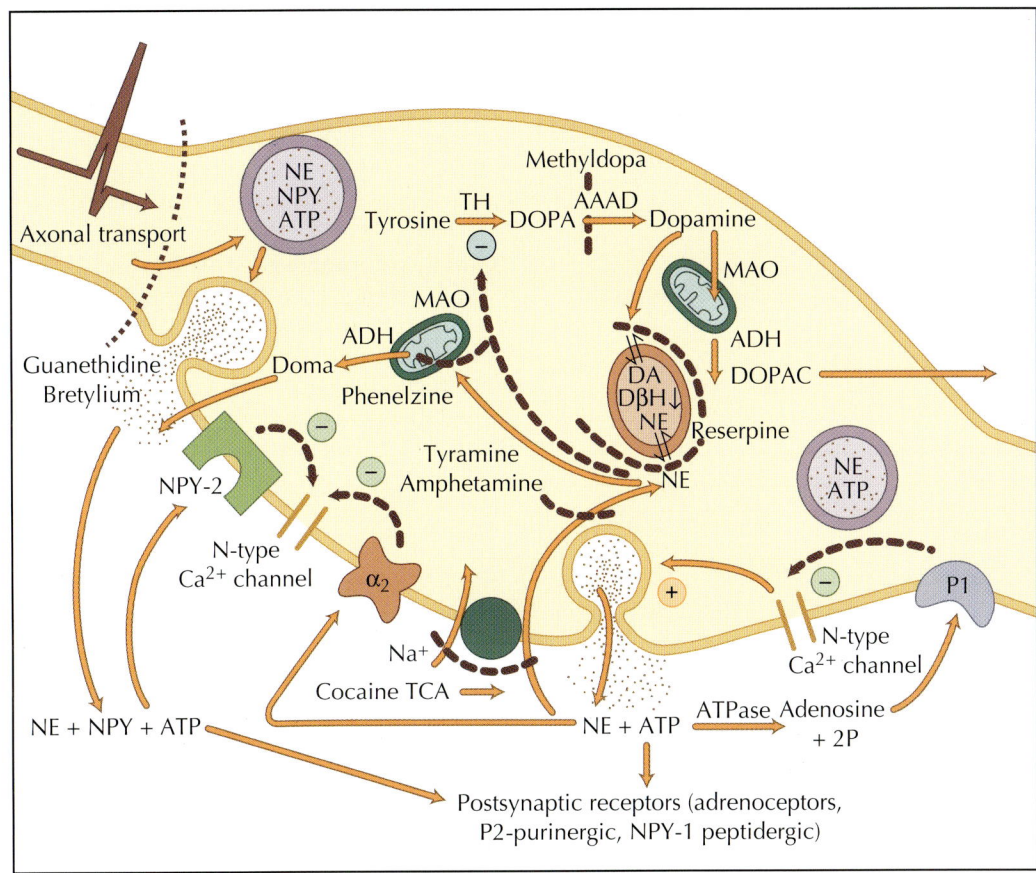

FIGURE 11-3. Neurotransmitter synthesis and release at adrenergic nerve terminals. Mechanisms controlling transmitter synthesis and release at adrenergic nerve terminals. Transmitters are stored in two types of synaptic vesicles, small vesicles containing only the principal transmitter norepinephrine (NE) and cotransmitter adenosine triphosphate (ATP) (each synthesized within the nerve terminal itself), and larger dense-core vesicles containing the polypeptide cotransmitter neuropeptide Y (NPY) and chromogranin (both of which are exclusively synthesized in the cell soma) as well as NE and ATP. The rate-limiting step for NE synthesis in the nerve terminal is tyrosine hydroxylase (TH) enzyme activity, which is negatively controlled by the cytoplasmic concentration of NE. The TH enzymatic product dopa is decarboxylated to dopamine by (unspecific) aromatic L-amino acid decarboxylase (AAAD) in a step subject to therapeutic interference by provision of the "false" substrate methyldopa (resulting in the eventual formation of the "false transmitter" -methyl-NE). Dopamine is to equal proportions either deaminated and excreted as DOPAC (3,4-dihydroxyphenylacetic acid) or taken up into dopamine–hydroxylase (DH)-containing storage vesicles via a reserpine-sensitive active uptake process and hydroxylated to NE. The cytoplasmic concentration of NE is determined by a dynamic equilibrium established between diffusion (leakage) out of storage vesicles, reserpine-sensitive (active) reuptake into storage vesicles, cytoplasmic displacement and extrusion by indirect sympathomimetics such as tyramine and amphetamine, reuptake from the extracellular space via a Na^+-dependent cotransport mechanism sensitive to inhibition by cocaine or tricyclic antidepressants, and elimination after metabolizing to 3,4-dihydroxymandelic acid (DOMA) by mitochondrial monoamine oxidase (MAO) and aldehyde dehydrogenase (ADH), a pathway sensitive to inhibition by MAO inhibitors such as phenelzine. In adrenal medullary neurons, 80% of cytoplasmic NE is methylized by N-methyl transferase into epinephrine before being packaged into storage vesicles. Nerve stimulation-evoked physiologic transmitter release occurs via fusion of synaptic storage vesicles with the cell membrane after the invasion of the nerve terminal by propagated action potentials (sensitive to blockade by guanethidine or bretylium) and the resulting increase in cytoplasmic Ca^{2+} through activation of voltage-sensitive (predominantly N-type) Ca^{2+} channels. Upon release, ATP, NE, and NPY produce neuroeffector responses through actions on postsynaptic membrane receptors. In addition, all three transmitters inhibit further release through action on presynaptic (P1, 2-adrenergic, NPY-2) receptors [52,53]. Transmitter actions are terminated by hydrolysis (ATP), reuptake into nerve terminals (NE), uptake into nonneuronal tissue and metabolism by catechol-O-methyl transferase (COMT) (NE), and diffusion away from the terminal and into the bloodstream (NE, NPY). ADH—aldehyde dehydrogenase; TCA—tricyclic antidepressants; TH—tyrosine hydroxylase. (*Adapted from* Nicholls *et al.* [54].)

RADIOPHARMACEUTICALS

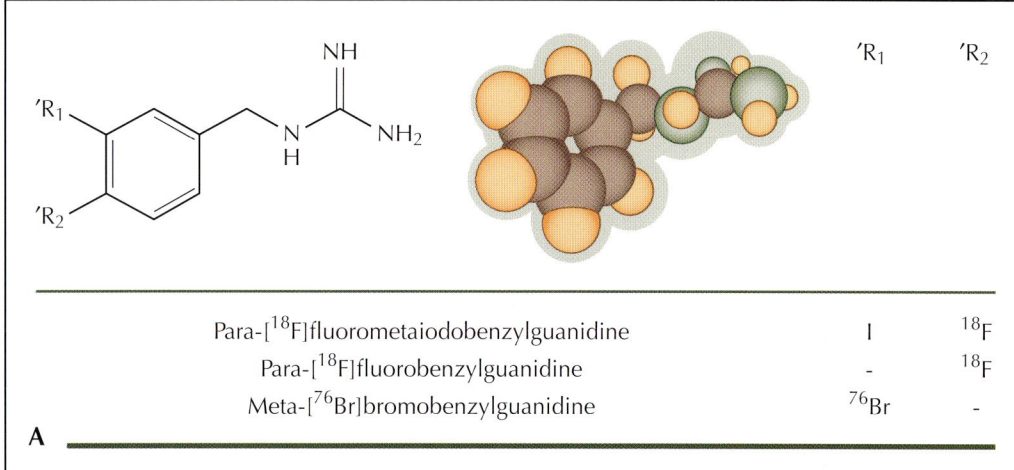

		'R₁	'R₂
Para-[^{18}F]fluorometaiodobenzylguanidine		I	^{18}F
Para-[^{18}F]fluorobenzylguanidine		-	^{18}F
Meta-[^{76}Br]bromobenzylguanidine		^{76}Br	-

A

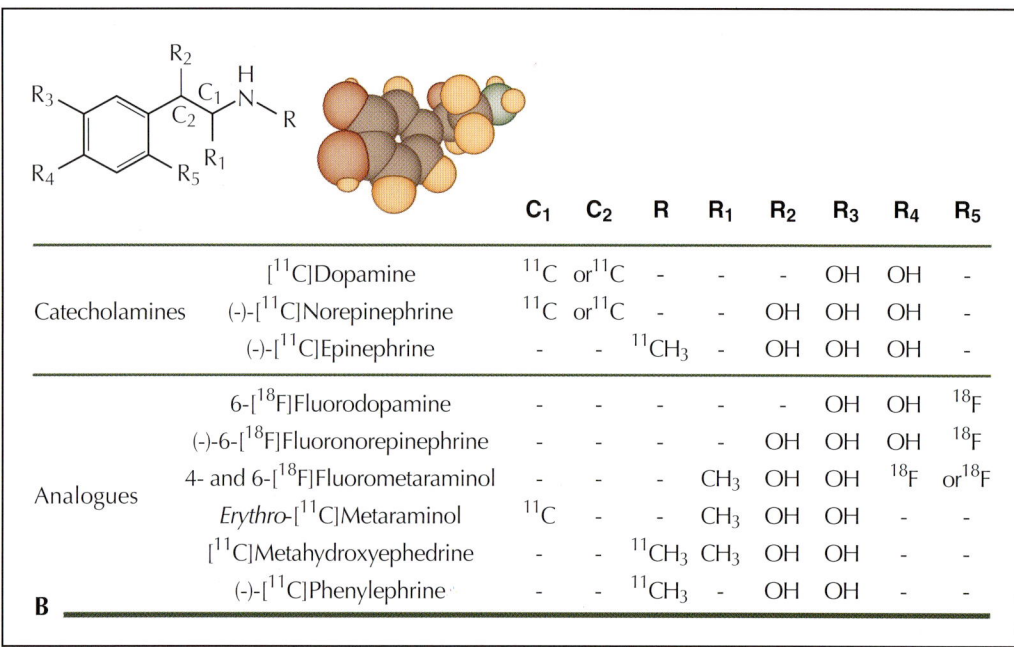

		C₁	C₂	R	R₁	R₂	R₃	R₄	R₅
Catecholamines	[^{11}C]Dopamine	^{11}C or^{11}C		-	-	-	OH	OH	-
	(-)-[^{11}C]Norepinephrine	^{11}C or^{11}C		-	-	OH	OH	OH	-
	(-)-[^{11}C]Epinephrine	-	-	^{11}CH₃	-	OH	OH	OH	-
Analogues	6-[^{18}F]Fluorodopamine	-	-	-	-	-	OH	OH	^{18}F
	(-)-6-[^{18}F]Fluoronorepinephrine	-	-	-	-	OH	OH	OH	^{18}F
	4- and 6-[^{18}F]Fluorometaraminol	-	-	-	CH₃	OH	OH	^{18}F	or^{18}F
	Erythro-[^{11}C]Metaraminol	^{11}C	-	-	CH₃	OH	OH	-	-
	[^{11}C]Metahydroxyephedrine	-	-	^{11}CH₃	CH₃	OH	OH	-	-
	(-)-[^{11}C]Phenylephrine	-	-	^{11}CH₃	-	OH	OH	-	-

B

FIGURE 11-4. PET radiotracers for mapping of cardiac sympathetic neurons. The radiotracers used for the evaluation of the sympathetic nervous system can be classified in three categories: radiolabeled analogues of benzylguanidine (**A**), radiolabeled catecholamines or catecholamine analogues (**B**), and β-adrenoceptor ligands (**C**). The common lead structure and a computed model of the prototypic compounds are provided. The ^{11}C-carbon position in *panel A* are indicated by 'R₁ and 'R₂ and in *panel C* by C₁ and C₂. The radiolabeled compounds are listed under the lead structures and computed models.

[structures shown: [^{11}C]CGP 12177, [^{11}C]CGP 12388, [^{18}C]Fluorocarazolol]

C

TRACER RETENTION IN NORMAL MYOCARDIUM

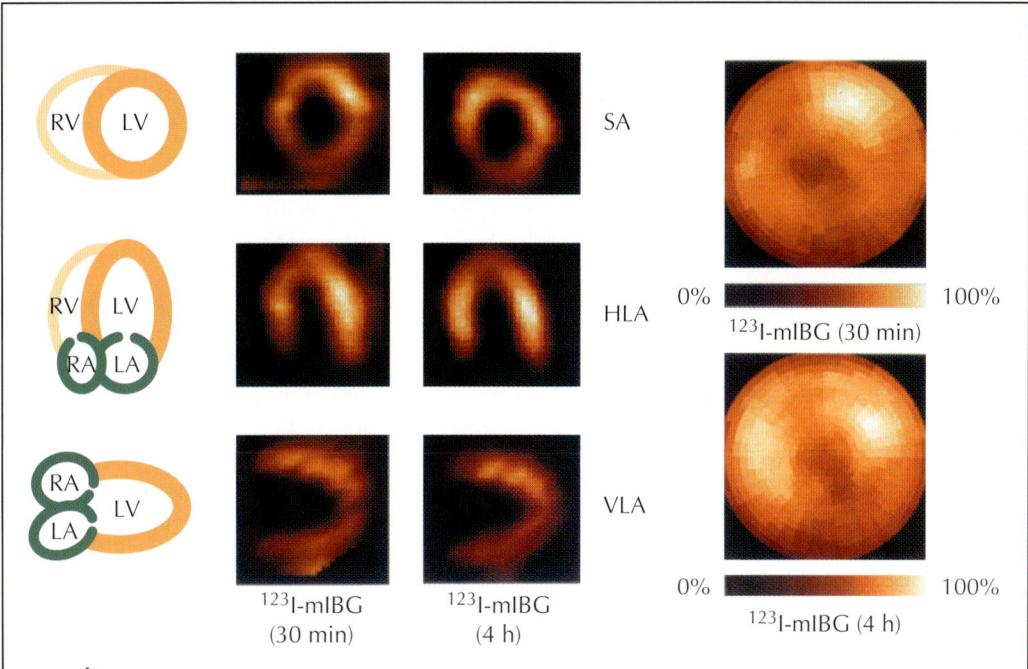

FIGURE 11-5. Metaiodobenzylguanidine (mIBG) distribution in normal myocardium. SPECT images were obtained at 180° in a normal healthy volunteer 30 minutes after intravenous injection of 10 mCi ^{123}I-mIBG. Data acquisition was repeated 4 hours later. Regional myocardial tracer retention is displayed in short-axis (SA), horizontal long-axis (HLA), and vertical long-axis (VLA) views. There is homogeneous uptake of the tracer throughout the myocardium of the left ventricle (LV). The right ventricle (RV), right atrium (RA), and left atrium (LA) are not seen due to their thin walls. Polar maps represent the 3-D distribution of the tracer within the left ventricle. The activity at the apex is displayed at the center of the map while the basal parts of the left ventricle represent the outer rings. The activity is normalized to maximal activity within the left ventricle. The regional tracer retention was determined by circumferential radial search for activity maxima. The individual circumferential profiles of several myocardial slices are then combined into one representative polar map. Note the relatively low activity of ^{123}I-mIBG in the inferior and inferoseptal areas, showing the known heterogeneity of neuronal distribution. The same distribution pattern can be found in the 4-hour images, which are also normalized to their own maxima. The relative washout of activity between 30 minutes and 4 hours averages around 20% to 30% in healthy people [15]. The late images are considered specific for the relative distribution of sympathetic nerve terminals, while the washout has been used as a marker of neuronal integrity or sympathetic tone.

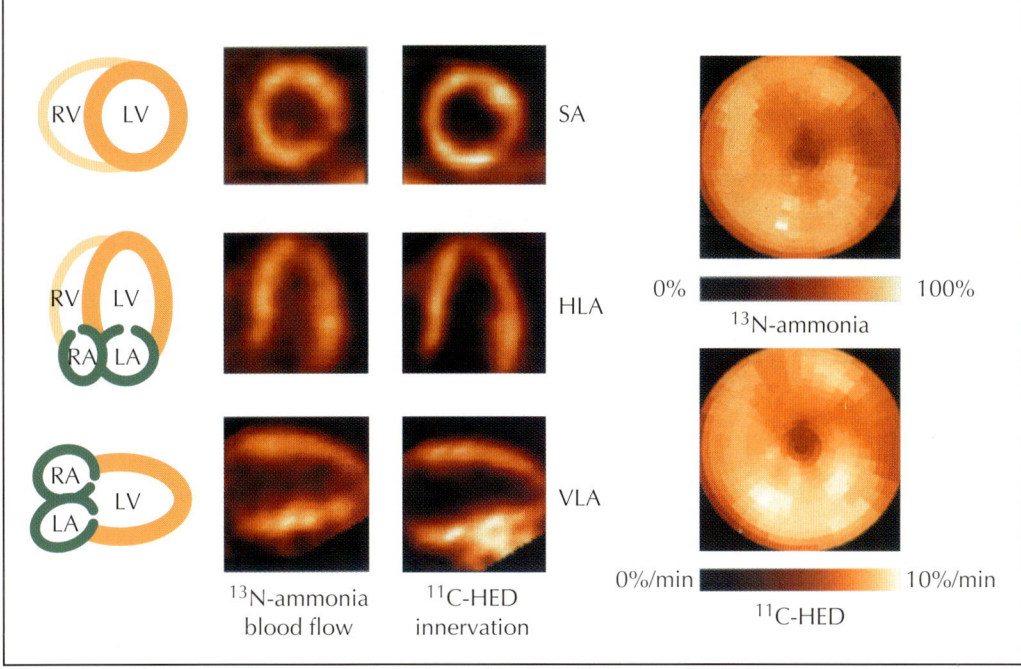

FIGURE 11-6. C-11 hydroxyephedrine (^{11}C-HED) distribution in normal myocardium. PET images in short-axis (SA), horizontal long-axis (HLA), and vertical long-axis (VLA) views were obtained following an injection of 20 mCi ^{13}N-ammonia as blood flow marker and about 40 minutes after the intravenous injection of 20 mCi ^{11}C-HED. The myocardial blood flow is homogeneous throughout the left ventricle (LV), paralleled by homogeneous uptake of ^{11}C-HED in all segments of the LV. Polar maps using circumferential profile analysis display homogeneous distribution of ^{13}N-ammonia and ^{11}C-HED. The polar maps of flow are normalized to their own maxima, while the ^{11}C-HED data are expressed by retention index. This index represents the activity at 40 minutes normalized to arterial input function, derived from a region of interest placed over left ventricular activity. Dynamic PET images allow for generation of myocardial and blood time activity curves. LA—left atrium; RA—right atrium; RV—right ventricle.

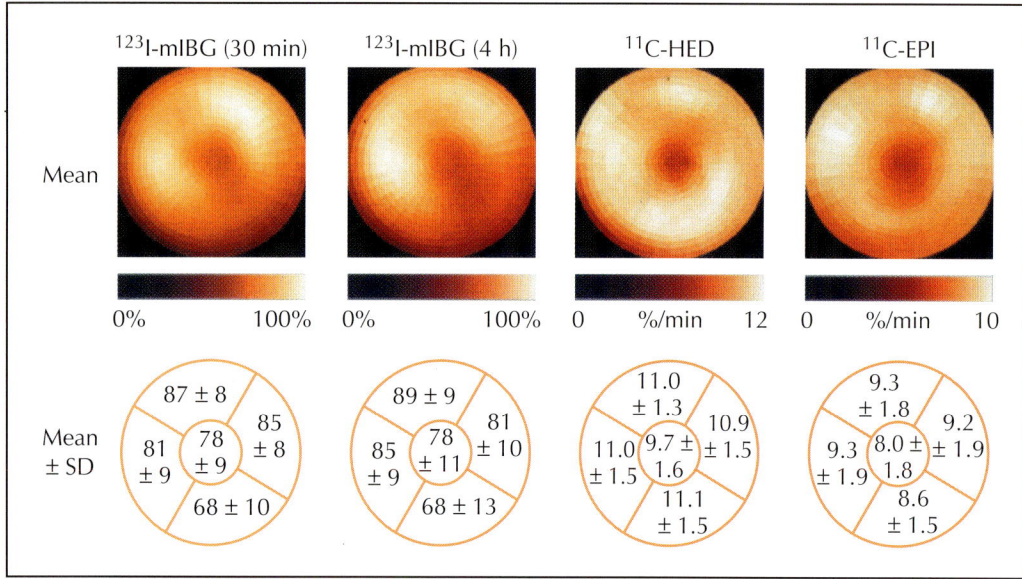

FIGURE 11-7. Comparison of normal tracer distribution of I-123 metaiodobenzylguanidine (^{123}I-mIBG), C-11 hydroxyephedrine (^{11}C-HED), and C-11 epinephrine (^{11}C-EPI) in normal myocardium. For each tracer distribution, 10 patients were imaged following intravenous injection of 10 mCi ^{123}I-mIBG, 20 mCi ^{11}C-HED, and 20 mCi ^{11}C-EPI. The relative tracer distribution normalized to the individual maximum in each patient is displayed in the lower panel. Note the slight heterogeneity of tracer retention at 30 minutes and 4 hours after ^{123}I-mIBG injection. The relative activity in the inferior segments of the left ventricle including the apex show significantly lower values as compared to the anteroseptal and anterolateral segments. This may represent an attenuation artifact, but inhomogeneous density of sympathetic nerve terminals in normal myocardium cannot be ruled out. The C-11 tracer retention is expressed as retention index, which represents tracer activity 40 minutes after tracer injection, normalized to the arterial input function obtained after placing a region of interest over the cavity of the left ventricle [19]. The retention index is expressed as %/min. ^{11}C-EPI retention was obtained 30 minutes after tracer injection and expressed as myocardial retention index. These measurements of myocardial PET tracer uptake display greater homogeneity compared with mIBG data. The lower retention index in the apex of the left ventricle most likely represents partial volume effect during nongated PET data acquisition. PET data are acquired with attenuation correction. However, there may be biologic differences in affinity for uptake I between mIBG and HED.

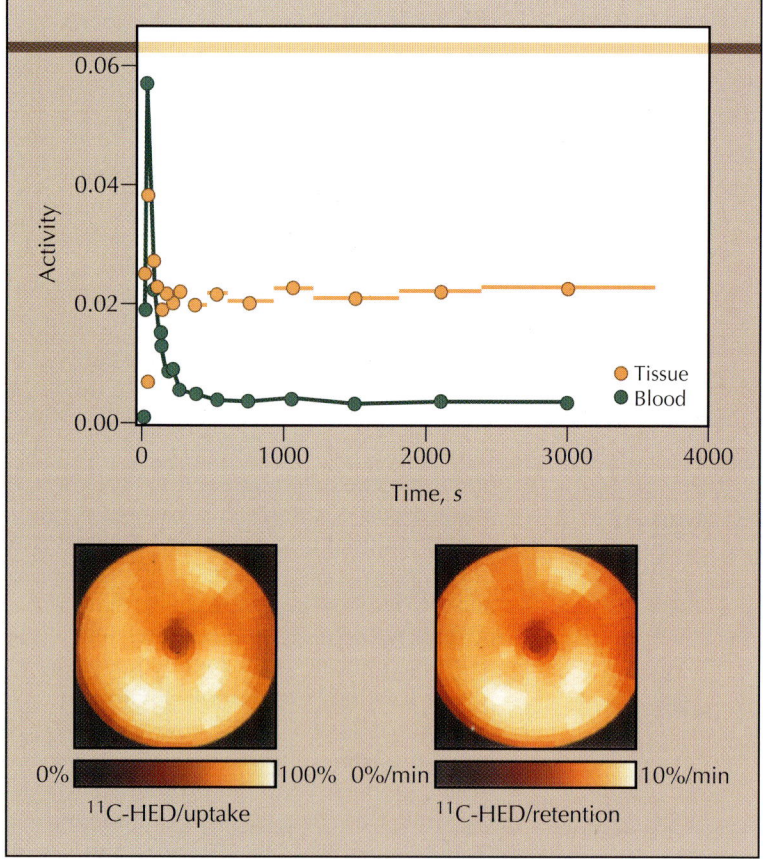

FIGURE 11-8. Time-activity curve obtained after intravenous injection of 20 mCi of the tracer C-11 hydroxyephedrine (^{11}C-HED) in a healthy volunteer. Dynamic PET imaging with short framing rate allows the determination of tracer time-activity curves of tissue and blood pool. The time-activity curves were determined using regions of interest placed over the chamber of the left ventricle for the determination of blood activity and placed over the left ventricular myocardium for the tissue activity distribution. The tracer rapidly clears from the blood, resulting in little residual blood activity minutes after tracer injection. In contrast, the activity obtained from the myocardial region of interest shows stable retention in the myocardium over the time of observation. The initial peak of myocardial tracer activity measured reflects contamination by blood pool activity. Dividing this activity measured 30 to 40 minutes after tracer injection by the integral of the input function, which reflects the available tracer to the myocardium during this time, yields the calculation of the myocardial retention index. This index averages over 12% in the normal heart.

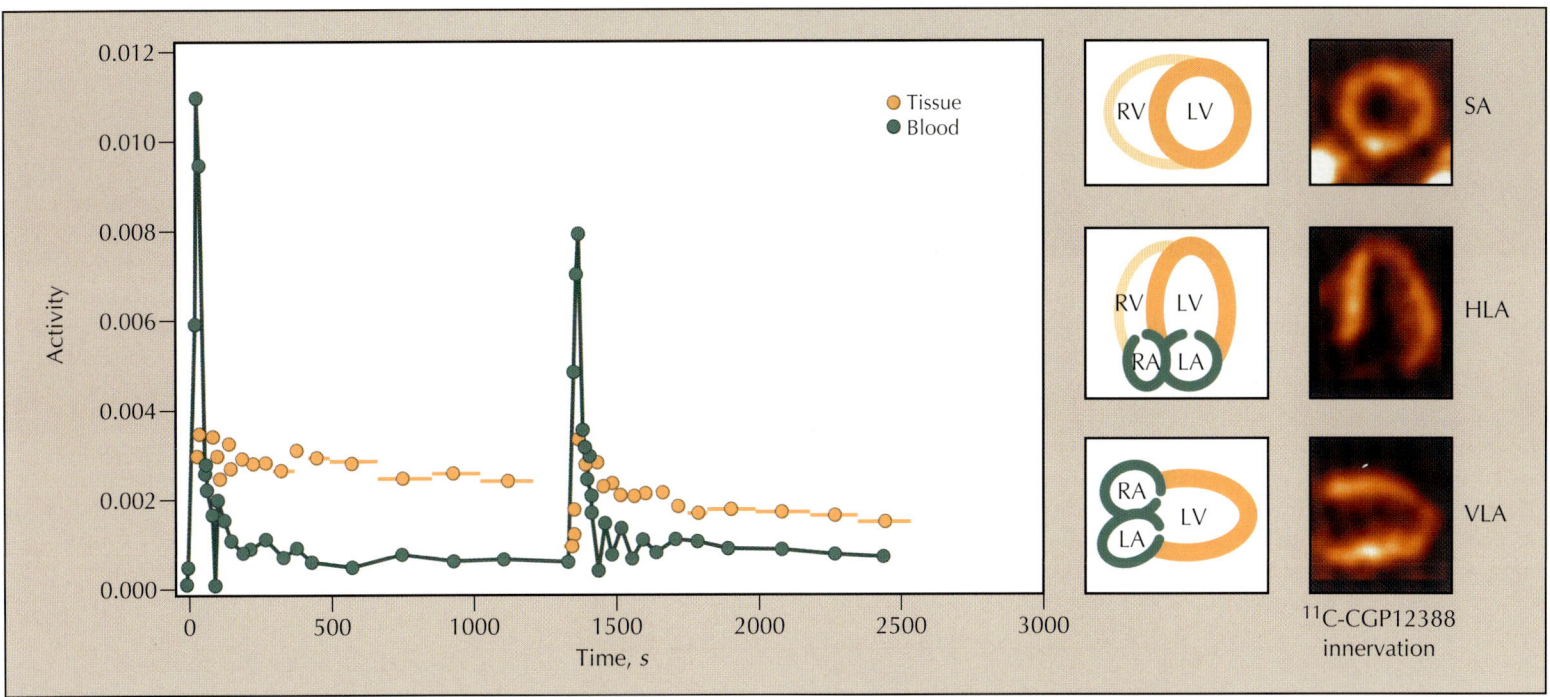

FIGURE 11-9. β receptor distribution in normal myocardium. PET images following the intravenous injection of β-receptor antagonist ^{11}C-CGP12388 are shown in short-axis (SA), horizontal long-axis (HLA), and vertical long-axis (VLA) images. Images were obtained 40 minutes after tracer injection and show high contrast between myocardial and nonmyocardial tissue. Pretreatment of patients with cold β-blocker β-receptor antagonists showed reduced tracer retention, suggesting high specific binding to the receptors. However, the shown retention images at 40 minutes primarily represent the delivery of tracer to the myocardium, which is determined by blood flow. To calculate the density of β receptors in the myocardium, a tracer kinetic model has been proposed by Delforge et al. [55]. A comparison of ^{11}C-CGP measurements with β-receptor density measured in vitro resulted in a linear correlation with high correlation coefficients. Using a tracer kinetic model consisting of two tracer injections with different specific activities, the receptor density can be calculated by curve-fitting procedures of tissue and blood pool–time-activity curves [55]. LA—left atrium; LV—left ventricle; RA—right atrium; RV—right ventricle.

MYOCARDIAL INFARCTION

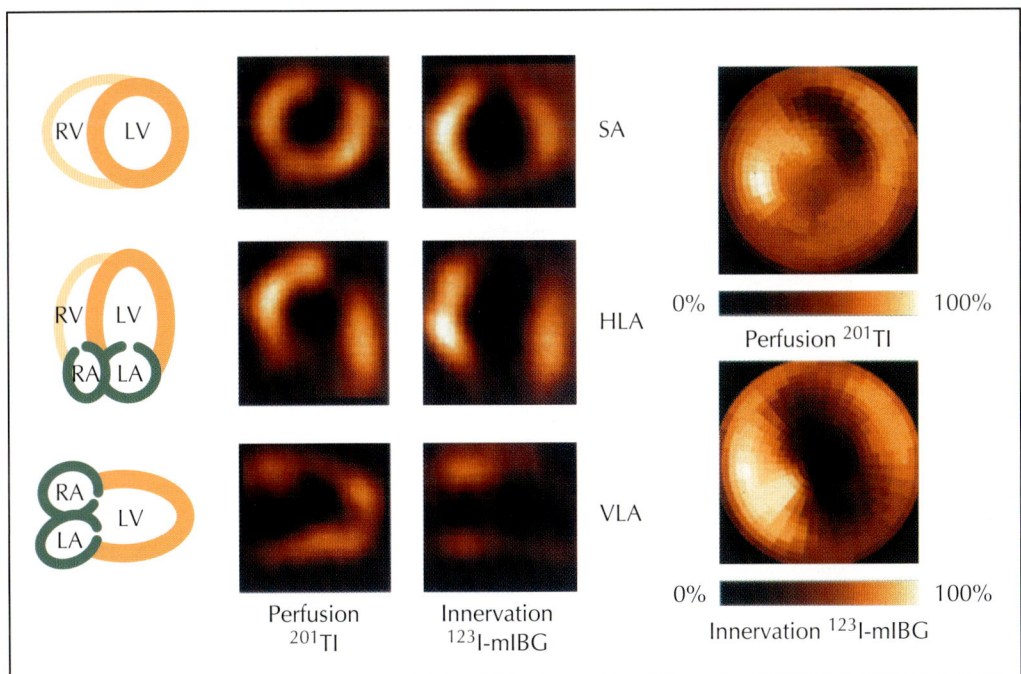

FIGURE 11-10. Assessment of neuronal function in the infarct zone. SPECT images were obtained in a patient within 14 days of an anterior myocardial infarction. The tomographic slices are displayed in short-axis (SA), horizontal long-axis (HLA), and vertical long-axis views (VLA). Regional retention of 10 mCi I-123 metaiodobenzylguanidine (^{123}I-mIBG) after 4 hours was compared with the myocardial perfusion as assessed from images acquired 20 minutes after injection of 2 mCi of ^{201}Tl. There is a perfusion abnormality in the ^{201}Tl images involving the anterolateral wall of the left ventricle. The images obtained after ^{123}I-mIBG injection reveal a markedly larger area of reduced ^{123}I-mIBG retention involving the anterolateral wall as well as the distal inferior wall. Polar maps display the disparity of perfusion and neuronal abnormality, reflecting the infarct size and area of denervation. This mismatch between perfusion and ^{123}I-mIBG retention indicates denervation of areas that survived the ischemic event. The mismatch between infarct size and denervation is present in almost 80% of patients after acute myocardial infarction. Although there is no clear correlation between extent and severity of myocardial denervation following myocardial infarction and clinical outcome, this disparity between denervation and infarct size has been linked to perioperative complications. Several studies have investigated the incidence of reinnervation following myocardial infarction [56–58]. The results are controversial because some studies show no reinnervation for up to 6 months, while others show that reinnervation takes place within few a months after the acute event. About 40% of infarcted segments show some degree of reinnervation, most likely reflecting a different degree of neuronal injury [15]. LA—left atrium; LV—left ventricle; RA—right atrium; RV—right ventricle.

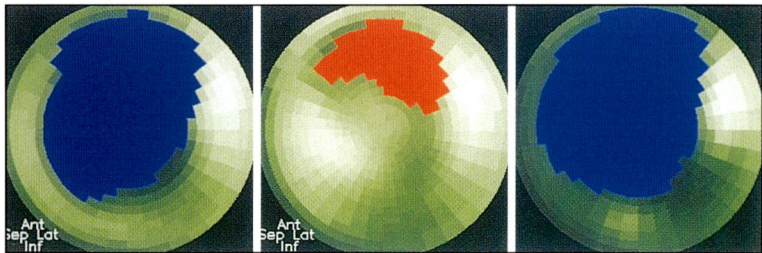

FIGURE 11-11. Neuronal damage in ischemic myocardium. ^{99m}Tc-sestamibi and ^{123}I-metaiodobenzylguanidine (^{123}I-mIBG) images were acquired in a 78-year-old man with anterior myocardial infarction, and polar maps were plotted to evaluate the area of risk, area of infarct, and neuronal integrity. After injection of the first sestamibi dose in the emergency room, the patient was transferred to the cardiac catheterization laboratory and percutaneous intervention of the left anterior descending artery was performed. Several hours after the intervention, SPECT images were taken. Using a 50% threshold of regional ^{99m}Tc-sestamibi activity, the area of risk was determined to be 58% of the left ventricle (*left*). The SPECT imaging was repeated at rest 14 days after the acute event. Based on the relative retention of ^{99m}Tc-sestamibi, the final infarct size was calculated again using a 50% threshold. The final infarct size was determined to be 15% of the left ventricle, documenting considerable salvage of myocardium following reperfusion therapy (*center*). The ^{123}I-mIBG images obtained on the 15th day following myocardial infarction display a large area of denervation within the left ventricle (59.3% of the left ventricle) comparable to the area at ischemic risk (*right*). These data indicate that the area of denervation, as determined by ^{123}I-mIBG images of tracer retention in the myocardium, is considerably larger than the infarct size, suggesting a mismatch between denervation and final infarct size. Interestingly, the area of denervation accurately matches the area of risk determined early during the ischemic event. This example confirms animal data, which indicate the higher sensitivity of neuronal activities to myocardial ischemia. Therefore, the ^{123}I-mIBG images obtained at 14 days after the ischemic event still reflect the area of risk as evidence of the extent and severity of the initial ischemic area [40,59–61].

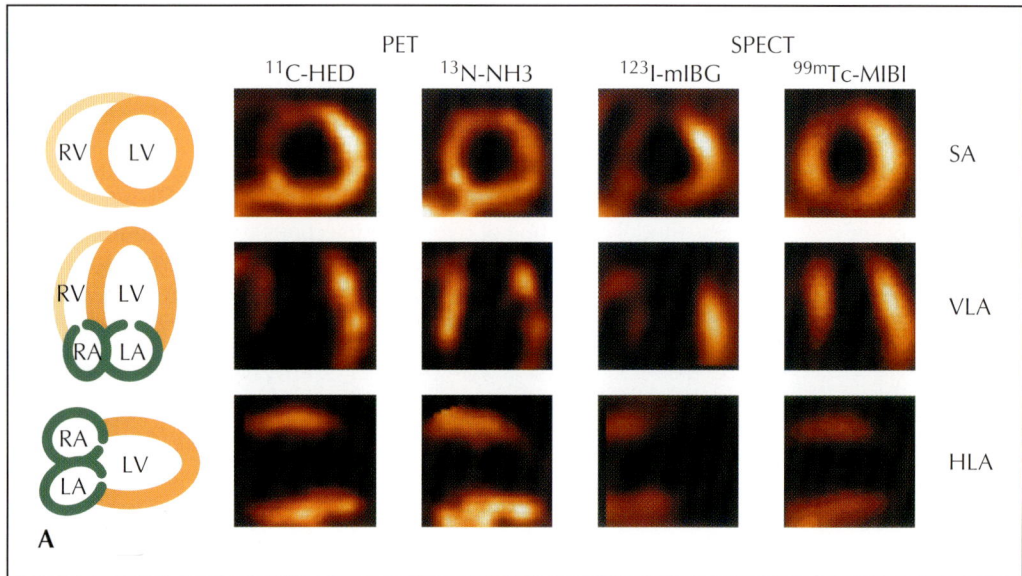

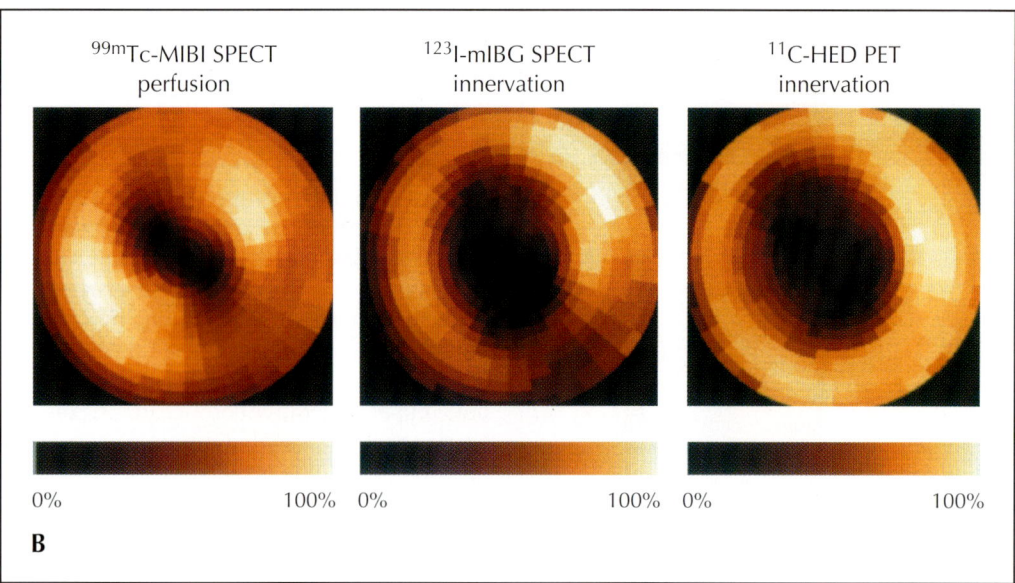

FIGURE 11-12. Comparison of SPECT and PET imaging of neural integrity. PET and SPECT images were obtained about 1 week after acute anterior myocardial infarction. **A**, The tomographic slices are displayed in short-axis (SA), vertical long-axis (VLA), and horizontal long-axis (HLA) views. The neuronal PET tracer C-11 hydroxyephedrine (^{11}C-HED) is compared with the regional myocardial perfusion as determined by ^{13}N-ammonia (^{13}N-NH$_3$). The SPECT images display the myocardial retention of ^{123}I-metaiodobenzylguanidine (^{123}I-mIBG) compared with the retention of ^{99m}Tc-sestamibi as blood flow marker. In both cases, there are perfusion abnormalities in the distal anterior wall and apex of the left ventricle (LV), best seen in the VLA and HLA views. The images of the presynaptic nerve terminals with ^{11}C-HED and ^{123}I-mIBG show tracer retention in the apex and anterior wall exceeding the area of perfusion abnormalities, especially in the septal areas of the LV. However, the ^{123}I-mIBG images show a larger defect involving also the inferior wall of the LV, which cannot be appreciated in the ^{11}C-HED images. This may represent an attenuation artifact of SPECT imaging or differences in the biologic behavior of ^{123}I-mIBG compared with ^{11}C-HED.

B, Quantitative analysis of PET and SPECT images are shown in polar maps. *Left*, Perfusion data obtained following ^{99m}Tc-sestamibi injection; *center*, the polar map derived from the ^{123}I-mIBG images; and *right*, the polar map following ^{11}C-HED injection. The area of myocardial infarction in the distal anterior septal wall and apex is denervated on both PET and SPECT maps. However, the area of denervation is larger than the final infarct size. The area of denervation appears largest in the ^{123}I-mIBG SPECT data involving not only the anterior, anteroseptal, and apical areas, but also the inferolateral wall, which is not present in the ^{11}C-HED data.

CARDIOMYOPATHY AND ARRHYTHMIAS

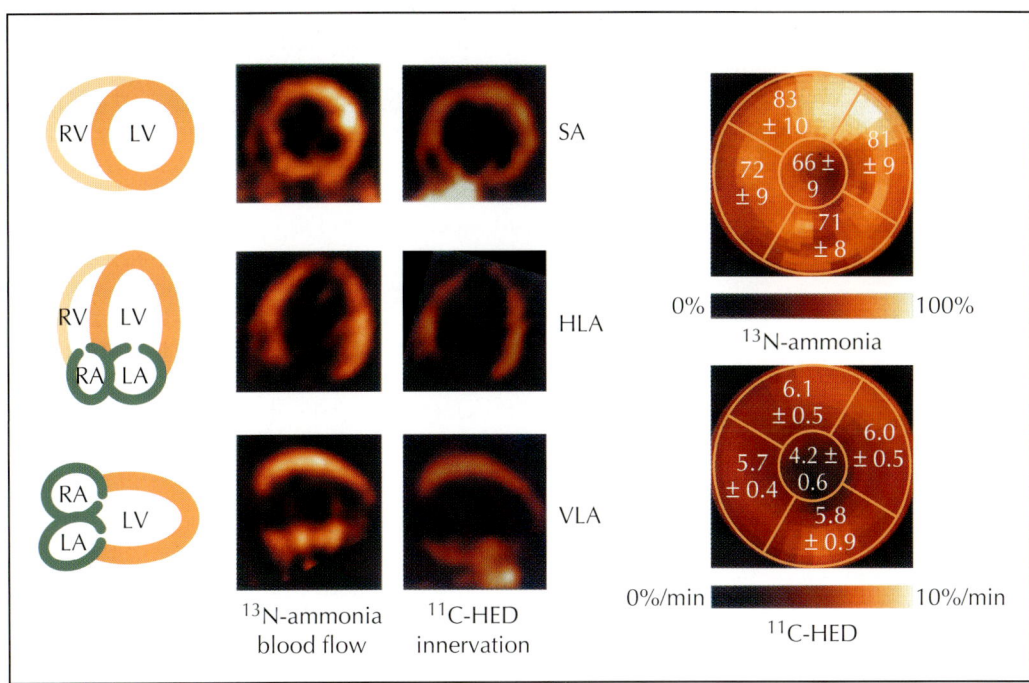

FIGURE 11-13. Role of neuronal imaging in cardiomyopathy. PET images were obtained in a patient with dilated cardiomyopathy and reduced left ventricular (LV) function following the injection of ^{13}N-ammonia and 40 minutes after the injection of C-11 hydroxyephedrine (^{11}C-HED). The tomographic slices are displayed in short-axis (SA), horizontal long-axis (HLA), and vertical long-axis (VLA) views. There is relatively homogeneous distribution of ^{13}N-ammonia, indicating integrity of myocardial perfusion. However, there is markedly reduced retention of ^{11}C-HED, indicating partial denervation of the LV in this patient with dilated cardiomyopathy. The retention index is reduced to 6% (normal values > 12%). The area of denervation is most evident in the distal anterior wall and apical area of the LV, confirming reports that injury of the autonomic nervous system is a heterogeneous process in patients with congestive heart failure [23]. This PET example confirms several reports, which have shown reduced ^{123}I-metaiodobenzyl-guanidine (^{123}I-mIBG) retention in the myocardium of patients with congestive heart failure. The SPECT ^{123}I-mIBG retention, however, can only be assessed semiquantitatively by placing regions of interest over the mediastinum and the myocardium and calculating a relative retention ratio. A ratio over 2 is considered normal. Patients with denervation display a reduced ratio of tracer retention. Values below 1.2 identify patients at high risk for subsequent cardiovascular complications [49]. There are data indicating the prognostic value of ^{11}C-HED in patients with congestive heart failure confirming the ^{123}I-mIBG observations [62]. The advantage of PET is that it provides an absolute quantification of ^{11}C-HED tracer retention in the myocardium of patients with heart failure. LA—left atrium; RA—right atrium; RV—right ventricle.

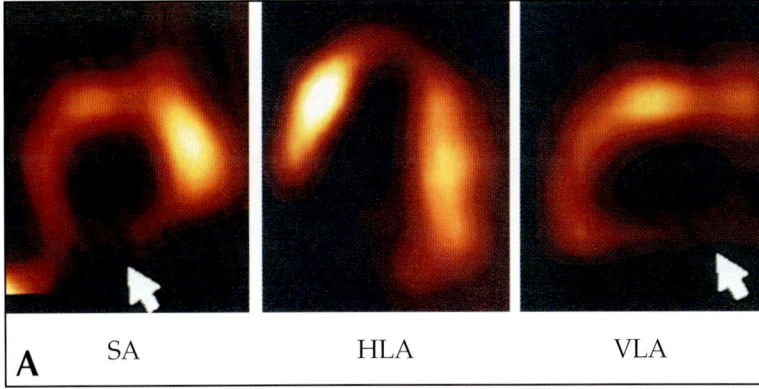

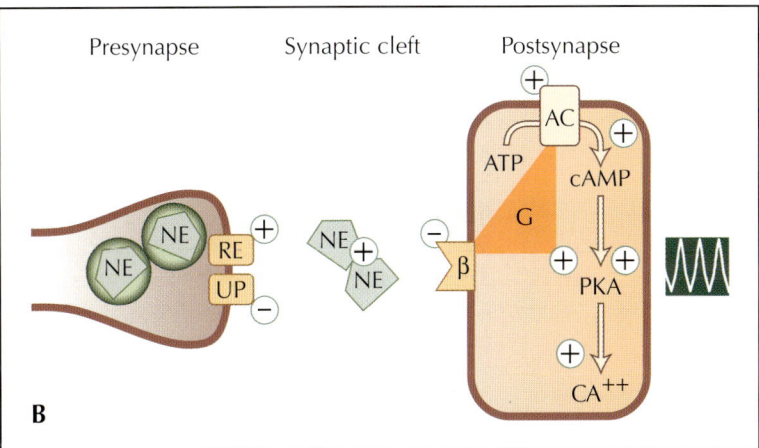

FIGURE 11-14. Neuronal imaging and cardiac arrhythmias. A, ^{123}I-metaiodobenzylguanidine (^{123}I-mIBG) SPECT images were obtained in a 54-year-old man with idiopathic right ventricular outflow tract tachycardia. The tomographic slices are displayed in short-axis (SA), horizontal long-axis (HLA), and vertical long-axis (VLA) views. ^{123}I-mIBG images acquired 4 hours following injection show a marked ^{123}I-mIBG retention defect in the midventricular and basal inferior walls (arrows), suggesting regional sympathetic denervation. Unfortunately, the right ventricle cannot be imaged by radionuclide techniques due to thin myocardial walls.

B, Schematic display illustrating a proposed pathophysiologic mechanism of tachycardia in patients with idiopathic right ventricular outflow tract tachycardia. Reduced re-uptake (UP) of norepinephrine (NE) into the nerve terminal or increased release (RE) into the synaptic cleft (assessed by the ^{123}I-mIBG defect) leads to an increase in local norepinephrine concentration in the synaptic cleft with down-regulation of postsynaptic β adrenoceptors [63]. Assuming that stimulatory G proteins (G) are up-regulated in connection with down-regulated β adrenoceptors, an acute increase in synaptic norepinephrine concentration would increase cAMP via activation of adenylyl cyclase (AC). The increase in cAMP will produce a rise in intracellular Ca^{2+} levels by activation of protein kinase A (PKA), and will eventually trigger ventricular tachycardia.

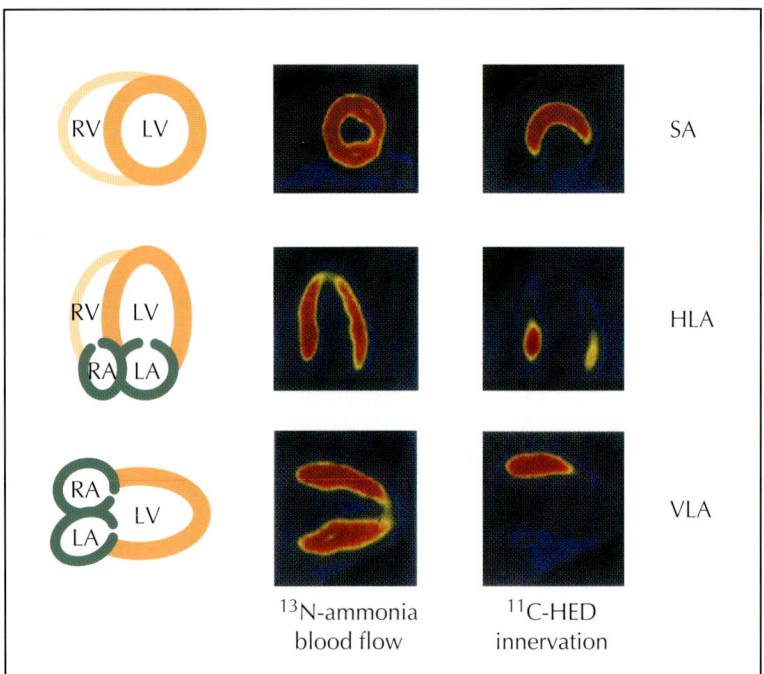

Figure 11-15. Myocardial denervation in diabetes. PET images were obtained in a patient with advanced diabetic neuropathy as defined by functional testing. Following the injection of C-11 hydroxyephedrine (^{11}C-HED), short-axis (SA), horizontal long-axis (HLA), and vertical long-axis (VLA) views were obtained. The regional retention of ^{11}C-HED is compared with the regional perfusion as assessed by ^{13}N-ammonia. There is heterogeneous denervation in patients with diabetic neuropathy. The ^{11}C-HED retention is reduced most prominently in the distal aspects of the anterior wall, apex, and inferior wall of the left ventricle (LV). As the process of neuropathy proceeds, denervation starts at the apex and extends to the basal aspects of the left ventricle. The proximal, anterior, and anterolateral wall segments are most protected from the disease process. This heterogeneity of denervation has been linked to the increased incidence of sudden cardiac death in patients with diabetic neuropathy of the heart [64]. However, no prospective data are available defining the prognostic value of neuronal imaging for detection of patients with increased incidence of cardiovascular complications [37,38,64–66]. LA—left atrium; RA—right atrium; RV—right ventricle.

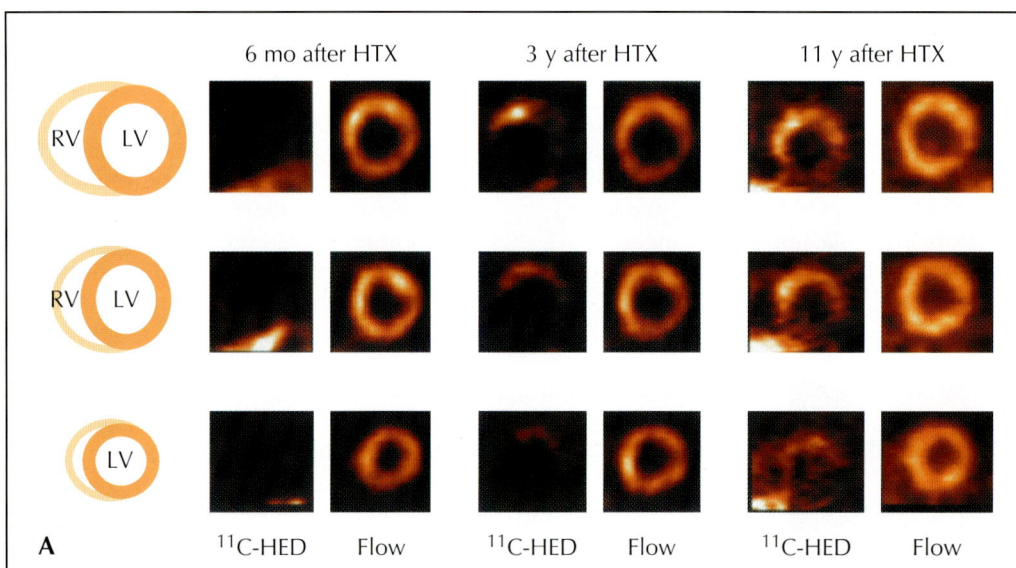

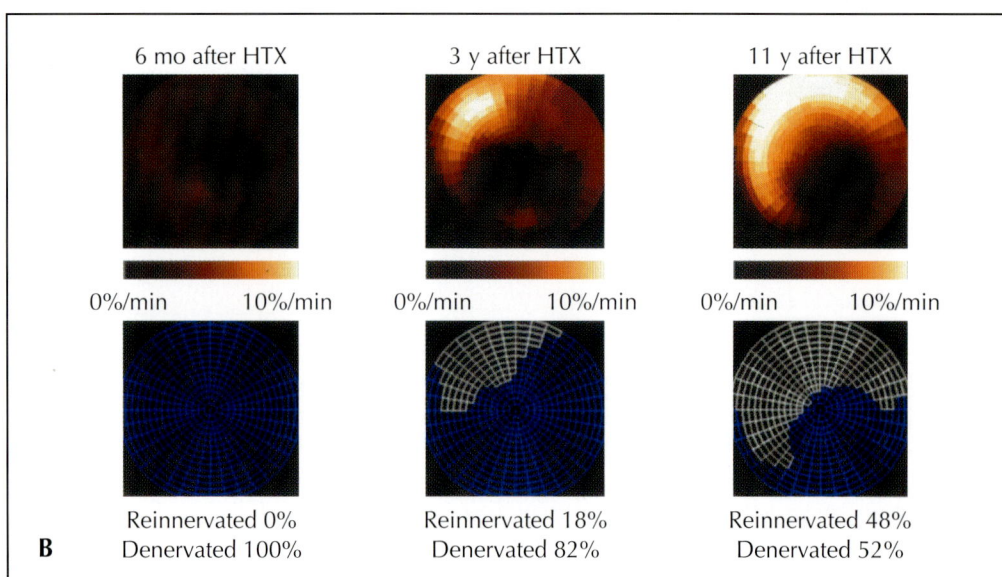

Figure 11-16. Reinnervation of cardiac allograft. Cardiac transplantation (HTX) represents the best model of cardiac denervation because the neuronal fibers are cut during the transplantation surgery. **A,** Neuronal imaging with C-11 hydroxyephedrine (^{11}C-HED) obtained 6 months after transplantation shows little retention of the tracer in the myocardium 40 minutes after tracer injection in comparison to the myocardial perfusion assessed with ^{13}N-ammonia. In a patient studied 3 years after heart transplantation, myocardial perfusion is homogeneous throughout the left ventricle (LV), but the ^{11}C-HED images obtained 40 minutes after injection reveal reappearance of regional ^{11}C-HED retention in the anteroseptal area of the LV. The area of reinnervation appears larger in a patient studied 11 years after transplantation, but regional denervation remains detectable in the inferior aspects of the LV that display normal perfusion. These examples of PET images at different time points after transplantation depict the reinnervation process occurring in about 40% to 50% of the patients. The reinnervation process does not result in complete reinnervation, but shows regional reappearance of sympathetic nerve terminals. Functional studies have shown that patients with reinnervation show greater heart rate variability, better exercise tolerance, and improved LV function with exercise [48].

B, PET–^{11}C-HED polar maps of cardiac transplantation patients at various time points after surgery. Early after transplantation, the retention index is reduced throughout the entire left ventricular myocardium. Using a threshold of 7%/min retention index, no reinnervated area can be detected. At 3 years after transplantation, the anteroseptal areas show reinnervated territories (about 18% of the left ventricle). The PET images obtained 11 years after transplantation show a reinnervated area of 48% of the left ventricle, illustrating the progress of the reinnervation process in the anterior septal wall towards the apex. However, the inferior inferolateral wall remains denervated as seen in most of the patients undergoing neuronal imaging late after cardiac transplantation [44,48,67].

References

1. Levy M: Sympathetic-parasympathetic interaction in the heart. New York: Futura; 1988.

2. Bristow MR, Minobe W, Rasmussen R, et al.: Beta-adrenergic neuroeffector abnormalities in the failing human heart are produced by local rather than systemic mechanisms. *J Clin Invest* 1992, 89:803–815.

3. Bristow MR, Anderson FL, Port JD, et al.: Differences in beta-adrenergic neuroeffector mechanisms in ischemic versus idiopathic dilated cardiomyopathy. *Circulation* 1991, 84:1024–1039.

4. Gill JS, Hunter GJ, Gane G, Camm AJ: Heterogeneity of the human myocardial sympathetic innervation: in vivo demonstration by iodine 123-labeled meta-iodobenzylguanidine scintigraphy. *Am Heart J* 1993, 126:390–398.

5. Momose M, Tyndale-Hines L, Bengel FM, Schwaiger M: How heterogeneous is the cardiac autonomic innervation? *Basic Res Cardiol* 2001, 96:539–546.

6. Langer O, Halldin C: PET and SPECT tracers for mapping the cardiac nervous system. *Eur J Nucl Med* 2002, 29:416–434.

7. Sisson JC, Shapiro B, Meyers L, et al.: Metaiodobenzylguanidine to map scintigraphically the adrenergic nervous system in man. *J Nucl Med* 1987, 28:1625–1636.

8. Wieland DM, Rosenspire KC, Hutchins GD, et al.: Neuronal mapping of the heart with 6-[18F]fluorometaraminol. *J Med Chem* 1990, 33:956–964.

9. Rosenspire KC, Haka MS, Van Dort ME, et al.: Synthesis and preliminary evaluation of carbon-11-meta-hydroxyephedrine: a false transmitter agent for heart neuronal imaging. *J Nucl Med* 1990, 31:1328–1334.

10. Raffel DM, Corbett JR, del Rosario RB, et al.: Clinical evaluation of carbon-11-phenylephrine: MAO-sensitive marker of cardiac sympathetic neurons. *J Nucl Med* 1996, 37:1923–1931.

11. Fischer JE, Weise VK, Kopin IJ: False adrenergic transmitter release from the isolated cat heart. *Am J Med Sci* 1968, 255:158–162.

12. Degrado TR, Zalutsky MR, Vaidyanathan G: Uptake mechanisms of meta-[123I]iodobenzylguanidine in isolated rat heart. *Nucl Med Biol* 1995, 22:1–12.

13. Nakajima K, Taki J, Tonami N, Hisada K: Decreased 123I-MIBG uptake and increased clearance in various cardiac diseases. *Nucl Med Commun* 1994, 15:317–323.

14. Bengel FM, Barthel P, Matsunari I, et al.: Kinetics of 123I-MIBG after acute myocardial infarction and reperfusion therapy. *J Nucl Med* 1999, 40:904–910.

15. Patel A, Iskandrian A: MIBG imaging. *J Nucl Cardiol* 2002, 9:75–94.

16. Farahati J, Bier D, Scheubeck M, et al.: Effect of specific activity on cardiac uptake of iodine-123-MIBG. *J Nucl Med* 1997, 38:447–451.

17. DeGrado TR, Zalutsky MR, Coleman RE, Vaidyanathan G: Effects of specific activity on meta-[(131)I]iodobenzylguanidine kinetics in isolated rat heart. *Nucl Med Biol* 1998, 25:59–64.

18. Schwaiger M, Kalff V, Rosenspire K, et al.: Noninvasive evaluation of sympathetic nervous system in human heart by positron emission tomography. *Circulation* 1990, 82:457–464.

19. Schwaiger M, Hutchins GD, Kalff V, et al.: Evidence for regional catecholamine uptake and storage sites in the transplanted human heart by positron emission tomography. *J Clin Invest* 1991, 87:1681–1690.

20. Bengel FM, Ueberfuhr P, Ziegler SI, et al.: Serial assessment of sympathetic reinnervation after orthotopic heart transplantation. A longitudinal study using PET and C-11 hydroxyephedrine. *Circulation* 1999, 99:1866–1871.

21. Schafers M, Dutka D, Rhodes CG, et al.: Myocardial presynaptic and postsynaptic autonomic dysfunction in hypertrophic cardiomyopathy. *Circ Res* 1998, 82:57–62.

22. Bohm M, La Rosee K, Schwinger RH, Erdmann E: Evidence for reduction of norepinephrine uptake sites in the failing human heart. *J Am Coll Cardiol* 1995, 25:146–153.

23. Hartmann F, Ziegler S, Nekolla S, et al.: Regional patterns of myocardial sympathetic denervation in dilated cardiomyopathy: an analysis using carbon-11 hydroxyephedrine and positron emission tomography. *Heart* 1999, 81:262–270.

24. Merlet P, Valette H, Dubois-Rande JL, et al.: Prognostic value of cardiac metaiodobenzylguanidine imaging in patients with heart failure. *J Nucl Med* 1992, 33:471–477.

25. Nakata T, Miyamoto K, Doi A, et al.: Cardiac death prediction and impaired cardiac sympathetic innervation assessed by MIBG in patients with failing and nonfailing hearts. *J Nucl Cardiol* 1998, 5:579–590.

26. Fukuoka S, Hayashida K, Hirose Y, et al.: Use of iodine-123 metaiodobenzylguanidine myocardial imaging to predict the effectiveness of beta-blocker therapy in patients with dilated cardiomyopathy. *Eur J Nucl Med* 1997, 24:523–529.

27. Suwa M, Otake Y, Moriguchi A, et al.: Iodine-123 metaiodobenzylguanidine myocardial scintigraphy for prediction of response to beta-blocker therapy in patients with dilated cardiomyopathy. *Am Heart J* 1997, 133:353–358.

28. Schwartz PJ: The autonomic nervous system and sudden death. *Eur Heart J* 1998, 19:F72–F80.

29. Meredith IT, Broughton A, Jennings GL, Esler MD: Evidence of a selective increase in cardiac sympathetic activity in patients with sustained ventricular arrhythmias. *N Engl J Med* 1991, 325:618–624.

30. Wichter T, Schafers M, Rhodes CG, et al.: Abnormalities of cardiac sympathetic innervation in arrhythmogenic right ventricular cardiomyopathy: quantitative assessment of presynaptic norepinephrine reuptake and postsynaptic beta-adrenergic receptor density with positron emission tomography. *Circulation* 2000, 101:1552–1558.

31. Yukinaka M, Nomura M, Ito S, Nakaya Y: Mismatch between myocardial accumulation of 123I-MIBG and 99mTc-MIBI and late ventricular potentials in patients after myocardial infarction: association with the development of ventricular arrhythmias. *Am Heart J* 1998, 136:859–867.

32. Lerch H, Bartenstein P, Wichter T, et al.: Sympathetic innervation of the left ventricle is impaired in arrhythmogenic right ventricular disease. *Eur J Nucl Med* 1993, 20:207–212.

33. Hattori N, Schwaiger M: Metaiodobenzylguanidine scintigraphy of the heart: what have we learnt clinically? *Eur J Nucl Med* 2000, 27:1–6.

34. Langer A, Freeman MR, Josse RG, Armstrong PW: Metaiodobenzylguanidine imaging in diabetes mellitus: assessment of cardiac sympathetic denervation and its relation to autonomic dysfunction and silent myocardial ischemia. *J Am Coll Cardiol* 1995, 25:610–618.

35. Schnell O, Muhr D, Dresel S, et al.: Autoantibodies against sympathetic ganglia and evidence of cardiac sympathetic dysinnervation in newly diagnosed and long-term IDDM patients. *Diabetologia* 1996, 39:970–975.

36. Schnell O, Muhr D, Weiss M, et al.: Reduced myocardial 123I-metaiodobenzylguanidine uptake in newly diagnosed IDDM patients. *Diabetes* 1996, 45:801–805.

37. Allman KC, Stevens MJ, Wieland DM, et al.: Noninvasive assessment of cardiac diabetic neuropathy by carbon-11 hydroxyephedrine and positron emission tomography. *J Am Coll Cardiol* 1993, 22:1425–1432.

38. Stevens MJ, Raffel DM, Allman KC, et al.: Cardiac sympathetic dysinnervation in diabetes: implications for enhanced cardiovascular risk. *Circulation* 1998, 98:961–968.

39. Zipes DP: Influence of myocardial ischemia and infarction on autonomic innervation of heart. *Circulation* 1990, 82:1095–1105.

40. Matsunari I, Schricke U, Bengel FM, *et al.*: Extent of cardiac sympathetic neuronal damage is determined by the area of ischemia in patients with acute coronary syndromes. *Circulation* 2000, 101:2579–2585.

41. Allman KC, Wieland DM, Muzik O, *et al.*: Carbon-11 hydroxyephedrine with positron emission tomography for serial assessment of cardiac adrenergic neuronal function after acute myocardial infarction in humans. *J Am Coll Cardiol* 1993, 22:368–375.

42. Minardo JD, Tuli MM, Mock BH, *et al.*: Scintigraphic and electrophysiological evidence of canine myocardial sympathetic denervation and reinnervation produced by myocardial infarction or phenol application. *Circulation* 1988, 78:1008–1019.

43. Hartikainen J, Kuikka J, Mantysaari M, *et al.*: Sympathetic reinnervation after acute myocardial infarction. *Am J Cardiol* 1996, 77:5–9.

44. De Marco T, Dae M, Yuen-Green MS, *et al.*: Iodine-123 metaiodobenzylguanidine scintigraphic assessment of the transplanted human heart: evidence for late reinnervation. *J Am Coll Cardiol* 1995, 25:927–931.

45. Guertner C, Krause BJ, Klepzig H, Jr., *et al.*: Sympathetic re-innervation after heart transplantation: dual-isotope neurotransmitter scintigraphy, norepinephrine content and histological examination. *Eur J Nucl Med* 1995, 22:443–452.

46. Dae MW, Herre JM, O'Connell JW, *et al.*: Scintigraphic assessment of sympathetic innervation after transmural versus nontransmural myocardial infarction. *J Am Coll Cardiol* 1991, 17:1416–1423.

47. Odaka K, von Scheidt W, Ziegler SI, *et al.*: Reappearance of cardiac presynaptic sympathetic nerve terminals in the transplanted heart: correlation between PET using (11)C-hydroxyephedrine and invasively measured norepinephrine release. *J Nucl Med* 2001, 42:1011–1016.

48. Bengel FM, Ueberfuhr P, Schiepel N, *et al.*: Effect of sympathetic reinnervation on cardiac performance after heart transplantation. *N Engl J Med* 2001, 345:731–738.

49. Merlet P, Benvenuti C, Moyse D, *et al.*: Prognostic value of MIBG imaging in idiopathic dilated cardiomyopathy. *J Nucl Med* 1999, 40:917–923.

50. Bannister R, Mathias CJ: Introduction and classification of autonomic disorders. In *Autonomic Failure*. Edited by Bannister R, Mathias CJ. New York: Oxford University Press; 1992:1–12.

51. Milner P, Burnstock G: Neurotransmitters in the autonomic nervous system. In *Handbook of Autonomic Nervous System Dysfunction*. Edited by Korczyn AD. New York: Marcel Dekker; 1995:5–32.

52. Lipscombe D, Kongsamut S, Tsien RW, *et al.*: Adrenergic inhibition of sympathetic neurotransmitter release mediated by modulation of N-type calcium-channel gating. *Nature* 1989, 340:639–642.

53. Toth PT, Bindokas VP, Bleakman D, *et al.*: Mechanism of presynaptic inhibition by neuropeptide Y at sympathetic nerve terminals. *Nature* 1993, 364:635–639.

54. Nicholls JG, Martin AR, Wallace BG, *et al.*: *From Neuron to Brain*. Sunderland, MA: Sinauer Associates; 1992.

55. Delforge J, Syrota A, Lancon JP, *et al.*: Cardiac beta-adrenergic receptor density measured in vivo using PET, CGP 12177, and a new graphical method [published erratum appears in *J Nucl Med* 1994, 35(5):921]. *J Nucl Med* 1991, 32:739–748.

56. Allman KC, Wieland DM, Muzik O, *et al.*: Carbon-11 hydroxyephedrine with positron emission tomography for serial assessment of cardiac adrenergic neuronal function after acute myocardial infarction in humans. *J Am Coll Cardiol* 1993, 22(2):368–375.

57. Fallen EL, Coates G, Nahmias C, *et al.*: Recovery rates of regional sympathetic reinnervation and myocardial blood flow after acute myocardial infarction. *Am Heart J* 1999, 137(5):863–869.

58. Simula S, Lakka T, Kuikka J, *et al.*: Cardiac adrenergic innervation within the first 3 months after acute myocardial infarction. *Clin Physiol* 2000, 20(5):366–373.

59. Schwaiger M, Guiborg H, Rosenspire K, *et al.*: Effect of regional myocardial ischemia on sympathetic nervous system as assessed by fluorine-18-metaraminol. *J Nucl Med* 1990, 31:1352–1357.

60. Schwaiblmair M, von Scheidt W, Uberfuhr P, *et al.*: Functional significance of cardiac reinnervation in heart transplant recipients. *J Heart Lung Transplant* 1999, 18:838–845.

61. Wolpers H, Nguyen N, Rosenspire K, *et al.*: C-11 hydroxyephedrine as marker for neuronal catecholamine retention in reperfused canine myocardium. *Coronary Artery Disease* 1991, 2:923–929.

62. Elsinga PH, Doze P, van Waarde A, *et al.*: Imaging of beta-adrenoceptors in the human thorax using (S)-[(11)C]CGP12388 and positron emission tomography. *Eur J Pharmacol* 2001, 433:173–176.

63. Schafers M, Lerch H, Wichter T, *et al.*: Cardiac sympathetic innervation in patients with idiopathic right ventricular outflow tract tachycardia. *J Am Coll Cardiol* 1998, 32:181–186.

64. Langen KJ, Ziegler D, Weise F, *et al.*: Evaluation of QT interval length, QT dispersion and myocardial m-iodobenzylguanidine uptake in insulin-dependent diabetic patients with and without autonomic neuropathy. *Clin Sci* 1997, 93:325–333.

65. Ziegler D, Weise F, Langen KJ, *et al.*: Effect of glycaemic control on myocardial sympathetic innervation assessed by [123I]metaiodobenzylguanidine scintigraphy: a 4-year prospective study in IDDM patients. *Diabetologia* 1998, 41:443–451.

66. Wei K, Dorian P, Newman D, Langer A: Association between QT dispersion and autonomic dysfunction in patients with diabetes mellitus. *J Am Coll Cardiol* 1995, 26:859–863.

67. Estorch M, Camprecios M, Flotats A, *et al.*: Sympathetic reinnervation of cardiac allografts evaluated by 123I-MIBG imaging. *J Nucl Med* 1999, 40:911–916.

CHAPTER 12

IMAGING MYOCARDIAL NECROSIS AND APOPTOSIS

Jagat Narula and Leo Hofstra

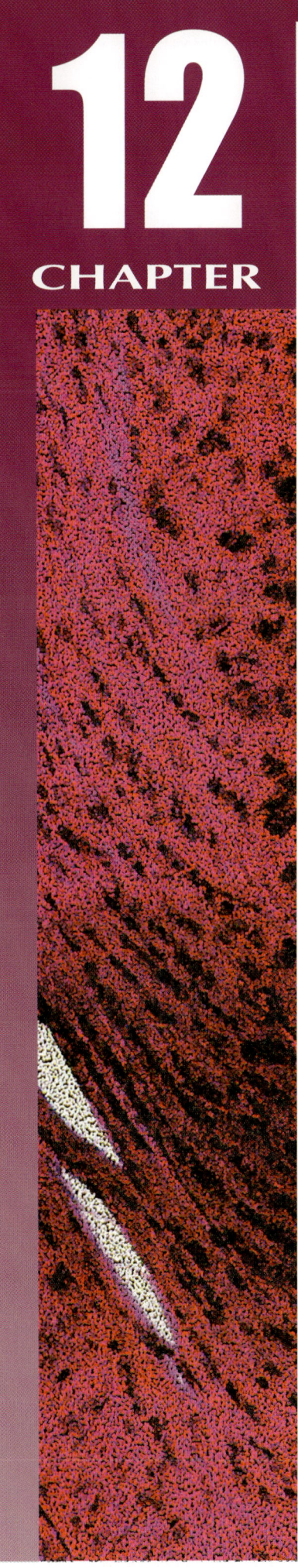

Necrosis and apoptosis are distinct forms of cell death, although their boundaries in heart muscle cell death are relatively hazy. Injured cardiomyocytes, depending upon their cellular energy reserves, may shuffle between necrotic and apoptotic cascades and may result in classic apoptosis, orthodox necrosis, or a hybrid thereof [1].

Necrosis is a common type of cell death that occurs after exogenous noxious insults, such as ischemic injury [2]. It is manifested by cell swelling and cell rupture, denaturation and coagulation of cytoplasmic proteins, and disintegration of cell organelles. Apoptosis occurs when a cell dies through activation of an internally controlled suicide program to eliminate unwanted cells normally during embryogenesis and various insidious physiologic processes. The dominant morphologic features include chromatin condensation and fragmentation. The cell shrinks and fragments into small apoptotic bodies. Doomed cells are removed with minimum disruption of the surrounding tissue architecture. Apoptosis may also occur under pathologic conditions in the heart. Although the mechanisms of necrosis and apoptosis differ, there is considerable overlap between the two processes. Oncosis defines the prelethal changes preceding necrotic cell death, which are characterized by cell swelling, and can be distinguished from the prelethal changes in apoptosis, associated largely with cell shrinkage [3].

Radionuclide imaging of necrosis and apoptosis has exploited the alterations in cell membrane characteristics [4]. In necrosis, the cell membrane is disrupted and intracellular constituents (normally precluded from accessibility) are targeted. ^{99m}Tc pyrophosphate, glucarate, and glucoheptonate target intracellular proteins, or intranuclear constituents, and have been used to detect acute myocardial infarction. On the other hand, ^{111}In-antimyosin antibody specifically targets myosin heavy chain, which remains in the necrotic myocyte carcass until removed by phagocytes [5]. Antimyosin imaging has been used for the detection of necrosis associated with myocardial infarction, myocarditis, and heart transplant rejection. Imaging with antimyosin antibody in acute infarction can help estimate the mass of myocardium lost. In patients with myocarditis, antimyosin imaging demonstrates diagnostic accuracy superior to endomyocardial biopsy and offers prognostic information. Similarly, antimyosin imaging in transplant recipients can contribute to therapeutic planning, can obviate the need for biopsies after the first year of transplantation, and can help assess the efficacy of immunosuppressive strategies.

During apoptosis, there is a loss of asymmetry of distribution of phospholipids in the cell membrane lipid bilayer, and phosphatidylserine is abnormally expressed on the outer surface of cell membrane [6,7]. Annexin V, a naturally occurring endogenous protein, has a high affinity for phosphatidylserine; labeled with ^{99m}Tc, it has been used for noninvasive detection of apoptosis. Annexin V imaging has been performed in acute myocardial infarction, myocarditis, and acute transplant rejection [8].

Since death by any means is a loss of functional tissue, should morphologic nuances in the type of cell death at all be important? It is conceivable that the overlapping process of myocyte death may produce various morphologic hybrids of the two cell death types. It also may be logical to presume that interventions to abrogate any one process may produce preventative benefits that exceed expectations [4].

Imaging Necrotic Cell Death

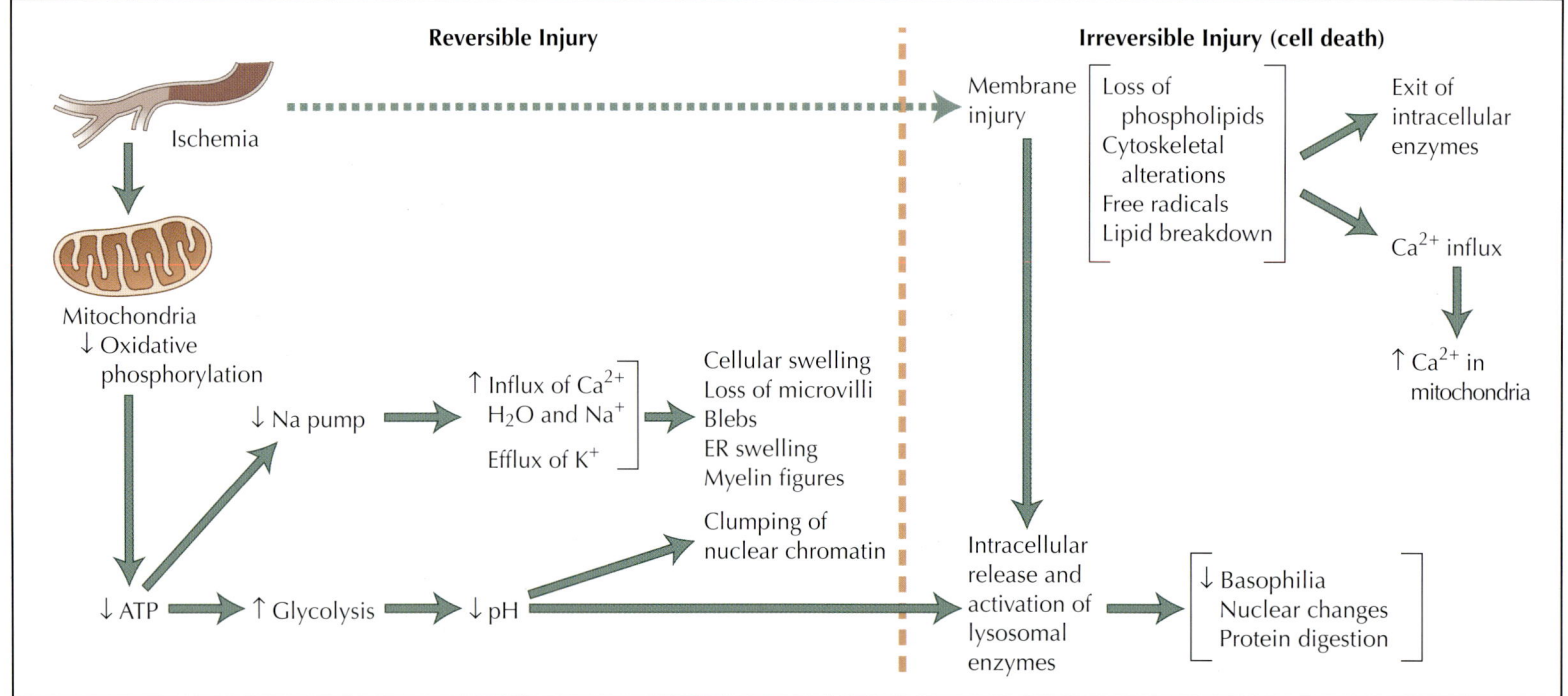

Figure 12-1. Pathogenetic basis of necrotic myocellular death. The causes of necrotic cell death are multiple. Ischemia is the most common cause and infringes on aerobic oxidative respiration. Infective agents, postinfective immune processes (myocarditis, rheumatic carditis, and Chagas' disease), hypersensitivity phenomenon, and autoimmune diseases result in predominantly inflammatory injury. Physical insults (*eg*, radiation) and chemical insults (*eg*, alcohol, doxorubicin) are infrequent causes of myocardial damage. Regardless of inciting agent, several common biochemical pathways mediate cell death by necrosis. The most important is ATP depletion that occurs commonly during ischemia. Partially reduced reactive oxygen forms, which are produced as unavoidable by-products during oxidative phosphorylation, are exaggerated during reperfusion injury and commonly are associated with cellular damage. In addition to ATP depletion and oxidative stress, a distinct increase is observed in intercellular calcium with loss of calcium homeostasis that activates potentially deleterious enzymes, such as phospholipases, proteases, ATPase, and endonucleases. All these biochemical events contribute to mitochondrial damage by formation of a high conductance channel (or mitochondrial permeability transition pores) in the inner mitochondrial membrane. Although reversible in its early stages, the nonselective pores become permanent upon persistence of inciting stimuli, precluding maintenance of mitochondrial membrane potential, which is otherwise critical for mitochondrial oxidative phosphorylation. The biochemical alterations, including mitochondrial damage, lead to loss of integrity of cell membrane, which is the hallmark of necrotic cell death. (*Adapted from* Kumar [2].)

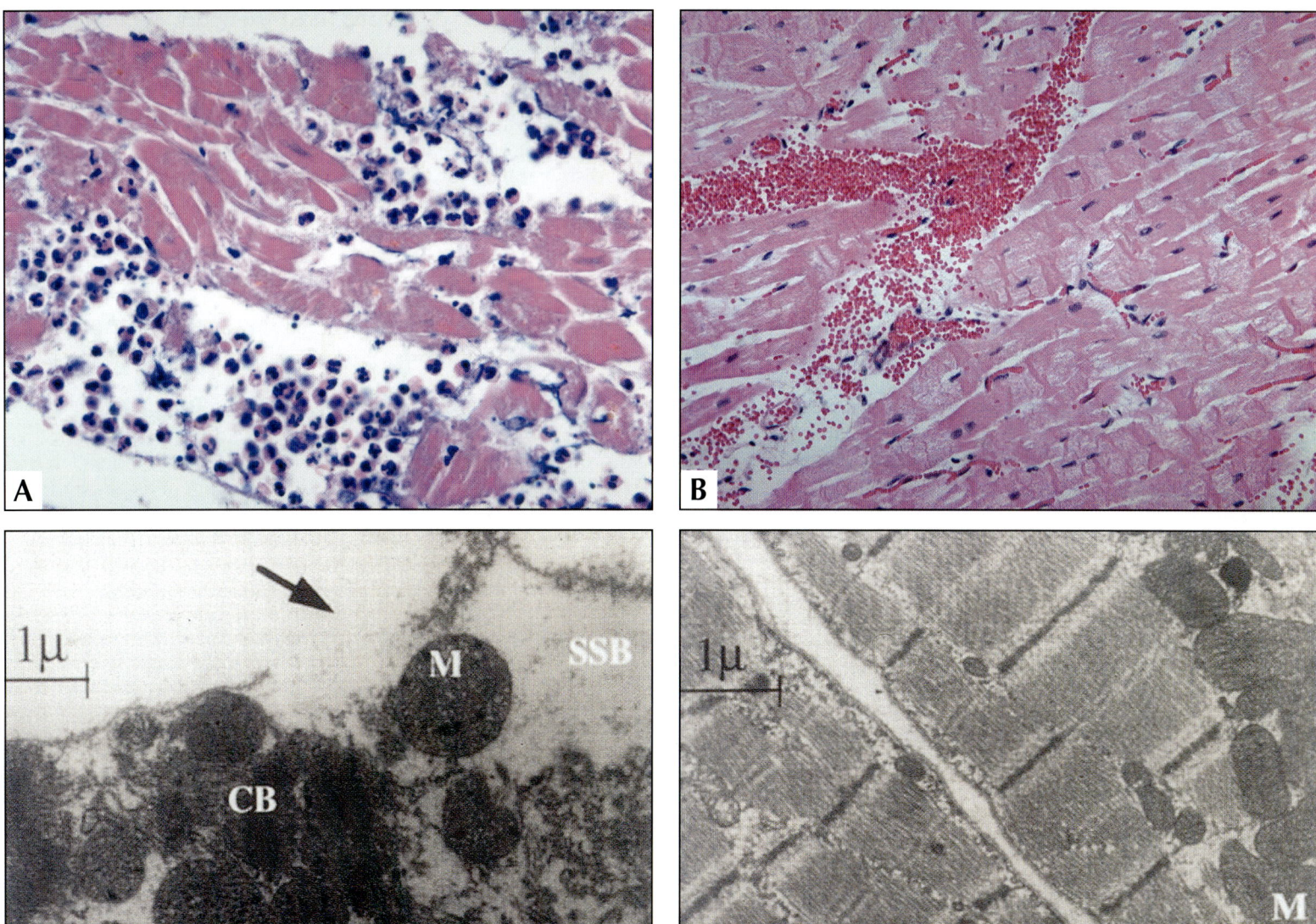

FIGURE 12-2. Morphologic characteristics of necrotic myocytes. **A**, Morphologically, the necrotic cells in acute myocardial infarction demonstrate increased eosinophilia with loss of striations and nuclei and neutrophilic infiltration, followed by gradually increasing macrophage infiltration. **B**, Upon reperfusion, interstitial hemorrhage and contraction bands are prominently seen. **C**, Ultrastructurally, necrotic cells are characterized by overt breach in the plasma membrane (*arrow*), dilation of mitochondria with appearance of large amorphous densities, intracytoplasmic myelin figures, and accumulation of fluffy material representing denatured protein. Nuclear changes (not shown) occur due to nonspecific breakdown of DNA and may present as karyolysis (loss of the chromatin), pyknosis (nuclear/DNA shrinkage), or karyorrhexis (fragmentation of pyknotic nuclei). Most necrotic cells and their debris are removed by a combined process of digestion and fragmentation, with phagocytosis of the particulate debris. If not destroyed and removed, they attract calcium salts and other minerals and develop dystrophic calcification. **D**, The electron micrograph of a normal cardiomyocyte shows intact sarcolemma for comparison. (*Panels A and B courtesy of* Navneet Narula, MD, University of Pennsylvania Medical Center, Philadelphia, PA; *panels C and D from* Kim *et al.* [9]; with permission.)

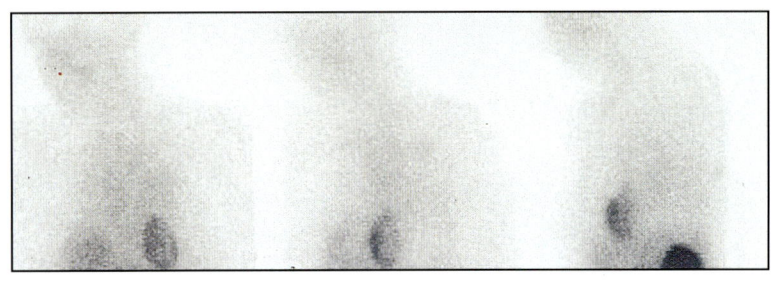

FIGURE 12-3. Noninvasive imaging of ischemic myocardial necrosis. All radionuclide imaging strategies, including ^{99m}Tc-labeled infarct-avid agents and ^{111}In-labeled antimyosin antibody, have exploited the loss of sarcolemmal integrity for noninvasive detection of myocardial necrosis. Several chelates of ^{99m}Tc (*eg*, pyrophosphate) have been used for imaging acute myocardial infarcts. The electron microscopic study suggested formation of calcium phosphate complexes, possibly with hydroxyapatite in mitochondria of infarcted myocardial cells. Thus, the bone-scanning agents (such as pyrophosphate) were thought to localize by surface adsorption to calcium phosphate deposited in the mitochondria of the necrotic cell. However, equally efficient infarct localization of non–bone scanning chelates (*eg*, tetracycline, glucarate, and gluco-heptonate) and studies using pyrophosphates labeled with beta-emitters (^{45}Ca, ^{3}H, ^{32}P) suggest extensive association of ^{99m}Tc-chelates to proteinaceous macromolecules in dying muscle cells. ^{99m}Tc chelates may also bind to serum proteins, which may gain access to necrotic myocytes through the breaches in sarcolemmal integrity [10]. On the other hand, Tc chelates, such as glucarate, localize in the infarcted tissue on the basis of electrostatic association; negatively charged glucarate is shown to target positively charged histones [11]. The mechanism of localization of Tc chelates, although not fully understood, may determine the length of imaging window for that tracer. For instance, the histones may disintegrate within hours after infarction, allowing only very early infarct imaging. On the other hand, calcium phosphate complexes in necrotic myocardium may not form for 24 to 48 hours after initiation of cell death and may allow detection of 2- to 8-day-old infarcts. Whatever the mechanism of localization, it is facilitated by breach of cell membrane integrity.

This figure demonstrates the role of ^{99m}Tc-glucarate imaging in a 69-year-old woman with a 2-hour history of retrosternal chest pain associated with nausea and sweating. The ECG showed early myocardial injury in precordial leads. Neither myoglobin (< 50 μg/L) nor creative kinase (CK) (22 U/L) were elevated at this time. Troponin I (0.50 μg/L) and CK (921 U/L) rose 6 hours later, and CK peaked at 12 hours (1629 U/L). The patient received the standard thrombolytic regimen. Glucaric acid (12.5 mg) labeled with ^{99m}Tc (15 mCi) was injected. Images (in anterior [*left*], left anterior oblique [*center*], and lateral [*right*] views) showed extensive uptake in anterior, anteroseptal, and apical left ventricular myocardium. Subsequent coronary angiography showed a 90% mid left anterior descending coronary artery stenosis. (*Courtesy of Ignasi Carrio, MD, Sant Pau Hospital, Barcelona, Spain.*)

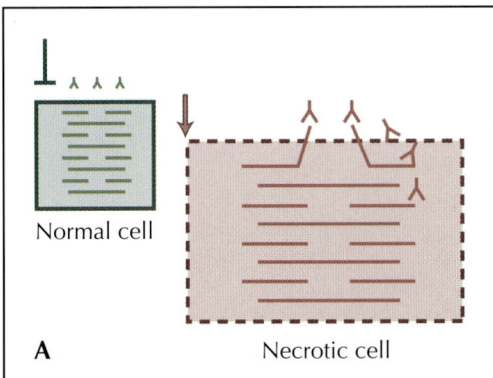

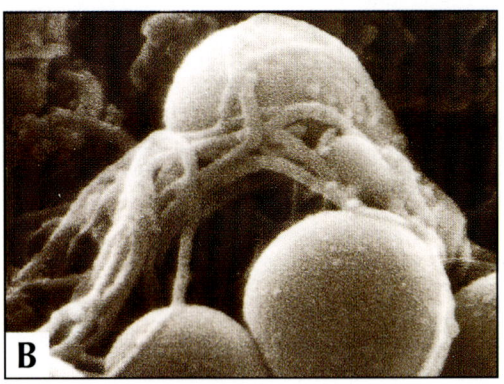

FIGURE 12-4. Pathogenetic basis of antimyosin antibody imaging. A viable cell with an intact cell membrane does not allow the passage of macromolecules and maintains an osmotic gradient between intracellular and extracellular milieu [12]. **A**, During necrosis of cardiomyocytes, loss of sarcolemma allows soluble intracellular macromolecules (*eg*, troponins, creatine kinase, myosin light chains) to wash out in the bloodstream, which can be measured as an indicator of severity of necrosis. On the other hand, the insoluble macromolecules (such as heavy chains of myosin) remain in situ until removed by the scavenger cells. An antibody specifically directed against the heavy chain of myosin (antimyosin antibody) allows differentiation of necrotic cells (with disintegrated sarcolemma) from viable cells (with intact sarcolemma). The necrotic myocardial regions, which allow binding of antimyosin antibody to the exposed myosin heavy chain, can be noninvasively localized by radionuclide imaging if the antibody is appropriately labeled with a gamma emitter and is administered intravenously [13].

B, The principle of antimyosin uptake is demonstrated in scanning electron micrographs of murine neonatal primary myocytes in culture subjected to anoxia and incubated with antimyosin antibody-coated fluorescent polystyrene beads. Normal myocytes with an intact cell membrane did not bind to antimyosin beads. On the other hand, necrotic myocytes with regions of sarcolemmal disruption showed antimyosin bead binding in those regions. A higher magnification (×100,000) of a region of sarcolemmal disruption shows binding of antimyosin beads to myofilaments that contains myosin. Antimyosin antibody Fab fragments labeled with ^{111}In have been used for clinical imaging of myocardial necrosis. The antibody uptake in infarction occurs discretely in the myocardial territory served by the occluded coronary artery [14]. The cardiovascular disorders characterized by multifocal myocardial necrosis, such as myocarditis and cardiac allograft rejection, demonstrate diffuse antibody uptake in the cardiac region. (*Panel B from Khaw et al.* [12]; *with permission.*)

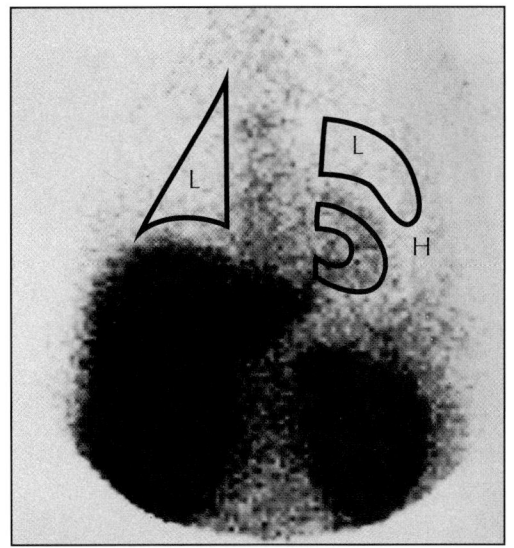

FIGURE 12-5. Antimyosin imaging: technique, interpretation and quantitation of uptake. Antimyosin Fab fragments (0.5 mg) are labeled with 2 mCi of ^{111}In and administered intravenously. Planar scans are obtained using a large field of view gamma camera fitted with a medium energy collimator and linked to a dedicated computer. A 20% symmetric window is centered on both peaks of ^{111}In (173 and 247 KeV), and a preset acquisition time of 10 minutes usually is used to collect at least 500,000 counts per frame. Generally, one anterior and two left anterior oblique views at 40° and 70° are acquired in a 128×128 frame format. SPECT images occasionally are acquired over 360° on 64×64 matrix frames. Tomograms of the heart along the three main axes are then reconstructed. The images are often intense and localized in acute myocardial infarction, and can be acquired within 6 to 12 hours after radiotracer administration. In diffuse myocardial necrosis, the images are acquired at 48 hours, when antibody has cleared from the blood pool. Since there is no focal uptake, a semiquantitative method of antibody uptake is employed in diffuse uptake to calculate heart-to-lung uptake per pixel ratio (HLR). This method delineates a region of interest in the heart (H) and regions on the lungs (L) on the anterior view of the thorax. A cutoff point of 1.55 or higher (2 SD greater than normal value, 1.46 ± 0.04) is used to define abnormal studies. The interobserver variability of this technique is less than 6% [15].

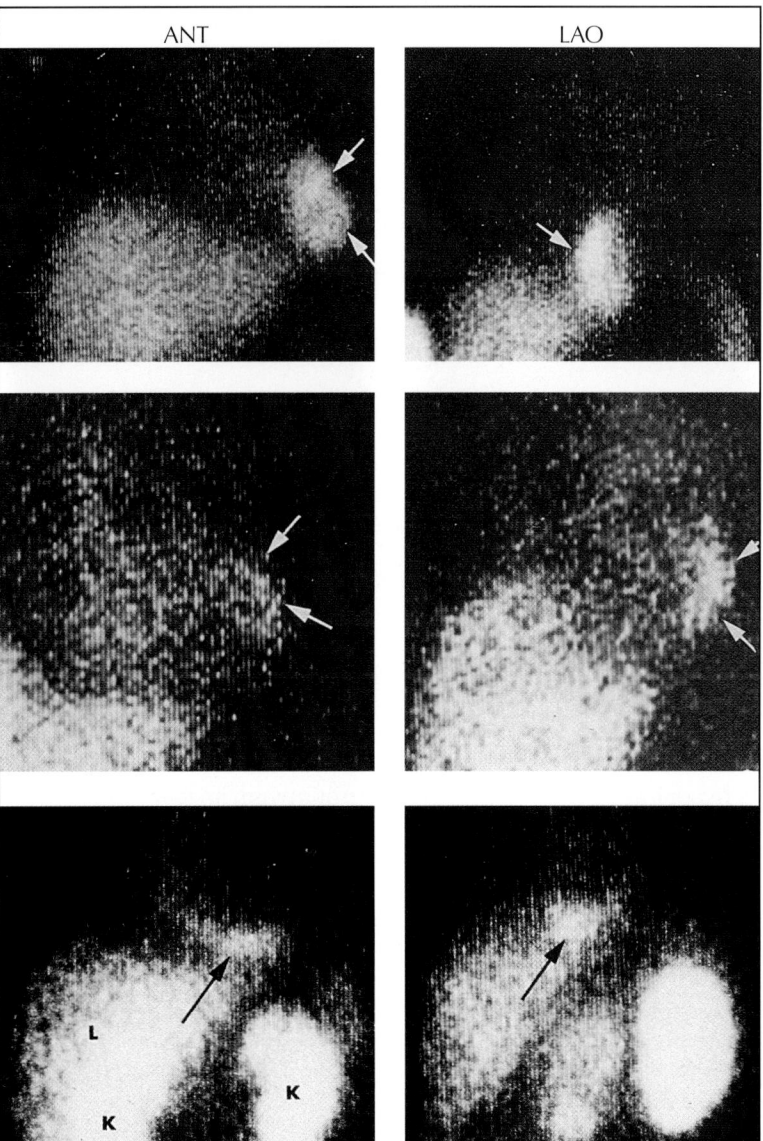

FIGURE 12-6. Antimyosin scintigraphy in acute myocardial infarction (MI). The uptake of antibody in MI conforms to a coronary artery territorial distribution, as depicted in three patients with acute anterior (*top panels*), posterolateral (*middle panels*), and inferior (*bottom panels*) MIs. *Left panels* demonstrate anterior views (ANT), and *right panels* show left anterior oblique views (LAO). The first patient (*top panels*) had occlusion of the proximal left anterior descending coronary artery, which could not be reperfused by thrombolytic therapy. Intense myocardial uptake of antimyosin antibody is seen in anteroapical and anteroseptal regions. Other cardiac regions are clearly negative for antibody uptake. The second patient with occlusion of the left circumflex (*middle panels*) demonstrates posterolateral wall antimyosin uptake in LAO view. Antibody uptake shine-through in the anterior image is observed as well. The third patient (*bottom panels*) had an occluded right coronary artery. There is a discrete uptake of antimyosin antibody in the inferior region. No antimyosin uptake is visible in the left anterior descending or circumflex coronary territories. Antibody localization in the liver (L) and kidney (K) represents normal route of catabolism and excretion of antibody. (*From* Strauss *et al.* [16]; with permission.)

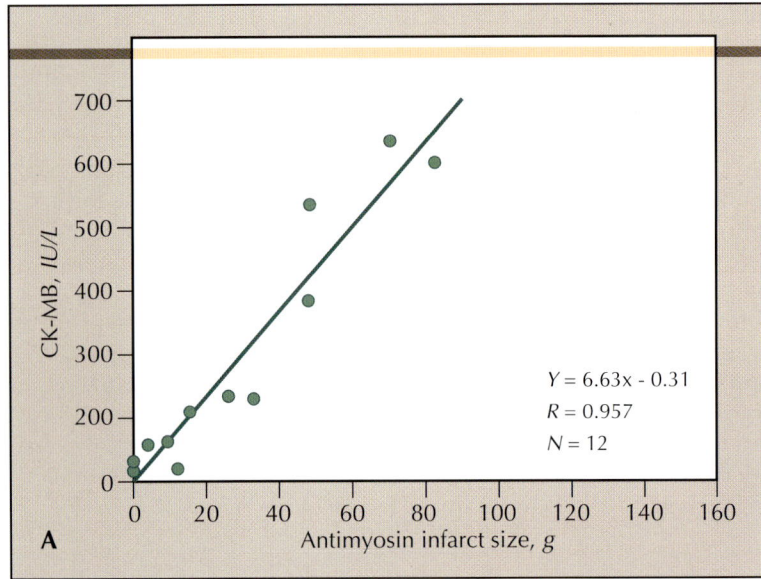

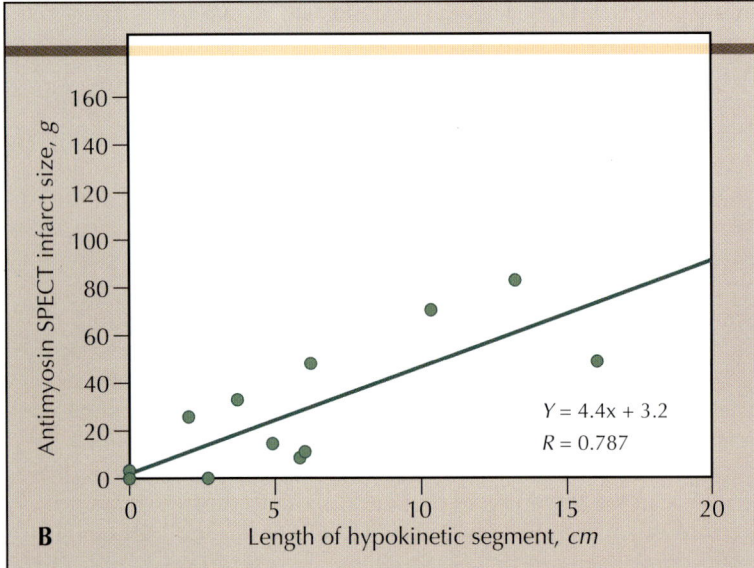

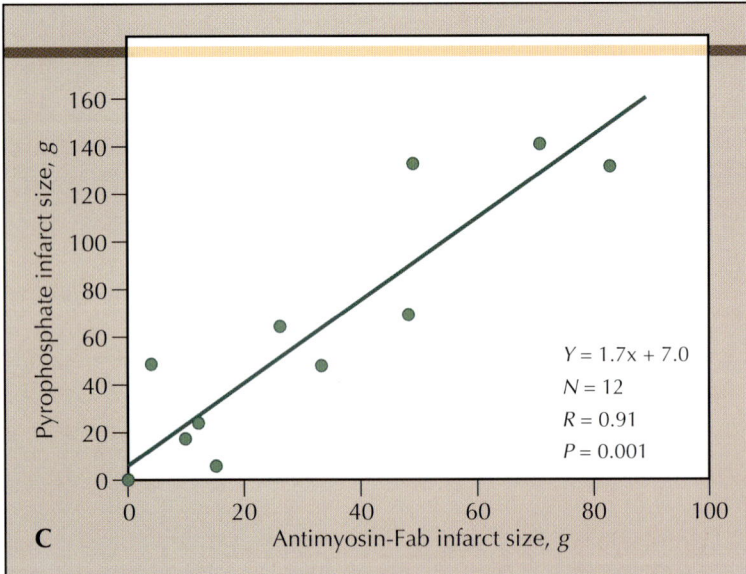

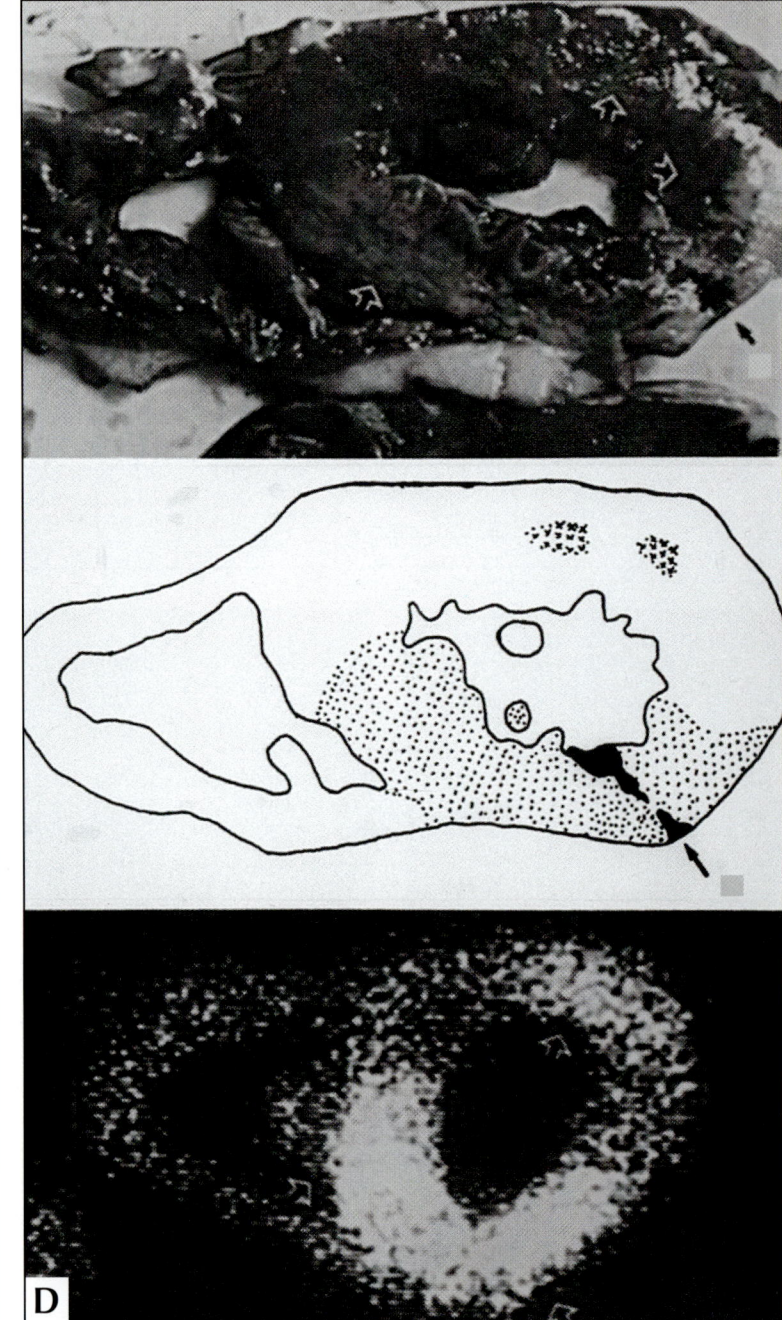

FIGURE 12-7. Diagnostic accuracy of antimyosin scintigraphy in acute myocardial infarction (MI). Antimyosin antibody imaging has demonstrated a high accuracy (96% sensitivity, 100% specificity) for the diagnosis of acute Q wave MI. Precise infarct weight can be calculated from the SPECT images. **A**, Antimyosin infarct weights correlate significantly with serum concentrations of MB isoenzyme fraction of creatinine kinase ($R = 0.96$), and **B**, angiographically determined lengths of hypokinetic segments ($R = 0.79$). **C**, Antimyosin imaging also demonstrates significant and proportional correlation with pyrophosphate infarct size ($R = 0.91$); however, tomographic pyrophosphate images are consistently larger than antimyosin images by a factor of 1.7 in the same set of patients. The larger pyrophosphate infarct size has been explained by the propensity of pyrophosphate uptake in severely ischemic myocardial regions. The specificity and accuracy of antimyosin uptake for the necrotic myocardium clearly has been demonstrated in histopathologic correlations in experimental studies. **D**, Additional confirmation is available from a postmortem examination of heart in a patient who had received radiolabeled antimyosin antibody before dying of myocardial rupture. *Top panel*, Postmortem gross specimen of a heart slice shows an anterior wall infarct with rupture of the free anterior wall and, *middle panel*, its schematic representation; the site of rupture is indicated by an *arrow*. The area of the infarct is delineated by triphenyl-tetrazolium as the pale area in anterior and anteroseptal walls. Focal area of damage was incidentally observed in the posterior wall as well. *Bottom panel*, The corresponding gamma image shows localization of radiolabeled antimyosin precisely in the region of myocardial infarct. Focal uptake of the tracer in the posterior wall also corresponded to histologic evidence of necrosis. (*Panels A through C adapted from* Khaw *et al.* [17]; *panel D from* Jain *et al.* [18]; with permission.)

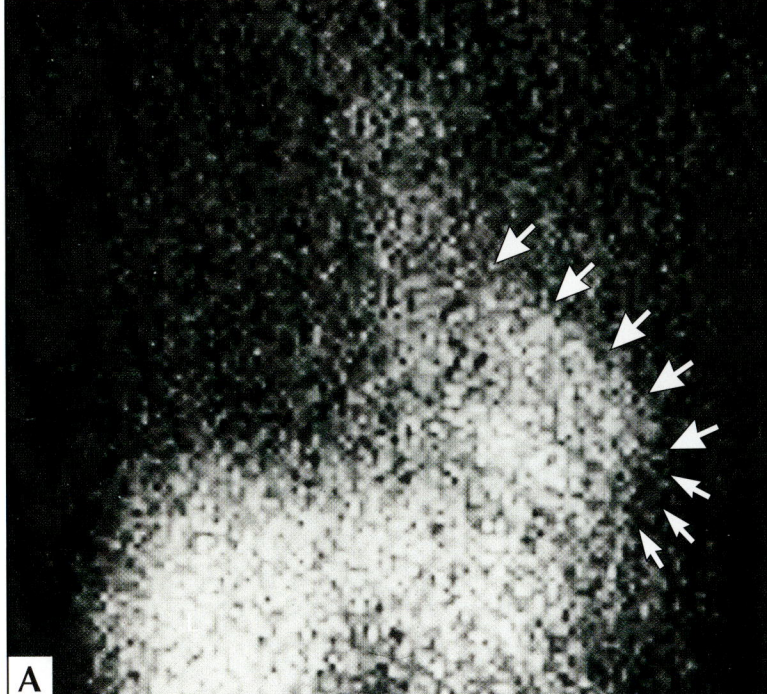 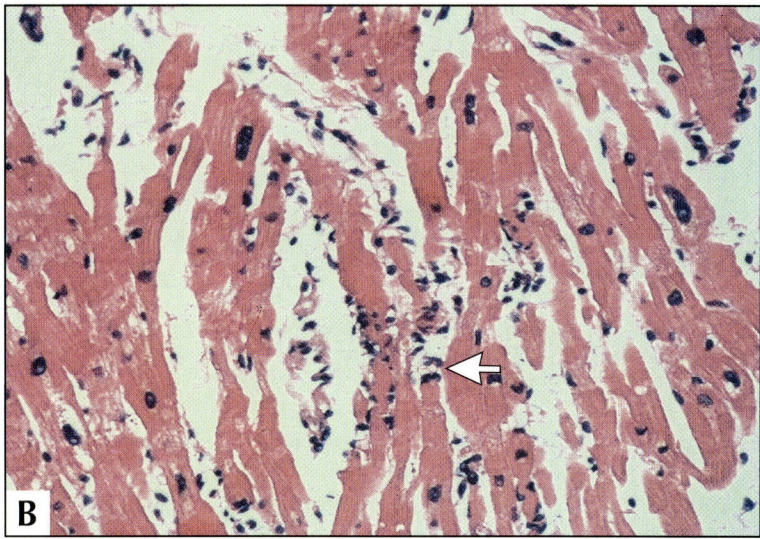

FIGURE 12-8. Clinical role for antimyosin imaging in acute myocardial infarction (MI). No imaging techniques usually are required for the diagnosis of acute MI because clinical presentation with ECG and biochemical alterations provide a definitive diagnosis. Further, antibody imaging requires at least a 6- to 48-hour wait for imaging, precluding immediate intervention for reperfusion. Apart from documentation purposes, imaging may be used in presentations suggestive of acute infarction when coronary atherosclerotic disease is not discovered. For instance, myocarditis occasionally can masquerade as acute MI. In this context, diffuse myocyte necrosis beyond a coronary territory detected by antimyosin scintigraphy indicates a strong likelihood of myocarditis, diagnosis of which would otherwise require performing an endomyocardial biopsy [14]. On the other hand, a pattern of antimyosin antibody uptake conforming to an individual coronary vascular distribution despite the presence of normal coronary arteries would indicate acute MI due to other causes of nonatherosclerotic coronary artery disease, such as spasm or coronary embolism [19]. A normal myocardial scan will exclude both myocardial infarct and myocarditis.

A, An antimyosin scan from a 44-year-old woman who sustained severe substernal chest pain and developed cardiogenic shock. She was placed on an intraortic balloon pump but continued to have chest pain. Her ECG revealed T-wave inversions in leads I, aVL, and V3-6, and peak creatine kinase was 269 U/L. Coronary angiogram revealed normal coronary arteries, and left ventricular angiogram showed impairment of the whole ventricle ranging from akinesia to dyskinesia, except for a normally contracting base and apex. The antimyosin scan showed diffuse, global uptake of radiotracer within the left ventricle (*large arrows*). The apical region was spared (*small arrows*). L—liver.

B, Endomyocardial biopsy demonstrated the central focus (*arrow*) of interstitial mononuclear inflammatory infiltrate associated with necrotic myocytes confirming the diagnosis of myocarditis (hematoxylin and eosin, ×60). (*From* Narula *et al.* [14]; with permission.)

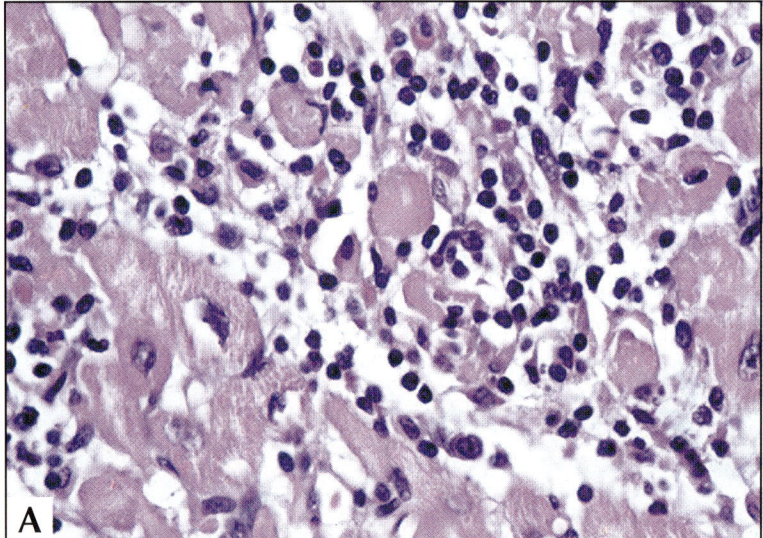
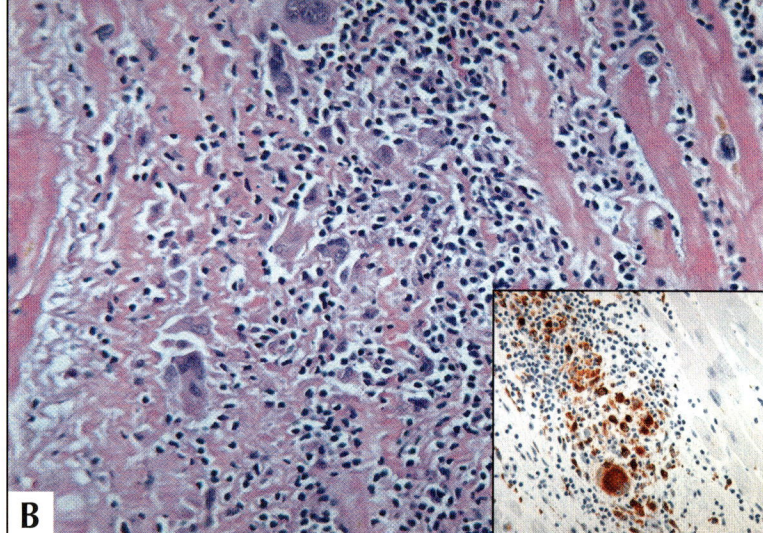

FIGURE 12-9. Necrosis in inflammatory myocardial disease. Myocardial dysfunction and cell death can be induced both by humoral and cellular immune mechanisms in inflammatory disease. Clinically, the inflammatory process is encountered most commonly in patients with acute myocarditis and cardiac allograft rejection. The inflammatory cell infiltrates predominantly comprise lymphocytes and macrophages. Polymorphonuclear leukocytes generally constitute a smaller fraction of the inflammatory infiltrate; occasionally eosinophils and giant cells are found [20]. **A**, Lymphocytic myocarditis is characterized by perivascular and interstitial lymphomononuclear cell infiltration. To define myocarditis by the Dallas criteria, it is imperative to demonstrate the presence of cellular infiltrates clustered around necrotic myocytes. Since myocardial necrosis is an obligatory component of the definition of myocarditis, the likelihood of finding diffuse positive antimyosin scans is high.

B, In comparison with *panel A*, an endomyocardial biopsy from a patient with giant cell myocarditis reveals inflammatory infiltrate comprising giant cells, lymphocytes, macrophages, and eosinophils. *Inset,* The giant cells (stained brown) are derived from macrophage-monocytic lineage, as shown in the immunohistochemical characterization with antimacrophage antibody. (*Panels A and B courtesy of* Navneet Narula, MD, Philadelphia.)

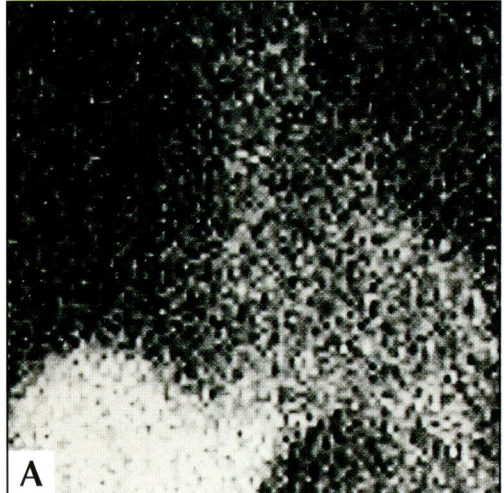
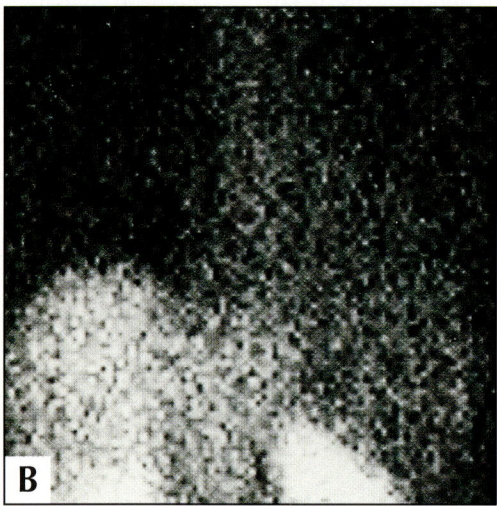

FIGURE 12-10. Antimyosin scintigraphy in myocarditis. Positive antimyosin scans in patients presenting with acute onset of dilated cardiomyopathy have been proposed as a sensitive indicator of myocarditis. In fact, almost all patients with a biopsy positive for myocarditis demonstrate an abnormal antimyosin scan (sensitivity, ≈ 95%), and almost all normal scans exclude the possibility of myocarditis in endomyocardial biopsy (EMB) (negative predictive value, ≈ 95%).

A 36-year-old woman presented with sudden onset of dilated cardiomyopathy. She had normal coronary arteries and her left ventricular ejection fraction was 27%. The antimyosin scan was diffusely positive, **A**, and concomitant EMB (not shown) confirmed the diagnosis of myocarditis. The patient was treated with immunosuppressive therapy including azathioprine and prednisone for 3 months. **B**, Repeat antimyosin scan at this time demonstrated significant resolution of antibody uptake, and the EMB (not shown) showed resolved myocarditis. Left ventricular ejection fraction had increased to 44% in this interval. Although abnormal antimyosin scan demonstrates high sensitivity, it is found in a large number of patients in whom diagnosis of myocarditis is not confirmed on EMB (specificity and positive predictive value, ≈ 50%). The high false-positive rate of antimyosin scan has been explained on the basis of low sensitivity of biopsy for the detection of myocarditis due to sampling error as well as by possible myocardial damage in cardiomyopathic hearts, even in the absence of inflammatory state. (*From* Narula *et al.* [21]; with permission.)

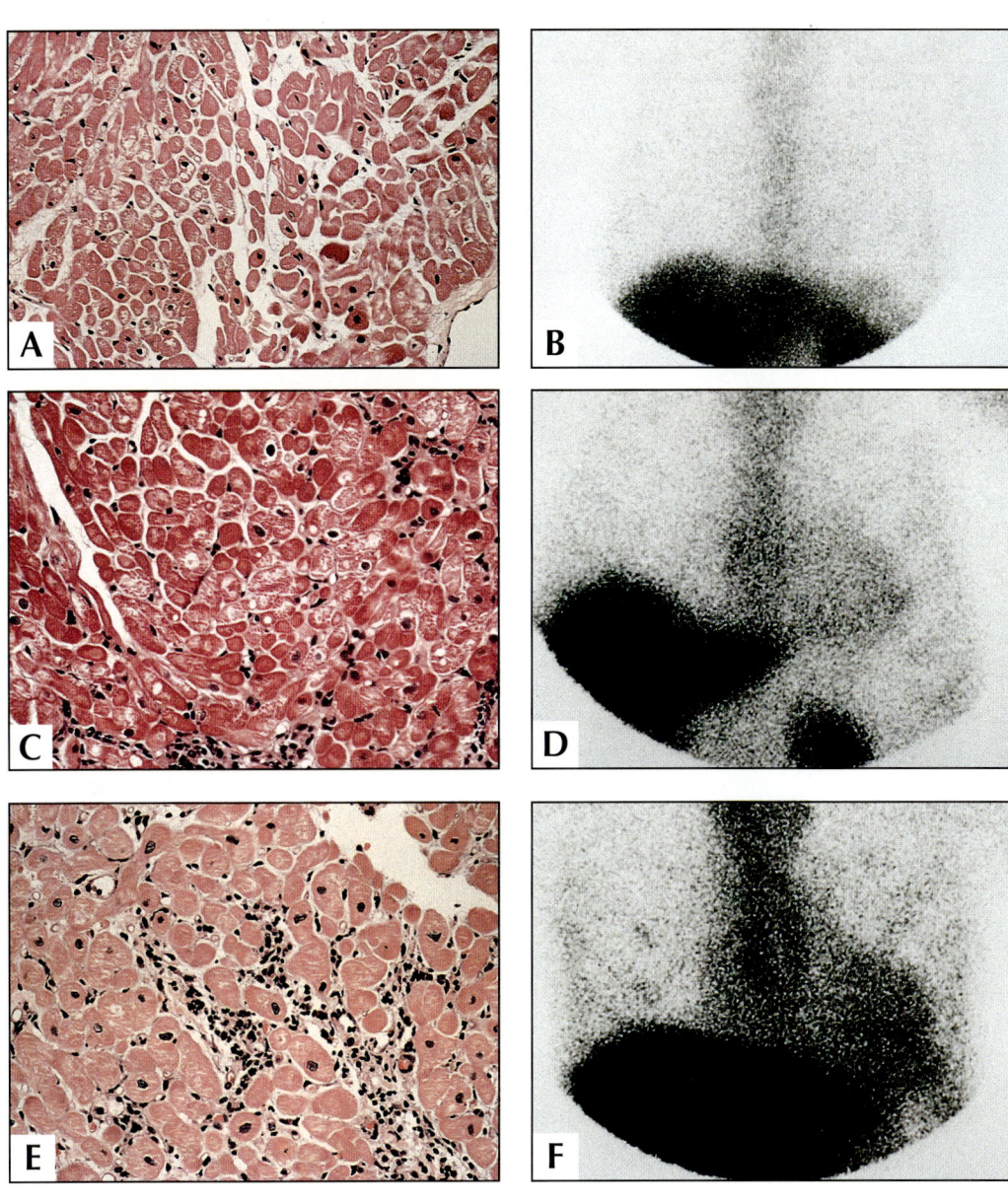

FIGURE 12-11. Noninvasive detection of myocardial damage in cardiac allograft rejection. The endomyocardial biopsy (EMB) remains the gold standard for the diagnosis of cardiac allograft rejection [22]. The International Society of Heart and Lung Transplantation (ISHLT) have classified allograft rejection on the severity scale of 0 to 4, wherein grade 0 represents absence of rejection. Transplant rejection higher than ISHLT grade 2 is associated with progressively increasing myocardial necrosis and necessitates augmentation of immunosuppressive treatment. Since the presence of myocardial necrosis determines the need for therapeutic intervention, antimyosin positivity should allow triage of patients and obviate the need for EMB in transplant recipients. EMB are performed 12 to 15 times in allograft recipients in the first year after transplantation, so a potential reduction in the need for EMB would be an immense contribution to the management of these patients.

The concomitant antimyosin scintigraphy and EMB studies performed in cardiac allograft recipients demonstrated that the magnitude of myocardial uptake increased proportionately to the degree of severity of transplant rejection. **A**, EMB from a patient with no histologic evidence of transplant rejection (ISHLT grade 0) demonstrated no antimyosin antibody uptake, **B**, with a heart to lung ratio (HLR) of 1.46 (anterior image). **C**, EMB from another patient demonstrated mild transplant rejection, showing diffuse lymphomononuclear infiltration (but no myocardial damage) and was classfied as ISHLT grade 1B rejection. **D**, Modest antimyosin uptake was reported with HLR of 1.65. **E**, In a patient with ISHLT grade 3A rejection, evidence of more than two foci of myocyte necrosis and mononuclear cellular infiltration in an allograft recipient corresponds to significant antimyosin uptake (HLR, 1.98) (**F**).

Continued on next page

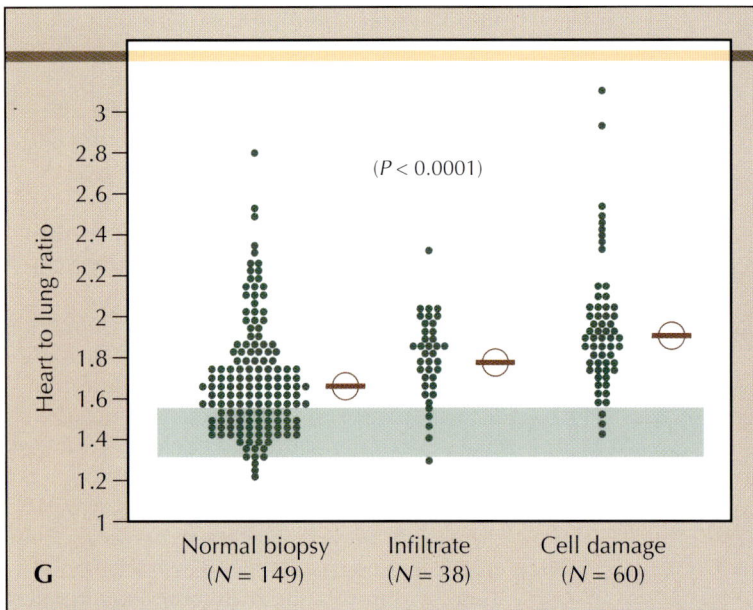
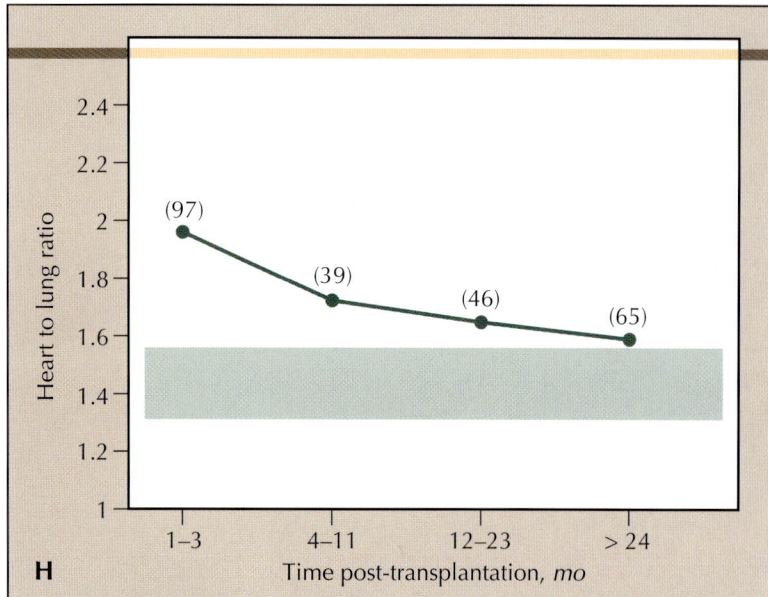

FIGURE 12-11. (*Continued*) **G**, On collective interpretation of results, antimyosin uptake was significantly higher in patients who had evidence of myocardial damage in their EMB specimens (HLR, 1.95 ± 0.38) compared with those who demonstrated only interstitial infiltration (1.88 ± 0.31) or had normal biopsy (1.78 ± 0.26). Although the magnitude of antimyosin uptake increases proportionally with the histologic severity of rejection, the uptake was highly variable and no definite range of antimyosin uptake could be established that predicted a higher likelihood of detecting histologic evidence of myocyte necrosis. Furthermore, antimyosin studies were usually positive during the first month after transplantation, reflecting myocardial damage from ischemic injury, and precluded the role of antimyosin scintigraphy as a test for detection of transplant rejection.

The natural course of rejection-related myocardial damage has been assessed through serial antimyosin studies [23]. **H**, The antimyosin antibody HLR uptake at 1 to 3, 4 to 12, 13 to 24, and longer than 24 months gradually declined from 1.93 ± 0.3, 1.73 ± 0.23, and 1.65 ± 0.22 to 1.58 ± 0.2, respectively. Analysis of sequential studies in the same patients suggested that resolution of antimyosin uptake may represent the development of partial immunologic tolerance, and may determine a favorable long-term course. Such an evolving trend differs substantially from the abrupt histologic evidence of acute rejection observed in EMB interspersed among intervals of normal biopsy results. Serial studies also demonstrate that the resolution of antimyosin uptake significantly varies from patient to patient, suggesting that the rate of development of tolerance to the graft is highly variable. In general, once a negative scan had developed, recurrent rejection was not observed in the absence of a change in immunosuppressive regimen. Complications related to rejection have been shown to be associated with intense antibody uptake. Patients who develop complications, *eg*, congestive heart failure, acute infarction, accelerated vasculopathy, require retransplantation, or die have higher antimyosin uptake (HLR, 2.1 ± 0.16) compared with those who did not suffer complications (HLR, 1.74 ± 0.3) ($P < 0.0001$) [23]. In fact, an HLR above 2.0 seemed to imply a substantial risk for the development of complications. (*Panels A through F from* Ballester *et al.* [24]; with permission; *panels G and H adapted from* Ballester *et al.* [22].)

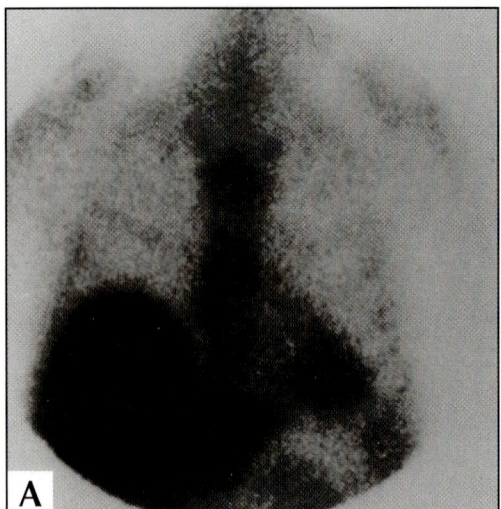
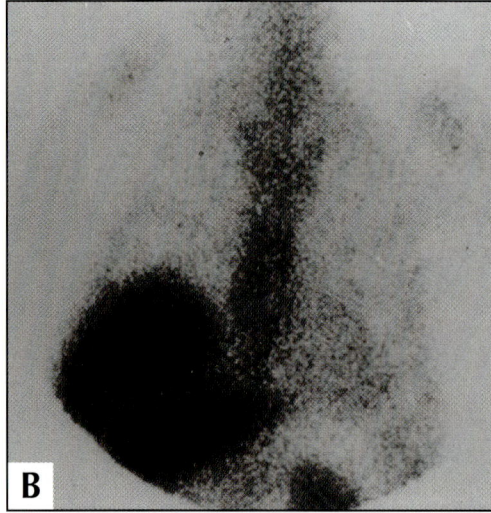

FIGURE 12-12. Algorithms for allograft management with antimyosin imaging. In antimyosin scans performed at 1, 2, and 3 months after transplantation, two evolving patterns of antibody uptake were detected [23]. In two thirds of patients, a decreasing pattern was observed whereby the intensity of antibody uptake at 3 months, **B**, was lower than the first month, **A**.

Continued on next page

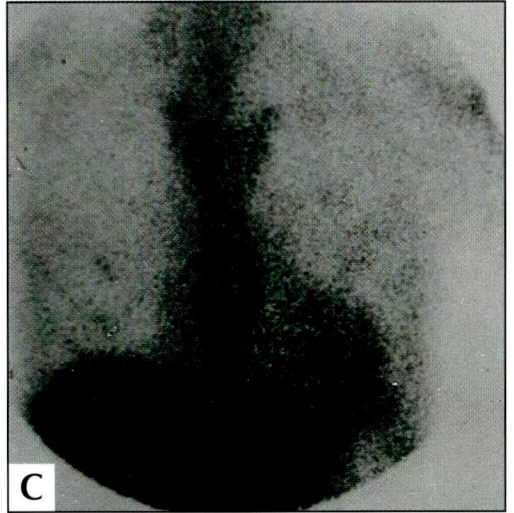
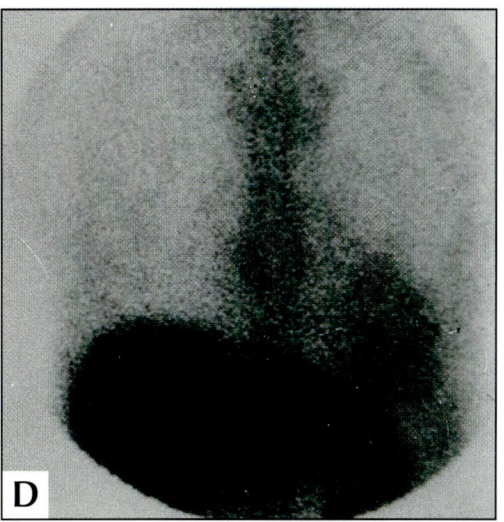
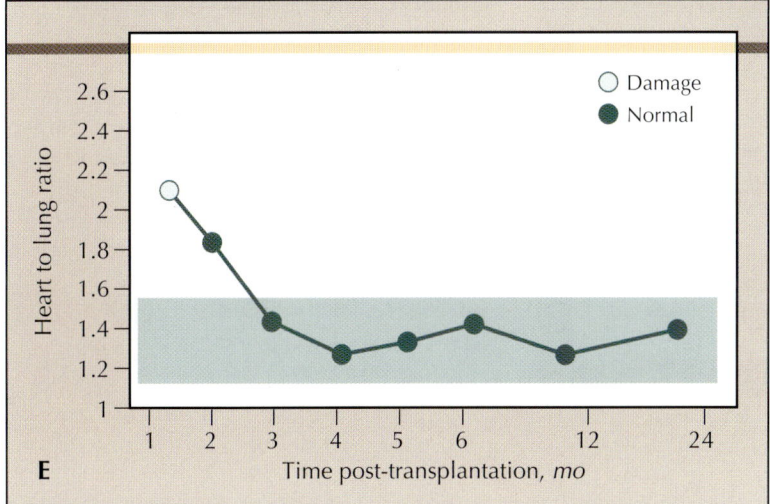
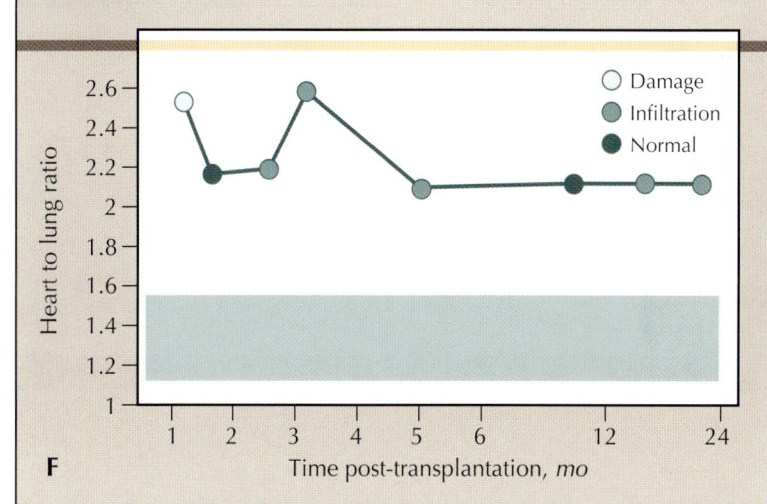

Figure 12-12. *(Continued)* In these patients, no rejection-related complications were seen during the first year. **C, D,** The remaining patients showed persistent uptake during the first 3 months, and 60% of that group developed complications. It is likely that persistent myocyte damage represented ongoing rejection activity regardless of histologic exacerbations of disease in the endomyocardial biopsy (EMB).

E, F, Trends of the heart to lung ratio (HLR) in resolving (*panel E*) and persistent (*panel F*) uptake groups, and their comparison with EMB results. Within the trend charts, EMB results demonstrate no consistency, and prognostic information provided by the evolution of scans was not obtained from EMB performed during the same time. In fact, patients who demonstrated either a decreasing or persistence pattern showed a similar prevalence of biopsy-verified rejection, 37% and 43%, respectively. Therefore, a decreasing 3-month pattern may allow a more rapid decrement in immunosuppression and a decrease in frequency of EMB. Conversely, high persistent antimyosin uptake during this period requires closer surveillance for rejection, and may warrant additional EMB and more aggressive immunosuppression regimens. The shaded HLR area represents normal antimyosin uptake. (*Panels A through D from* Ballester *et al.* [22]; *with permission; panels E and F adapted from* Ballester *et al.* [22].)

Apoptotic Cell Death

Characteristics of Cellular Necrosis and Apoptosis

CHARACTERISTICS	APOPTOSIS	NECROSIS
Topography		
Distribution	Scattered	Adjacent cells
Cellular involvement	Usually single	Group of cells
Morphology		
Cell volume	Decreased	Increased
Organelle structure	Intact	Swollen
Cell membrane	Intact	Ruptured
Cell integrity	Small fragments	Ruptured cells
Nucleus		
Chromatin pattern	Large crescentic	Small crescentic
DNA pattern	Fragmented, laddering on electrophoresis	Fragmented, laddering Absent, smearing
Disposition		
Inflammation	Absent	Marked
Removal	Cellular phagocytosis	Intracellular contents released

FIGURE 12-13. Characteristics of cellular necrosis and apoptosis. Apoptosis is markedly different from necrosis. Necrosis is a disorderly process that involves a group of cells and results in local inflammation; apoptosis is a genetically programmed and energy-requiring complex series of events that permits the cell to die without inducing an inflammatory response [25]. Apoptosis is believed to play a complementary but opposite role to mitosis or cellular proliferation. Apoptosis is an integral component of embryologic development and regulation of the immune system, and a cause of cell death in viral illness [26]. Excessive apoptosis or lack of appropriate apoptosis plays a role in many diseases. In oncogenesis, loss of normal apoptosis results in excessive cellular proliferation; in end-stage heart failure, apoptosis is related to progressive loss of functioning myocytes; and in autoimmune disorders, diminished apoptosis permits immunologically competent cells to survive and continue inappropriate damage to target organs.

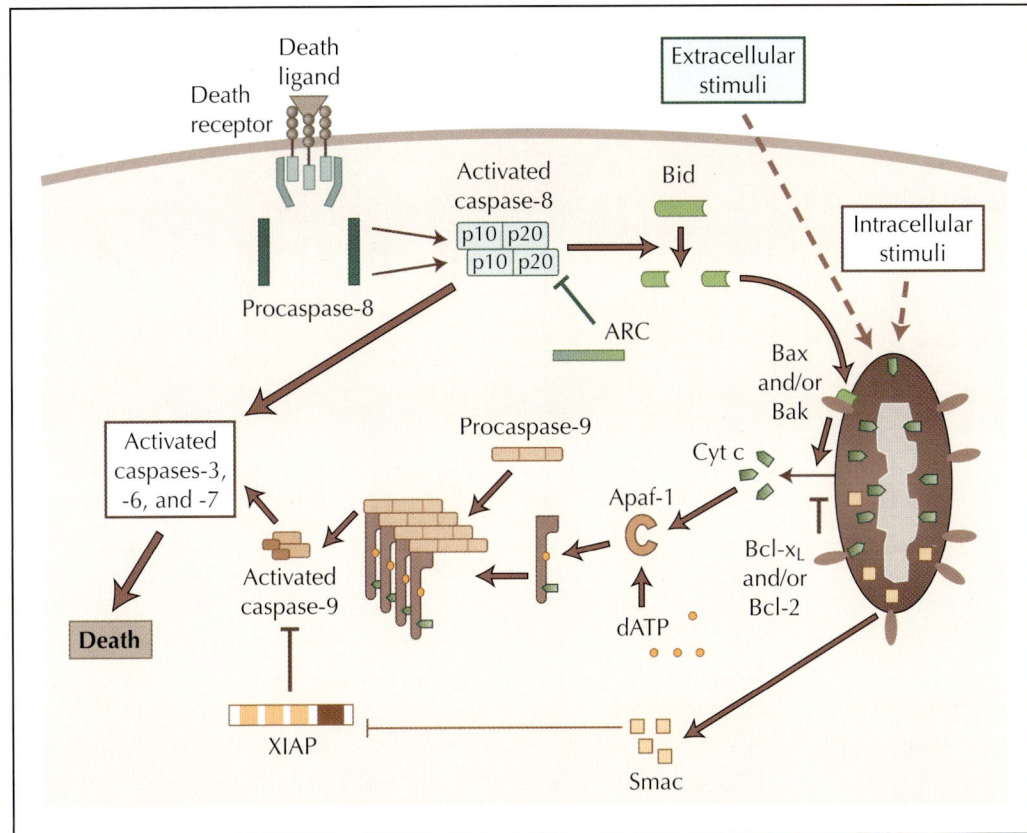

FIGURE 12-14. Signaling pathways in apoptotic cell death. Two distinct, but mutually not exclusive, pathways have been described in apoptotic cell death, one occurring through death receptors and the other through the mitochondria [27]. In the death receptor pathway, soluble or cell surface death ligands, *eg*, tumor necrosis factor-α and the Fas ligand, bind their corresponding receptors inducing the recruitment and activation of caspase-8, followed by cleavage and activation of downstream procaspases, *eg*, caspases-3, -6, and -7. Once activated, these "effector" caspases fragment cellular proteins resulting in the orderly deconstruction of the cell. The effector caspases also activate DNAses and lead to fragmentation of nuclear DNA [28]. In the mitochondrial pathway, the central event is the translocation of cytochrome c (Cyt c) from the inner mitochondrial membrane to the cytoplasm [29]. This pathway is initiated by death stimuli that include ischemia, oxidative stress, genotoxic stress, UV radiation, chemotherapeutic agents, and calcium excess. The signaling pathways that transduce these signals to the mitochondria are poorly understood. Once in the cytoplasm, cytochrome c and dATP/ATP (already present in the cytoplasm) bind Apaf-1, stimulating its oligomerization and the subsequent recruitment of procaspase-9 into a large complex termed the *apoptosome*. Following its activation, caspase-9 cleaves and activates downstream effector caspases. The death receptor and mitochondrial pathways are linked by Bid, which is cleaved by caspase-8 following death receptor activation [30]. Subsequently, the carboxy fragment of Bid, tBid, translocates to the mitochondria where it inserts into the outer mitochondrial membrane and stimulates cytochrome c release through its interactions with Bax and/or Bak, which are pro-apoptotic proteins. Bcl-2 and Bcl-x_L, anti-apoptotic proteins, which also reside in the outer mitochondrial membrane, inhibit cell death by competing with Bax and Bak for tBid, and possibly through their direct interactions with Bax and Bak [31]. These death pathways are inhibited by several other prosurvival pathways, which include ARC or FLIP (inhibitors of caspase-8), and XIAP or related proteins (inhibitors of caspases-3 and -9) [32]. When apoptosis is induced, in addition to cytochrome c, SMAC is also released from the mitochondria that binds to XIAP, precluding its inhibition of caspases. (*Courtesy of* Richard Kitsis, MD, Albert Einstein College of Medicine, Bronx, NY.)

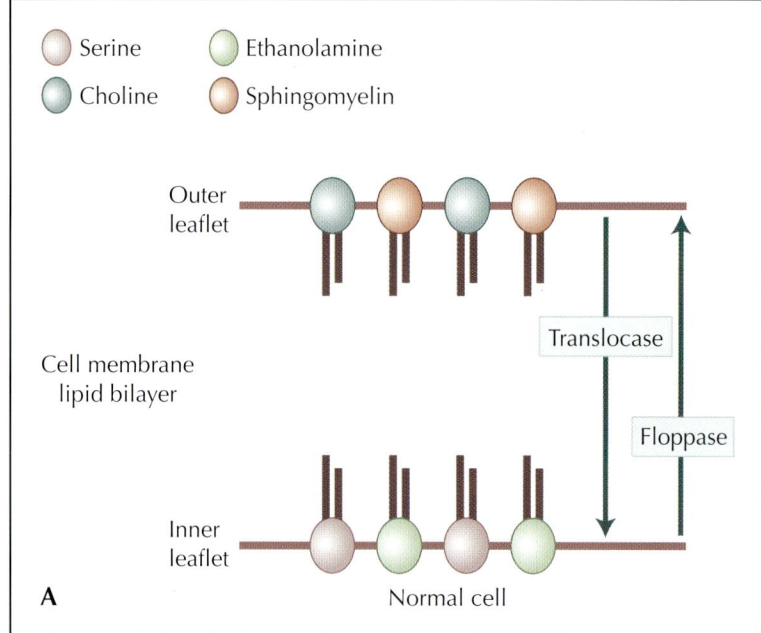 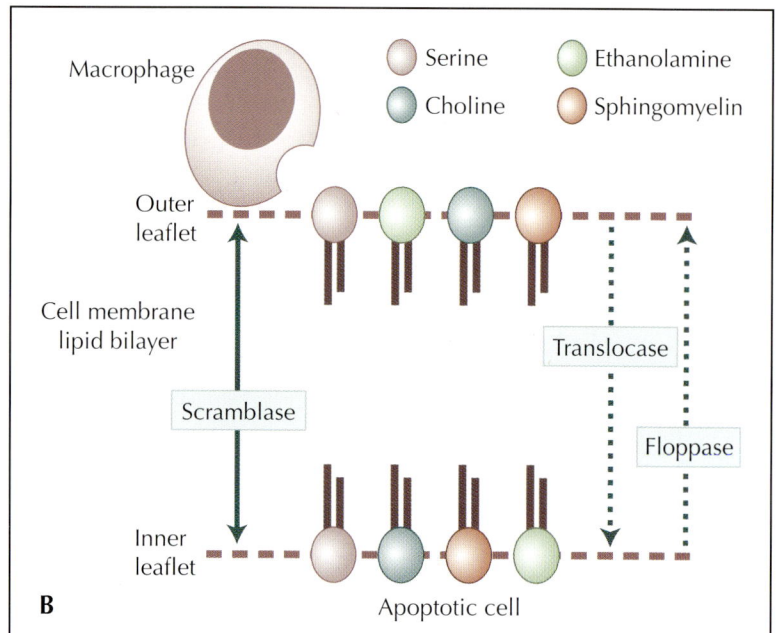

FIGURE 12-15. Molecular basis of imaging of apoptosis. All major morphologic alterations in apoptosis are intracellular. For noninvasive radionuclide imaging, it is preferable to target extracellular surface alterations [6,7]. Cell membrane changes predominantly are brought about by disorderly distribution of phospholipids in the lipid bilayer. Exposure of phosphatidylserine (PS) on the cell surface constitutes the most important cell membrane alteration during apoptosis. A, PS is actively restricted to the inner leaflet of the lipid bilayer by an ATP-dependent enzyme, *translocase*; PS is virtually absent from the surface of normal cells. Translocase in concert with a second energy-dependent enzyme, *floppase*, which actively pumps cationic phospholipids such as phosphatidylcholine and sphingomyelin to the outer leaflet of the lipid bilayer, maintains an asymmetric distribution of anionic (acidic, inner) and cationic (basic, outer) phospholipids across the plasma membrane. B, During apoptosis, translocase and floppase enzymes are deactivated, and in addition, yet another enzyme, *scramblase*, is activated. The latter enzyme facilitates bidirectional movement of phospholipids within the lipid bilayer. The ubiquitous exposure of PS during apoptosis makes it an attractive target for the detection of apoptotic cells. Annexin V, an endogenous human protein with a molecular weight of 35 kD, has a nanomolar affinity for PS bound to the cell membrane. Annexin complexed to membrane-bound PS may be the principal signal for phagocytosis of cells undergoing apoptosis [4]. Annexin V labeled with fluorescein has been used in conjunction with flow cytometry to identify apoptotic cells. Recombinant human annexin V has been radiolabeled with ^{99m}Tc, and has been used for noninvasive imaging of apoptosis following intravenous injection.

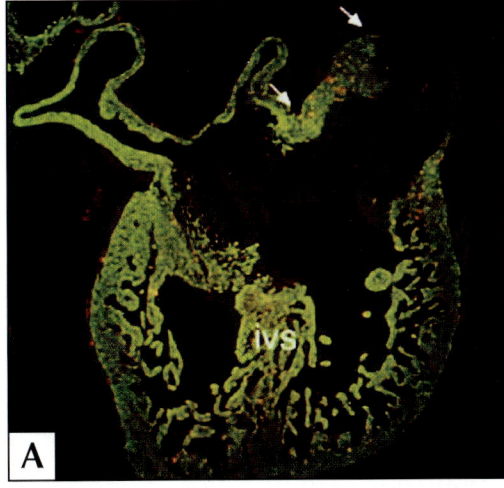 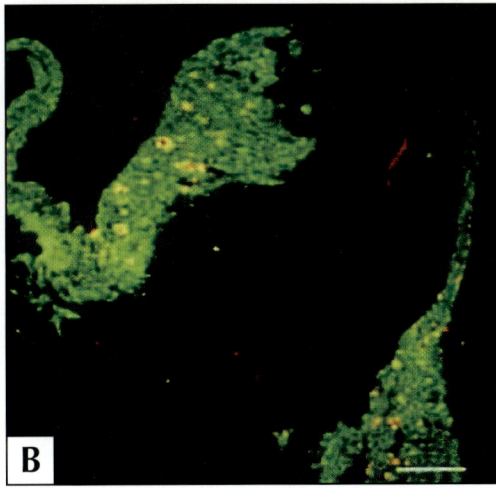 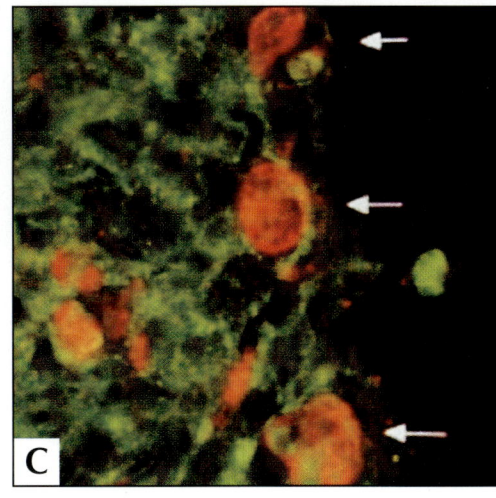

FIGURE 12-16. Apoptosis during development of the heart. During morphogenesis of the heart, apoptosis regulates the development of atrial and ventricular cavities and valves and routing of great vessels [33,34]. Failure to control apoptosis during morphogenesis of the heart may result in congenital cardiac diseases, such as bicuspid aortic valve, ventricular dysplasias, congenital heart block, and outflow tract abnormalities. **A**, Apoptosis is detected in the developing chicken heart at embryonic day 8 in the outflow tract region using fluorescent annexin V to detect apoptotic cells (*arrows*). **B**, Higher magnification of outflow tract region. **C**, High magnification with confocal microscopy shows three apoptotic cells in different stages of apoptosis. The frequency of apoptosis correlated with outflow tract remodeling and shortening, suggesting that critically timed removal of myocardial cells is crucial for proper development of the outflow tract.

Although apoptosis is very important for appropriate embryologic development of the heart, it does not occur in adult cardiomyocytes, which are terminally differentiated and have lost the capability to proliferate. However, various pathologic insults may induce apoptotic cell death. Apoptosis may occur when necrotic stimuli are not severe enough to result in cell death or when the injury is interrupted. Slow, ongoing apoptosis in chronic myocardial disease has also been reported, especially during growth factor excess in cardiomyopathy and heart failure [34]. (*From* Watanabe *et al.* [35]; with permission.)

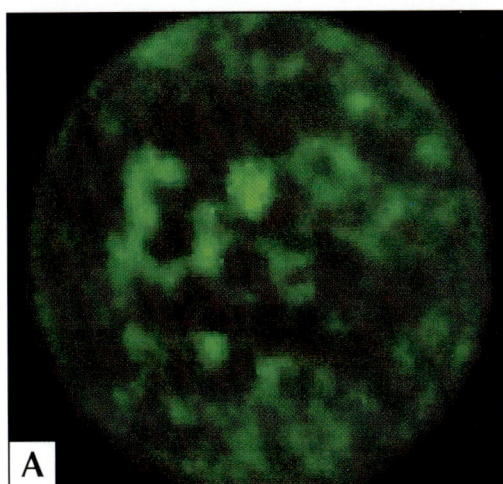 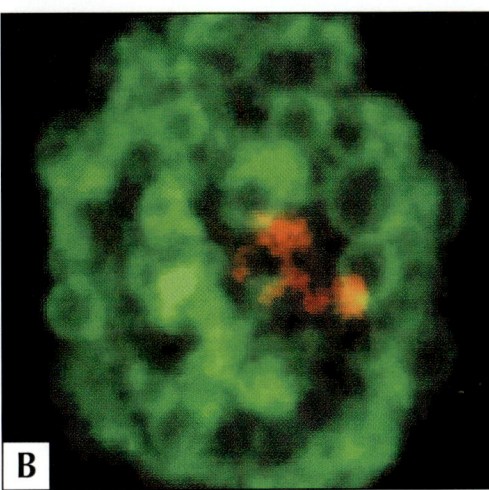 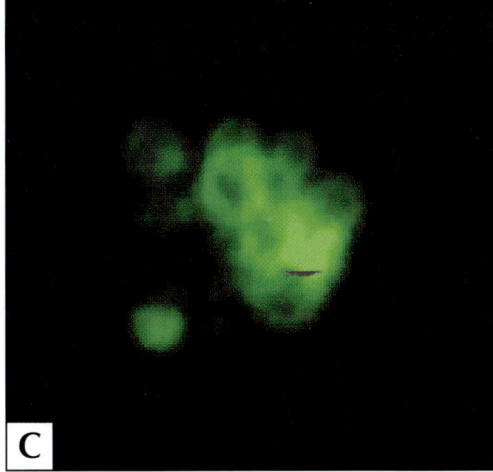

FIGURE 12-17. Specificity of annexin V binding to apoptotic cells. Cell death detection studies in vitro have shown the specificity of annexin V binding to apoptotic cells in all phases of the apoptotic process, from very early to the final stages [36]. **A**, Binding of annexin V to a Jurkatt cell in the early phase of apoptosis indicated by green fluorescence on the cell surface. The cell was stimulated with Fas antibody, resulting in activation of the death receptor pathway. Although the binding of annexin V to the Jurkatt cell surface is observed, the shape and integrity of the cell are still intact. **B**, Binding of annexin V to a Jurkatt cell in the late phase of apoptosis, when the cell has started to show blebbing and shrinkage. Note binding of propidium iodide to the cell nucleus (red) due to plasma membrane leakage, which indicates secondary necrosis. This illustrates the plasticity among the various forms of cell death. **C**, Binding of annexin V in the last stage of apoptosis characterized by the formation of apoptotic bodies. It is believed that phosphatidylserine exposure (and hence the annexin V binding) occurs downstream to the caspase-3 activation. (*Courtesy of* C. Reutelingsperger, the Netherlands.)

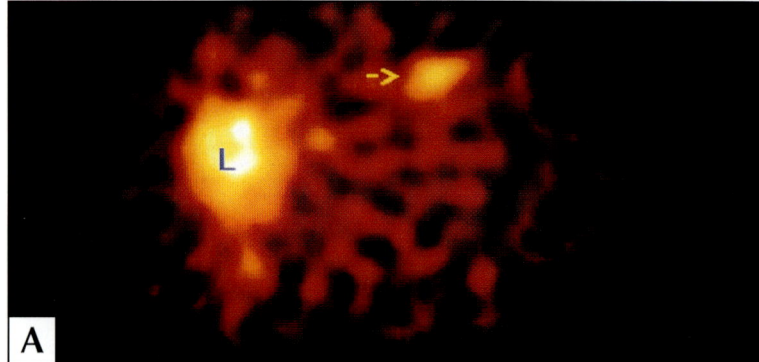
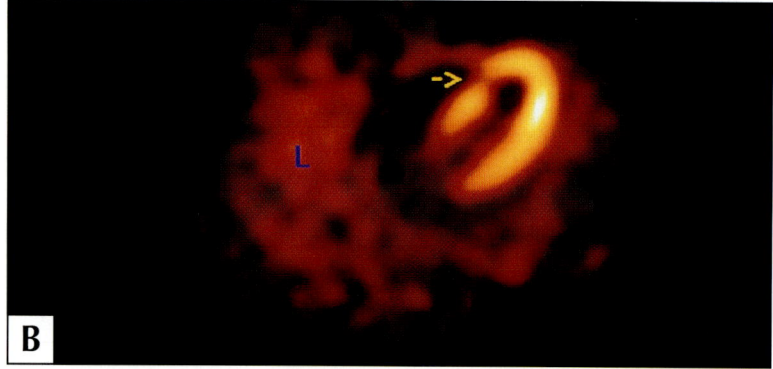

FIGURE 12-18. Noninvasive detection of apoptosis in acute myocardial infarction. Post-mortem studies in patients with acute myocardial infarction have shown high frequency of apoptotic cell death program in the infarct area. The apoptotic cells predominantly are seen in the infarct periphery, where the severity of ischemic insult is milder. However, upon reperfusion the infarct center shows an extensive admixture of apoptotic and necrotic cells as the doomed cells are rescued from necrosis but die by apoptosis. Further, reperfusion injury may accelerate apoptosis in the cells in the center of the infarct. Accordingly, annexin V studies have been performed in patients with acute myocardial infarction [37].

A, Patient with acute antero-apical infarction was injected with annexin V labeled with ^{99m}Tc immediately following reperfusion; the transverse SPECT image shows enhanced uptake of annexin V in the apical region of the heart (*arrow*). **B,** The sestamibi perfusion scan obtained 48 hours later shows a perfusion defect that corresponds to the region of annexin uptake. The defect on the sestamibi SPECT indicates that cells that bound annexin V on day 1 must have undergone cell death. One intriguing possibility is that the binding of annexin V in the infarct area may indicate that cell death in this region may be preventable through intervention in the cell death program (*see* Fig. 12-22). (*From* Hofstra *et al.* [37]; with permission.)

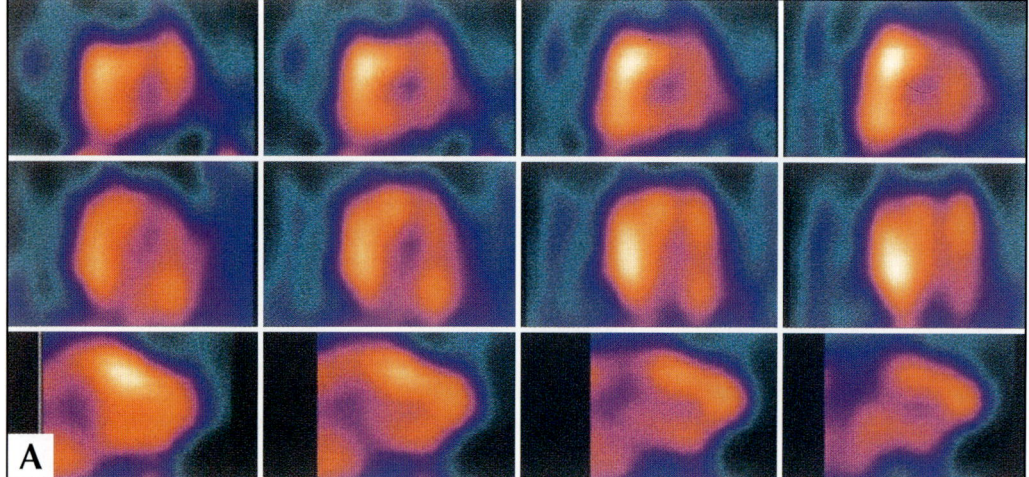
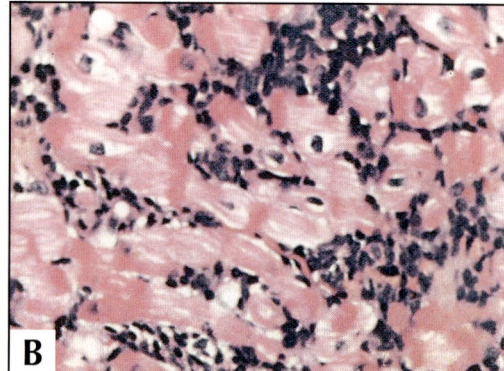
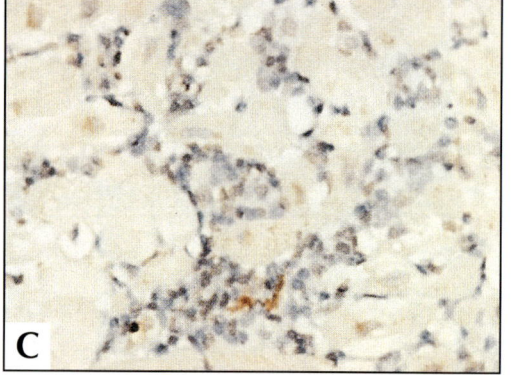
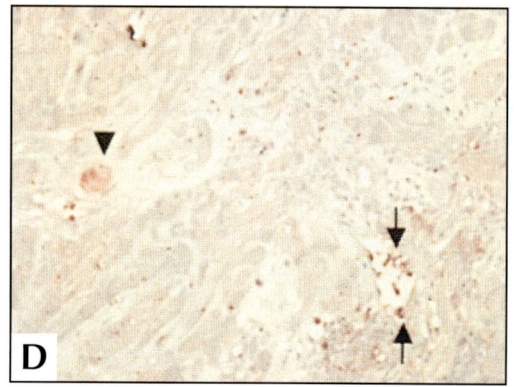

FIGURE 12-19. Detection of cell death in patients with cardiac transplant rejection. The process of rejection is initiated by the invasion of inflammatory cells in the heart, which subsequently leads to myocardial damage. Myocardial cell death at least in part may occur by activation of the apoptotic program. The severity of apoptosis in allograft rejection increases in proportion to severity of rejection, and therefore, visualization of cell death with ^{99m}Tc-labeled annexin V may provide a means for noninvasive detection of transplant rejection [38].

A, Short-axis (*top row*), vertical long-axis (*middle row*), and horizontal long-axis (*bottom row*) resting SPECT myocardial perfusion images showing enhanced uptake of annexin V in the heart of a cardiac transplant recipient, indicating the presence of apoptosis.

B, Histologic analysis of a biopsy taken from this patient shows International Society of Heart and Lung Transplantation (ISHLT) grade 3A/4 rejection exemplified by the presence of two foci of myocardial damage surrounded by lymphomononuclear cell infiltrate; one focus of myocyte damage is demonstrated here. **C,** In situ end-labeling staining and **D,** caspase-3 staining of subjacent sections reveal numerous apoptotic cells. Treatment of the patient with augmented immunosuppressive drugs resulted in abrogation of annexin V uptake on a follow-up annexin V study [38]. Of the 18 patients studied, 13 patients had negative annexin V scans; biopsy revealed no evidence of significant transplant rejection. Of the remaining five patients, three had nondiffuse annexin V uptake and biopsy evidence of ISHLT grade 2 rejection, whereas two patients demonstrated diffuse annexin V uptake and histologic evidence of ISHLT grade 3A or higher rejection. Since patients with grade 2 or higher rejection require augmented immunosuppressive treatment, it is conceivable that the need for endomyocardial biopsies may be obviated if larger clinical trials confirm the initial findings. (*From* Narula *et al.* [38]; with permission.)

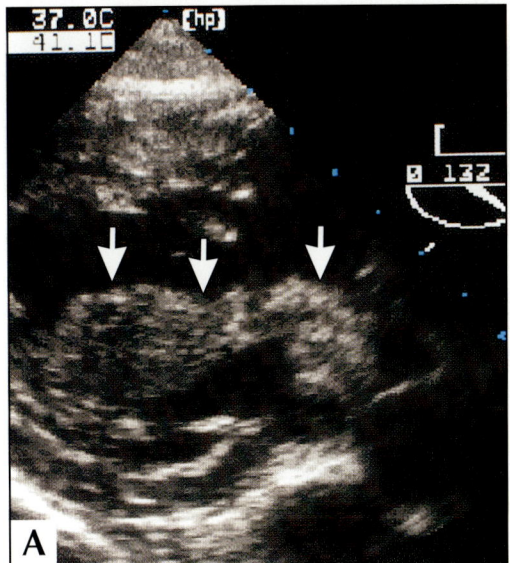 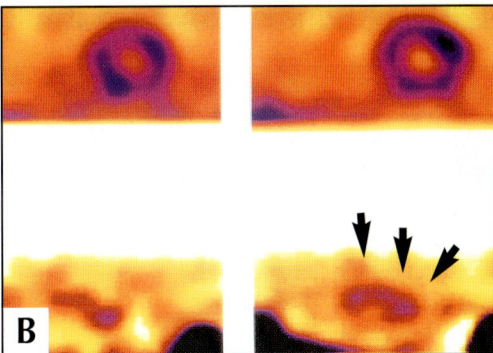 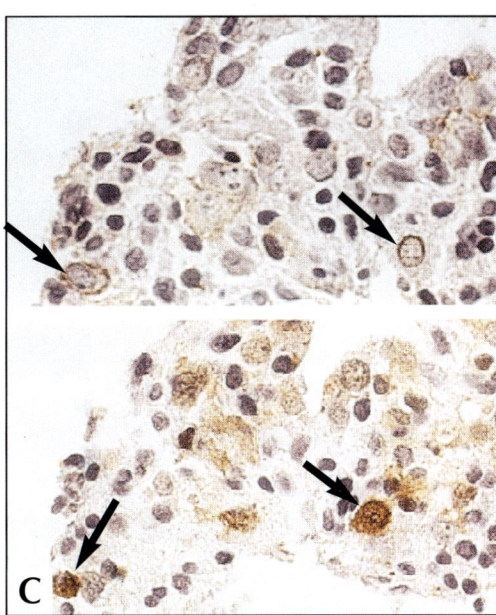

FIGURE 12-20. Detection of cell death in a patient with an intracardiac tumor. It is often difficult to obtain diagnostic information on tumors that cannot be biopsied prior to treatment, such as intracardiac tumors. Pathologic studies have demonstrated that malignant tumors not only possess high proliferation rates, but also high apoptosis rates. Therefore, noninvasive imaging of cell death with annexin V may offer means to obtain diagnostic information [39]. **A,** Transesophageal echocardiographic image of a patient who presented with symptoms of fatigue and syncope showing a large mass originating from the anterolateral left ventricular wall (*arrows*). **B,** Radionuclide ^{201}Tl imaging study demonstrates normal perfusion of the left ventricle (LV) (*top panel*). Simultaneous annexin V study (*bottom panel*) demonstrated enhanced uptake of radiotracer within the contour of the LV, with a morphology resembling the echocardiographic image (*arrows*). **C,** Histologic analysis of the tumor revealed an undifferentiated malignant angiosarcoma, showing annexin V binding (brown staining, *top, arrows*) to cells with apoptosis also indicated by positive staining for caspase-3 (CM1 antibody, *bottom, arrows*). Annexin uptake has not been observed in benign intracardiac tumors such as atrial myxomas. (*From* Hofstra *et al.* [39]; with permission.)

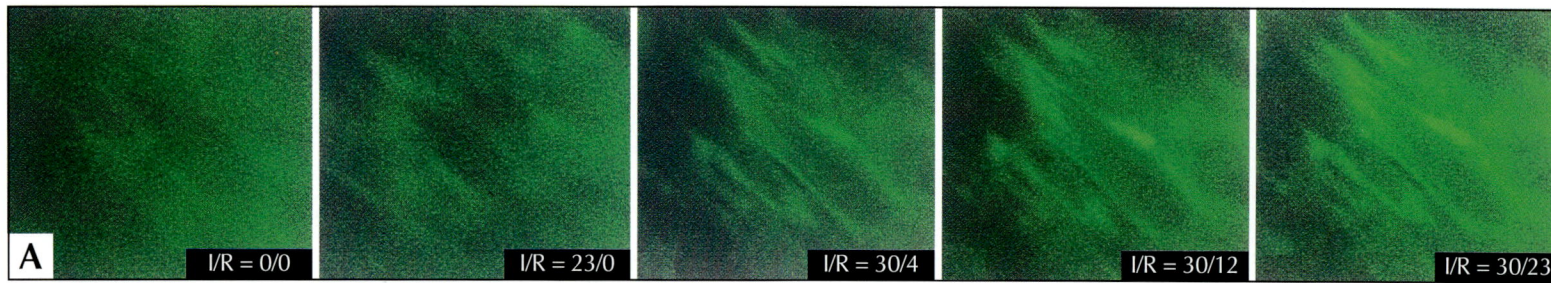

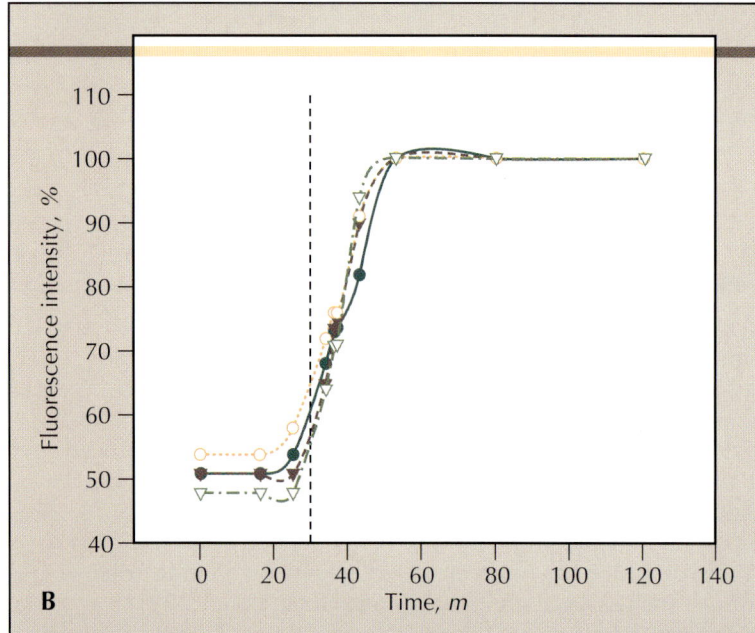

Figure 12-21. Dynamics of annexin V binding within myocardial infarction in a beating heart mouse model. Novel optical imaging technology and the development of photostable fluorescent probes have allowed detection of the binding of annexin V to single cells in the beating heart of the living mouse and to clarify the kinetics of annexin V binding [40]. These experiments facilitate development of noninvasive radionuclide imaging protocols. **A**, Extensive binding of annexin V to the myocytes occurs in the myocardial region at ischemic risk at various time points. I/R represents ischemia and reperfusion times, respectively, in minutes. Kinetic studies at the level of the single cell show that binding of annexin V starts at the time of reperfusion and rapidly progresses, resulting in a complete saturation of the cell within 20 minutes after the onset of reperfusion. **B**, Schematic representation of the kinetics of annexin V binding to single cardiomyocytes from different experiments. *Dotted vertical line* denotes the onset of reperfusion. Within 15 to 20 minutes following the onset of reperfusion, complete saturation of the cells can be seen. (*Panel A from* Dumont *et al.* [40]; with permission; *panel B adapted from* Dumont *et al.* [40].)

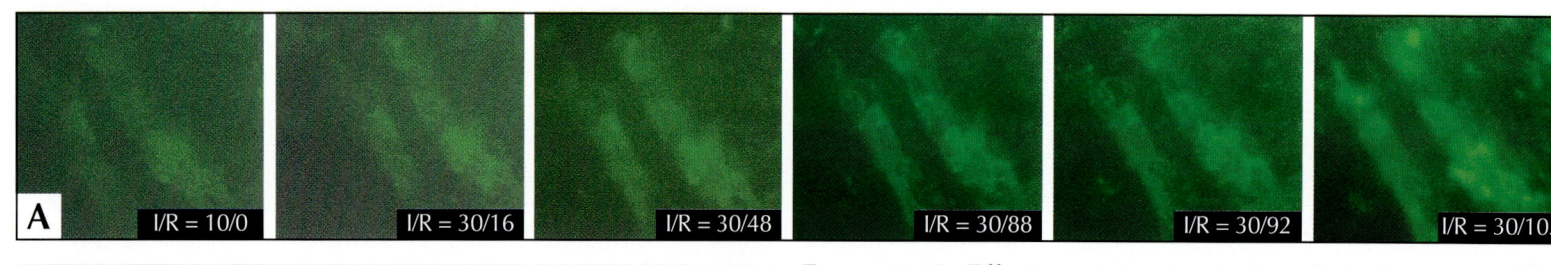

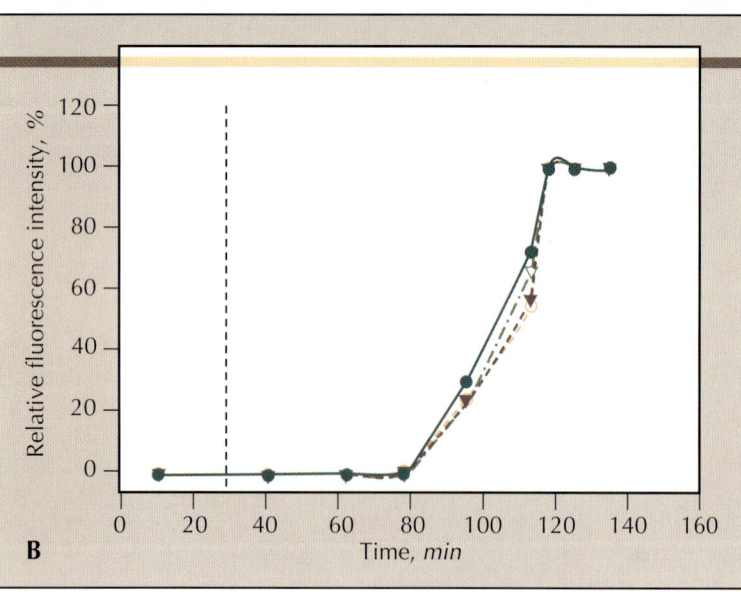

Figure 12-22. Effective intervention in the cell death program. The possibility of detecting apoptotic cell membrane changes in the heart of the living mouse allows for the rapid screening of novel cell death-inhibiting compounds, such as caspase inhibitors. This also offers the possibility of the development of novel strategies for intervention in early ischemic periods, including acute myocardial infarction. **A**, The effect of a caspase inhibitor on the binding of annexin V in vivo [40]. Pretreatment of the mouse with a caspase blocker (IDUN `965; Idun Pharmaceuticals, San Diego, CA) results in almost complete abrogation of binding of annexin V to the injured area, indicating rescue of the cells (compare with Fig. 12-21). The cells that still take up annexin V show a delay in the onset of binding and a slower saturation curve. In addition, the morphology of the cell looks different. I/R represents ischemia and reperfusion times, respectively, in minutes. These data indicate that caspase activation is a crucial step in the cell death program following ischemia and reperfusion, at least in the acute phase.

B, Schematic representation of delayed annexin V binding to cardiomyocytes. Different symbols indicate individual cells. (*Panel A from* Dumont *et al.* [40]; with permission; *panel B adapted from* Dumont *et al.* [40].)

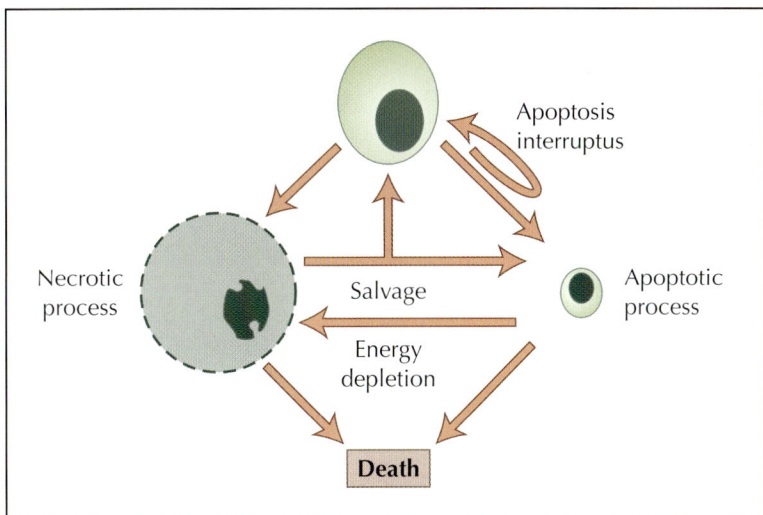

Figure 12-23. Future directions. Researchers recognize that cell death may not be divisible into classic apoptosis and necrosis, and the doomed cells may defect from necrotic to apoptotic process and vice versa based on the available energy content [41,42]. This may be especially true during acute insults and particularly in terminally differentiated cells (*eg*, heart muscle and neuronal cells). During the process of apoptosis, the cells may exhaust energy stores and die by necrosis. Unlike necrosis, apoptosis is an active energy-requiring process, and energy consumption increases enormously if repair of the apoptotic DNA is undertaken, such as by the help of poly-ADP-ribose polymerase [43]. On the other hand, the cells may be exposed to necrotogenic stimuli (such as during acute myocardial infarction) but interruption of injury (such as by reperfusion) may prevent the necrotic process, and partially damaged cells may progress to death through apoptotic cascade [44]. Similarly, milder necrotogenic stimuli may also induce cell death by apoptosis [45]. It is conceivable that the pendular process of cell death may produce various morphologic hybrids of the two cell death types, and interventions to abrogate any one process may produce benefits that exceed expectations. The cell death, at least in terminally differentiated cells, may therefore allow multiple avenues of intervention and the importance of appropriate recognition of the death programs can hardly be overemphasized.

REFERENCES

1. Narula J, Baliga R: What's in a name? Would that which we call death by any other name be less tragic? *Ann Thorac Surg* 2001, 72:1454–1456.

2. Kumar V: Cellular pathology I: Cell Injury and Cell Death. In *Robbins Pathologic Basis of Disease*, edn 6. Edited by Cotran RS, Kumar V, Collins T, *et al*. Philadelphia: WB Saunders Company; 1999:8.

3. Majno J, Joris I: Apoptosis, oncosis, and necrosis: an overview of cell death. *Am J Pathol* 1995, 146:3.

4. Narula J, Zaret BL: Noninvasive detection of cell death: from tracking epitaphs to counting coffins. *J Nucl Cardiol* 2002, 9:554–560.

5. Khaw BA, Narula J: Antimyosin scintigraphy in cardiovascular disease. *Trends Cardiovasc Med* 1992, 2:197–204.

6. Fadok VA, Laszlo DJ, Noble PW, *et al*.: Particle digestibility is required for induction of the phosphatidylserine recognition mechanism used by murine macrophages to phagocytose apoptotic cells. *J Immunol* 1993, 151:4274–4285.

7. Koopman G, Reutelingsperger CP, Kuijten GA, *et al*.: Annexin V for flow cytometric detection of phosphatidylserine expression on B cells undergoing apoptosis. *Blood* 1994, 84:5–20.

8. Strauss HW, Narula J, Blankenberg FG: Radioimaging to identify myocardial cell death and probably injury. *Lancet* 2000, 356:180–181.

9. Kim RJ, Chen EL, Lima JA, Judd RM: Myocardial Gd-DTPA kinetics determine MRI contrast enhancement and reflect extent of and severity of myocardial injury after acute reperfused infarction. *Circulation* 1996, 94:3318–3326.

10. Dewanjee MK, Kahn PC: Mechanism of localization of ^{99m}Tc-labeled pyrophosphate and tetracycline in infarcted myocardium. *J Nucl Med* 1976, 17:639–646.

11. Khaw BA, Nakazawa A, O'Donnell SM, *et al*.: Avidity of technetium 99m glucarate for the necrotic myocardium: in vivo and in vitro assessment. *J Nucl Cardiol* 1997, 4:283–290.

12. Khaw BA, Scott J, Fallon JT, *et al*.: Myocardial injury: quantitation by cell sorting initiated with anti-myosin fluorescent spheres. *Science* 1982, 217:1050–1053.

13. Khaw BA, Fallon FT, Strauss HW, *et al*.: Myocardial infarct imaging of antibodies to canine cardiac myosin with indium-111-diethylene-triamine pentaacetic acid. *Science* 1980, 209:295–297.

14. Narula J, Khaw BA, Dec GW Jr, *et al*.: Recognition of acute myocarditis masquerading as acute myocardial infarction. *N Engl J Med* 1993, 328:100–104.

15. Carrio I, Estorch M, Berna L, *et al*.: Assessment of anthracycline-induced myocardial damage by quantitative indium 111 myosin-specific monoclonal antibody studies. *Eur J Nucl Med* 1991, 18:806–812.

16. Strauss HW, Narula J, Khaw BA: Acute myocardial infarct imaging with Tc-99m and In-111 antimyosin Fab. In *Monoclonal Antibodies in Cardiovascular Disease*. Edited by Khaw BA, Narula J, Strauss HW. Philadelphia: Lea & Febiger; 1994:30–42.

17. Khaw BA, Fallon JT, Beller GA, *et al*.: Specificity of localization of myosin specific antibody fragments in experimental myocardial infarction: histologic, histochemical, autoradiographic and scintigraphic studies. *Circulation* 1979, 60:1527–1531.

18. Jain D, Lahiri A, Crawley JCW, *et al*.: Indium-111 antimyosin imaging in a patient with acute myocardial infarction: postmortem correlation between histopathologic and autoradiographic extent of myocardial necrosis. *Am J Cardiac Imaging* 1988, 2:158–161.

19. Jain D, Lahiri A, Raferty EB: Immunoscintigraphy for detecting acute myocardial infarction without electrocardiographic changes. *BMJ* 1990, 300:151–153.

20. Aretz HT: Myocarditis: the Dallas criteria. *Hum Pathol* 1987, 18:619–624.

21. Narula J, Khaw BH, Dec GW: Diagnostic accuracy of antimyosin scintigraphy in suspected myocarditis. *J Nucl Cardiol* 1996, 3:371–381.

22. Ballester M, Carrio I, Narula J: Algorithms for management of heart transplant rejection based on surveillance of myocardial damage by antimyosin antibody imaging. In *Cardiac Allograft Rejection*. Edited by Dec GW, Narula J, Ballester M, Carrio I. Boston: Academic Publishers; 2001:381–398.

23. Ballester M, Obrador D, Carrio I, *et al*.: Early postoperative reduction of monoclonal antimyosin antibody uptake is associated with absent rejection-related complications after heart transplantation. *Circulation* 1992, 85:61–68.

24. Ballester M, Bordes R, Tazelaar HD, *et al*.: Evaluation of biopsy classification for rejection: relation to detection of myocardial damage by monoclonal antimyosin antibody imaging. *J Am Coll Cardiol* 1998, 31:1357–1361.

25. Horvitz HR: Genetic control of programmed cell death in the nematode *Caenorhabditis elegans*. *Cancer Res* 1999, 59(Suppl 7):S1701–S1706.

26. Thompson CB: Apoptosis in the pathogenesis and treatment of disease. *Science* 1995, 267:1456–1462.

27. Green DR: Apoptotic pathways: the roads to ruin. *Cell* 1998, 94:695–698.

28. Green DR: Apoptotic pathways: paper wraps stone blunts scissors. *Cell* 2000, 102:1–4.

29. Zamzami N, Kroemer G: The mitochondrion in apoptosis: how Pandora's box opens. *Nat Rev Mol Cell Biol* 2001, 2:67–71.

30. Gross A, Yin XM, Wang K, *et al.*: Caspase cleaved BID targets mitochondria and is required for cytochrome c release, while BCL-XL prevents this release but not tumor necrosis factor-R1/Fas death. *J Biol Chem* 1999, 274:1156–1163.

31. Gross A, McDonnell JM, Korsmeyer SJ: BCL-2 family members and the mitochondria in apoptosis. *Genes Dev* 1999, 13:1899–1911.

32. Salvesen GS, Duckett CS: Apoptosis: IAP proteins: blocking the road to death's door. *Nat Rev Mol Cell Biol* 2002, 3:401–410.

33. Watanabe M, Jafri A, Fisher SA: Apoptosis is required for the proper formation of the ventriculo-arterial connections. *Dev Biol* 2001, 240:274–288.

34. Narula J, Haider N, Virmani R, *et al.*: Apoptosis in myocytes in end-stage heart failure. *N Engl J Med* 1996, 335:1182–1189.

35. Watanabe M, Choudhry A, Berlan M, *et al.*: Developmental remodeling and shortening of the cardiac outflow tract involves myocyte programmed cell death. *Development* 1998, 125:3809–3820.

36. Reutelingsperger CP, Dumont E, Thimister PW, *et al.*: Visualization of cell death in vivo with the annexin A5 imaging protocol. *J Immunol Methods* 2002, 265:123–132.

37. Hofstra L, Liem IH, Dumont E, *et al.*: Visualisation of cell death in vivo in patients with acute myocardial infarction. *Lancet* 2000, 356:209–212.

38. Narula J, Acio ER, Narula N, *et al.*: Annexin V imaging for noninvasive detection of cardiac allograft rejection. *Nat Med* 2001, 7:1347–1352.

39. Hofstra L, Dumont EA, Thimister PW, *et al.*: In vivo detection of apoptosis in an intracardiac tumor. *JAMA* 2001, 285:1841–1842.

40. Dumont EA, Reutelingsperger CP, Smits JF, *et al.*: Real-time imaging of apoptotic cell-membrane changes at the single-cell level in the beating murine heart. *Nat Med* 2001, 7:1352–1355.

41. Leist M, Single B, Naumann H, *et al.*: Inhibition of mitochondrial ATP generation by nitric oxide switches apoptosis to necrosis. *Exp Cell Res* 1999, 249:396–403.

42. Leist M, Nicotera P: The shape of cell death. *Biochem Biophys Res Commun* 1997, 236:1–9.

43. Blankenberg F, Narula J, Strauss HW: In vivo detection of apoptotic cell death: a necessary measurement for evaluating therapy for myocarditis, ischemia, and heart failure. *J Nucl Cardiol* 1999, 6:531–539.

44. Gottlieb RA, Burleson KO, Kloner RA, *et al.*: Reperfusion injury induces apoptosis in rabbit cardiomyocytes. *J Clin Invest* 1994, 94:1621–1628.

45. Tanaka M, Ito H, Adachi S, *et al.*: Hypoxia induces apoptosis with enhanced expression of Fas antigen messenger RNA in cultured neonatal rat cardiomyocytes. *Circ Res* 1994, 75:426–433.

CHAPTER 13

RADIONUCLIDE IMAGING OF ATHEROSCLEROTIC LESIONS

Jagat Narula, Renu Virmani, and Barry L. Zaret

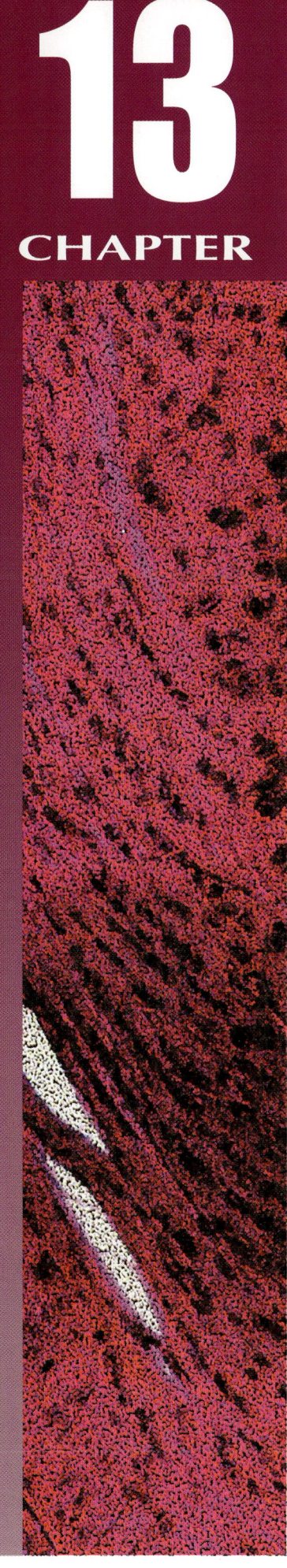

Coronary artery disease is the most important cardiovascular health problem of the past century [1,2], and threatens to continue to be the major cause of morbidity and mortality in the 21st century, both in developing and developed nations, and in men and women. The management of coronary artery disease has traditionally been based on assessment of the severity of stenosis of the vascular lumen [3]. Although the degree of luminal encroachment by the plaque may determine the severity of anginal symptoms, it does not predict the outcomes such as likelihood of development of acute coronary syndromes including sudden cardiac death. Limited success has been achieved by the use of angioscopy and intravascular ultrasonography or more recently with optical coherence tomography and MRI in the assessment of plaque morphology [4–7]. Appropriate targeting strategies with radionuclide imaging techniques could identify the predominant cellular population and biochemistry of the atherosclerotic plaque and help predict the likelihood of clinical events [8].

Approximately 13 million people in the United States suffer from coronary artery disease [1]. Although recognition of each one of them should constitute the ultimate diagnostic goal, it is most desirable to identify the subset of patients who are likely to develop acute coronary events. Of the 13 million people arriving at emergency departments, 1.1 million have acute coronary events, and nearly 45% of these people die every year. It is well recognized that thrombotic occlusion of the vessel wall usually occurs as a result of plaque rupture or plaque surface erosion [9]. The plaques that are vulnerable to rupture have large lipid cores, attenuated fibrous caps, and intense macrophage infiltration [9,10]. Macrophages release metalloproteinases that digest matrix and induce fibrous cap rupture [11]. Plaque rupture exposes the thrombogenic lipid core, leading to thrombotic luminal obstruction. Therefore, if the plaques vulnerable to rupture are to be identified, radionuclide strategies should be developed that target either macrophages or large lipid cores. It is conceivable that only modified lipids of the plaque should be targeted that are not present in the circulation, and similarly those macrophage epitopes should be targeted that are expressed on the lesional macrophages and are not expressed by the circulating monocytes [8].

In addition to identification of vulnerable plaques, radionuclide imaging can be exploited for noninvasive recognition of postangioplasty restenosis because the pathologic substrate of the complication is often characteristic. At least 700,000 coronary artery angioplasties are performed every year with or without stent placement. Although the newer stents have demonstrated a significant promise of reduction in restenotic complications, approximately 15% to 40% of the patients develop postinterventional restenosis [12]. Restenosis results from aggressive proliferation of smooth muscle cells, extracellular matricial growth, and vascular remodeling [13,14]. Targeting strategies will require identification of the rate of proliferation of smooth muscle cells, and it will be expected that we target those characteristics of smooth muscle cells that are acquired by the proliferating ones and are not present on quiescent cells [8].

This chapter provides a simplified scheme of pathogenetic events in atherosclerosis. The diagrams and their descriptions are by no means complete, but they offer necessary information for development of novel molecular techniques for the noninvasive detection of atherosclerotic lesions. Clinical imaging studies have not been performed in the coronary arteries owing to the inadequate resolution capabilities of the gamma camera; only a few studies have been performed in the peripheral arteries, including femoral and carotid arteries, with limited success. Most of the data presented here are derived from studies performed in common experimental models of atherosclerosis. These models include New Zealand White rabbits subjected to balloon de-endothelialization of their abdominal aorta followed by high-lipid, high-cholesterol diet; Watanabe heritable hypercholesterolemic rabbits; and ApoE-deficient mice. To improve the resolution for obtaining clinically useful information on particularly vulnerable but less occlusive plaques, new intravascular β-detectors are undergoing experimental validation.

EVOLUTION OF ATHEROSCLEROTIC LESIONS

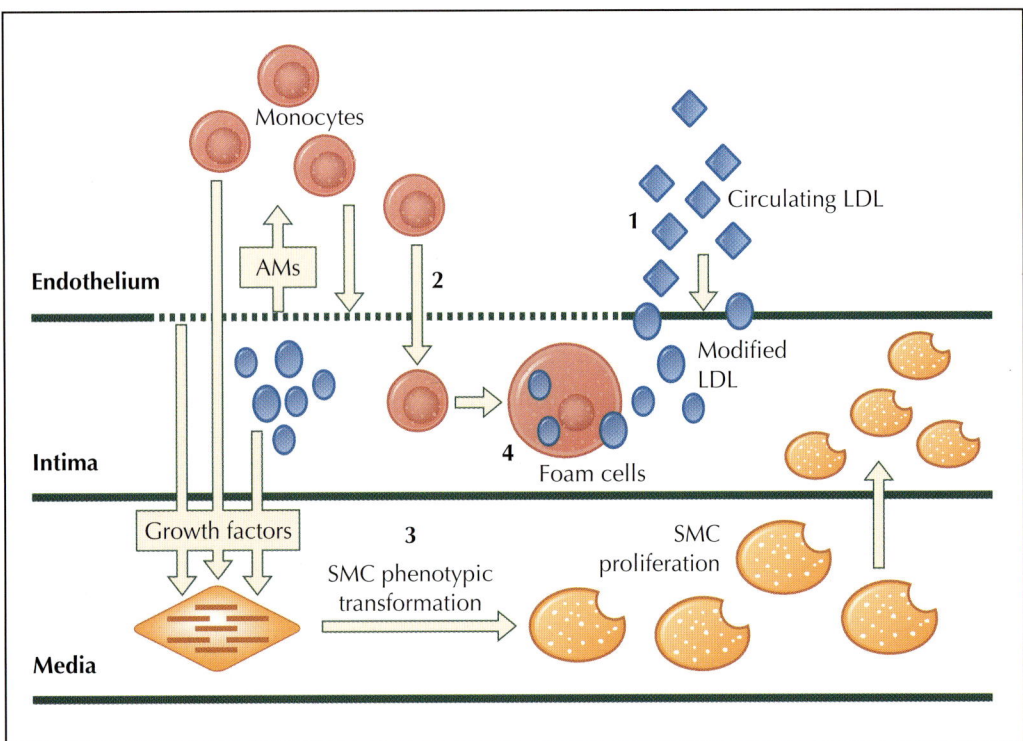

FIGURE 13-1. Pathogenesis of atherosclerosis. Although the pathogenesis of atherosclerosis is not well understood, it is currently considered to be an immunoinflammatory response of the endothelium to the injury. The damage to the intima is initiated by various standard risk factors of coronary atherosclerotic disease, most importantly hyperlipidemia. The intimal reaction initiates a complex interplay of blood vessel wall components with blood elements [15,16]. A consequent expression of adhesion molecules (AMs) on the endothelium leads to recruitment of monocytes, which migrate to the subendothelial layer. The tempered release of vasoactive substances from the injured endothelium induces a phenotypic alteration of medial smooth muscle cells (SMCs). At this time, the constellation of injured intimal cells, monocyte-derived macrophages, and modified lipids leads to release of growth factors that induce proliferation of phenotypically transformed SMCs and ultimately their migration to the neointima.

Macrophages and SMCs in the subendothelial space ingest modified low-density lipoprotein (LDL) cholesterol and evolve into foam cells. The uptake of modified lipid in the monocytes occurs through scavenger LDL receptors (SRA; see Fig. 13-3), which are not inhibited by intracellular lipid contents, and these foam cells are restricted from departing the subintimal space. (Courtesy of Jeffrey Bender and Jagat Narula).

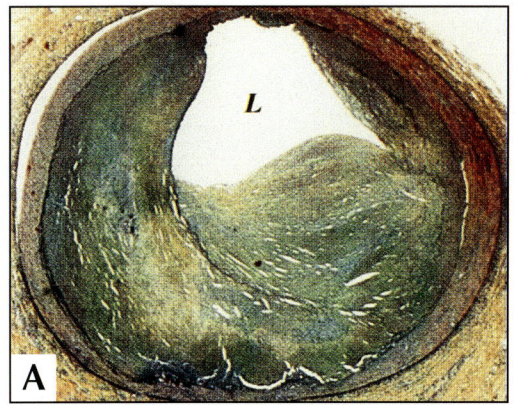
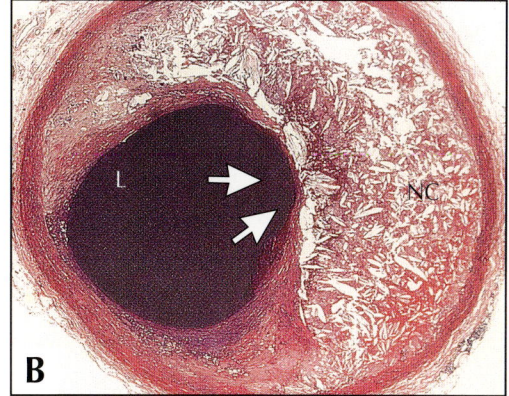
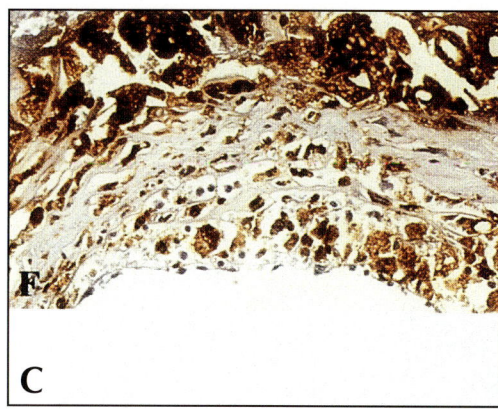

FIGURE 13-2. Pathologic basis of radionuclide imaging of atherosclerotic lesions. Radionuclide imaging of atherosclerotic lesions targets one of the three major components of the plaque, including lipid cores, macrophage infiltration, or proliferating smooth muscle cells (SMCs) [8]. The presence of a large necrotic lipid core and a thin overlying fibrous cap contributes to vulnerability of plaque to rupture. In addition, intense macrophage infiltration in the fibrous cap leads to release of cytokines and matrix metalloproteinases (MMPs), and thereby renders the plaque prone to rupture [17,18]. Histopathologic characteristics of vulnerable or unstable plaques dictate targeting macrophages (or cytokines and MMPs) or large lipid cores for noninvasive imaging. On the other hand, prevalence of SMCs provides stability to plaque, but their rapid proliferation is associated with progressive luminal stenosis such as in postangioplastic restenosis [13,14] and is also seen in sudden coronary death in the young. It should be possible to selectively target any one of these components by radionuclide imaging.

This figure demonstrates morphologic characteristics of stable plaque (**A**) and vulnerable plaque (**B, C**). The stable plaque in **A** consists almost exclusively of fibrous tissue. The vulnerable plaque in **B** comprises a necrotic core (NC), a thin (< 65 μ) overlying fibrous cap (*arrows*), and heavy infiltration by macrophages, which has stained brown after immunohistochemical staining with anti-macrophage KP-1 antibody (**C**). **A, B,** Movat pentachrome stain; **C,** KP1-1/CD68 antibody staining with avidin-biotin peroxidase complex method. L—lumen. (*From* Narula *et al.* [8]; with permission.)

TARGETING MACROPHAGE INFILTRATION IN ATHEROSCLEROTIC LESIONS

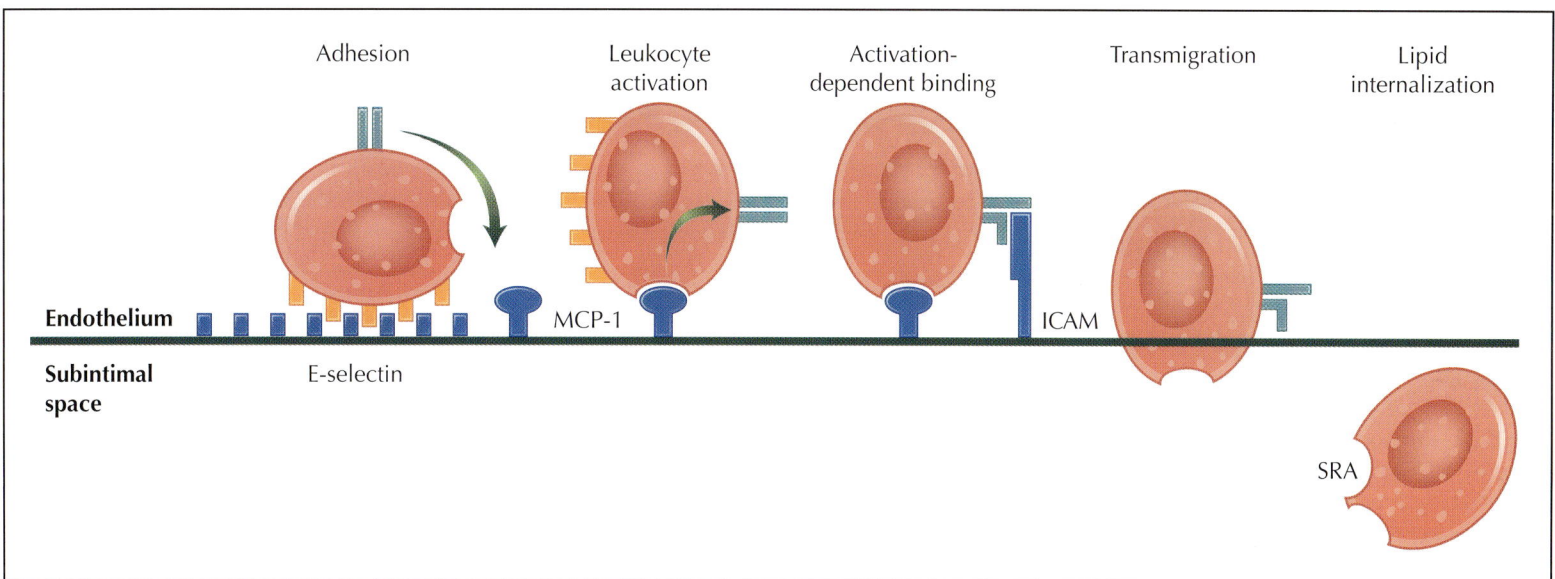

FIGURE 13-3. Potential molecular targets of infiltrating macrophages. Macrophage infiltration in the vessel wall follows a systematic process that includes phases such as leukocyte rolling, leukocyte and endothelial activation, and activation-dependent adhesion of leukocytes [19]. The initial endothelial cell activation results in expression of selectin molecules such as E- or P-selectin. Corresponding monocyte selectins such as L-selectin facilitate monocyte-endothelial interactions. This interaction induces a potentially reversible monocyte "rolling," and slows the otherwise rapidly moving circulating monocytes, providing a greater opportunity for subsequent monocyte arrest. Monocytes adhere avidly and thus firmly to the endothelium if chemotactic peptides such as monocyte chemoattractant protein-1 (MCP-1) are expressed on the endothelial surface. If the endothelial injury is not significant and chemoattractants have not been expressed, the selectins are shed, and the monocytes roll back to the blood stream. The interaction of the endothelial chemoattractants and their receptors on monocytes lead to a G protein–coupled receptor-mediated activation of β_1- or β_2-integrins (*eg*, VLA-4, LFA-1, or Mac-1). These integrins bind firmly to endothelial-expressed adhesion molecules of the immunoglobulin gene superfamily such as VCAM-1 and ICAM (intercellular adhesion molecule)-1 or -2. The multipronged attachment of monocytes to the endothelium commits them to transendothelial migration. This is also a dynamic process mediated, in part, by endothelial cell junctional molecules including PECAM-1, cadherins, and the newly described β_2-integrin ligand DNAM-1. (*Courtesy of* Jeffrey Bender and Jagat Narula).

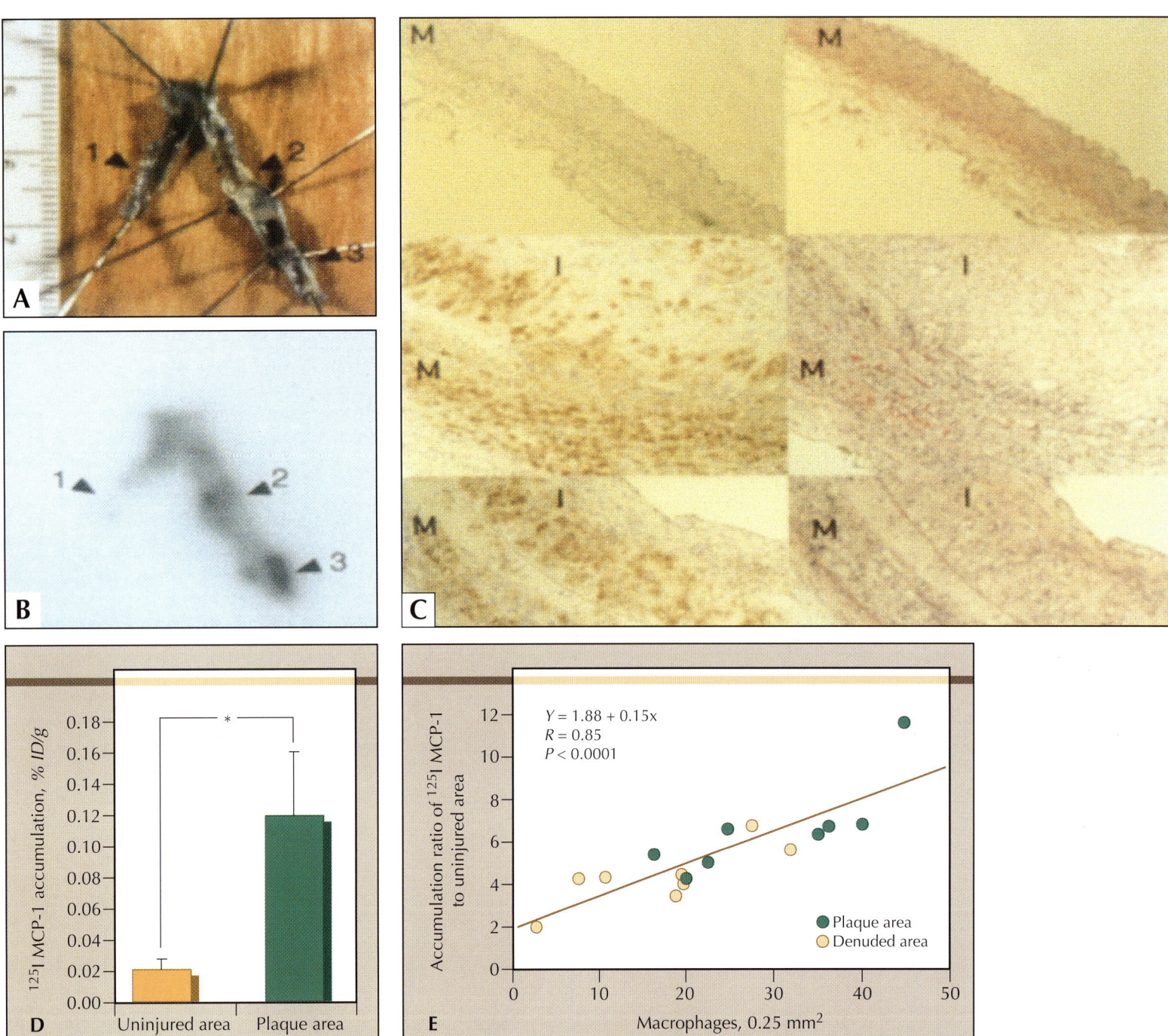

FIGURE 13-4. Radionuclide imaging of inflammation in the atherosclerotic plaques. As the first proof of the principle, ^{111}In oxine-labeled autologous monocytes were used in the patients with angiographic evidence of peripheral vascular disease [20]. After transition through the lungs during dynamic acquisition, the major site of the in vivo uptake of radiolabeled monocytes was the spleen. Focal sites of uptake were visible over the carotid or femoral arteries only in 40% of patients with proven atherosclerotic disease.

Because the receptors for chemoattractants or adhesion molecules are only expressed by infiltrating monocytes, radiolabeled MCP-1 (monocyte chemoattractant protein-1) and ICAM (intercellular adhesion molecule) have been used for the noninvasive detection of atherosclerotic lesions. ^{131}I-labeled MCP-1 has been shown to selectively accumulate in lipid-rich, macrophage-rich regions of experimental atherosclerosis model in rabbits by macroautoradiography [21]. **A,** Gross lesions of an explanted aorta from an atherosclerotic rabbit. **B,** The macroautoradiographic results closely correlate with the severity of lesions, with no uptake in uninjured part of aorta (1), moderate uptake with atherosclerotic lesions (2), and maximum uptake in the area with significant lesions (3). **C,** The histopathologic (*right*, hematoxylin and eosin) and immunohistochemical characterization (*left*, antimacrophage antibody-RAM-11) of the aortic specimens from sites 1 through 3 demonstrated proportionally increasing prevalence of macrophages. The autoradiographic uptake of MCP-1 closely correlated to the prevalence of macrophages in the lesions. **D,** The percent injected dose per gram uptake of the radiolabeled MCP-1 was significantly higher in the diseased aorta than in the nonatherosclerotic regions. **E,** Further, quantitative estimates of the number of macrophages per unit area correlated with percent injected dose per gram accumulation of ^{125}I-MCP-1 in the atherosclerotic lesions.

After subendothelial migration, monocytes develop scavenger receptors and ingest oxidized LDL more avidly (than native LDL). Scavenger receptors are not downregulated with an increase in the cholesterol content of the cell. At least four types of macrophage scavenger receptors for oxidized LDL uptake have been recognized [22]. These include scavenger receptor I or II (SRA), CD36, CD68, and FcγRII. Up to 50% of cholesterol uptake may occur via CD36 and 30% via SRA. These receptors are unique to the recruited macrophages and are not borne by circulating monocytes; the radiolabeled ligands for these receptors may constitute attractive targets for noninvasive imaging. Only Fc receptors have been targeted with limited success by radiolabeled nonspecific IgG imaging of the peripheral arterial lesions in four patients (data not shown) [23]. (*Panels A–C from* Ohtsuki *et al.* [21]; with permission; *panels D and E adapted from* Ohtsuki *et al.* [21].)

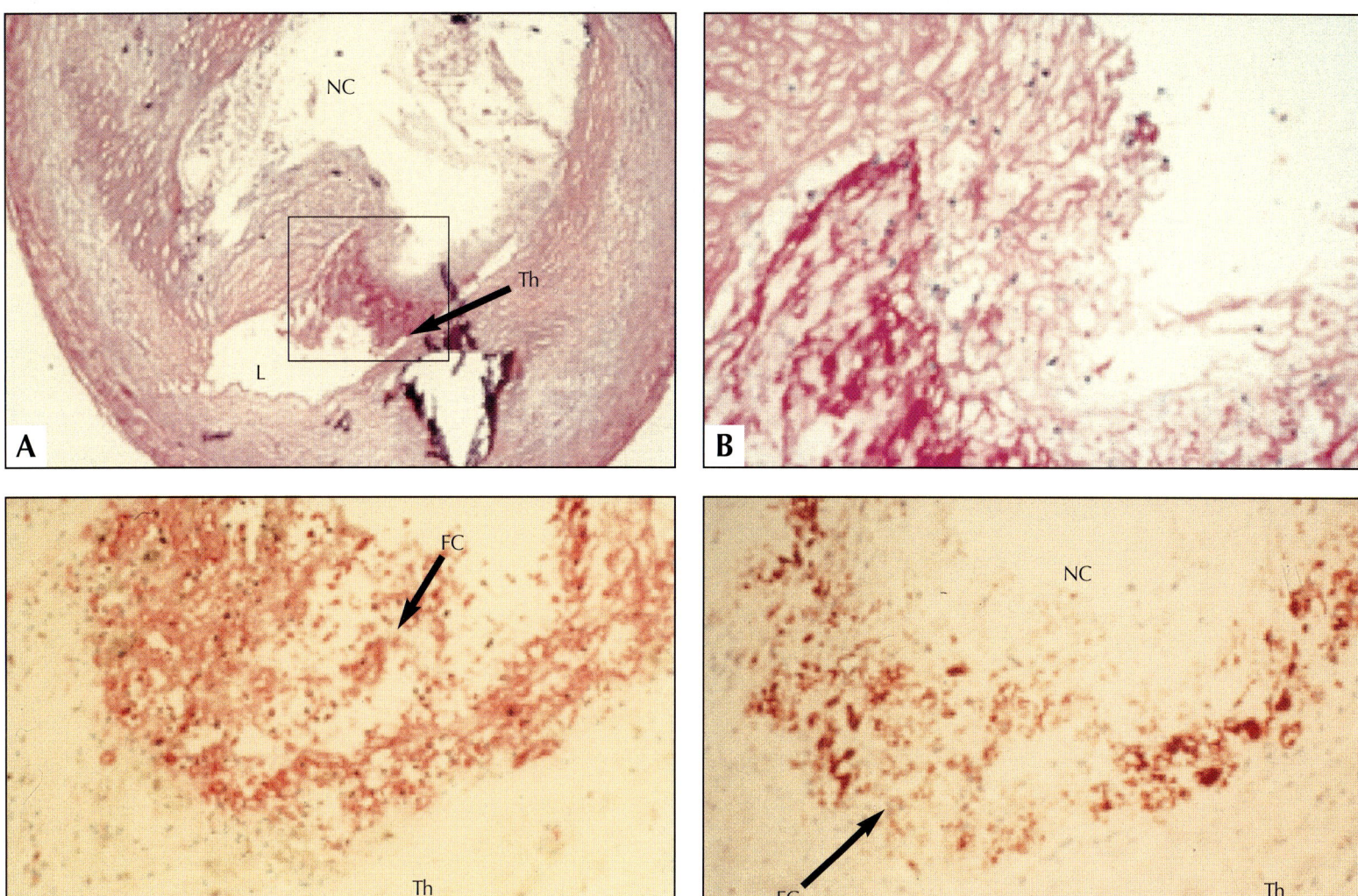

FIGURE 13-5. Potential relationship between inflammation and plaque vulnerability. Although the mechanisms that convert a stable plaque into a vulnerable plaque are not well understood, recent literature supports the theory that cell death in neointima may contribute to vulnerability of plaque to rupture. In a study of nonulcerated atheromatous plaques [24], a high incidence of apoptosis was observed in inflammatory cells, predominantly in macrophages surrounding the lipid core. This finding is corroborated by other studies of human plaques [25–27], suggesting that macrophage cell death is perhaps responsible for core formation and/or expansion. Other studies have proposed that the chronic loss of smooth muscle cells (SMCs) in atherosclerotic plaques in the human aorta [28] may lead to fibrous cap (FC) thinning and vulnerability. Plaque-derived SMCs in culture appear to possess an innate susceptibility to cell death, which may be associated with a defect in the phosphorylation of the tumor suppressor gene (*eg, p105rb*) [29,30], or an excess of cyclin-dependent kinase inhibitor (*eg, p21*) [31]. In addition to direct cap thinning, SMC apoptosis may also contribute to plaque vulnerability by massive recruitment of inflammation in the fibrous cap, by induction of expression of MCP-1 (monocyte chemoattractant protein-1) and IL (interleukin)-8 [32].

In addition to plaque vulnerability, apoptosis of macrophages may contribute to the actual process of plaque rupture. In our study in the hearts of victims of sudden death secondary to plaque rupture [27], we observed a strikingly high prevalence of apoptotic nuclei at the rupture sites by in situ end-labeling (ISEL). **A,** Micrograph of a cross-section of an epicardial coronary artery showing a plaque rupture with an acute luminal (L) thrombus (Th). The acute rupture is represented by a connection between luminal platelet-fibrin thrombus and the necrotic core (NC) through the disrupted fibrous cap (hematoxylin and eosin, ×30). **B,** Serial section of the magnified boxed area of **A** after DNA fragmentation staining by ISEL at the site of plaque rupture and adjoining thin fibrous cap. Numerous apoptotic cells (*blue nuclear staining*) are identified at the plaque rupture site (eosin counterstain × 150). Further characterization demonstrated that the apoptotic cells in the culprit lesions stained for combination of ISEL (dark-brown reaction product) and specific antibody for macrophages (KP-1/CD-68, red reaction product) (**C**). Subsequent immunohistochemical characterization revealed that the apoptotic macrophages predominantly expressed caspase-1 (**D,** stained brown × 150). *Continued on next page*

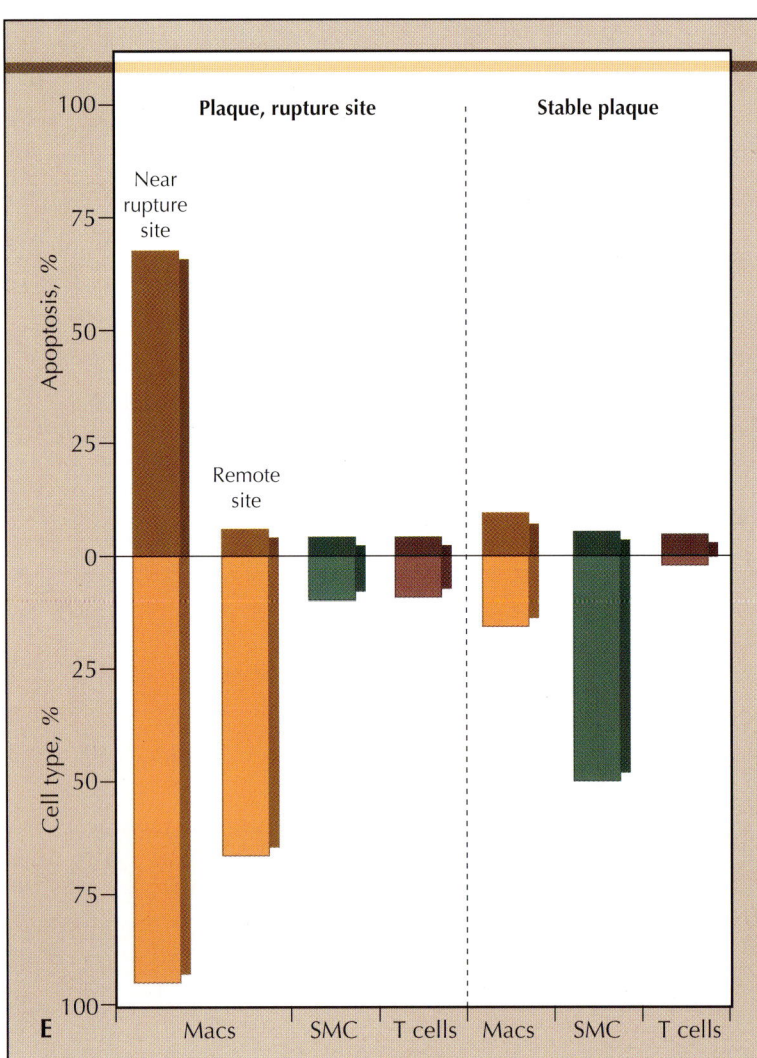

FIGURE 13-5. *(Continued)* **E,** On quantitative analysis of the prevalence of cells (*bottom*) and incidence of apoptosis in various cell types (*top*), apoptotic cells were observed predominantly at the rupture site and only occasionally encountered in the regions of the same plaque remote from the site of rupture; apoptosis was most prevalent in macrophages. Stable plaques demonstrated minimal evidence of apoptotic cells, which was predominantly confined to SMCs. (*Panels A–D from* Kolodgie *et al.* [27]; with permission; *panel E adapted from* Kolodgie *et al.* [27].)

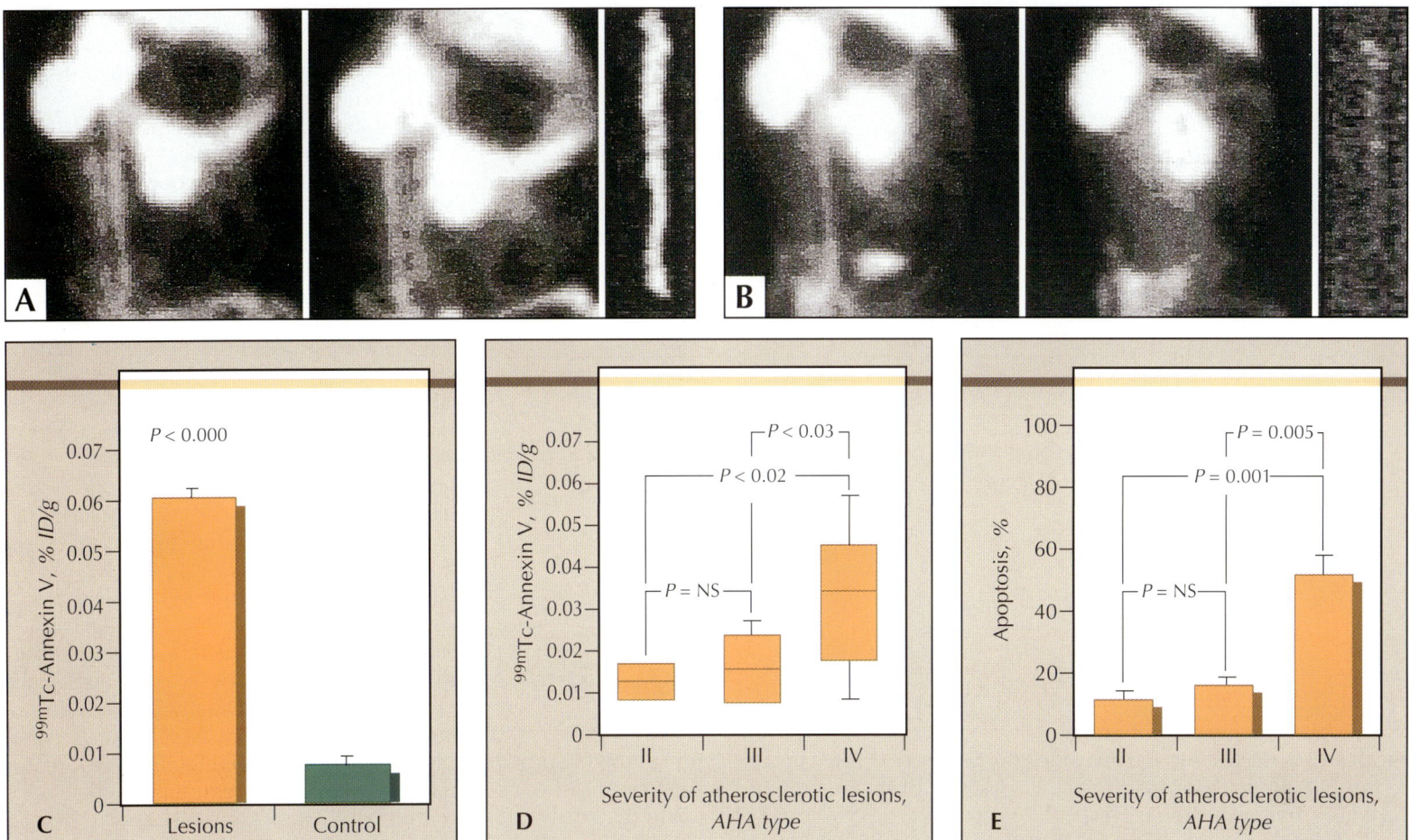

FIGURE 13-6. Noninvasive detection of apoptosis of macrophages in atherosclerotic plaques. Because annexin V can identify the cell membrane alterations associated with apoptosis and the process of apoptosis contributes to plaque vulnerability and plaque rupture, we used radiolabeled annexin V for the detection of experimental atherosclerotic lesions [33]. Atherosclerotic lesions were induced in New Zealand White rabbits by de-endothelialization of the infradiaphragmatic aorta followed by 12 weeks of a high-fat, high-cholesterol diet. All animals received 0.5 to 1 mg annexin V labeled with 7 to 10 mCi ^{99m}Tc intravenously for in vivo imaging studies. **A,** The left lateral decubitus gamma images showed primarily blood pool activity shortly after radiotracer administration (*left*), and there was clear delineation of radiolabel within the abdominal aorta after 2 hours (*center*). Ex vivo images of the explanted aorta showed a robust uptake of radiotracer in the infradiaphragmatic aorta within the lesion distribution corresponding to the in vivo images (*right*). In contrast, the uptake of radiotracer was absent in areas without grossly visible atherosclerotic lesions; these areas were localized (not shown) predominantly to the nondenuded descending thoracic aorta. **B,** The left lateral decubitus images of unmanipulated control animals showed blood pool activity similar to those animals with balloon injury and a high-fat diet (*left*). In contrast to vessels with plaques, at 2 hours after administration there was no localization of radiotracer in presumably normal vessel wall (*center*); ex vivo imaging confirmed the lack of radiotracer uptake (*right*). The accumulation of ^{99m}Tc annexin V in atherosclerotic lesions in the balloon-denuded region of the aorta was approximately tenfold greater than in the corresponding control abdominal aortic region (**C**). The mean ± SEM percent-injected dose per gram uptake in the specimens with lesions (95% CI, 0.054 ± 0.00) was significantly higher than the background activity in the normal specimens (0.0058 ± 0.001; $P< 0.000$). Histopathologic correlation of the severity of atherosclerotic lesions and the radiotracer uptake demonstrated that annexin V accumulation predominantly occurred in American Heart Association (AHA) type IV lesions with only minimal uptake in types II and III lesions (**D**). A large proportion of the cells stained positively for the presence of apoptosis in type IV lesions, which had shown the maximal radiotracer uptake (**E**). (*Panels A and B from* Kolodgie *et al.* [33]; with permission.)

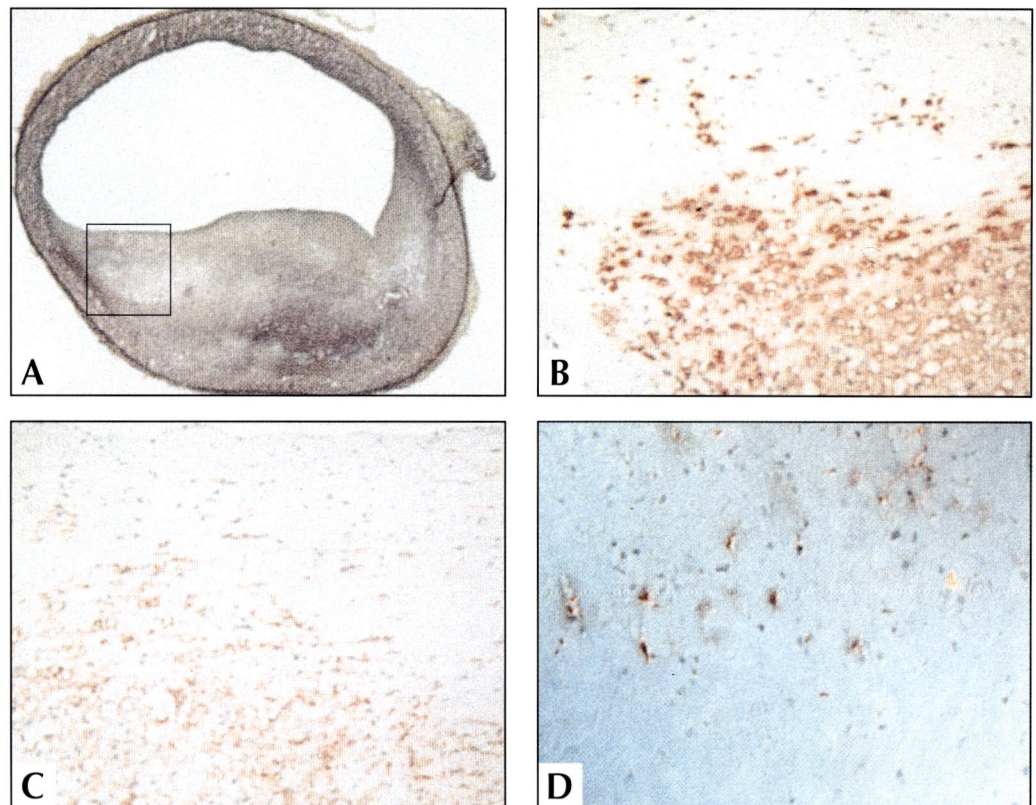

FIGURE 13-7. Detection of matrix metalloproteinase (MMP) upregulation in atherosclerotic lesions. Inflammation within the atherosclerotic plaque may further perpetuate plaque instability by production of MMP. When activated by cytokines (TNF-α, interleukin-1), macrophages secrete inactive MMP, including interstitial collagenases (MMP-1), gelatinase B (MMP-9), stromolysins 1–3 (MMP-3, -10, -11), and a membrane type. When activated by plasmin or by inactivation of intrinsic inhibitors in tissue, MMP can degrade the connective tissue matrix [34]. Mechanical testing in vitro of fibrous cap tissue shows that an increase in the number of macrophages and a reduction in collagen and glycosaminoglycans content reduce the amount of stress needed to fracture the tissue [35]. Sections of plaques laid on a gelatin substrate in vitro show active degeneration of collagen in lipid-rich plaques [36]. Plaque cap rupture can therefore be seen resulting from a destructive process initiated by macrophages that gains ascendancy over the repair process of collagen deposition by smooth muscle cells.

The MMP production can be seen in the vicinity of macrophage predominance in human coronary atherosclerotic lesions. This figure demonstrates serial cryostat sections of an American Heart Association type IV lesion within the left circumflex artery. **A,** A low-power view of a Movat pentachrome–stained section ($\times 20$). The *area outlined by the box* is the shoulder region (magnified in **B–D**). **B,** Immunostaining demonstrates numerous macrophages (KP-1/CD-68 staining, brown color product, $\times 200$). **C,** MMP-1 colocalizes mostly to macrophage-rich regions. **D,** Higher power view of **C** demonstrates apoptosis using in situ end-labeling (ISEL) and interference contrast microscopy (reddish-brown nuclei, *arrowheads*, $\times 400$; counterstain is methyl green).

Because active digestion of fibrous cap by MMP upregulation and activation may be an important event in plaque instability, noninvasive detection of MMP should allow better prediction of clinical outcomes in coronary artery disease patients. To demonstrate proof of this principle, a broad-spectrum MMP inhibitor (specificity for MMP-1 to -3 and 7 to 9 and 13, Ki 1–15 nM; Bristol-Myers Squibb, North Billerica, MA) radiolabeled with ^{111}In was used for imaging experimental atherosclerotic lesions in New Zealand White rabbits [37]. By noninvasive γ-imaging, the abdominal atherosclerotic lesions were visualized at 3 hours in atherosclerotic lesions. The percent injected dose per gram uptake of radiolabeled MMP inhibitor was maximum in lesions (0.033 ± 0.019; lesion-to-nonlesion ratio, 11:1), and significantly higher than control animals (0.003 ± 0.001). The radiotracer uptake was significantly resolved after diet interruption or diet withdrawal. Threshold analysis of histologic sections after immunostaining showed a significant increase of MMP in plaque segments demonstrating a high radiolabeled MMP inhibitor uptake (MMP-1, 12.5 ± 2.1; MMP-3, 14.3 ± 1.8; MMP-9, 1.3 ± 0.5 mm^2) relative to those with low uptake (MMP-1, 7.7 ± 0.2; MMP-3, 9.1 ± 1.5, MMP-9, 0.2 ± 0.05 mm^2; $P < 0.03$). These preliminary observations suggest that in vivo quantitation of MMP in atherosclerotic plaques is feasible, and correlates with their pathologic distribution in the plaque. The observations have also confirmed the previous belief [38–40] that withdrawal of the hyperlipidemic diet (and use of statins) abrogates MMP upregulation in the plaque.

Targeting Large Lipid Cores in Atherosclerotic Lesions

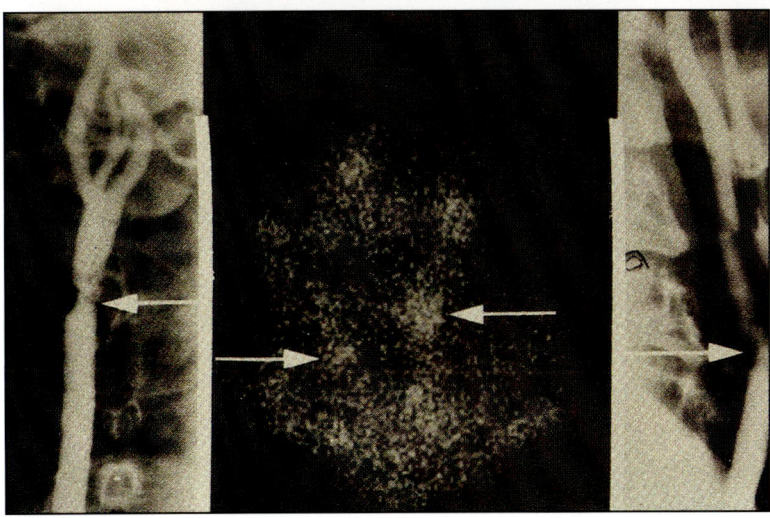

FIGURE 13-8. Noninvasive imaging with radiolabeled lipids. Besides intense inflammation of the fibrous caps, large lipid (or necrotic) cores contribute to the vulnerability of the plaque. Therefore, methods that evaluate lipid burden within the plaque should provide a useful prognostic marker in the atherosclerotic disease. Circulating LDL cholesterol undergoes oxidative modification during deposition in atherosclerotic plaques [41]. Ingestion occurs through scavenger receptors [41]. Modified LDL (mLDL) limits the egress of the lipid-laden monocytes from the intima; some of these lipid-laden macrophages that are able to escape from the subendothelial space cause additional endothelial injury and thrombogenesis. In addition, modified LDL induces release of tissue factor from macrophages, thereby initiating thrombosis. Modified LDL has also been demonstrated to impair vasorelaxation by directly diminishing endothelial nitric oxide synthase levels or activity. Reduced vasodilator (and elevated vasoconstrictor) levels may in turn stimulate SMC alteration in the vascular medial layer.

Iodinated LDL was used for the first ever imaging of atherosclerotic lesions in patients with angiographically confirmed carotid vessel disease [42]. Images of carotid artery lesions were successfully obtained in all patients 36 hours after intravenous injection of iodine ^{125}I-LDL (*center*); the site of uptake (*arrows*) corresponds to the angiographically confirmed atherosclerotic lesions in bilateral internal carotid arteries (*left, right*). No focal LDL accumulation occurred in the vertebral arteries. The coronary and renal vessels, as well as the adrenal glands, were not visualized. No LDL uptake was reported in the carotid arteries of the control subjects. The concentration of ^{125}I-LDL in the areas of focal accumulation was assessed to be 0.01% to 0.1%, which was 1.5 to three times higher than the concentration in the surrounding vessel. Although the poor-quality spatial resolution of images may be attributable to the use of ^{125}I, results obtained with subsequent use of ^{99m}Tc-labeled LDL were no better [43]. Despite a suboptimal contrast between the carotid lesion and the surrounding vessel activities, peripheral lesions such as tendon xanthomas were easily visualized [44].

Other components of the LDL cholesterol complex such as cholesteryl esters and apolipoprotein B have also been targeted in experimental models. ^{125}I-labeled nonhydrolyzable ester analogue, cholesteryl iopanoate, has been used in New Zealand White rabbits fed a cholesterol-enriched diet [45]. Scintigraphic and autoradiographic studies demonstrated tissue distribution of cholesteryl ester and localization in the thoracic and abdominal aorta atherosclerotic lesions. Use of hypolipidemic drugs such as colestipol and clofibrate reduced the cholesteryl ester accumulation in the atherosclerotic lesions. Similarly, an oligopeptide fragment of apolipoprotein B, SP4, labeled with either ^{123}I or ^{99m}Tc has been used successfully for imaging of ascending aorta atherosclerotic lesions in Watanabe heritable hyperlipidemic rabbits [46]. These studies have indicated the feasibility of use of radiolabeled lipids, lipoproteins, or apolipoproteins for imaging of atherosclerotic plaques. In all these studies, however, the tracer uptake in the lesions was reported to be low and background activity was high, which limited potential clinical utility of targeting lipid deposits for the noninvasive detection of atherosclerotic plaques. (*From* Lees *et al.* [42]; with permission.)

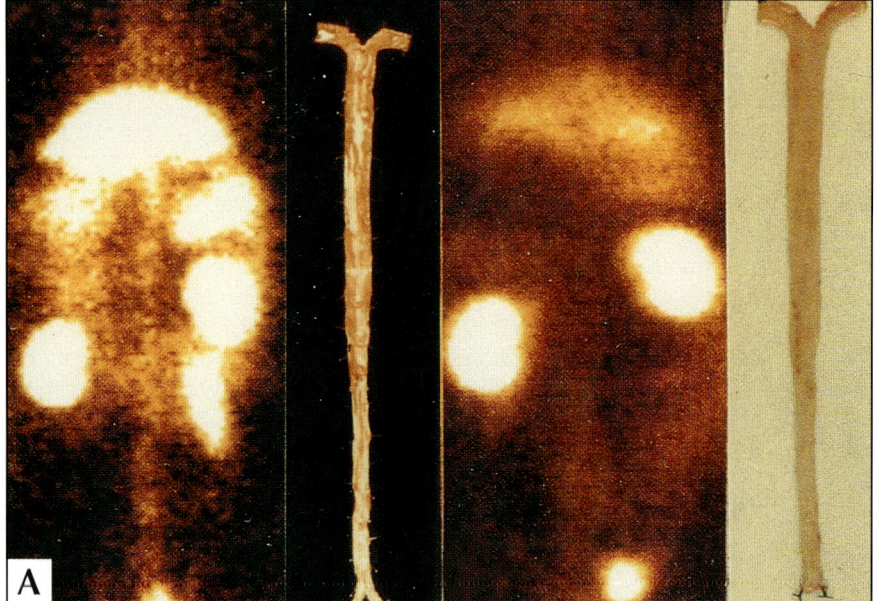
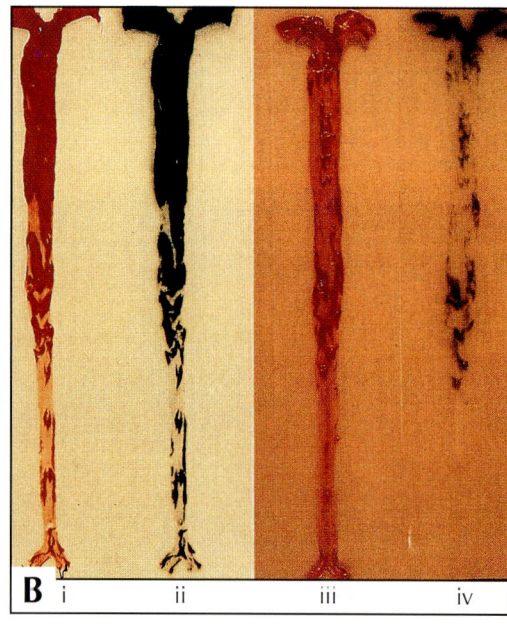
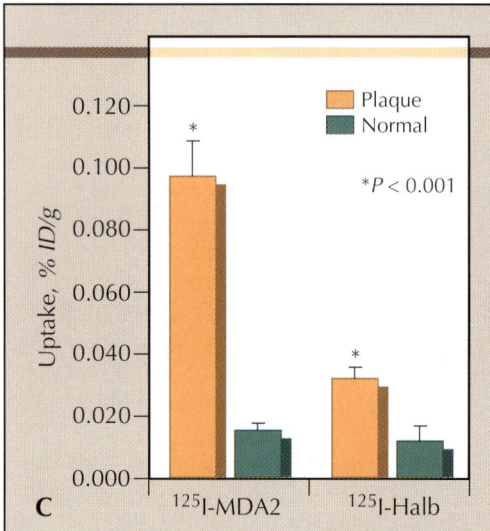

FIGURE 13-9. Recognition of plaque-specific lipids in atherosclerotic lesions. It has been proposed that the antigenic moieties, which are exclusively present in the atherosclerotic lipids, can be selectively targeted by radionuclide imaging [47]. It is conceivable that lack of these specific moieties on the circulating lipids should allow development of high target-to-background ratios. A monoclonal antibody (MDA2) directed against an epitope of oxidized low-density lipoprotein (LDL) has been developed that does not cross-react with the native LDL. Biodistribution, autoradiography, and in vivo imaging studies performed with ^{125}I-, ^{131}I-, or ^{99m}Tc-labeled antibodies have demonstrated the ability of MDA2 to localize at the site of atheroma. **A**, In vivo gamma camera images of Watanabe heritable hyperlipidemic (WHHL) (*left*) and control (*right*) rabbits injected with ^{99m}Tc MDA2. There is a significant uptake of radiotracer in the atherosclerotic lesions at 14 hours after injection (*left*), which corresponds to gross atheromatous lesions identified by Sudan-IV in the explanted aorta (laid on the side). In vivo gamma image in the normal rabbit shows no uptake, and Sudan-IV staining of the explanted aorta shows no lesion. For further confirmation, ^{125}I-MDA2 was compared with ^{125}I-Halb (human albumin) in WHHL rabbits. **B**, Sudan staining (*red; i, iii*) and corresponding autoradiographs (*black; ii, iv*) of WHHL rabbit aortas injected with ^{125}I-MDA2 (*i, ii*) and control radiotracer ^{125}I-Halb (*iii, iv*). The uptake of MDA2 is exceedingly superior to the Halb uptake and conforms to the gross distribution of atherosclerotic lesions. The quantitative assessment (**C**) of the test and control radiotracers in the plaque tissue versus adjacent grossly normal tissue in same rabbit aortas demonstrate that there was a much higher uptake of MDA2 in the plaque tissue as compared to the Halb ($P < 0.01$), but no difference in uptake in normal tissue ($P = $ NS). (*Panels A and B from* Tsimikas *et al.* [47]; with permission; *panel C adapted from* Tsimikas *et al.* [47].)

TARGETING PROLIFERATING SMOOTH MUSCLE CELLS

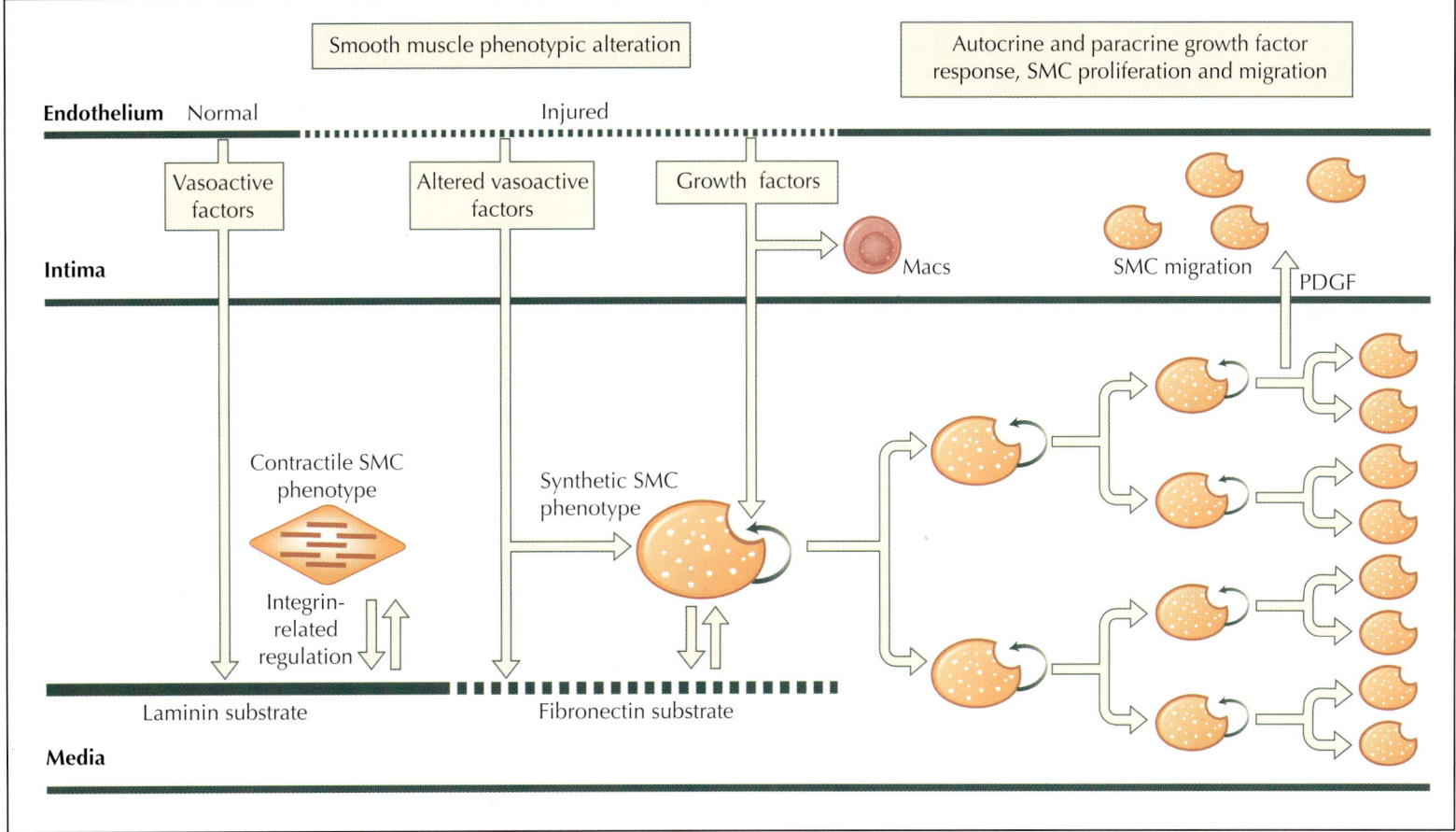

FIGURE 13-10. Molecular basis of vascular smooth muscle cell (SMC) proliferation. Unlike predominance of macrophages (Macs) and lipid cores in vulnerable atherosclerotic lesions, rapidly proliferating SMCs leading eventually to inward (constrictive) remodeling largely explains the postangioplasty phenomenon of restenosis. For selective targeting of replicating SMCs, those cell surface characteristics that are upregulated during phenotypic transformation of SMCs need to be defined [8,48]. In adult vasculature, SMCs retain a contractile phenotype, thereby contributing to maintenance of vascular tone. They are differentiated, contain abundant contractile apparatus and a heterochromatic nucleus, and are not capable of proliferation [49]. The extracellular matrix surrounding normal SMCs facilitates maintenance of contractile phenotype. Endothelial injury leads to altered release of vasoactive substances (from NO and prostaglandin I_2 to angiotensin II and endothelin-1), leading to alteration in extracellular matrix substrate and induced transformation of the SMCs, mediated both through membrane integrins, and direct cellular effects of vasoconstrictor soluble factors. The phenotypic change is associated with loss of myofilaments, development of abundant rough endoplasmic reticulum and Golgi complex, and is referred to as synthetic phenotype [49]. Altered SMCs develop modified cell surface characteristics that include enhanced growth factor receptor expression. The growth factors are derived from components of the pathologic lesion (altered endothelium, activated macrophages, and phenotypically transformed smooth muscle cells). In addition to driving proliferation, SMC autocrine production of growth factors is stimulated, resulting in amplification of the pathologic cascade. PDGF—platelet-derived growth factor. (*Courtesy of* Jeffrey Bender and Jagat Narula).

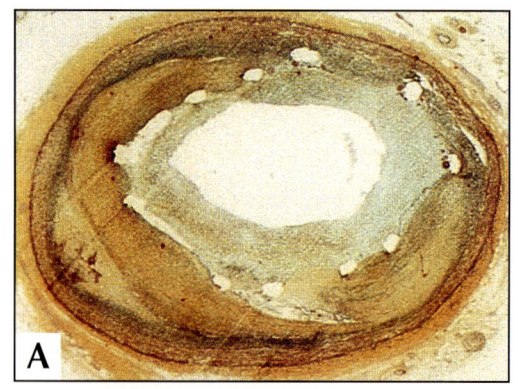
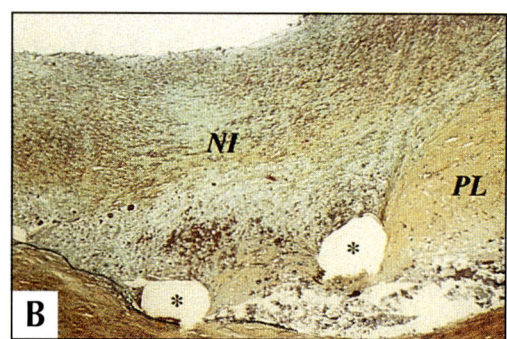
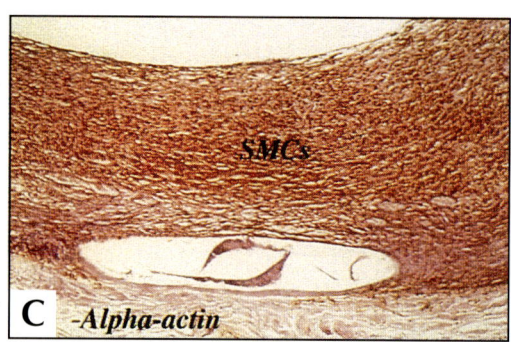
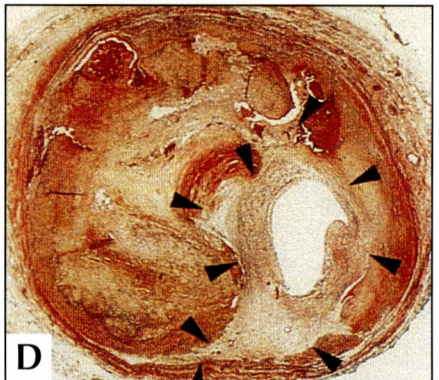
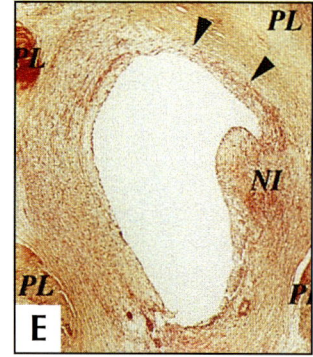
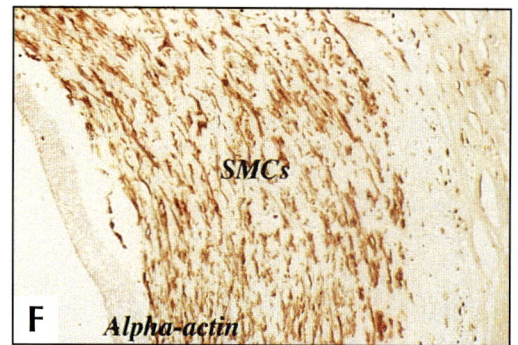

FIGURE 13-11. Morphologic characteristics of postangioplastic restenosis. **A, B,** Photomicrographs of right coronary artery section from a 59-year-old man who died suddenly 4 months after balloon angioplasty and Palmaz-Schatz (Cordis Corp., Miami, FL) stent placement. **A** demonstrates cross-section of artery (empty spaces represent sites of stent struts) with neointimal thickening or restenosis developing inside stent. **B** shows higher magnification of two stent struts with compressed plaque (PL) and overlying neointima (NI) consisting of spindle-shaped smooth muscle cells in proteoglycan-rich matrix (green). Area close to struts (asterisk) shows presence of fibrin (magenta) and foam cells. **C** shows high-power view of Gianturco-Rubin (Cook, Bloomington, IN) stent after staining for α-actin to identify smooth muscle cells that are major components of restenotic lesions. **D–F,** Sections of coronary artery from a patient who underwent balloon angioplasty 3 months before death; note neointima (**D,** *inside arrowheads*). **E** is higher magnification of *panel D*, showing area of neointimal (NI) growth consisting of smooth muscle cells in proteoglycan-collagen matrix and surrounding plaque (PL). **F** shows higher magnification of section staining brown after α-actin antibody staining to identify smooth muscle cells. (*Panels A, B, D, and E*, Movat pentachrome stain; *panels C and F*, α-actin antibody staining with avidin-biotin peroxidase complex method). (*From* Narula *et al.* [8]; with permission.)

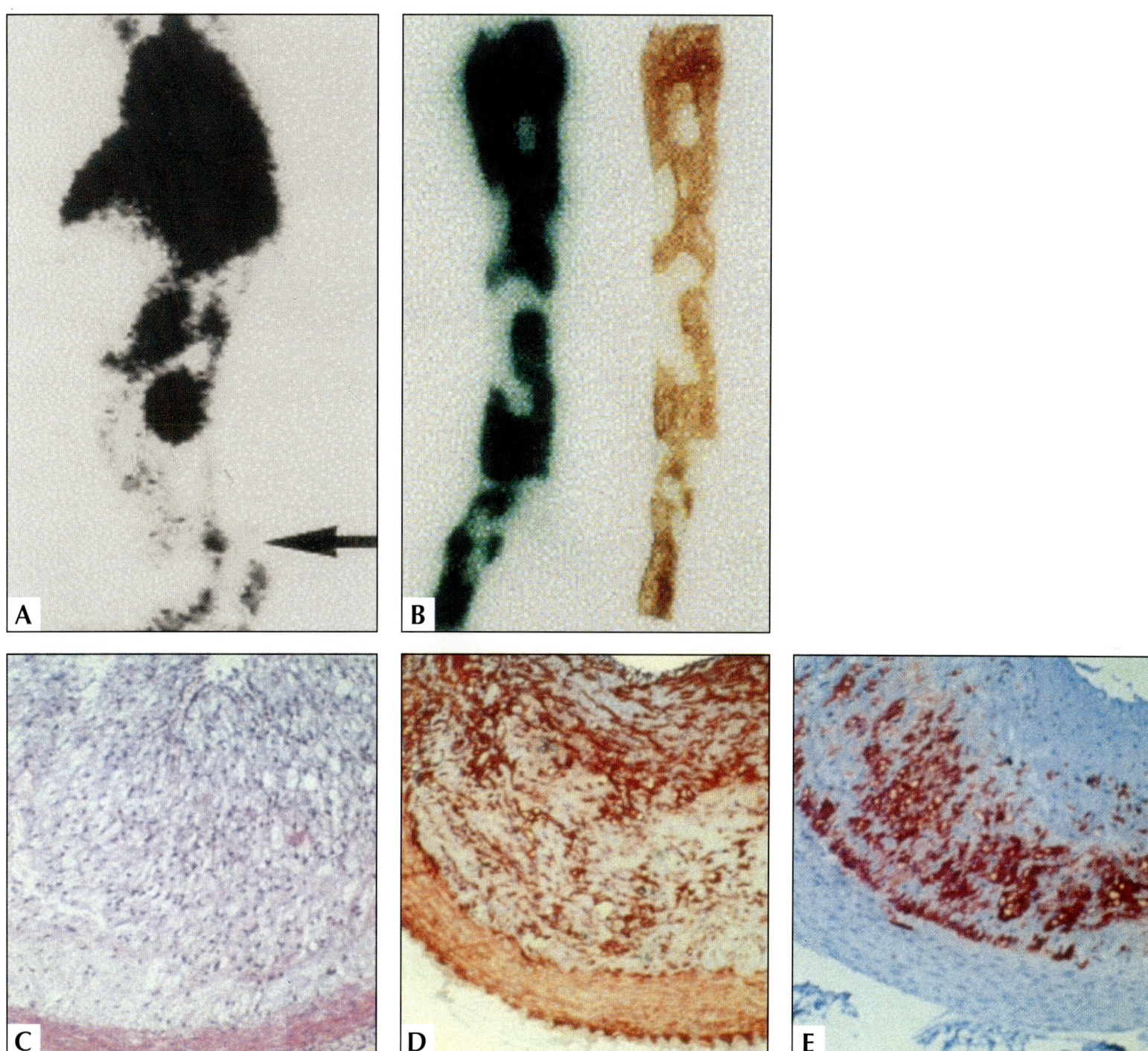

FIGURE 13-12. Targeting of growth factor receptors. Growth factors induce tissue proliferation by two discrete signal transduction pathways [50]. Polypeptide growth factors such as platelet-derived growth factor, epidermal growth factor, and endothelin-1 bind to receptors with tyrosine kinase activity. The second class of receptors for growth factors on proliferating smooth muscle cells (SMCs) are coupled with G protein–signaling pathways. Such growth factors are calcium-mobilizing mitogens, and the prototypic ATP induces significant proliferation of human and murine vascular SMCs.

Endothelin-1 derivatives have been used for the noninvasive targeting of experimental atherosclerotic lesions. The imaging with ^{99m}Tc-labeled ZK 167054, a tridecapeptide of endothelin, was reported to accumulate in the balloon–de-endothelialized aortic atherosclerotic lesions as early as 15 minutes after intravenous administration in New Zealand White rabbits by noninvasive imaging (*arrow*) (**A**) [51,52]; the lesion-to-background uptake ratio was 7:1. The uptake corresponded to the gross distribution of atherosclerotic lesions as demonstrated in the comparison of abdominal aorta autoradiograph (*black*) and the Sudan-IV–stained explanted aorta (**B**). The histologic (**C**; hematoxylin and eosin) and immunohistochemical (**D,E**) characterization demonstrated that the endothelin uptake occurred predominantly in the SMC-rich areas (**D,** α-actin, reddish-brown reaction product), but not in macrophage-rich lesions (**E;** RAM-11, red reaction product). Quantitative assessment demonstrated a direct and close correlation between the radiolabeled endothelin uptake and the number of SMCs in the lesion   *Continued on next page*

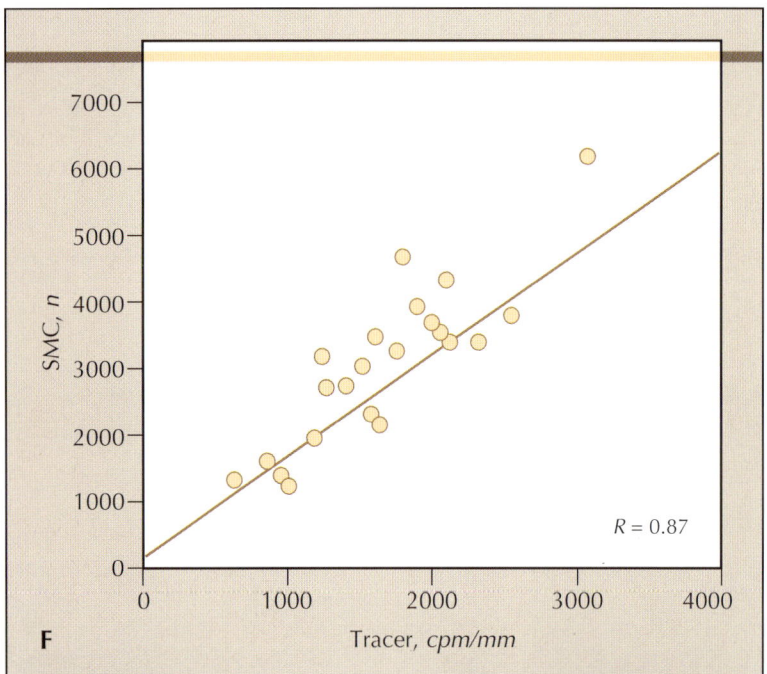

Figure 13-12. *(Continued)* (**F**); no correlation was observed between endothelin uptake and the amount of macrophages in plaque. *(Panels A and B from Dinkelborg et al. [51]; with permission; panels C, D, and E from Tepe et al. [52]; with permission.)*

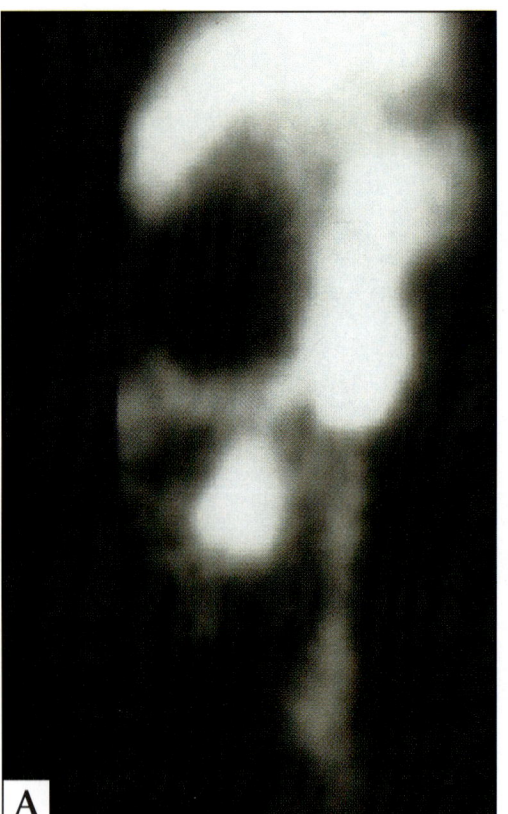
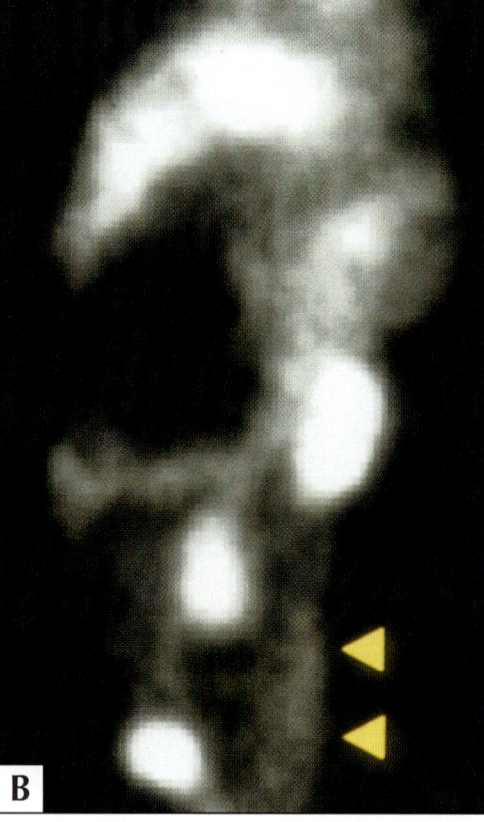
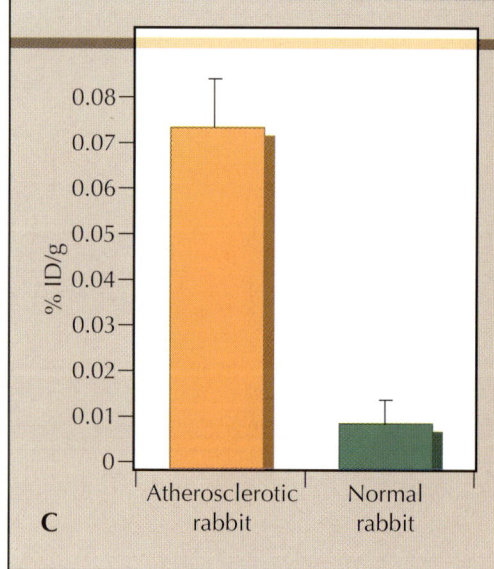

Figure 13-13. Targeting of growth factor purinoceptors. Endogenous diadenosine polyphosphates share membrane purinoceptors with ATP [53] and exert mitogenic effects on vascular smooth muscle cells (SMCs) that are as potent as ATP [54]. Accordingly, we have used diadenosine tetraphosphate (AP4A) for noninvasive detection of SMC-rich atherosclerotic lesions [55]. The ^{99m}Tc-labeled AP4A intravenous injection (**A**) in New Zealand White rabbits allowed precise localization of atherosclerotic lesions in abdominal aorta within 17 to 20 minutes (**B**, *arrowheads*). Radiotracer uptake in the ex vivo image corresponded to the radiotracer uptake and gross distribution of the lesions (not shown). There was no uptake of radiotracer in the control unmanipulated animal, both in in vivo and ex vivo images (data not shown). The radiotracer uptake in the lesions was sevenfold higher than the background or uptake in abdominal aortas from normal rabbits (**C**).

After the growth factors bind to their surface targets, they generate secondary messengers to upregulate proto-oncogenes and transcription factors that induce genes leading to cells growth [56]. The generation of mRNA for various transcription factors can be detected in the proliferating cells by developing radiolabeled probes that are complementary to the mRNA. These probes (termed *antisense nucleotides*) bind to the mRNA irreversibly and can be scintigraphically localized. Although no antisense probes so far have been used for imaging of atherosclerotic lesions, numerous studies have demonstrated upregulation of proto-oncogenes such as c-myb or cdK2 in proliferating smooth muscle cells [57]. Antisense probes to these mRNAs can be conveniently labeled with radioisotopes. No data are available for targeting of atherosclerotic lesions, but proto-oncogenes have been investigated for noninvasive diagnosis of tumors and offer a conceptual proof of such as imaging technology and may be used in the imaging of proliferating smooth muscle cells. *(Panels A and B from Elmaleh et al. [55]; with permission.)*

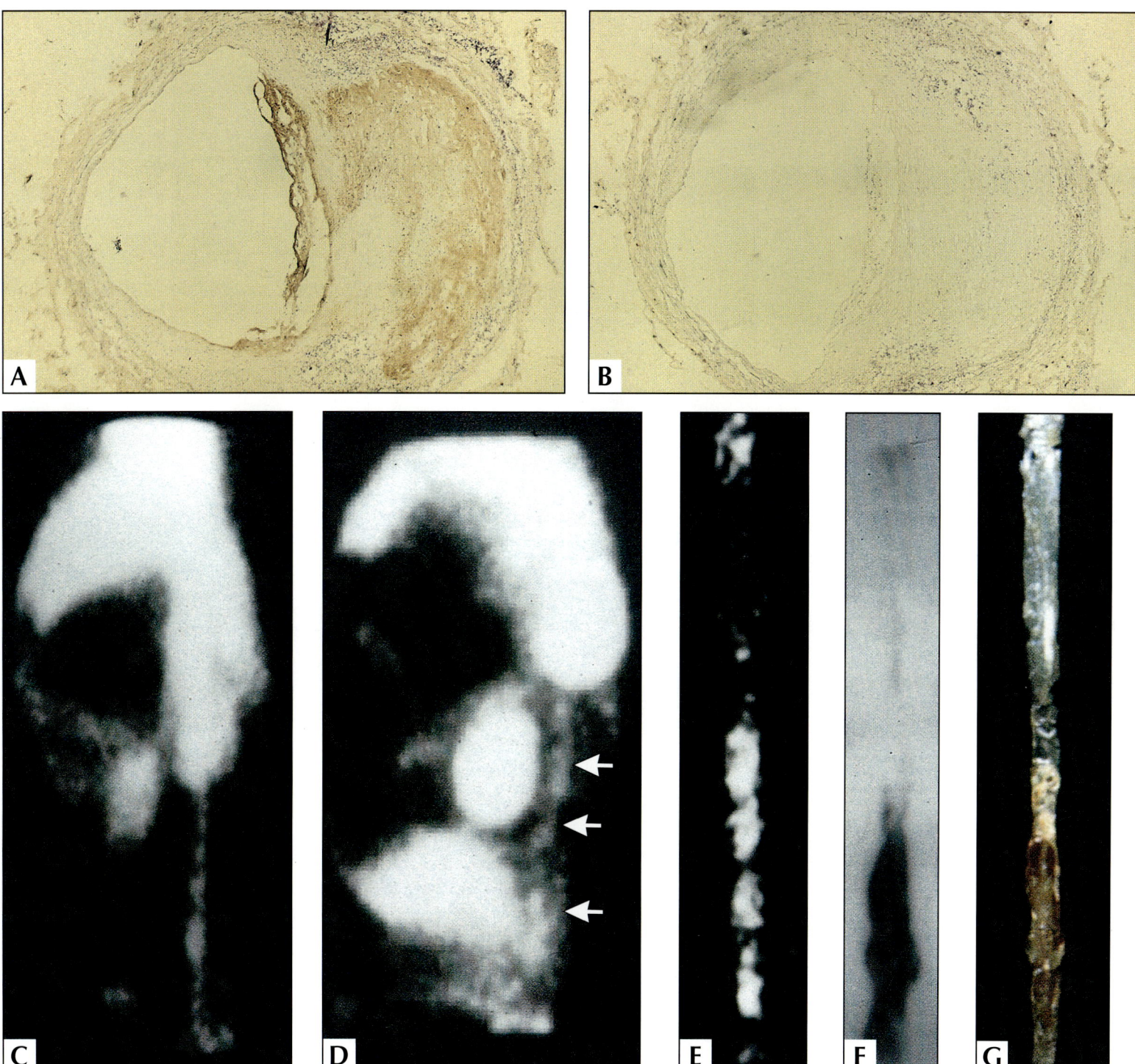

FIGURE 13-14. Radionuclide imaging of synthetic phenotype of smooth muscle cells (SMCs) in experimental atherosclerotic lesions. During proliferation of SMCs, apart from upregulation of receptors for diverse growth factors, new antigenic moieties may become expressed on the cell surface. The targeting of such molecules can allow differentiation of quiescent medial SMCs from proliferating neointimal SMCs. Expression of a heterodimeric protein with characteristic sterol moiety has been described on the proliferating SMCs [58]. An antibody directed against this antigen (called Z2D3) recognizes neointimal proliferating SMCs in a human coronary artery atherosclerotic lesion and does not react with quiescent medial SMC layers (**A**); control experiment in the subjacent section omitted the primary antibody (**B**). A comparative immunohistochemical study showed that Z2D3-positive SMC areas corresponded to the areas of nuclear staining with an antibody specific for proliferating cell nuclear antigen (data not shown). Radiolabeled Z2D3 has allowed localization of atherosclerotic lesions in experimental rabbit atherosclerotic models [58–61] and the advanced atherosclerotic plaques in carotid arteries in patients undergoing endarterectomy [62]. The uptake of the antibody is directly proportional to the rate of proliferation of SMCs [63]. Accordingly, only modest uptake of antibody is seen in the atherosclerotic plaques in Watanabe rabbits where SMC proliferation is very slow. On the other hand, rapid proliferation of SMCs occurs in balloon–de-endothelialized New Zealand White rabbits, and the Z2D3 antibody uptake is significantly higher. It is therefore presumed that the magnitude of antibody uptake will predict the likelihood of restenotic complications after angioplasty procedures [48]. **C**, Left lateral oblique gamma images of rabbits injected with ^{111}In-Z2D3 for noninvasive visualization of experimental atherosclerotic lesions. **D**, Imaging performed at 48 hours reveals focal accumulation of Z2D3 in aortic atherosclerotic lesions (*arrows*). No localization of the radiolabeled nonspecific antibody was seen in similar experiments (data not shown). **E**, In vivo localization of Z2D3 in **D** corresponds to the regions of tracer accumulation observed in the ex vivo image. Nonspecific antibody did not localize in the lesions in the ex vivo image despite the presence of significant atherosclerosis (not shown). **F**, Macroautoradiograph of the aorta in the animal injected with ^{111}In-Z2D3 shows localization of the radioactivity corresponding to the pathologic lesions (**G**). (*From* Narula *et al.* [58]; with permission.)

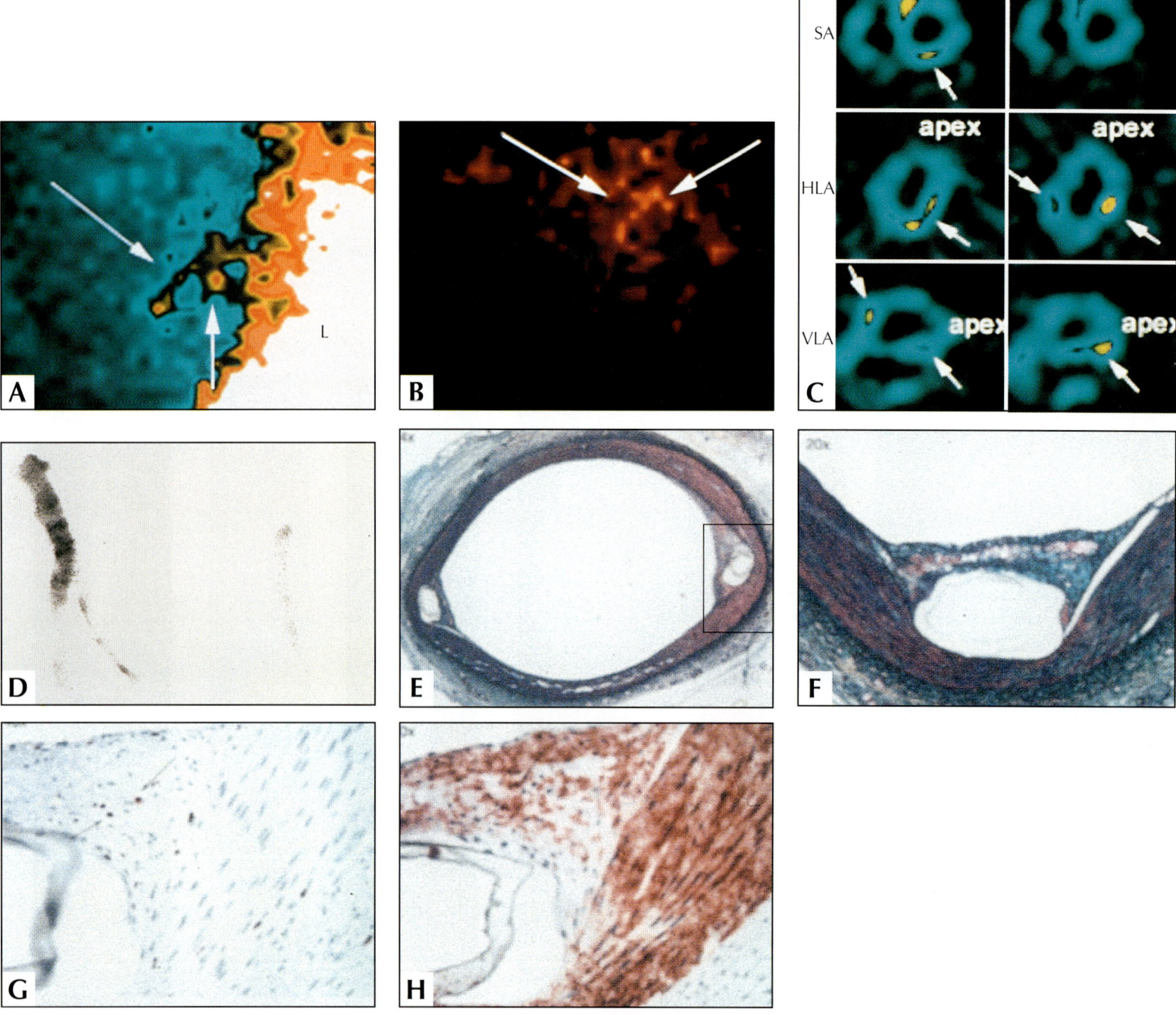

FIGURE 13-15. Feasibility of imaging smooth muscle cells in experimental coronary atherosclerotic lesions in swine. Z2D3 antibody radiolabeled with ^{111}In was used in a swine model of coronary artery restenosis. Z2D3 uptake correlated with the replication rates of smooth muscle cells (SMCs) as well as the volume of neointimal tissue proliferation [64]. In this study, 16 stents were placed using balloon over-expansion technique in the coronary arteries of 10 juvenile domestic swine. A mean of 9 days later, animals received 2.0 mCi of ^{111}In-Z2D3. The rate of replication of SMC was identified by premortem administration of bromodeoxyuridine (BrDU, 50 mg/kg); BrDU is incorporated in the nucleus of replicating cells. Animals were killed after coronary angiography and SPECT imaging. Ex vivo images of the explanted hearts were acquired in planar and SPECT views, followed by dissection of stented vessels for autoradiography and pathologic characterization. Percent vessel stenosis was calculated from Movat-stained sections, and medial and neointimal areas and BrDU labeling–based cell proliferation indices were quantified. Sagittal, coronal, and transverse reconstructed SPECT images were interpreted for tracer uptake in coronary vessels using the stent locations on angiograms to aid in localization. Twelve of 16 stented vessels showed focal uptake on in vivo imaging. The mean count ratio (stented:control) for visualized vessels was 2.2 and for nonvisualized vessels was 1.0. Z2D3 uptake was significantly higher in severely stenotic lesions with higher rates of cellular proliferation. When counts per gram in the stented vessels were corrected for stent weight and plotted versus BrDU positive cells/m^2, there was a significant correlation (r = 0.558).

A, In vivo left anterior oblique image after Z2D3 administration shows focal antibody uptake in the mid right coronary artery and proximal left anterior descending coronary artery (LAD) corresponding to stent positions in an animal 1 week post–double stent placement (*arrows*). Increased Z2D3 uptake is confirmed in the ex vivo planar (*arrows*) (**B**) and SPECT (*arrows*) (**C**) images of the explanted heart and macroautoradiograph of explanted LAD artery. No uptake is seen in explanted circumflex (**D**, *right*). **E,** Histopathologic characterization is performed with Movat-pentachrome (magnification of *E* in **F**), BrDU (**G**), and a-actin (**H**) staining. There is significant in-stent restenosis; empty spaces in the histologic section denote stent struts. The a-actin staining demonstrates abundance of SMCs in the restenotic lesion; positive staining for BrDU represents evidence of proliferation. (*Panels A, B, and D adapted from* Johnson *et al.* [64]; with permission; *panels C, E–H courtesy of* Lynne Johnson.)

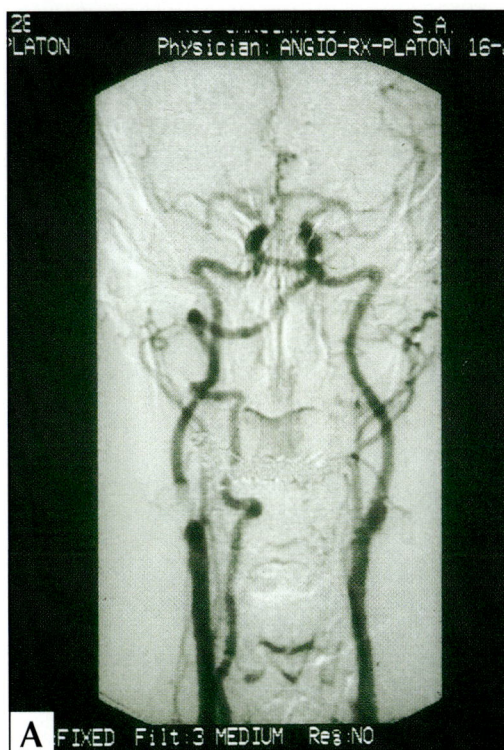
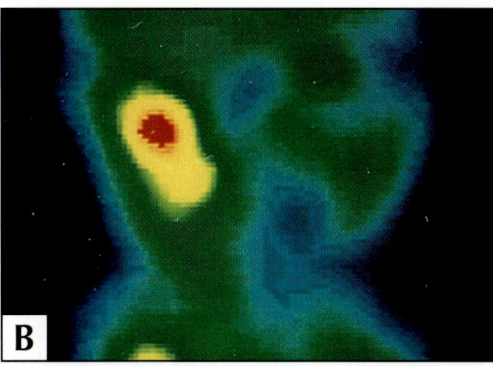
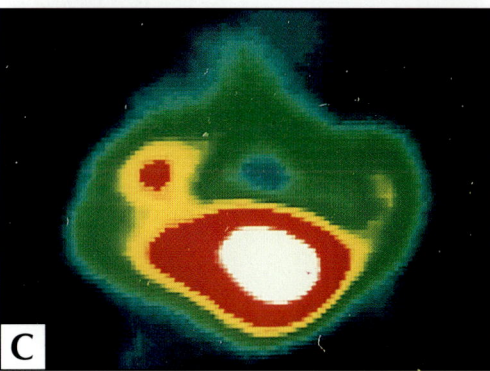

FIGURE 13-16. Clinical imaging of smooth muscle cell proliferation in carotid atherosclerosis. After the successful demonstration of the feasibility of imaging of proliferating smooth muscle cells (SMCs), the safety, biodistribution, accumulation, and elimination of Z2D3 were assessed in 11 patients who were candidates for carotid endarterectomy [62]. Arteriographic and Doppler echographic studies demonstrated significant stenosis in one carotid bed of all 11 patients; nine patients had bilateral disease. The arteriographic degree of stenosis ranged between 70% and 90% in the vessel on which endarterectomy was going to be performed, and between 10% and 70% in the contralateral sides of patients with bilateral disease. Z2D3 (250 µg) labeled with 5 mCi of ^{111}In was administered by slow intravenous injection. Planar and SPECT images were obtained 4, 24, 48, and 72 hours later. Positive antibody uptake was observed in all of the 11 carotid arteries that underwent endarterectomy. Positive uptake also was seen in five contralateral sites with minimal evidence of stenosis in the arteriograms. A, Significant obstructive lesion is observed in the carotid angiogram (*arrow*). Uptake of ^{111}In-Z2D3 at the site of the carotid plaques was seen in the planar and SPECT views at 4 hours (B, sagittal; C, transverse). The antibody uptake was localized discretely in the stenotic artery and corresponded with the angiographic location of the disease. The antibody uptake in planar images occasionally resulted in diffuse increase in radioactivity on the affected side compared with the contralateral normal carotid artery. SPECT images demonstrated the atherosclerotic plaques with more intense focal uptake in the majority of lesions, providing better delineation of the lesion sites. The intensity of uptake at the site of the plaques reached a maximum at 4 hours and decreased at subsequent time intervals. The target-to-control ratios were 2.20 ± 0.3, 1.98 ± 0.3, 1.60 ± 0.2, and 1.45 ± 0.2 at 4, 24, 48, and 72 hours, respectively. Comparison of the pattern of antibody uptake with the appearance of the plaques on arteriography revealed that the region with severe stenosis did not always correspond precisely with the site of more intense antibody uptake. In addition, the pattern of uptake was frequently more extended than the stenotic regions as delineated by the angiograms. Pathologic examination of the specimens by direct avidin-biotin-peroxidase immunocytochemistry revealed staining of neointimal SMC in scan-positive plaques (data not shown). Endarterectomy specimens were intensely radioactive, and the mean percent of the injected dose per gram localization in the specimens was 0.0475 ± 0.007. (*From* Carrio *et al.* [62]; with permission.)

FUTURE DIRECTIONS

The future of vascular imaging is dependent upon two factors: new radioligand development and new imaging and detection technology. It is clear that the explosion of information in vascular biology and atherosclerosis research will be translated ultimately into effective imaging strategies. As shown in this chapter, the initial approaches have already yielded exciting results. However, detection of radioligand uptake in small vascular lesions is a significant technologic undertaking. Whether this challenge will be best met by higher resolution imaging cameras or by intravascular radiation detectors comparable to intravascular ultrasound remains to be determined. In any event, the future appears extremely promising as imaging moves toward molecular paradigms in defining its next phase.

References

1. Coronary Heart Disease and Angina Pectoris. In *American Heart Association: 2002 Heart and Stroke Statistical Update*. Dallas: American Heart Association; 2001:11–13.
2. Levy DL, Wilson PWF: Atherosclerotic cardiovascular disease: an epidemiological perspective. In *Textbook of Cardiovascular Medicine*. Edited by Topol EJ. Philadelphia: Lippincott-Raven; 1998:13–30.
3. Pepine CJ: Coronary angiography and cardiac catheterization. In *Textbook of Cardiovascular Medicine*. Edited by Topol EJ. Philadelphia: Lippincott-Raven; 1998:1935–1956.
4. Mizumo K, Satomura K, Miyamoto A, *et al.*: Angioscopic evaluation of coronary-artery thrombi in acute coronary syndrome. *N Engl J Med* 1992, 326:287–291.
5. Waller BF, Pinkerton CA, Stack JD: Intravascular ultrasound: a histologic study of vessels during life: the new gold standard of vascular imaging. *Circulation* 1992, 85:2305–2309.
6. Hodgson JM, Reddy KG, Suneja R, *et al.*: Intracoronary ultrasound imaging correlation of plaque morphology with angiography, clinical syndrome and procedural results in patients undergoing coronary angioplasty. *J Am Coll Cardiol* 1993, 21:35–44.
7. Yabushita H, Bouma BE, Houser SL, *et al.*: Characterization of human atherosclerosis by optical coherence tomography. *Circulation* 2002, 106:1640–1645.
8. Narula J, Virmani R, Iskandrian AE: Strategic targeting of atherosclerotic lesions. *J Nucl Cardiol* 1999, 6:81–90.
9. Burke A, Farb A, Malcolm GT, *et al.*: Coronary risk factors and plaque morphology in men with coronary artery disease who died suddenly. *N Engl J Med* 1997, 336:1276–1282.
10. Kolodgie FD, Burke AP, Farb A, *et al.*: The thin-cap fibroatheroma: a type of vulnerable plaque: the major precursor lesion to acute coronary syndromes. *Curr Opin Cardiol* 2001, 16:285–292.
11. Lee RT, Libby P: The unstable atheroma. *Arterioscler Thromb Vasc Biol* 1997, 17:1859–1867.
12. Holmes DR Jr, Vietstra RE, Smith HC, *et al.*: Restenosis after percutaneous transluminal coronary angioplasty (PTCA): a report from PTCA registry of the National Heart, Lung and Blood Institute. *Am J Cardiol* 1984, 53:77C–81C.
13. Farb A, Virmani R, Atkinson JB, Kolodgie FD: Plaque morphology and pathologic outcome after coronary balloon angioplasty. *J Am Coll Cardiol* 1990, 16:1421–1429.
14. Farb A, Sangiorgi G, Carter AJ, *et al.*: Pathology of acute and chronic coronary stenting in humans. *Circulation* 1999, 99:44–52.
15. Davies MJ, Woolfe N: Atherosclerosis: what is it and why does it occur? *Br Heart J* 1993, 69:S3–S11.
16. Narula J, Ditlow C, Chen FW, Khaw BA: Monoclonal antibodies for the detection of atherosclerotic lesions. In *Monoclonal Antibodies in Cardiovascular Disease*. Edited by Khaw BA, Narula J, Strauss HW. Philadelphia: Lea & Febiger; 1994:206.
17. Libby P: Molecular basis of acute coronary syndromes. *Circulation* 1995, 91:2844–2850.
18. Libby P: Atherosclerosis: the new view. *Sci Am* 2002, 286:46–55.
19. Butcher EC: Leukocyte-endothelial cell recognition: three (or more) steps to specificity and diversity. *Cell* 1991, 67:1033–1066.
20. Virgolini I, Muller C, Fitscha P, *et al.*: Radiolabeling autologous monocytes with ^{111}In oxine for reinjection in patients with atherosclerosis. *Prog Clin Biol Res* 1990, 355:271–280.
21. Ohtsuki K, Hayase M, Akashi K, *et al.*: Detection of monocyte chemoattractant protein-1 receptor expression in experimental atherosclerotic lesions: an autoradiographic study. *Circulation* 2001, 104:203–208.
22. Steinberg D, Witzum JL: Lipoproteins, lipoprotein oxidation, and atherogenesis. In *Molecular Basis of Cardiovascular Disease*. Edited by Cheien KR. Philadelphia: WB Saunders; 1998:458–476.
23. Fischman AJ, Rubin RH, Delvecchio A, Strauss HW: Imaging of atheromatous lesions in the iliac and femoral vessels: preliminary experience with [111]In IgG in human subjects. *J Nucl Med* 1989, 30:817.
24. Bjorkerud S, Bjorkerud B: Apoptosis is abundant in human atherosclerotic lesions, especially in inflammatory cells (macrophages and T cells) and may contribute to the accumulation of gruel and plaque instability. *Am J Pathol* 1996, 149:367–380.
25. Cai W, Devaux B, Schaper W: The role of Fas/APO 1 and apoptosis in the development of human atherosclerotic lesions. *Atherosclerosis* 1997, 131:177–186.
26. Crisby M, Kallin B, Thyberg J: Cell death in human atherosclerotic plaques involves both oncosis and apoptosis. *Atherosclerosis* 1997, 130:17–27.
27. Kolodgie FD, Narula J, Burke AP, *et al.*: Localization of apoptotic macrophages at the site of plaque rupture in sudden coronary death. *Am J Pathol* 2000, 157:1259–1268.
28. Geng YJ, Libby P: Evidence for apoptosis in advanced human atheroma: colocalization with interleukin-1 beta-converting enzyme. *Am J Pathol* 1995, 147:251–266.
29. Bennett MR, Evan GI, Schwartz SM: Apoptosis of human vascular smooth muscle cells derived from normal vessels and coronary atherosclerotic plaques. *J Clin Invest* 1995, 95:2266–2274.
30. Bennett MR, Littlewood TD, Schwartz SM, *et al.*: Increased sensitivity of human vascular smooth muscle cells from atherosclerotic plaques to p53-mediated apoptosis. *Circ Res* 1997, 81:591–599.
31. Chang BD, Watanabe K, Broude EV: Effects of p21Waf1/Cip1/Sdi1 on cellular gene expression: implications for carcinogenesis, senescence, and age-related diseases. *Proc Natl Acad Sci U S A* 2000, 97:4291–4296.
32. Schaub FJ, Han DK, Conrad Liles W, *et al.*: Fas/FADD-mediated activation of a specific program of inflammatory gene expression in vascular smooth muscle cells. *Nat Med* 2000, 6:790–796.
33. Kolodgie FD, Petrov A, Fasseas P, *et al.*: ^{99m}Tc-Annexin-V imaging for noninvasive detection of experimental atherosclerotic lesions. *Circulation* 2000, 102:II-404.
34. Galis ZS, Sukhova GK, Libby P: Increased expression of MMPs and matrix degrading activity in vulnerable human atherosclerotic plaques. *J Clin Invest* 1994, 94:2493–2503.
35. Lendon CL, Davies MJ, Born GV: Atherosclerotic plaque caps are locally weakened when macrophages density is increased. *Atherosclerosis* 1991, 87:87–90.
36. Sukhova GK, Schonbeck U, Libby P, *et al.*: Evidence for increased collagenolysis by interstitial collagenases 1 and 3 vulnerable human atherosclerotic plaques. *Circulation* 1999, 99:2503–2509.
37. Kolodgie FD, Edwards S, Petrov A, *et al.*: Noninvasive detection of matrix metalloproteinase upregulation in experimental atherosclerotic lesions and its abrogation by dietary modification. *Circulation* 2001, 104:II-694.
38. Aikawa M, Rabkin E, Libby P, *et al.*: Cerivastatin suppresses growth of macrophages expressing MMP and TF in vivo and in vitro. *Circulation* 2001, 103:276–283.
39. Aikawa M, Rabkin E, Libby P, *et al.*: Lipid lowering by diet reduces MMP activity and increases collagen content of rabbit atheroma. *Circulation* 1998, 97:2433–2444.
40. Fukumoto Y, Libby P, *et al.*: Statins alter SMC accumulation and collagen content in established atheroma of WHHL rabbits. *Circulation* 2001, 103:993–999.
41. Witztum J: The oxidation hypothesis of atherosclerosis. *Lancet* 1994, 344:793–795.
42. Lees RS, Lees AM, Strauss HW: External imaging of human atherosclerosis. *J Nucl Med* 1983, 24:154–156.

43. Lees AM, Lees RS, Schoen FJ, et al.: Imaging human atherosclerosis with ^{99m}Tc-labeled LDL. *Atherosclerosis* 1988, 8:461–470.

44. Ginsberg HN, Goldsmith SJ, Vallabhajosula S: Noninvasive imaging of ^{99m}Tc-labeled LDL, uptake by tendon xanthomas in hypercholesterolemic patients. *Arteriosclerosis* 1990, 10:256–262.

45. DeFore LE, Schwendner SW, DeGalan MR, et al.: Noninvasive assessment of lipid disposition of treated and untreated atherosclerotic rabbits. *Pharm Res* 1989, 6:1011–1016.

46. Hardoff R, Braegelmann F, Zanzonico P, et al.: External imaging of atherosclerosis in rabbits using an 123I-labeled synthetic peptide fragment. *J Clin Pharmacol* 1993, 33:1039–1047.

47. Tsimiakis S, Palinski W, Halpern SE, et al.: Radiolabeled MDA2, an oxidation-specific monoclonal antibody, identifies native atherosclerotic lesions in vivo. *J Nucl Cardiol* 1999, 6:41–53.

48. Narula J, Strauss HW: Predicting post angioplastic restenosis; a proliferating challenge for nuclear medicine. *J Nucl Med* 2000, 41:1541–1544.

49. Thyberg J, Heidin U, Sjolund M, et al.: Regulation of differentiated properties and proliferation of arterial smooth muscle cells. *Arteriosclerosis* 1990, 10:966–990.

50. Narula N, Haider N, Narula J: Cell biology for the nuclear cardiologist. *J Nucl Cardiol* 1998, 5:426–437.

51. Dinkelborg LM, Duda SH, Hanke H, et al.: Molecular imaging of atherosclerosis using a technetium-99m-labeled endothelin derivative. *J Nucl Med* 1998, 39:1819–1822.

52. Tepe G, Duda SH, Meding J, et al.: Tc-99m-labeled endothelin derivative for imaging of experimentally induced atherosclerosis. *Atherosclerosis* 2001, 157:383–292.

53. Pintor J, Miras-Portugal MT: Diadenosine polyphosphages (APXA) as new neurotransmitters. *Drug Dev Res* 1993, 28:259–262.

54. Erlinge D, You J, Wahlestedt C, Edvinsson L: Diadenosine polyphosphates as new neurotransmitters. *Eur J Pharmacol* 1995, 289:135–149.

55. Elmaleh D, Narula J, Petrov A, et al.: Tc-99m-Ap4A for early gamma scintigraphic visualization of experimental atherosclerotic lesions. *Proc Natl Acad Sci U S A* 1998, 95:691–695.

56. Dewanjee MK, Haider N, Narula J: Imaging with radiolabeled antisense oligonucleotides for the detection of intracellular messenger RNA and cardiovascular disease. *J Nucl Cardiol* 1999, 6:345–356.

57. Tanner FC, Yang ZY, Duckers E, et al.: Expression of cyclin-dependent kinase inhibitors in vascular disease. *Circ Res* 1998, 82:396–403.

58. Narula J, Bianchi C, Petrov A, et al.: Noninvasive localization of experimental atherosclerotic lesions with mouse/human chimeric Z2D3 antibody specific for the proliferating smooth muscle cells of human atheroma. *Circulation* 1995, 92:474–484.

59. Narula J, Petrov A, Ditlow C, et al.: Technetium-99m-based imaging of experimental atherosclerotic lesions by selective localization of proliferating smooth muscle cells of atheroma. *Chest* 1997, 111:1684–1690.

60. Narula J, Petrov A, O'Donnell SM, Ditlow C, et al.: Gamma imaging of atherosclerotic lesions: the role of antibody affinity in the in vivo target localization. *J Nucl Cardiol* 1997, 4:226–233.

61. Narula J, Petrov A, Ditlow C, et al.: Maximizing radiotracer delivery for scintigraphic localization of experimental atherosclerotic lesions with high-dose negative-charge-modified Z2D3 antibody. *J Nucl Cardiol* 1997, 4:226–233.

62. Carrio I, Pieri P, Narula J, et al.: Noninvasive localization of human atherosclerotic lesions with indium-111-labeled monoclonal Z2D3 antibody specific for proliferating smooth muscle cells. *J Nucl Cardiol* 1998, 5:551–557.

63. Narula J, Kolodgie FD, Virmani R, et al.: Should assessment of the rate of smooth muscle cell proliferation by indium-111-Z3D3 antibody imaging allow for predicting postangioplastic restenosis? *J Nucl Med* 1997, 38:3.

64. Johnson LL, Schofield LM, Verdesca SA, et al.: In vivo uptake of radiolabeled antibody to proliferating smooth muscle cells in a swine model of coronary stent restenosis. *J Nucl Med* 2000, 41:1535–1540.

INDEX

A

ACE
  [^{18}F]Fluorobenzyl-linsinopril binding to, 144
  activity of in tissue renin-angiotensin system, 143
ACE inhibitors
  for ischemic cardiomyopathy, 131
  in left ventricular remodeling, 142
Acetylcholine, 185
  stimulation of, 98
Acetylcholine and papaverine (PAPA) doses, 64
Acute coronary syndromes
  assessment of, 117–121
  development of, 217
  diagnosis of, 115–116
  initial classification of, 117
  perfusion imaging for, 127
  risk assessment in, 117–128
Acute ischemic syndromes
  absence of myocardial perfusion abnormalities in, 118
  diagnostic and therapeutic decision points in, 116
  predictors of, 98
Adenosine
  continuous coronary Doppler flow wire tracing with, 54
  direct and indirect action of on vascular smooth muscle cells, 50
  hyperemic stress effects of, 50
  infusion protocol for, 52
  peripheral hemodynamic responses to, 52
  side effects of intravenous imaging with, 53
Adenosine-induced myocardial hyperemia, 84, 86
  determinants of, 85
Adenosine SPECT imaging, 124–125
Adenosine stress testing
  characteristics of, 51
  cumulative test accuracy data from, 55
  in ST segment depression, 108
Adenosine-^{201}Tl tomography, 58
Adenosine triphosphate (ATP), 187
  depletion of, 198
Adhesion molecules, 218
Adrenergic nerve terminals, 187
Allografts
  algorithms for management of, 205–207
  severity of apoptosis in rejection of, 212
Ambulatory left ventricular function monitoring, 15
American College of Physicians/American College of Cardiology/American Heart Association practice guidelines, 47
Analog computer-smoothed display, 151
Anger cameras, 8, 10
  restricted spatial resolution of, 148
Angina
  exercise-induced, post-ischemic myocardial metabolic alterations with, 138
  unstable
    continuous left ventricular function monitoring in, 164–165
    risk stratification in, 128

Angiographic coronary artery disease, 76
Angiographic stenosis
  coronary, 87
  PET quantitation of, 79
Angiographic territory score, ^{99m}Tc-sestamibi risk area and, 64
Angioscopy, 217
Angiotensin II, 142
Angiotensin II type I receptors, 143
  immunolabeling of, 144
Annexin V, 210, 223
  binding of in infarct area, 212, 214
  delayed binding of to cardiomyocytes, 214
  specificity of binding to apoptotic cells, 211
Annexin V imaging, 197
  of cell death, 213
Anteroseptal defect
  quantification of SPECT images of, 71
  reversible, 73
Anti-ischemic therapy, 158
Antimyosin
  Fab fragments of, 200, 201
  uptake of, 200
Antimyosin imaging, 197
  with algorithms for allograft management, 205–207
  in myocardial infarction, 203
  pathogenetic basis of, 200
  technique, interpretation and quantitation of uptake in, 201
Antimyosin scintigraphy, 201
  in cardiac allograft rejection, 205–206
  diagnostic accuracy of, 202
  in myocarditis, 204
Antisense nucleotides, 230
Aortic regurgitation
  aortic valve replacement for, 160
  prognostication in, 159
  radionuclide angiography for, 158–159
Aortic stenosis, 160
Aortic valve replacement, 159
  left ventricular ejection fraction after, 160
Apical defect
  quantification of SPECT images of, 71
  reversible, 73
Apolipoprotein B, 225
Apoptosis
  characteristics of, 208
  detection of in intracardiac tumor, 213
  future research on, 215
  imaging of, 197, 208–215
  molecular basis of imaging of, 210
  noninvasive detection of, 223
  in various cell types, 222
Apoptotic cells
  annexin V binding to, 211
  signaling pathways in death of, 209
Arrhythmias, innervation in, 193–194
Arterial radiotracer input function, 82
Aspirin, 127
Atheromatous plaques, 16
Atherosclerosis, pathogenesis of, 218
Atherosclerotic lesions
  evolution of, 218–219

  future research on, 233
  matrix metalloproteinase upregulation in, 224
  plaque-specific lipids in, 226
  radionuclide imaging of, 217–233
  targeting large lipid cores in, 225–226
  targeting macrophage infiltration in, 219–224
  targeting proliferating smooth muscle cells in, 227–233
Atherosclerotic plaques
  inflammation and vulnerability of, 220, 221–222
  lipid cores of, 217
  morphologic characteristics of, 219
  noninvasive detection of apoptosis in, 223
  rupture of, 217, 222
  vulnerable, identification of, 217–218
Attenuation artifact, 12
Attenuation correction devices, 63
Autonomic nervous system, 185–186

B

Backprojection, 14
Balloon angioplasty, 228
Beat length acceptance window, setting, 169
Becquerel, 4
Benzylguanidine analogues, radiolabeled, 188
Beta decay, 2
β-adrenergic blockers, 131
β-adrenoceptor ligands, 188
β-blockers, 127
β-methyliodopentadecanoic acid, 38
β-receptor, distribution of, 191
Blood flow velocity, 87
Blood pool imaging, 163
BMIPP SPECT imaging, 128
Bone-scanning agents, 200
Breast attenuation
  artifacts of, 68
  with history of shortness of breath, 175

C

C-11 epinephrine, 190
C-11 hydroxyephedrine, 184
  myocardial distribution of, 189, 190
  in neural integrity imaging, 192
  time-activity curve after injection of, 190
^{11}C-acetate, 39
^{11}C-palmitate, 38
Cadherins, 219
Cardiac allograft
  myocardial damage in rejection of, 205–206
  reinnervation of, 194
Cardiac blood pool studies, 147
Cardiac death
  as function of amount of ischemia, 110
  prediction of, 102
Cardiac disease, function severity of, 155
Cardiac event rate
  post-myocardial infarction inducible ischemia and, 122
  resting ^{99m}Tc-sestamibi SPECT myocardial perfusion imaging and, 119
Cardiac imaging, clinical role of, 55
Cardiac rate-pressure product, 53

Cardiac risk
  dipyridamole-^{201}Tl imaging for preoperative assessment of, 57–58
  stratification of, 57–58
    for noncardiac surgical procedures, 55
Cardiac testing, for perioperative risk, 56
Cardiac transplantation
  reinnervation of, 194
  rejection of, 212
Cardiac troponin I, serial analysis of, 119
Cardiomyocytes
  injured, 197
  subcellular changes of in hibernating myocardium, 139
Cardiomyopathy
  ECG-gated SPECT of, 75
  innervation in, 193–194
  ischemic
    gross cardiac pathology in, 140
    histomorphologic confirmation of, 26
    mean volume fraction of collagen in, 142
    myocardial reperfusion in, 131
  metoprolol for, 37
  myocardial perfusion defects in, 75
  nonischemic, 74
  nonischemic with atypical chest pain, 178
  radionuclide angiography in, 162–165
  restrictive, 162
  SPECT perfusion imaging for, 74–75
Cardiospecific enzymes, 119
Cardiovascular conditioning, 91
Cardiovascular disease, 87–94
Cardiovascular mortality, post-myocardial infarction, 122
Cardiovascular nuclear imaging, principles of, 1–16
Cardiovascular research, 15–16
Carotid atherosclerosis, 233
Caspase-3, 212
Caspase-3 antibody, 213
Caspase inhibitors, 214
Catecholamine analogues, radiolabeled, 183, 188
Catecholamines
  infusion of, 47
  radiolabeled, 183, 184, 188
  release of, 185
Catheterization rate, 104
Cell death
  apoptotic, 208–215
  effective intervention in, 214
  forms of, 197
  future research on, 215
  necrotic, 198–207
Cell membrane integrity, 20, 131–132
Cellular necrosis, 208
Cellular viability, 132
Chelates, non-bone scanning, 200
Chemistry, nuclear imaging, 2–5
Chest pain
  absence of myocardial perfusion abnormalities in, 118
  atypical in nonischemic cardiomyopathy, 178
  clinical studies involving myocardial perfusion in, 119
  myocardial perfusion abnormalities in, 117
  myocardial perfusion imaging in assessing, 120–121

Chest pain center protocol, 121
Chest pain syndrome, 117
Chromatin, condensation and fragmentation of, 197
Chromogranin, 187
Cineangiogram, equilibrium radionuclide, 152
Clinical imaging, SPECT perfusion, 65–68
Clinical outcome, 104
Clinical risk predictors, 47
Cloud chamber detector, 9
Coincidence detection, 10, 12
Cold pressor testing
  coronary flow responses to, 91
  flow responses to, 90–91
Collagen, mean volume fraction of, 142
Collagen weave, 139
Collimator, 10
  gamma ray detection by, 11–12
  high-energy designs, 44
Computer and electronics process, 10
Computer technology
  in cardiac blood pool studies, 147
  in SPECT imaging, 167
Contraction-perfusion match, 137
Contraction-perfusion mismatch, 135–138
Contrast, 11
Coronary angiography
  contrast, 63
  normal, 64
Coronary artery
  diffuse luminal narrowing of, 93
  restenosis of, 1, 217–218
  severity of ischemic heart disease with obstruction of, 156–157
  stenosis of
    blood flow velocity and, 87
    in coronary artery disease risk, 98
    Doppler flow wire crossing, 54
    function reductions in, 135
    myocardial blood flow in, 79, 135
    severity of, 87, 167–168
Coronary artery bypass grafting (CABG)
  myocardial viability and outcome of, 43
  prognosis for, 157
  radionuclide angiography in assessment of, 158
  risk stratification for, 97–98
Coronary artery disease
  cardiovascular nuclear imaging in, 1–2
  clinical morbidity of, 64
  diagnostic tools of, 47
  in heart failure, 131
  integration of test results in risk assessment in, 112
  myocardial blood flow distribution in, 80
  myocardial tracer activity in, 83
  myocardial viability testing in prognosis of, 45
  noninvasive imaging for, 1
  nuclear cardiology for risk stratification in, 106
  patient management decisions in, 97
  pharmacologic stressors in, 47–59
  prevalence of, 217
  radionuclide angiography in diagnosis of, 148–149
  risk stratification for, 97–98
  scintigraphic findings in, 6–7
  SPECT perfusion tracers for, 63–76
  transient ischemic dilation and extent of, 107

Coronary artery territories, 69
Coronary blood flow, 6
  velocity of, 54
Coronary circulation, 86
Coronary driving pressure, 85
Coronary plaques, pre-myocardial infarction, 98
Coronary revascularization, 58
Coronary risk factors
  base to apex perfusion gradient with, 94
  coronary vasomotor function and, 89
  diminished hyperemic myocardial blood flow with, 88
  vasodilator capacity and, 88
Coronary stenting, 106
Coronary vasodilation, 50
Coronary vasomotor function
  coronary risk factors and, 89
  in long-term smokers, 89
Cost-benefit relationship, stress imaging techniques, 59
COURAGE trial, 106
Cox regression models, 122
Curie, 4

D

Decision analysis, 48
Diabetes
  myocardial denervation in, 194
  prognostic value of summed stress score in, 105
DIAD trial, 106
Diagnostic imaging, 1
  accuracy of with gated SPECT imaging, 174
  in acute coronary syndromes, 115–128
  antimyosin scintigraphy in, 202
  pharmacologic stress imaging for, 49
  radionuclide angiography in, 148–149
  SPECT perfusion imaging in, 76
Diaphragmatic attenuation, 68
  with hypertension, hypercholesterolemia, and nonanginal chest discomfort, 176
Diastolic function, 172
Diastolic imaging, gated SPECT, 178–179
Dipyridamole
  continuous coronary Doppler flow wire tracing with, 54
  direct and indirect action of on vascular smooth muscle cells, 50
  hyperemic stress effects of, 50
  intravenous
    hemodynamic responses to, 51
    myocardial perfusion imaging protocol for, 51
    side effects of, 53
  in pharmacologic vasodilation, 63
Dipyridamole-induced myocardial hyperemia, 84
  determinants of, 85
  myocardial blood flow during with coronary risk factors, 94
Dipyridamole stress testing
  characteristics of, 51
  cumulative test accuracy data from, 55
  prognostic value of, 55, 59
  with stable chest pain, 59
Dipyridamole-^{201}Tl imaging
  predictive accuracy of, 58
  for preoperative cardiac risk assessment, 57–58
DNAM-1, 219
DNAses, 209

Dobutamine adenosine stress testing, 55
Dobutamine stress testing
  characteristics of, 51
  intravenous infusion protocol for, 52
  peripheral hemodynamic responses to, 52
Dopamine, 187
Doppler flow wire
  continuous coronary tracing of with hyperemic agents, 54
  schematic illustration of, 54
Doxorubicin, 163
Drug boluses, intracoronary, 54
Drug stress pharmacology. See also Pharmacologic stressors
  evidence-based evolution in, 47
  target populations for, 47
Drug therapy assessment, 157
Dual-isotope injection, 33
Duke University treadmill score
  in chronic coronary artery disease, 112
  long-term outcome and, 104
  in risk assessment, 110, 112
  summed stress score and, 103–104

E

E-selectin, 219
ECG, 120
ECG-gated imaging, breast artifact, 68
ECG-gated SPECT, 71, 72
  in cardiomyopathy, 75
Echocardiography, 150
Effector caspases, 209
Ejection fraction. See also Left ventricular ejection fraction; Right ventricular ejection fraction
  incremental prognostic power of, 123
  mapping, 152
Electromagnetic radiation, 3
Electromagnetic waves, spectrum of, 3
Electron capture, 2
Electron emission, 2
End-diastolic imaging, 152
  gated SPECT, 178–179
End-organ innervation, 185
  determinants of, 186
End-systolic images, 152
Endarterectomy, 233
Endless loop cineing, 173
Endomyocardial biopsy, 203
  in cardiac allograft rejection, 205–206
  in giant cell myocarditis, 204
Endothelial cells
  activation of, 219
  junctional molecules of, 219
Endothelial function, 90–91
Endothelin-1, 229
Epidermal growth factor, 229
Epinephrine, 185
Exercise-induced myocardial ischemia, 138
  scintigraphic imaging of, 8
Exercise SPECT imaging
  normal, 67
  prognostic value of, 65
Exercise stress ^{99m}Tc-sestamibi imaging
  myocardial defect size changes in, 32
  of severe and extensive stress perfusion defect, 100
  of small stress perfusion defect, 99

Exercise stress testing
  basic concepts of, 63
  characteristics of, 51
  prognostic value of with stable chest pain, 59
  submaximal, with drug stress, 47
Exercise tolerance, 161
Extracardiac activity, hypertension-related, 177

F

False adrenergic neurotransmitters, 183
Fatty acid imaging, 38
  for risk stratification in unstable angina, 128
Fission, 3
Floppase, 210
Flow tracers
  first-pass extraction and retention fractions of, 81
  myocardial tissue kinetics of, 80
  net myocardial uptake of, 81
[^{18}F]Fluorobenzyl-linsinopril, 144
[^{18}F]-Fluorodeoxyglucose, 131–132
  biodistribution of, 44
  mismatch patterns with, 42
  myocardial metabolism assessment by, 33
  in PET imaging, 40
  standardization schemes for optimizing, 41
Fourier transformation, 13
Functional capacity, perioperative, 56

G

G protein-signaling pathways, 229
Gamma cameras
  Anger-type, 63
  scintigraphic work with, 19–20
  single-crystal, 8
  single-photon, 9
  structure of, 10
Gamma decay, 2
Gamma rays, 2, 3, 19
  detection of, 11–12
Gas-filled detectors, 9
Gated blood pool imaging, 1
Gated blood pool SPECT, 168, 179
  quantitation of, 180
Gated perfusion SPECT imaging, 167–180
  acquisition in, 168
  as percentage of all myocardial SPECT, 168
  in risk assessment, 108
Gated post-stress ^{99m}Tc-sestamibi SPECT imaging, 175
  function component of, 176
Gated rest ^{99m}Tc-sestamibi SPECT imaging, 177
Gated SPECT imaging
  clinical research on, 167
  clinical value of, 174
  in coronary artery disease management, 110
  diastolic, 178–179
  incremental prognostic value of, 112
  measuring left ventricular ejection fraction, 109
  modified protocols of, 168
  normal, 67
  partial volume effects in, 11
  quality control in, 169
  quantitation of, 170
  technique of, 167–180
  three-dimensional display of, 173
  two-dimensional display of, 172

  validation of left ventricular ejection fraction in, 170
Gated SPECT volumes, 171
Gating devices, 147
Gating errors, 169
Gating technique, 8
Geiger-Mueller counter, 5, 9
Giant cell myocarditis, 204
Glucarate, 200
Glucose-loading, 41
Glycolysis, 40
Gray, 4
Growth factor receptors, 229–230

H

Half-life, 2
Hard event rate, 103
Heart development, apoptosis during, 211
Heart failure
  angiotensin II in, 142
  with coronary artery disease, 131
  metoprolol for, 37
  radionuclide angiography in diagnosis of, 148
Heart rate, continuous trend of, 15
Heart to lung ratio trends, 207
Heparin, 127
Hibernating myocardium, 134, 136
  experimental model for, 137
  subcellular cardiomyocyte changes in, 139
HMG CoA-reductase inhibitors, 92–93
Hypercholesteremia, 93
Hyperemia
  adenosine-stimulated, 86
  pharmacologic stress and, 84
Hyperemic agents
  continuous coronary Doppler flow wire tracing with, 54
  development of, 47
Hyperemic myocardial blood flow
  coronary driving pressure and, 85
  diminished with coronary risk factors, 88
  insulin and pharmacologically induced, 86
Hyperemic stress, 50
Hyperinsulinemic-euglycemic clamping, 41
Hyperlipidemia, Watanabe heritable, 226
Hypertension, extracardiac activity in, 177

I

I-123 metaiodobenzylguanidine
  myocardial distribution of, 190
  in myocardial imaging, 126
  in neural integrity imaging, 192
  retention of in myocardial infarction, 191
Image
  acquisition of, 12–13
  interpretation of, 69–74
  processing of, 13–15
Infarct zone ischemia
  prognostic value of, 58
  residual, 123
Inflammatory myocardial disease, 204
Instrumentation, 9–12
  advances in, 1
Insulin, 41
Insulin-induced hyperemic myocardial blood flow, 86

239

Intercellular adhesion molecules (ICAMs), 219, 220
Interleukin-8, 221
International Society of Heart and Lung Transplantation (ISHLT) grades, 205–206, 212
Interstitial fibrosis, 25
Intracardiac tumor, 213
Intravascular detectors, 10
Intravascular radiation probe, 16
Ionizing radiation, 2
Ischemic heart disease. *See also* Acute ischemic syndromes; Myocardial ischemia
  assessing severity of, 156–157
  cardiac death rate and, 110
  left ventricular dysfunction and, 141
  oxygen supply/demand imbalance in, 132
  structural damage in, 25
Ischemic myocardial necrosis, 200
Isobaric transition, 2

K
Karyorrhexis, 199

L
L-selectin, 219
LDL cholesterol
  in atherosclerotic lesions, 225–226
  uptake of, 220
Left bundle branch block, 105
Left ventricle time-activity curves, 151
Left ventricular diastolic function, 156
Left ventricular dysfunction
  contractile, 140
  extent of myocardial infarction inducible ischemia and, 122–123
  histomorphologic and structural changes underlying, 139–140
  left ventricular ejection fraction with, 134
  myocardial viability testing in prognosis of, 45
  reversible myocardial viability in, 131–144
  stable chronic ischemic heart disease and, 141
  survival in, 133
Left ventricular ejection fraction, 15
  accuracy of with equilibrium radionuclide angiography, 155
  after aortic valve replacement, 160
  in aortic regurgitation, 159
  changes in with left ventricular dysfunction, 134
  with doxorubicin therapy, 163
  equilibrium radionuclide angiography for, 157
  gated SPECT, validation of, 170
  life-table cumulative survival in, 133
  nonfatal myocardial infarction and, 109
  quantitation of, 180
  regional, determination of, 154
  subnormal, 150
Left ventricular end-diastolic volume, 153
Left ventricular end-systolic volume, 111
Left ventricular function
  continuous monitoring of, 164–165
  gated SPECT quantitation of, 171
  myocardial perfusion and in hibernating and stunned myocardium, 136
  validation of monitoring devices for, 164
Left ventricular remodeling, 131
  ACE inhibitor impact on, 142
Leg swinging, 53
Lipid cores, atherosclerotic lesion, 225–226
Low-pass filtering, 13–14

M
Macrophages
  infiltration of in atherosclerotic lesions, 219–224
  metalloproteinase release by, 217
  potential molecular targets of, 219
Magnetic resonance imaging, 217
MAO inhibitors, 187
Matrix metalloproteinase, 224
MCP-1
  expression of, 221
  radiolabeled, 220
MDA2, 226
Mcgabccqucrel, 4
Metabolic equivalents (METs), 65
Metaiodobenzylguanidine (mIBG), 183–184
  myocardial distribution of, 189, 190
Metalloproteinases, 217, 224
Metoprolol, 37
Microsphere technique, radiolabeled, 7
Millicurie, 4
Mitochondrial permeability transition pores, 198
Mitral regurgitation
  exercise tolerance with, 161
  first-pass radionuclide angiography for, 151
  prognostication in, 160–161
Mitral stenosis, 150
^{99}Mo-^{99m}Tc generator, 4
Monocyte chemoattractant protein-1, 219
Mortality rate, Duke treadmill score and, 104
Multicrystal camera, 10
Myocarditis, 197
Myocardial blood flow
  angiographic coronary stenoses and, 87
  cardiovascular conditioning and, 91
  in cardiovascular disease, 87–94
  in coronary artery disease, 80
  dependency of at rest on cardiac work, 84
  with diffuse coronary artery luminal narrowing, 93
  distribution of, 79–90
  HMG CoA-reductase inhibitors and, 92, 93
  metoprolol effect on, 37
  ^{13}N-ammonia uptake in assessing, 36
  net myocardial tracer uptake and, 81
  nitric oxide synthase inhibition and, 86
  in normal heart, 80
  normal values of, 84
  PET applications and radiotracers for, 34
  PET quantitation of, 79–94
  reduction of in coronary artery stenosis, 135
  regional, polar map estimation of, 83
  validation of PET-based measurement of, 82
Myocardial ^{11}C-acetate tissue time-activity curve, 39
Myocardial flow reserve, 85
Myocardial infarction
  annexin V binding in, 212, 214
  antimyosin imaging in, 201–202, 203
  histomorphologic analysis of, 141
  infarct size and clinical outcomes of, 125
  innervation in, 191–192
  left ventricular ejection fraction and, 109
  left ventricular end-systolic volume in survival after, 111
  prediction of, 102
  prediction of cardiac events after, 58
  risk of, 98
  scar tissue after, 140
Myocardial infarction inducible ischemia, 122
Myocardial ischemia
  myocardial viability and, 132
  neuronal damage in, 192
  oxygen supply/demand imbalance in, 132
  suppression of, 124–125
Myocardial perfusion
  abnormalities of with chest pain, 117
  in acute chest pain, 119
  assessment of, 7
  direct measurement of, 6
  early scintigraphic detection of, 6–7
  left ventricular function and, 136
  quantitation of severity of reduction in, 33
  severity of reduction in, 20
  ventricular function and, 131
Myocardial perfusion defects
  large, fixed and irreversible, 70
  large, reversible, 72
  quantification of, 70
  size of, 32, 71, 73, 75
    left ventricular ejection fraction and, 123
    during repeat SPECT imaging, 124–125
Myocardial perfusion imaging
  for acute ischemic coronary syndromes, 115
  assessment of role of in chest pain, 120–121
  characterization of equivocal results of, 120
  with chest pain, 119
  development of, 1
  evolution of, 8
  in non-ST elevation acute coronary syndrome, 128
  for non-ST segment elevation myocardial infarction, 127
  with nondiagnostic ECG changes, 120
  role of, 126
  U.S. and Canadian protocols for, 50
Myocardial perfusion scintigraphy
  incremental prognostic value of, 101
  in prognosis, 149
Myocardial perfusion SPECT imaging
  cumulative test accuracy data from, 55
  long-term prognostic value of after coronary stenting, 106
  in optimized risk stratification strategy, 102
  in prediction of myocardial infarction versus cardiac death, 102
  quantification of, 71, 73
Myocardial perfusion tracers, 28
Myocardial tissue response, 82

Myocardial viability
  assessment of, 131
  in ischemic left ventricular dysfunction and heart failure treatment, 132
  ^{15}O-water in assessment of, 35
  perfusion tracers in assessment of, 28
  PET techniques for, 34, 38–45
  preoperative assessment of and clinical outcome, 43
  reversible, 131–144
  testing of
    prognostic implications of, 45
    before surgical revascularization, 135
  underestimation of, 33
Myocardial wall
  maximum count value and thickness of, 173
  perfusion defect and motion of, 175
  thickening of, 172
Myocarditis, 204
Myocardium. *See also* Hibernating myocardium; Stunned myocardium
  angiotensin II type I receptors in remodeling of, 143
  contractile reserve of, 20
  denervation of in diabetes, 194
  extent and severity of hypoperfusion of, 98
  function of
    assessment of, 8
    metoprolol effect on, 37
    semiquantitative scoring of, 174
  injury of in ischemic cardiomyopathy, 140
  innervation of, 183–194
  left ventricular contractile dysfunction and extent of injury in, 140
  metabolism of
    ^{13}N-ammonia uptake and, 36
    PET applications and radiotracers for, 34
    PET techniques for, 38–43
  necrosis of, 197–207
  perfusion, function and metabolism of, 20
  regional function patterns in, 173
  thallium redistribution in, 23
  tracer retention in, 189–191
Myocytes
  metabolic pathways and regulatory steps of, 40
  necrotic, 199
Myopathy, restrictive, 162

N

^{13}N-ammonia
  mechanism of uptake of, 36
  myocardial tissue kinetics of, 80
  myocardial uptake of, 81
  in PET imaging, 36
  transit of through central circulation, 82
Na-K ATPase pump, 65
Necrotic cell death
  future research on, 215
  imaging of, 197–207
Necrotic myocellular death, 198
Nervous system, myocardial, 183–194
Neural integrity, 192
Neuronal function, 191

Neuronal imaging
  of cardiac allograft reinnervation, 194
  cardiac arrhythmias and, 193
  in cardiomyopathy, 193
Neuropeptide Y, 187
Neurostimulation, 183
Neurotransmitters, 183
  nonclassic systems of, 186
  synthesis and release of, 187
Neutrino, 3
Nicotinic acid derivative, 41
Nitrates
  for acute coronary syndrome, 127
  before rest ^{99m}Tc-sestamibi or ^{99m}Tc-tetrofosmin injection, 32
Nitric oxide synthase inhibition, 86
Nitroglycerin
  effectiveness of, 157
  radionuclide angiography in assessment of, 158
NOET
  in myocardial viability assessment, 28
  in SPECT imaging, 30
Noise, 11
Non-ST segment elevation myocardial infarction, 127–128
Nonexercise stress testing, 49
Nonimaging detectors, 10
Noninvasive imaging techniques, 97
  first, 1
Nonionizing radiation, 2
Norepinephrine, 184, 185, 187
Norepinephrine transporter, 183
Nuclear cardiology
  historical perspective on, 5–8
  instrumentation for, 9–12
  in patient management decisions, 97
  for risk stratification, 106
  in risk stratification, 97–98

O

^{15}O-water
  myocardial uptake of, 81
  in PET imaging, 35
Oncosis, 197
Open Artery Trial (OAT), 123
Optical coherence tomography, 217
Oxygen supply/demand imbalance, 132

P

Palmaz-Schatz stent placement, 228
Papaverine, 54
Parasympathetic nervous system, 183, 185
Partial volume effect, 11
  in gated SPECT images, 172–173
Patient management
  gated SPECT in, 110
  risk stratification in, 97–112
Patient outcome, 27
PECAM-1, 219
Percutaneous coronary intervention, 121
Percutaneous transluminal coronary angioplasty, 123–124

Perfusable tissue fraction (PTF), 35
Perfusion defects. *See* Myocardial perfusion defects; Stress perfusion defects
Perfusion-metabolism mismatch
  PET scan demonstrating, 138
  prognosis and pattern of, 43
Pericardial constriction, 162
Perioperative events, clinical predictors of, 56
PET camera, 10
  photon detection by, 12
  in small animal imaging systems, 16
Pharmacologic stress imaging
  cumulative test accuracy data from, 55
  indications for, 48
  in moderate and severe coronary artery occlusion, 31
  myocardial perfusion, 47
  patient protocol selection algorithm for, 48
Pharmacologic stress testing characteristics, 49
Pharmacologic stressors, 47–59
Phenelzine, 187
Phosphatidylserine, 197, 210
Phospholipids, cationic, 210
Photomultiplier tube, 1, 10
Photon detection, 12
Physics, basic concepts of, 2–5
Planar imaging technique, 12
Platelet-derived growth factor, 229
Point spread function, 11
Polar maps
  of late ^{201}Tl redistribution, 22
  of myocardial tracer activity with coronary artery disease, 83
  of regional myocardial blood flow, 83
Polypeptide growth factors, 229
Positron decay, 3
Positron emission, 2
Positron-emission tomographic (PET) imaging
  applications of, 34
  in cardiovascular disease, 87–94
  diagnostic capabilities of, 79
  methodology of, 80–83
  mismatch patterns in, 42
  of myocardial denervation in diabetes, 194
  of neural integrity, 192
  normal, mismatch, and match patterns under glucose-loading in, 41
  normal findings in, 84–86
  of post-ischemic myocardial metabolic alterations with exercise-induced angina, 138
  techniques of, 19–20, 20
  techniques of for myocardial metabolism and viability assessment, 38–45
Positron-emission tomographic (PET) mismatch, 43
Positron-emission tomographic (PET) quantitation, 79–94
Positron-emitting (PET) radiotracers, 80, 183
  in cardiac sympathetic neuron mapping, 188
  PET applications and, 34
Positron-emitting radioisotopes, 19–20
Postangioplastic restenosis, 228
Procaspase-9, 209

Prognosis
  after coronary stenting, 106
  for aortic regurgitation, 159
  determinants of in coronary artery disease, 98
  dipyridamole stress myocardial imaging in, 59
  equilibrium radionuclide angiography in, 157
  gated SPECT imaging in, 112, 167
  for mitral regurgitation, 160–161
  ^{99m}Tc-sestamibi imaging in, 59
  myocardial perfusion imaging in, 101, 106
  myocardial viability testing in, 45
  PET mismatch and, 43
  pharmacologic stress imaging for, 49
  preoperative peripheral vascular disease assessment in, 55
  radionuclide angiography in, 148, 149
  rest-redistribution ^{201}Tl SPECT imaging in, 27
  resting reversibility in, 107
  stress myocardial perfusion imaging in, 63, 65
  summed stress score in, 105
  ^{201}Tl reinjection in, 26
  ^{201}Tl SPECT scanning in, 102
  thallium scintigraphy in, 22
  vasodilator SPECT in, 105
Prone imaging, SPECT, 176
Pulse-height analyzer, 12

Q

Quality control, 167, 169
Quantitative circumferential analysis programs, 12

R

Rad, 4
Radiation, 2
Radiation detectors, 9
Radiation exposure, natural, 5
Radioactive decay, 2
Radioactivity
  definition of, 2
  units of, 4
Radioactivity exposure units, 4
Radioiodine-labeled fatty acid analogues, 38
Radioisotopes, 1
  positron-emitting, 19–20
  production of, 3
  in SPECT imaging, 19–20
Radiolabeled albumin, 1, 5
Radiolabeled compounds, 183
Radionuclide angiocardiography, equilibrium, 1
Radionuclide angiography
  accuracy of, 155
  in cardiomyopathic disorders, 162–165
  clinical applications of, 148–149
  equilibrium, 147–149, 152–158
  first-pass, 147–149, 150–151
  relative advantages of first-pass and equilibrium, 154
  schematic diagram of role of, 150
  in valvular heart disease, 158–161
Radionuclide imaging
  of apoptosis, 197, 208–215
  of atherosclerotic lesions, 217–233
  clinical acceptance of, 63
  of necrosis, 197, 198–207
  novel applications of, 15–16
  pathologic basis of, 219
  pathophysiology underlying, 66
Radionuclide imaging devices, 10
Radionuclides
  first use of in humans, 5
  in in vivo circulation study, 1
  naturally occurring and manmade, 3
Radiopharmaceuticals
  in cardiac sympathetic and parasympathetic neuron mapping, 188–191
  development of, 63–64
  properties of, 1
  in SPECT and PET imaging, 19
Radiotracers
  for angiographic coronary artery disease, 76
  blood clearance of, 66
  development of, 131
  PET, 34, 80, 183, 188
  retention of in normal myocardium, 189–191
  for SPECT perfusion imaging, 65
Reactive fibrosis, 143
Rectilinear scanners, 9, 10
Rem (roentgen equivalent man), 4
Renin-angiotensin system, 142
  upregulation of components of, 143
Rest myocardial perfusion SPECT imaging, 177
Rest-redistribution short-axis ^{201}Tl tomography, 27
Rest-redistribution ^{201}Tl imaging, 27
  protocol for, 27
Rest ^{201}Tl imaging, 99–100
Resting ejection fraction, 122
Resting ^{99m}Tc-sestamibi SPECT myocardial perfusion imaging, 119
Revascularization
  benefits of, 45
  for inducible ischemia, 123–124
  myocardial viability testing before, 135
  potential benefit of, 123
  risk stratification for, 97–98
Right ventricular ejection fraction
  from equilibrium radionuclide angiograms, 153
  with mitral regurgitation, 161
  quantitation of, 180
  radionuclide angiography for, 150
Risk assessment
  in acute coronary syndromes, 117–128
  in chronic coronary artery disease, 112
  gated myocardial perfusion SPECT in, 108
Risk stratification
  in acute coronary syndromes, 115–128
  gated SPECT imaging in, 167
  myocardial perfusion SPECT data on, 106
  nuclear cardiology for, 106
  optimized strategy for, 102
  patient management and, 97–112
  stress myocardial perfusion in, 63
  in unstable angina, 128
Roentgen, 4
Rubidium-82, 34

S

Sarcolemma, 199
Sarcolemmal cell membrane integrity, 20
Scintigraphic indices, 99
Scintigraphy, 184
Scintillation detectors, 1, 5, 9, 10
Scramblase, 210
Selectin expression, 219
Semiconductor detectors, 9
Sievert, 4
Single-head planar projection imaging, 63
Single photon devices, 19
Small animal imaging systems, 10, 16
Smoking, 89
Smooth muscle cells (SMCs)
  chronic loss of, 221–222
  clinical imaging of proliferation of, 233
  feasibility of imaging, 232
  phenotypic alteration of, 218
  proliferating, 227–233
  synthetic phenotype of, 231
Sodium iodide crystal, 1
Sodium iodide scintillation crystal, 9
Sodium iodide scintillation detector, 5
Spatial resolution, 11
SPECT camera, 10
  head configuration of, 13
  in small animal imaging systems, 16
SPECT imaging
  in acute coronary syndrome diagnosis, 117–118
  for acute ischemic coronary syndromes, 115
  backprojection of, 14
  for cardiomyopathy, 74–75
  clinical indications for, 76
  coronary flow velocity reserve with, 54
  ECG-gated, 47
  filtering of, 13–14
  high- and low-risk, 74
  image interpretation and quantification in, 69–74
  of neuronal damage in ischemic myocardium, 192
  normal variations in, 68
  perfusion tracers in, 63–76
  post-myocardial infarction risk stratification, 124
  quantitative perfusion, 100
  radiotracers for, 65
  in risk stratification, 97
  standard nomenclature and segmentation for, 69
  ^{99m}Tc-labeled perfusion tracers in, 28–33
  techniques of, 19–20
  thallium-201, 21–27
  vertical long-axis, 126
  visual scoring for, 69
SPECT radionuclide angiography, 163
SPECT slices, display of, 15
SPECT tracers, 183
SPECT transient ischemic dilation ratio, 179
ST segment depression, 108
ST segment elevation myocardial infarction (STEMI)
  in acute coronary syndrome diagnosis, 116
  assessment of, 121–126
  therapeutic pathways with, 121
Stress myocardial perfusion imaging
  incremental prognostic value of, 65
  techniques of, 59
Stress myocardial perfusion SPECT
  abnormalities in, 98–99
  with high risk for coronary artery disease, 103
Stress perfusion defects
  abnormal summed stress score with, 99
  quantitative perfusion SPECT analysis of, 100
  severe and extensive, 100

Stress-redistribution-reinjection ^{201}Tl protocol, 26
Stress-redistribution ^{201}Tl imaging, 21–22
Stress-redistribution ^{201}Tl protocol, 21
Stress sestamibi SPECT scanning, 101
Stress testing, characteristics of, 51
Stunned myocardium, 136
  experimental evidence for, 137
  post-stress, 167–168
  scanning electron micrograph of, 139
Sudden cardiac death, 217
Summed difference score (SDS), 110
Summed rest late difference score (SRLDS), 107
Summed rest score (SRS), 99
Summed stress score (SSS), 99, 100
  catheterization rate and, 104
  hard event rate as function of, 103–104
  prognostic value of in diabetic patients, 105
Survival rates, 111
Sympathetic nerve fibers, 183
Sympathetic nerve terminals, 184
  density of, 183
Sympathetic nervous system, 183, 185

T

Tachycardia, 193
TACTICS, 127
Targeting strategies, 217–218
^{99m}Tc-glucarate imaging, 200
^{99m}Tc-labeled complexes, 28
^{99m}Tc-labeled sestamibi, 29
^{99m}Tc-labeled tracers, 65
  in SPECT imaging, 28–33
  in SPECT techniques, 28–33
^{99m}Tc-NOET, 30, 63–64
^{99m}Tc-sestamibi
  accuracy of, 28
  angiographic territory score and risk area of, 64
  blood clearance of, 66
  cellular kinetics of, 30
  changes in defect size of, 32
  in myocardial biopsies, 31
  in myocardial perfusion imaging, 65
  nitrate administration before injection of, 32
  prognostic value of, 59
  in severity of myocardial perfusion reduction, 33
  in SPECT imaging, 176
  in validation of infarct size, 125
^{99m}Tc-sestamibi myocardial perfusion defects, 31
^{99m}Tc-teboroxime, 28, 29
^{99m}Tc-tetrofosmin
  blood clearance of, 66
  hard event-free survival with, 103
  in myocardial perfusion imaging, 65
  nitrate administration before injection of, 32
  in severity of myocardial perfusion reduction, 33
  in SPECT imaging, 28–29, 176
Thallium-201
  cellular kinetics of, 30
  histomorphologic confirmation with, 26
  late redistribution protocol of, 22
  in moderate and severe coronary artery occlusion, 31
  in myocardial biopsies, 31
  regional activity of and interstitial fibrosis regional volume fraction, 25
  in SPECT techniques, 21–27
Thallium-201 radiotracers, 65
Thallium-201 reinjection, 23–24
  beneficial effect of, 24
  incremental prognostic value of, 26
Thallium scintigraphy, 22
Thallium SPECT imaging, 102
Therapeutic radiation, 1
Thrombolysis in myocardial infarction (TIMI), 127
Thrombolytic therapy, 121, 123–124
Time-activity curves, 147
  background-corrected, 152
  diastolic portion of, 162
  left ventricle, 151
Time to peak filling rate (TPFR), 156
Time to peak left ventricular filling rate (TTPFR), 162
Time-volume curves, 152
  in gated SPECT, 172
Tracer compartment model, 81
Transesophageal echocardiography, 213
Transient ischemic dilation, 107
Translocase, 210
Treadmill scores, 103–104, 110, 112
Triage, clinical risk predictors in, 47
Tyrosine hydroxylase activity, 187
Tyrosine kinase, 229

U

Ultrasonography, intravascular, 217
Upright submaximal treadmill walking, 53

V

Valvular heart disease
  diagnosis of, 148
  radionuclide angiography in, 158–161
Vascular imaging, future of, 233
Vascular smooth muscle cells
  adenosine and dipyridamole action on, 50
  molecular basis of proliferation of, 227
Vasodilator capacity, 88
Vasodilator stress imaging, 98
  indications for, 48
  SPECT, prognostic value of in left bundle branch block, 105
VCAM-1, 219
Ventricular function, 131
Visual scoring, SPECT myocardial, 69

W

Water perfusable tissue index (PTI), 35

Z

Z2D3, 231, 233
Z2D3 antibody, 232